PCAT*

2008–2009 Edition

The Staff of Kaplan Test Prep and Admissions

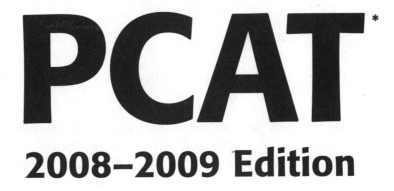

PUBLISHING

New York

Vice President and Publisher: Maureen McMahon
Editorial Director: Jennifer Farthing
Development Editor: Anne Kemper
Production Editor: Dominique Polfliet
Cover Designer: Carly Schnur

© 2007 by Kaplan , Inc.

Published by Kaplan Publishing, a division of Kaplan, Inc.
1 Liberty Plaza, 24th Floor
New York, NY 10006

Printed in the United States of America

June 2007
10   9   8   7   6   5   4   3

ISBN-13: 978-1-4195-5155-0

Kaplan Publishing books are available at special quantity discounts to use for sales promotions, employee premiums, or educational purposes. Please email our Special Sales Department to order or for more information at kaplanpublishing@kaplan.com, or write to Kaplan Publishing, 1 Liberty Plaza, 24th Floor, New York, NY 10006

TABLE OF CONTENTS

Section I: PCAT Strategies

Section II: Verbal Ability

Section III: Biology

Section IV: Reading Comprehension

Section V: Quantitative Ability

Section VI: Chemistry

Section VII: Writing

Section VIII: Self-Check: Are You Prepared?

Preface

If you are serious about going to Pharmacy school, you need to be serious about preparing for the PCAT. Although the PCAT is not the biggest factor for schools when determining admissions, you owe it to yourself to make sure that your performance on the PCAT accurately reflects your readiness to embark on a Pharmacy career.

The PCAT is a prospective, not a retrospective, examination: it isn't designed to assess what you've learned in college. Instead, it attempts to predict whether you'll be successful in the field of Pharmacy. The emphasis is on applying concepts rather than on regurgitating information. This means that the PCAT is not like your college examinations; in fact, it's probably unlike any exam you've ever taken. To do well, you'll need to make sure you have a solid understanding of the content tested, can apply your knowledge in the setting of PCAT-style passages, and have the strategic know-how and confidence to finish the examination in the allotted time under pressure.

We have designed the *PCAT 2008–2009 Edition* to help you prepare for the many challenges presented by the PCAT. Kaplan's *PCAT 2008–2009 Edition* is the best preparation you can find in any bookstore. Throughout the book, you'll be exposed to our proven methods and strategies. You'll learn to take control of the process. You can trust Kaplan. We've been preparing students for over 35 years in our comprehensive courses throughout North America.

We're confident that this guide can help you achieve your goals of PCAT success and admission into Pharmacy school.

Good luck!

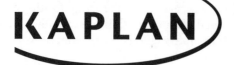

AVAILABLE ONLINE

Late-Breaking Developments

kaptest.com/publishing

The material in this book is up-to-date at the time of publication. However, the test makers may release more information on test changes after this book is published.

Be sure to read carefully the materials you receive when you register for the test. If there are any important late-breaking developments—or any changes or corrections to the Kaplan test preparation materials in this book—we will post that information online at **kaptest.com/publishing**.

Feedback and Comments

kaplansurveys.com/books

We would appreciate your comments and suggestions about this book. We invite you to fill out our online survey form at **kaplansurveys.com/books**. Your feedback is extremely helpful as we continue to develop high-quality resources to meet your needs.

A Special Note for International Students

If you are an international student hoping to attend a Pharmacy school in the United States, Kaplan can help you explore your options. Here are some things to think about.

- If English is not your first language, most Pharmacy schools will require you to take the TOEFL (Test of English as a Foreign Language) or provide some other evidence that you are proficient in English.
- Plan to take the PCAT. The majority of U.S. Pharmacy schools require it.
- Begin the process of applying to Pharmacy schools at least 18 months before the fall of the year you plan to start your studies. Most programs have only September start dates.
- You will need to obtain an I-20 Certificate of Eligibility from the school you plan to attend if you intend to apply for an F-1 Student Visa to study in the United States.
- If you've already completed a Pharmacy degree outside the United States, get information from U.S. schools—some may have special programs for international graduates of Pharmacy.

Kaplan English Programs

If you need more help with the process of Pharmacy school admissions; assistance preparing for the PCA or TOEFL; or help building your English language skills, you may be interested in Kaplan's programs for international students. These programs were designed to help students and professionals from outside the United States meet their educational and career goals. At locations throughout the United States, international students are improving their academic and conversational English skills, raising their scores on standardized exams, and gaining admission to the schools of their choice. Our staff and instructors give you the individualized attention you need to succeed. Here are some brief program descriptions:

General Intensive English

This class is designed to help you improve your skills in all areas of English and to increase your fluency in spoken and written English. Classes are available for beginning to advanced students, and the average class size is 12 students.

TOEFL and Academic English

This course provides you with the skills you need to improve your TOEFL score and succeed at an American school. It includes advanced reading, writing, listening, grammar, and conversational English. Your training will include use of Kaplan's exclusive computer-based practice materials.

English Language Structured-Study Program

This program allows you to improve your English at your own pace. The books, tapes, and videos provided are for students whose skills range from beginner to intermediate.

Medical English Communication Review Course

This program is for international doctors and medical professionals. Lessons include mastering pronunciation, building your medical vocabulary, and developing presentation and medical writing skills. Coursework also helps you develop the English skills you will need for the PCAT exam, professional interviews, and interactions with patients.

Other Kaplan Programs

Since 1938, more than 3 million students have come to Kaplan to advance their studies, prepare for entry to American universities, and further their careers. In addition to the above programs, Kaplan offers courses to prepare for the SAT, ACT, GMAT, GRE, LSAT, MCAT, DAT, USMLE, NCLEX, and other standardized exams at locations throughout the United States. For more information, contact us at:

Kaplan English Programs
700 South Flower, Suite 2900
Los Angeles, CA   90017
Phone outside of the USA: 1-213-452-5800
Phone inside of the USA: 1-800-818-9128
Fax: 1-213-892-1364

Website: kaplanenglish.com
Email: world@kaplan.com

Kaplan is authorized under federal law to enroll nonimmigrant alien students.

Kaplan is accredited by ACCET (Accrediting Council for Continuing Education and Training).

Test names are registered trademarks of their respective owners.

FREE Services for International Students

Kaplan now offers international students many services online—*free of charge*!
Students may assess their TOEFL skills and gain valuable feedback on their English
language proficiency in just a few hours with Kaplan's TOEFL Skills Assessment.
Log onto kaplanenglish.com today.

CHAPTER ONE

Introduction to the PCAT

Take out a No. 2 pencil...Do not make any stray marks on the grid...What is the acceleration due to gravity of a dime thrown from the Empire State Building if... You've faced these tests before, so you know the drill, right? Wrong. The Pharmacy College Admission Test, affectionately known as the PCAT, is different from any other test you've encountered in your academic career. It's not like the knowledge-based exams from high school and college, whose emphasis was on memorizing and regurgitating information. Pharmacy schools can assess your academic prowess by looking at your transcript. The PCAT isn't even like other standardized tests you may have taken, where the focus was on proving your general skills. Pharmacy schools use PCAT scores to assess whether you possess the foundation upon which to build a successful pharmacy career. Though you certainly need to know the content to do well, the stress is on thought process. The PCAT emphasizes reasoning, critical and analytical thinking, reading comprehension, data analysis, and problem-solving skills.

The PCAT's power comes from its use as an indicator of your abilities. Good scores can open doors. Your power comes from preparation and mindset because the key to PCAT success is knowing what you're up against. That's where this book comes in. We'll explain the philosophy behind the test, review the sections one by one, show you sample questions, share some of Kaplan's proven methods, and clue you in to what the test makers are really after. You'll get a handle on the process; find a confident, new perspective; and achieve your highest possible scores.

REGISTRATION

Talk to your prepharmacy advisor to find out about the latest PCAT administration schedule and how to register for the test. If you don't have an advisor, contact the PCAT Program Office. They'll send you a registration packet, which contains important information about PCAT fees and score reporting.

Registration for the current year generally opens around March 1. The PCAT is generally administered three times each year: June, November, and January. A test date in August has been added for 2007.

Psychological Corporation
PSE Customer Relations—PCAT
19500 Bulverde Road
San Antonio, Texas 78259
1-800-622-3231 or 1-210-339-8711
Email: scoring.services@harcourt.com

You can also find out about the PCAT and register to take the test on the PCAT website (pcatweb.info). You also can register online at tpc-etesting.com/PCAT. Note that submitting a paper registration form costs an additional $35.00.

Don't drag your feet gathering information. You'll need time not only to prepare and practice for the test but also to get all your registration paperwork done.

Plan Ahead

The PCAT is offered only a few times a year, so be sure to give yourself lots of lead time for getting information. Download a PCAT Candidate Information Booklet at pcatwweb.info.

Be a Control Freak

The PCAT should be viewed just like any other part of your application: as an opportunity to show the Pharmacy schools who you are and what you can do. Take control of your PCAT experience.

ANATOMY OF THE PCAT

Before mastering strategies, you need to know exactly what you're dealing with on the PCAT. Let's start with the basics. The PCAT is, among other things, an endurance test. It consists of seven sections and approximately 240 multiple-choice questions. Add in the administrative details at both ends of the testing experience, plus one break halfway through the test, and you can count on being in the test room for over four hours. It's a grueling experience, to say the least. If you can't approach it with confidence and stamina, you'll quickly lose your composure. That's why it's so important that you take control of the test.

June 2007 Test Changes

Several changes to the PCAT went into effect in June 2007. The test now contains two problem-solving essays instead of one, as well as fewer multiple-choice questions in Verbal Ability, Biology, Chemistry, and Quantitative Ability. Geometry is no longer tested, and questions on probability, statistics, and genetics appear more frequently.

The PCAT consists of seven timed sections—Verbal Ability, Biology, Reading Comprehension, Quantitative Ability, Chemistry—and two Writing sections. Later, we'll take an in-depth look at each PCAT section, including content, sample question types, and specific test-smart hints.

Writing

Time: 30 minutes

Format: problem-solving essay based on a given topic

What it tests: general composition skills and conventions of language, ability to communicate a solution to a problem

Verbal Ability

Time: 30 minutes

Format: 48 multiple-choice questions

What it tests: general, nonscientific word knowledge using analogies and sentence completion

Biology

Time: 30 minutes

Format: 48 multiple-choice questions

What it tests: the knowledge of the concepts and principles of basic biology with an emphasis on human biology, microbiology, and anatomy/physiology

Chemistry

Time: 30 minutes

Format: 48 multiple-choice questions

What it tests: the knowledge of the concepts and principles of inorganic and elementary organic chemistry

Writing

Time: 30 minutes

Format: problem-solving essay based on a given topic

What it tests: general composition skills and conventions of language, ability to communicate a solution to a problem

Reading Comprehension

Time: 50 minutes

Format: 48 multiple-choice questions; there are 6 passages with 6–9 questions to follow

What it tests: the ability of the student to comprehend, analyze, and interpret reading passages on scientific topics

Quantitative Ability

Time: 40 minutes

Format: 48 multiple-choice questions

What it tests: skills in arithmetic processes, including fractions, decimals, and percentages, and the ability to reason through and understand quantitative concepts and their relationships, including applications of algebra, probability and statistics, precalculus, and calculus.

Scoring

Each PCAT section receives its own score. Each section is scored on a scale ranging from 200 – 600, with 600 as the highest and a mean of 400.

The Writing section is scored numerically from 0 to 5. One of the Writing prompts will be experimental and will not count toward your score. Two Writing scores will be recorded: one reflecting use of appropriate grammar and style and the other reflecting ability to create and support a solution to a problem.

The number of multiple-choice questions that you answer correctly per section is your "raw score." Your raw score will then be converted to yield the "scaled score"—the one that will fall somewhere in that 200–600 range. These scaled scores are what are reported to Pharmacy schools as your PCAT scores. All multiple-choice questions are worth the same amount—one raw point—*so there's no penalty for guessing.* That means that *you should always fill in an answer for every question, whether you get to that question or not!* Never let time run out on any section without filling in an answer for every question on the grid. Your score report will tell you—and your potential Pharmacy schools—not only your scaled scores but also the national mean score for each section, as well as standard deviations, national scoring profiles for each section, and your percentile ranking.

Your Percentile

The percentile figure tells you how many other test takers scored at or below your level. In other words, a percentile figure of 80 means that 80 percent did as well or worse than you did and that only 20 percent did better.

WHAT'S A GOOD SCORE?

There's no such thing as a cut-and-dried good score. Much depends on the strength of the rest of your application (if your transcript is first-rate, the pressure to strut your stuff on the PCAT isn't as intense) and on where you want to go to school (different schools have different score expectations).

For each PCAT administration, the average scaled scores are approximately 400 for each section; this equates to the 50th percentile. You need scores of at least 450 to be considered competitive by most pharmacy schools, and if you're aiming for the top, you've got to do even better and score above 450.

It's important to maximize your performance on every question. Just a few questions one way or the other can make a big difference in your scaled score. You should make an extra effort to score well on a test section if you did poorly in a corresponding class. So the best revenge for getting a C in chemistry class is acing the Chemistry section of the PCAT.

WHAT THE PCAT REALLY TESTS

It's important to grasp not only the nuts and bolts of the PCAT so you'll know what to do on Test Day but also the underlying principles of the test so you'll know why you're doing what you're doing. We'll cover the straightforward PCAT facts later. Now it's time to examine the heart and soul of the PCAT to see what it's really about.

THE MYTH

Most people preparing for the PCAT fall prey to the myth that the PCAT is a straightforward science test. They think something like this:

> *It covers the two years of science I had to take in school: biology, chemistry, and basic organic chemistry, plus math and freshman English. The important stuff is the science, though. After all, we're going to be pharmacists.*

Well, here's the little secret no one seems to want you to know: the PCAT is not just a science test; it's also a thinking test. This means that the test is designed to let you demonstrate your thought process as well as your thought content. The implications are vast. Once you shift your test-taking paradigm to match the PCAT's modus operandi, you'll find a new level of confidence and control over the test. You'll begin to work with the nature of the PCAT rather than against it. You'll be more efficient and insightful as you prepare for the test, and you'll be more relaxed on test day. In fact, you'll be able to see the PCAT for what it is rather than for what it's dressed up to be. We want your Test Day to feel familiar, not awkward!

THE ZEN OF PCAT

Pharmacy schools do not need to rely on the PCAT to see what you already know. Admission committees can measure your subject-area proficiency using your undergraduate coursework and grades. Schools are most interested in the potential of your mind.

In recent years, many Pharmacy schools have shifted pedagogic focus away from an information-heavy curriculum to a concept-based curriculum. Currently more emphasis is placed on problem solving, holistic thinking, and cross-disciplinary study. Be careful not to dismiss this important point, figuring you'll wait to worry about academic trends until you're actually in Pharmacy school. This trend affects you right now because it's reflected in the PCAT. Every good tool matches its task. In this case, the tool is the test, which is used to measure you and other candidates, and the task is to quantify how likely it is that you'll succeed in Pharmacy school.

Your intellectual potential—how skillfully you annex new territory into your mental boundaries, how quickly you build "thought highways" between ideas, and how confidently and creatively you solve problems—is far more important to admission committees than your ability to recite Young's modulus for every material known to man. The schools assume they can expand your knowledge base. They choose applicants carefully because expansive knowledge is not enough to succeed in Pharmacy school or in the profession. There's something more, and it's this *something more* that the PCAT is trying to measure: every section on the PCAT tests essentially the same higher-order thinking skills: analytical reasoning, abstract thinking, and problem solving. Most test takers get trapped into thinking they are being tested strictly about biology, chemistry, etc. Thus, they approach each section with a new outlook on what's expected. This constant mental gear shifting can be exhausting, not to mention counterproductive. Instead of perceiving the test as parsed into radically different sections, you need to maintain your focus on the underlying nature of the test; each section presents a variation on the same theme. The PCAT is not just about what you know. It's also about how you think.

WHAT ABOUT THE SCIENCE?

With this perspective, you may be left asking the question: "What about the science? What about the content? Don't I need to know the basics?" The answer is a resounding Yes! You must be fluent in the different languages of the test. You cannot do well on the PCAT if you don't know the basics of general chemistry, biology, basic organic chemistry, and math. We recommend that you take one year each of biology and general chemistry and one semester of organic chemistry before taking the PCAT and that you review the content in this book thoroughly. Knowing these basics is just the beginning of doing well on the PCAT. That's a shock to most test takers. They presume that once they recall or relearn their undergraduate science, they are ready to do battle against the PCAT. Wrong! They merely have directions to the battlefield. They lack what they need to beat the test: a copy of the test maker's battle plan. You won't be drilled on facts and formulas on the PCAT. You'll need to demonstrate ability to reason based on ideas and concepts. The science questions are painted with a broad brush, testing your general understanding.

TAKE CONTROL: THE PCAT MINDSET

In addition to being a thinking test, as we've stressed, the PCAT is a standardized test. As such, it has its own consistent patterns and idiosyncrasies that can actually work in your favor. This is the key to why test preparation works. You have the opportunity to familiarize yourself with those consistent peculiarities and to adopt the proper test-taking mindset.

The PCAT Mindset is something you want to bring to every question, passage, and section you encounter. Being in the PCAT Mindset means reshaping the test-taking experience so that you are in the driver's seat:

- Answer questions *when* you want to; feel free to skip tough but feasible passages and questions, coming back to them only after you've racked up points on easy ones.
- Answer questions *how* you want to; use our shortcuts and methods to get points quickly and confidently, even if those methods aren't exactly what the test makers had in mind when they wrote the test.

Some overriding principles of the PCAT Mindset that will be covered in depth in the chapters to come are as follows:

- Read actively and critically.
- Translate prose into your own words.
- Save the toughest questions and passages for last.
- Know the test and its components inside and out.
- Do PCAT-style problems in each topic area after you've reviewed it.
- Allow your confidence to build on itself.
- Take full-length practice tests a week or two before the test to break down the mystique of the real experience.
- Learn from your mistakes—get the most out of your practice tests.
- Look at the PCAT as a challenge, the first step in your pharmacy career, rather than as an arbitrary obstacle.

That's what the PCAT Mindset boils down to: taking control, being proactive, and being on top of the testing experience so that you can get as many points as you can as quickly and as easily as possible. Keep this in mind as you read and work through the material in this book and, of course, as you face the challenge on Test Day.

CHAPTER TWO

Test Expertise

The first year of the professional phase of Pharmacy school is a frenzied experience for most students. To meet the requirements of a rigorous work schedule, students either learn to prioritize and budget their time or else fall hopelessly behind. It's no surprise, then, that the PCAT, the test specifically designed to predict success in the first year of Pharmacy school, is a high-speed, time-intensive test. It demands excellent time-management skills as well as that sine qua non of the successful physician—grace under pressure.

It's one thing to answer a Reading Comprehension question correctly; it's quite another to answer all 48 of them correctly in only 50 minutes. The same applies for the other sections. It's a completely different experience to move from handling an individual passage or problem at leisure to handling a full section under timed conditions. Time is a factor that affects every test taker, and the good news is that you can easily improve your scores by following the five basic principles outlined below.

A Matter of Time

For complete PCAT success, you've got to get as many correct answers as possible in the time you're allotted. Knowing the strategies is not enough. You have to perfect your time management skills so that you get a chance to use those strategies on as many questions as possible.

THE FIVE BASIC PRINCIPLES OF TEST EXPERTISE

On some tests, if a question seems particularly difficult, you spend significantly more time on it because you'll probably be given more points for correctly answering a hard question. Not so on the PCAT. Remember, every PCAT question, no matter how hard, is worth a single point. There's no partial credit or A for effort, and because there are so many questions to do in so little time, you'd be a fool to spend 10 minutes getting a point for a hard question and then not having time to get a couple of quick points from three easy questions later in the section.

Given this combination—limited time and all questions equal in weight—you've got to develop a way of handling the test sections to make sure you get as many points as you can as quickly and easily as you can. Here are the principles that will help you do that.

1. Feel Free To Skip Around

One of the most valuable strategies to help you finish the sections in time is to learn to recognize and deal first with the questions and passages that are easier and more familiar to you. That means temporarily skipping those that promise to be difficult and time consuming if you feel comfortable doing so. You can always come back to these at the end, and if you run out of time, you're much better off not getting to questions you may have had difficulty with, rather than potentially feasible material. Of course, because there's no guessing penalty, always fill in an answer to every question on the test, whether you get to it or not. Also, remember to work on those passages with the most questions so you maximize your points.

This strategy is difficult for most test takers; we're conditioned to do things in order. But give it a try when you practice. Remember, if you do the test in the exact order given, you're letting the test makers control you. But you control how you take this test. On the other hand, if skipping around goes against your moral fiber and makes you a nervous wreck—don't do it. Just be mindful of the clock, and don't get bogged down with the tough questions.

2. Learn to Recognize and Seek Out Questions You Can Do

Another thing to remember about managing the test sections is that PCAT questions and passages, unlike items on the SAT and other standardized tests, are not presented in order of difficulty. There's no rule that says you have to work through the sections in any particular order; in fact, the test makers scatter the easy and difficult questions throughout the section, in effect rewarding those who actually get to the end. Don't lose sight of what you're being tested for along with your reading and thinking skills: efficiency and cleverness. If general chemistry questions are your thing, head straight for them when you first turn to the General Chemistry section and save the organic chemistry questions until the end.

Be a Test Expert

To meet the stringent time requirements of the PCAT, you have to cultivate the following elements of test expertise:

- Feel free to skip around.
- Learn to recognize and seek out questions you can do.
- Use a process of answer elimination.
- Remain calm.
- Keep track of time.

Guess!

We've said it before, and we'll say it again: if you can't do a question or can't get to it, guess! Fill in an answer–any answer–on the answer grid. There's no penalty if you're wrong, but you score a point if you're right.

Don't waste time on questions you can't do. We know that skipping a possibly tough question is easier said than done; we all have the natural instinct to plow through test sections in their given order. But it just doesn't pay off on the PCAT. The computer won't be impressed if you get the toughest question right. If you dig in your heels on a tough question, refusing to move on until you've cracked it, well, you're letting your ego get in the way of your test score. A test section (not to mention life itself) is too short to waste on lost causes.

3. Use a Process of Answer Elimination

Using a process of elimination is another way to answer questions both quickly and effectively. There are two ways to get all the answers right on the PCAT. You either know all the right answers, or you know all the wrong answers. Because there are three times as many wrong answers, you should be able to eliminate some, if not all, of them. By doing so, you either get to the correct response or increase your chances of guessing the correct response. You start out with a 25 percent chance of picking the right answer, and with each eliminated answer, your odds go up. Eliminate one, and you'll have a 33 1/3 percent chance of picking the right one; eliminate two, and you'll have a 50 percent chance, and so on. Increase your efficiency by actually crossing out the wrong choices. Remember to look for wrong-answer traps when you're eliminating. Some answers are designed to seduce you by distorting the correct answer.

4. Remain Calm

It's imperative that you remain calm and composed while working through a section. You can't allow yourself to become so rattled by one hard reading passage that it throws off your performance on the rest of the section. Expect to find at least one killer passage in the reading comprehensive section, but remember, you won't be the only one having trouble with it. The test is curved to take the tough material into account. Having trouble with a difficult question isn't going to ruin your score, but getting upset about it and letting it throw you off track will. When you understand that part of the test maker's goal is to reward those who keep their composure, you'll recognize the importance of not panicking when you run into challenging material.

5. Keep Track of Time

Of course, the last thing you want to happen is to have time called on a particular section before you've gotten to half the questions. Therefore, it's essential that you pace yourself, keeping in mind the general guidelines for how long to spend on any individual question or passage. Have a sense of how long you have to do each question so you know when you're exceeding the limit and should start to move faster.

When working on a section, always remember to keep track of time. Don't spend a wildly disproportionate amount of time on any one question or group of questions. Also, give yourself 30 seconds or so at the end of each section to fill in answers for any questions you haven't gotten to.

Leave Your Ego at Home

Don't let your ego sabotage your score. It isn't easy for some of us to give up on a tough, time-consuming question, but sometimes it's better simply to move on. Remember that there's no point of honor at stake here, but there are PCAT points at stake.

Pop Quiz

Every question is worth exactly one point, but questions vary dramatically in difficulty level. Given a shortage of time, which questions should you work on—easy or hard?

Increase Your Chances of Success

If you don't know the right answer, eliminate as many wrong answers as you can. This way you'll either get to, or increase your chances of getting to, the right one.

SECTION-SPECIFIC PACING

Let's now look at the section-specific timing requirements and some tips for meeting them. Keep in mind that the times per question or passage are only averages; there are bound to be some that take less time and some that take more. Try to stay balanced. Remember, too, that every question is of equal worth, so don't get hung up on any one. Think about it: if a question is so hard that it takes you a long time to answer it, chances are you may get it wrong anyway. In that case, you'd have nothing to show for your extra time but a lower score.

Reading Comprehension

Allow yourself approximately seven or eight minutes per passage and respective questions. It may sound like a lot of time, but it goes quickly. Do the easiest passages first. Within a section, if you're deciding which passage to do based on time alone, do the one with the most questions. That way you maximize your reading efficiency. However, keep in mind that some passages are longer than others. On average, give yourself about two to three minutes to read and then four to five minutes for the questions.

Verbal Ability, Biology, Quantitative Ability, and Chemistry

Averaging over each section, you'll have about 37 seconds per question for Verbal, Biology, and Chemistry questions, and about 50 seconds for each Quantitatve question. Some questions, of course, will take more time and some less. Again, the rule is to do your best work first. Also, don't feel that you have to understand everything in a passage before you go on to the questions. You may not need that deep an understanding to answer questions because a lot of information may be extraneous. You should overcome your perfectionism and use your time wisely.

Answer Grid Expertise

An important part of PCAT test expertise is knowing how to handle the answer grid. After all, you not only have to get right answers, but you also have to transfer those right answers onto the answer grid in an efficient and accurate way. It sounds simple, but it's extremely important: **don't make mistakes filling out your answer grid!** When time is short, it's easy to get confused going back and forth between your test book and your grid. If you know the answer but misgrid, you won't get the point. Here are a few methods of avoiding mistakes on the answer grid.

Always Circle the Questions You Skip

Put a big circle in your test book around the number of any question you skip (you may even want to circle the whole question). When you go back, such questions will then be easy to locate. Also, if you accidentally skip an oval on the grid, you can easily check your grid against your book to see where you went wrong.

Always Circle the Answers You Choose

Circle the correct answers in your test booklet, but don't transfer the answer to the grid right away. Circling your answers in the test book will also make it easier to check your grid against your book.

Grid Five or More Answers at Once

As we said, don't transfer your answers to the grid after every question. Transfer your answers after every five questions or at the end of each passage in the reading comprehensive section (find the method that works best for you). That way, you won't keep breaking your concentration to mark the grid. You'll save time and improve accuracy. Just make sure you're not left at the end of the section with ungridded answers!

Save Time at the End for a Final Grid Check

Make sure you have enough time at the end of every section to make a quick check of your grid and to make sure you've got an oval filled in for each question in the section. Remember that a blank grid has no chance of earning a point, but a guess does.

CHAPTER THREE

Test Mentality

Now we will turn our attention to the often-overlooked attitudinal aspects of the test to put the finishing touches on your comprehensive PCAT approach.

What Makes for Good Test Mentality?

We're glad you asked. The important elements are:

- Test Awareness
- Stamina
- Confidence
- The Right Attitude

THE FOUR BASIC PRINCIPLES OF GOOD TEST MENTALITY

Knowing the test content arms you with the weapons you need to do well on the PCAT. But you must wield those weapons with the right frame of mind and in the right spirit. Otherwise, you could end up shooting yourself in the foot. This involves taking a certain stance toward the entire test. Here's what's involved:

1. Test Awareness

To do your best on the PCAT, you must always keep in mind that the test is like no other test you've taken before, both in terms of content and in terms of the scoring system. If you took a test in high school or college and got a number of the questions wrong, you wouldn't receive a perfect grade. However, on the PCAT, you can get a handful of questions wrong and still get a "perfect" score. The test is geared so that only the very best test takers are able to finish every section, but even these people rarely get every question right. What does this mean for you? Well, just as you shouldn't let one bad passage ruin an entire section, you shouldn't let what you consider to be a subpar performance on one section ruin your performance on the entire test. Often when you think you did not do well, you may be mistaken. Test takers tend to think they did poorly, only to find out they actually did well. If you allow a feeling of failure to rattle you, it can have a cumulative negative effect, setting in motion a downward spiral. That kind of thing could potentially do serious damage to your score. Losing a few extra points won't do you in, but losing your cool will. Remember, if you feel you've done poorly on a section, don't sweat it. Chances are it's just a difficult section, and that factor will already be figured into the scoring curve. The point is, remain calm and collected. Simply do your best on each section, and once a section is over, forget about it and move on.

2. Stamina

You must work on your test-taking stamina. Overall, the PCAT is a fairly grueling experience, and some test takers simply run out of gas on the last section. To avoid this, you must prepare by taking a few full-length practice tests in the weeks before the test so that on Test Day, seven sections will seem like a breeze. (Well, maybe not a breeze, but at least not a hurricane.) Take the full-length practice test included in this book. You'll be able to review answer explanations and assess your performance.

You can't be assured that your score on a practice test will predict your actual score. The score you get on a practice test is less important than the practice itself.

3. Confidence

Confidence feeds on itself, and unfortunately, so does the opposite of confidence—self-doubt. Confidence in your ability leads to quick, sure answers and a sense of well-being that translates into more points. If you lack confidence, you end up reading the sentences and answer choices two, three, or four times, until you confuse yourself and get off track. This leads to timing difficulties, which only perpetuate the downward spiral, causing anxiety and a tendency to rush to finish sections.

However, if you subscribe to the PCAT Mindset we've described, you'll gear all of your practice toward the major goal of taking control of the test. When you've achieved that goal—armed with the principles, techniques, strategies, and approaches set forth in this book—you'll be ready to face the PCAT with supreme confidence, and that's the one sure way to score your best on test day.

4. The Right Attitude

Those students who approach the PCAT as an obstacle, rail against the necessity of taking it, make light of its importance, or spend more time making fun of the Psychological Corporation than studying for the test usually don't fare as well as those who see the PCAT as an opportunity to show off the reading and reasoning skills that the Pharmacy schools are looking for. Don't waste time making value judgments about the PCAT. It's not going to go away. Deal with it. Those who look forward to doing battle with the PCAT—or, at least, who enjoy the opportunity to distinguish themselves from the rest of the applicant pack—tend to score better than do those who resent or dread it.

It may sound a little dubious, but take our word for it: attitude adjustment is a proven test-taking technique. Here are a few steps you can take to make sure you develop the right PCAT attitude:

- Look at the PCAT as a challenge but try not to obsess over it; you certainly don't want to psyche yourself out of the game.
- Remember that, yes, the PCAT is obviously important, but contrary to what some students think, this one test will not single-handedly determine the outcome of your life.

- Try to have fun with the test. Learning how to match your wits against the test makers can be a very satisfying experience, and the reading and thinking skills you'll acquire will benefit you in Pharmacy school as well as in your future Pharmacy career.
- Remember that you're more prepared than most people. You've trained with Kaplan. You have the tools you need plus the know-how to use those tools.

Get in Shape

You wouldn't run a marathon without working on your stamina well in advance of the race, would you? The same goes for taking the PCAT.

And now…

KAPLAN'S TOP TEN PCAT STRATEGIES

1. **Relax!**

2. **Remember: It's primarily a thinking test.**

   Never forget the purpose of the PCAT: it's designed to test your powers of analytical reasoning. You need to know the content because each section has its own particular "language," but the underlying PCAT intention is consistent throughout the test.

3. **Feel free to skip around within each section.**

   Attack each section confidently. You're in charge. Move around if you feel comfortable doing so. Work your best areas first to maximize your opportunity for PCAT points. Don't be a passive victim of the test structure!

4. **For passage-based questions in the Reading Comprehension section, choose an answer based on the information given.**

   Be careful not to be "too smart for your own good." Passages—especially those that describe experimental findings (a PCAT favorite, by the way)—often generate their own data. Your answer choices must be consistent with the information in the passage, even if that means an answer choice is inconsistent with the science of ideal theoretical situations.

5. **Avoid wrong-answer traps.**

   Try to anticipate answers before you read the answer choices. This helps boost your confidence and protects you from persuasive or tricky incorrect choices. Most wrong answer choices are logical twists on the correct choice.

6. **Think, think, think!**

   We said it before, but it's important enough to say again: Think. Don't Compute.

7. **Don't look back.**

   Don't spend time worrying about questions you had to guess on. Keep moving forward. Don't let your spirit start to flag, or your attitude will slow you down. You can recheck answers within a section if you have time left, but don't worry about a section after time has been called.

8. **Be careful transferring answers to your grid.**

   Be sure that you are very careful transcribing answers to your grid, especially if you do skip around within the test sections.

9. **Don't leave any blanks on your answer grid.**

   No points are taken off for wrong answers, so if you're not sure of an answer, guess, and guess quickly so you'll have more time to work through other questions.

10. **Call us! We're here to help! 1-800-KAP-TEST.**

Develop a PCATtitude

It sounds touchy-feely, we know, but your attitude toward the test really does affect your performance. We're not asking you to think nice thoughts about the PCAT, but we are recommending that you change your mental stance toward the test.

Diagnostic Exam
Answer Sheet

Remove (or photocopy) this answer sheet and use it to complete the practice test.

If a section has fewer questions than answer spaces, leave the extra spaces blank.

Verbal Ability

1 (A) (B) (C) (D)   11 (A) (B) (C) (D)   21 (A) (B) (C) (D)
2 (A) (B) (C) (D)   12 (A) (B) (C) (D)   22 (A) (B) (C) (D)
3 (A) (B) (C) (D)   13 (A) (B) (C) (D)   23 (A) (B) (C) (D)
4 (A) (B) (C) (D)   14 (A) (B) (C) (D)   24 (A) (B) (C) (D)
5 (A) (B) (C) (D)   15 (A) (B) (C) (D)
6 (A) (B) (C) (D)   16 (A) (B) (C) (D)
7 (A) (B) (C) (D)   17 (A) (B) (C) (D)
8 (A) (B) (C) (D)   18 (A) (B) (C) (D)
9 (A) (B) (C) (D)   19 (A) (B) (C) (D)
10 (A) (B) (C) (D)   20 (A) (B) (C) (D)

Biology

1 (A) (B) (C) (D)   11 (A) (B) (C) (D)   21 (A) (B) (C) (D)
2 (A) (B) (C) (D)   12 (A) (B) (C) (D)   22 (A) (B) (C) (D)
3 (A) (B) (C) (D)   13 (A) (B) (C) (D)   23 (A) (B) (C) (D)
4 (A) (B) (C) (D)   14 (A) (B) (C) (D)   24 (A) (B) (C) (D)
5 (A) (B) (C) (D)   15 (A) (B) (C) (D)
6 (A) (B) (C) (D)   16 (A) (B) (C) (D)
7 (A) (B) (C) (D)   17 (A) (B) (C) (D)
8 (A) (B) (C) (D)   18 (A) (B) (C) (D)
9 (A) (B) (C) (D)   19 (A) (B) (C) (D)
10 (A) (B) (C) (D)   20 (A) (B) (C) (D)

Chemistry

1 (A) (B) (C) (D)   11 (A) (B) (C) (D)   21 (A) (B) (C) (D)
2 (A) (B) (C) (D)   12 (A) (B) (C) (D)   22 (A) (B) (C) (D)
3 (A) (B) (C) (D)   13 (A) (B) (C) (D)   23 (A) (B) (C) (D)
4 (A) (B) (C) (D)   14 (A) (B) (C) (D)   24 (A) (B) (C) (D)
5 (A) (B) (C) (D)   15 (A) (B) (C) (D)   25 (A) (B) (C) (D)
6 (A) (B) (C) (D)   16 (A) (B) (C) (D)
7 (A) (B) (C) (D)   17 (A) (B) (C) (D)
8 (A) (B) (C) (D)   18 (A) (B) (C) (D)
9 (A) (B) (C) (D)   19 (A) (B) (C) (D)
10 (A) (B) (C) (D)   20 (A) (B) (C) (D)

Reading Comprehension

1 (A) (B) (C) (D)   11 (A) (B) (C) (D)
2 (A) (B) (C) (D)   12 (A) (B) (C) (D)
3 (A) (B) (C) (D)   13 (A) (B) (C) (D)
4 (A) (B) (C) (D)   14 (A) (B) (C) (D)
5 (A) (B) (C) (D)   15 (A) (B) (C) (D)
6 (A) (B) (C) (D)   16 (A) (B) (C) (D)
7 (A) (B) (C) (D)   17 (A) (B) (C) (D)
8 (A) (B) (C) (D)   18 (A) (B) (C) (D)
9 (A) (B) (C) (D)   19 (A) (B) (C) (D)
10 (A) (B) (C) (D)   20 (A) (B) (C) (D)

Quantitative Ability

1 (A) (B) (C) (D)   11 (A) (B) (C) (D)   21 (A) (B) (C) (D)
2 (A) (B) (C) (D)   12 (A) (B) (C) (D)   22 (A) (B) (C) (D)
3 (A) (B) (C) (D)   13 (A) (B) (C) (D)   23 (A) (B) (C) (D)
4 (A) (B) (C) (D)   14 (A) (B) (C) (D)   24 (A) (B) (C) (D)
5 (A) (B) (C) (D)   15 (A) (B) (C) (D)
6 (A) (B) (C) (D)   16 (A) (B) (C) (D)
7 (A) (B) (C) (D)   17 (A) (B) (C) (D)
8 (A) (B) (C) (D)   18 (A) (B) (C) (D)
9 (A) (B) (C) (D)   19 (A) (B) (C) (D)
10 (A) (B) (C) (D)   20 (A) (B) (C) (D)

CHAPTER FOUR

Diagnostic Exam

Instructions: This examination contains the following sections:

Section 1:	**Verbal Ability**	**15 minutes**
Section 2:	**Biology**	**15 minutes**
Section 3:	**Chemistry**	**15 minutes**
Section 4:	**Reading Comprehension**	**25 minutes**
Section 5:	**Quantitative Ability**	**20 minutes**

The actual PCAT will include two Writing Sections. Also, this Diagnostic Exam is approximately half as long as the actual PCAT. During the time allocated for a specific section, *you may work only on that section*. If you finish a section early, you may check your work only within that section, *but do not go back to a previous section or ahead to a forthcoming section*.

Place all your answers on the answer grid. Use a #2 pencil only. Blacken the space for each question that corresponds to the answer choice you have selected. Be sure your mark fills the answer choice completely. If you change your answer, be sure to erase the previous choice completely and leave no stray marks on the answer grid.

When you have completed the Diagnostic Exam, check your answers and read the explanations provided. Use these results to guide your study plan and concentrate on those sections you had the most trouble with.

Important Note:
This Diagnostic Exam does not test Calculus. For Calculus practice, go to **kaptest.com/booksonline**.

VERBAL ABILITY

Questions: 24
Time: 15 minutes

Sentence Completion

Directions: Each sentence below has one or two blanks, each blank indicating that something has been omitted. Beneath the sentence are five lettered words or sets of words. Choose the word or set of words for each blank that best fit the meaning of the sentence as a whole.

1. The _____ of the desert explains why so many Egyptian mummies are still intact, whereas the humidity of the tombs in tropical rain forests supports agents of decay so that few Aztec mummies have _____ .

   (A) heat ... survived
   (B) aridity ... endured
   (C) dehydration ... decayed
   (D) barrenness ... proliferated

2. They _____ until there was no recourse but to _____ a desperate, last-minute solution to the problem.

   (A) filibustered ... reject
   (B) delayed ... envision
   (C) procrastinated ... implement
   (D) debated ... maintain

3. The Wankel Rotary Engine was an engineering marvel that substantially reduced automobile exhaust emissions, but because it was less fuel-efficient than the standard piston-cylinder engine, it was _____ in the early 1970s when _____ pollution gave way to panic over fuel shortages.

   (A) needed ... disillusionment with
   (B) conceived ... attention on
   (C) modified ... opinion on
   (D) abandoned ... preoccupation with

4. Friendship, no matter how _____ , has its boundaries; _____ advice, when thrust insistently upon one, is rarely an act of friendship, regardless of the advisor's intent.

   (A) cool ... contradictory
   (B) enjoyable ... obverse
   (C) intimate ... unsolicited
   (D) distant ... marital

5. Despite generous helpings of _____ from a group of _____ critics, this iconoclastic poet's three volumes have sold steadily.

   (A) vitriol ... influential
   (B) mockery ... obscure
   (C) tedium ... respected
   (D) abuse ... ineffectual

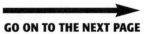

GO ON TO THE NEXT PAGE

KAPLAN

6. Because the different components of the film industry were "vertically" oriented—arranged so that all _____ , from production to projection, were held by one company—it was _____ that monopolistic practices would arise.

 (A) opportunities for control ... inevitable

 (B) burdens of business ... understandable

 (C) exercises of power ... appropriate

 (D) means of solicitation ... predictable

7. From the _____ that the peasants tried to conceal as they knelt before the body of the dictator's son, I concluded that, far from affection, it was _____ that had brought them to the wake.

 (A) hatred ... sarcasm

 (B) reticence ... violence

 (C) diligence ... adulation

 (D) trepidation ... fear

8. Despite the increased attention _____ juvenile delinquency, there has been a _____ in crimes committed by juveniles.

 (A) allotted to ... dip

 (B) offered to ... development

 (C) given to ... rise

 (D) spent on ... decrease

9. Much of the Beatles's music, as evidenced by "All You Need Is Love," was characterized by a superficial _____ subtly contradicted by an inherent, deeper cynicism.

 (A) competence

 (B) world-weariness

 (C) liveliness

 (D) naiveté

10. During their famous clash, Jung was ambivalent about Freud so he attacked the father of modern psychoanalysis even as he _____ him.

 (A) enlightened

 (B) chastened

 (C) revered

 (D) despised

GO ON TO THE NEXT PAGE

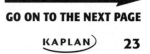

Analogies

Directions: Choose the word that **best** completes the analogy in capital letters.

11. DRAKE : DUCK :: BULL :
    (A) sheep
    (B) chicken
    (C) monkey
    (D) ox

12. PREAMBLE : DOCUMENT :: PROLOGUE :
    (A) interlude
    (B) letter
    (C) statement
    (D) play

13. SARTORIAL : TAILOR :: TONSORIAL :
    (A) student
    (B) barber
    (C) dentist
    (D) politician

14. RUMINATE : REFLECT :: BROOD :
    (A) heal
    (B) worry
    (C) ponder
    (D) store

15. PAEAN : PRAISE :: DIRGE :
    (A) marriage
    (B) mourning
    (C) irreverence
    (D) ceremony

16. RECTORY : CLERIC :: PALACE :
    (A) soldier
    (B) mendicant
    (C) potentate
    (D) monk

17. PEREGRINATION : TRAVEL :: GYRATION :
    (A) walk
    (B) depart
    (C) debate
    (D) revolve

18. ABSTRACT : ARTICLE :: SYNOPSIS :
    (A) statement
    (B) rule
    (C) summary
    (D) narrative

19. ABSTEMIOUS : BINGE :: FRUGAL :
    (A) escape
    (B) splurge
    (C) evade
    (D) satisfy

20. AUGUST : GRANDEUR :: CRASS :
    (A) indelicacy
    (B) volume
    (C) certitude
    (D) youth

21. WATER : POTABLE :: FOOD :
    (A) palatable
    (B) poisonous
    (C) edible
    (D) audible

22. PICAYUNE : ATTENTION :: LUDICROUS :
    (A) size
    (B) authority
    (C) respect
    (D) compassion

23. IMMUTABLE : CHANGE :: IMMOBILE :
    (A) stasis
    (B) childhood
    (C) mutation
    (D) movement

24. MAELSTROM : WATER :: TORNADO :
    (A) fire
    (B) air
    (C) earth
    (D) lightning

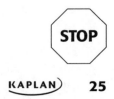

BIOLOGY

Questions: 24
Time: 10 minutes

Directions: Choose the **best** answer to each of the following questions.

1. If the hypothalamus were damaged, which of the following would probably be most affected?
   (A) Respiration rate
   (B) Appetite
   (C) Coordination
   (D) Memory

2. Which of the following is a function of the lymphatic system?
   (A) Transport of oxygen to the tissues
   (B) Absorption of carbohydrates from the gastrointestinal tract
   (C) Drainage of excess cerebrospinal fluid from the brain
   (D) Removal and destruction of foreign particles

3. Which of the following is the primary function of the human liver?
   (A) Conversion of waste to urea
   (B) Fat absorption
   (C) Protein storage
   (D) Red blood cell production

4. The RNA that functions as an amino acid carrier during translation is known as
   (A) hnRNA.
   (B) mRNA.
   (C) rRNA.
   (D) tRNA.

5. Fungal cells, unlike animal cells, do not contain:
   (A) mitochondria.
   (B) ribosomes.
   (C) centrioles.
   (D) a nucleus.

6. Which of the following stimulates the conversion of glycogen to glucose?
   (A) Insulin
   (B) Parathyroid hormone
   (C) Glucagon
   (D) Cortisol

7. Which of the following is a mechanism of heat conservation?
   (A) Piloerection
   (B) Perspiration
   (C) Secretion of aldosterone
   (D) Blood vessel dilation

8. Chromosomes condense, shorten, and coil during which phase of mitosis?
   (A) Telophase
   (B) Metaphase
   (C) Anaphase
   (D) Prophase

9. The basis for the pairing of the two strands of DNA in the double helix is
   (A) covalent bonding.
   (B) hydrogen bonding.
   (C) hydrophobic interactions.
   (D) ionic bonding.

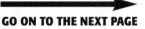

GO ON TO THE NEXT PAGE

10. The cellular organelles that are involved in the storage of materials are known as

    (A) mitochondria.
    (B) ribosomes.
    (C) centrioles.
    (D) vacuoles.

11. For a constant enzyme concentration, as the substrate concentration increases, the rate of enzyme action

    (A) decreases.
    (B) increases.
    (C) increases, then plateaus.
    (D) remains the same.

12. Which of the following contains RNA as its genetic material?

    (A) Retrovirus
    (B) Yeast cell
    (C) Muscle cell
    (D) Neuron

13. The major effect of ACTH is to cause the

    (A) adrenal cortex to release cortisone.
    (B) adrenal cortex to release norepinephrine.
    (C) adrenal medulla to release epinephrine.
    (D) adrenal medulla to release cortisone.

14. Which enzyme breaks down starch to disaccharides?

    (A) Amylase
    (B) Maltase
    (C) Lipase
    (D) Carboxypeptidase

15. Which of the following processes involves the uptake of genetic material from the environment?

    (A) Transformation
    (B) Conjugation
    (C) Transduction
    (D) Binary fission

16. In humans, the normal site of fertilization is the

    (A) ovary.
    (B) fallopian tube.
    (C) uterus.
    (D) vagina.

17. Muscle contraction results from

    (A) myosin and actin filaments simultaneously contracting.
    (B) myosin filament contraction only.
    (C) myosin and actin filaments sliding over each other.
    (D) myosin filaments expanding while actin filaments contract.

18. From which germ layer(s) do the kidneys arise?

    (A) Ectoderm
    (B) Mesoderm
    (C) Endoderm
    (D) Ectoderm and mesoderm

19. During glycolysis

    (A) $FADH_2$ is produced.
    (B) NADH is produced.
    (C) one molecule of glucose is converted into one molecule of pyruvate.
    (D) the end products always go on to form acetyl CoA.

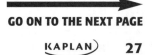

20. According to the endosymbiont hypothesis, mitochondria developed from aerobic prokaryotes that were engulfed by larger host prokaryotes. Many of the enzymes required for aerobic respiration are located on the inner membrane of the mitochondria. Where would these enzymes, or their precursors, most likely have been found prior to endosymbiosis?

    (A) In the cytoplasm of the anaerobic host cells

    (B) In the cytoplasm of the aerobic prokaryotic symbiont cells

    (C) On the plasma membrane of the anaerobic prokaryotic host cells

    (D) On the plasma membrane of the aerobic prokaryotic symbiont cells

21. Two organisms live in a close nutritional relationship where one organism benefits while the other is not harmed. This relationship is best defined as

    (A) predation.

    (B) mutualism.

    (C) commensalism.

    (D) parasitism.

22. Which of the following statements about respiration is TRUE?

    (A) O_2 and CO_2 are exchanged by active transport.

    (B) Hemoglobin is incapable of binding CO_2.

    (C) Gas exchange occurs in the trachea.

    (D) Contraction of the diaphragm results in inhalation.

23. Which of the following statements regarding photosynthesis is TRUE?

    (A) During the light cycle, sugar is produced.

    (B) The dark cycle occurs only in the absence of light.

    (C) During the dark cycle, ATP is produced.

    (D) The light cycle occurs only during exposure to light.

24. In humans, the allele for black hair (B) is dominant to the allele to brown hair (b). When a heterozygote is crossed against an individual with brown hair, what is the phenotypic ratio of the offspring?

    (A) 1 black hair: 1 brown hair

    (B) 3 black hairs: 1 brown hair

    (C) 3 brown hairs: 1 black hair

    (D) 2 brown hairs: 1 black hair

STOP

CHEMISTRY
Questions: 25
Time: 15 minutes

1. What is the molecular geometry of PH_2Cl?

   (A) Square planar

   (B) Trigonal planar

   (C) Tetrahedral

   (D) Trigonal pyramid

2. A rigid container holds 3.00 moles of an ideal gas at 298K. How many moles of gas would need to be added to the container at constant temperature to increase the pressure from 1.00 atm to 1.80 atm?

   (A) 73.4 moles

   (B) 24.4 moles

   (C) 22.4 moles

   (D) 2.4 moles

3. Determine the numerical value of the rate constant for the reaction $A + B \longrightarrow C$ from the experimental rate data given below.

Experiment	$[A]_0$ (M)	$[B]_0$ (M)	rate (Ms^{-1})
1	0.181	0.148	1.87
2	0.181	0.300	1.87
3	0.543	0.148	16.83

   (A) $k = \dfrac{1.87}{(0.181)^2}$

   (B) $k = \dfrac{1.87}{(0.181)(0.148)^2}$

   (C) $k = \dfrac{1.87}{(0.181)^2(0.323)}$

   (D) $k = \dfrac{(0.181)(0.148)}{1.87}$

4. The balanced equation below is for a nonspontaneous reaction ($\Delta H° = 131$ kJ/mol and $\Delta S° = 134$ J/mol·K). Assuming that ΔH and ΔS do not vary with temperature, at what temperature will the reaction become spontaneous?

   $C(s) + H_2O\ (l) \rightarrow CO(g) + H_2(g)$

   (A) 1,250°C

   (B) 1,022°C

   (C) 978°C

   (D) 749°C

5. At 0°C, a mixture of neon and argon gases occupies a volume of 44.8 liters with a total pressure of 1 atm. If the mixture contains 1.5 moles of argon, how many moles of neon are present?

   (A) 0.50

   (B) 0.75

   (C) 1.00

   (D) 1.50

6. What is the percentage of oxygen by mass in a 200-gram sample of $CuSO_4·5H_2O$? (atomic weights: Cu = 63.5, S = 32, O = 16, H = 1)

   (A) 30.1%

   (B) 32.1%

   (C) 36.1%

   (D) 57.7%

7. Which of the following could be the correct electron configuration for the ground state neutral atom of a nonmetallic element?

   (A) $1s^2 2s^2 2p^6 3s^2$

   (B) $1s^2 2s^2 2p^6 3s^2 4s^2$

   (C) $1s^2 2s^2 2p^6 3s^2 3p^4$

   (D) $1s^2 2s^2 2p^6 3s^2 3p^7$

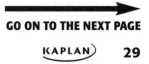

GO ON TO THE NEXT PAGE

8. How many grams of $Al_2(SO_4)_3$ are needed to make 87.5 g of 0.3 m $Al_2(SO_4)_3$ solution? (Atomic weights of Al = 27, S = 32, O = 16)

   (A) $(87.5 \times 102.6)/1,000$
   (B) $87.5/1,102.6$
   (C) $102.6/(87.5 \times 1,102.6)$
   (D) $(87.5 \times 102.6)/1,102.6$

9. Which of the following is the most polar molecular compound?

   (A) BF_3
   (B) CF_4
   (C) CBr_4
   (D) CH_2Cl_2

10. What volume of hydrogen gas, in liters, at 40°C and 763 torr can be produced by the complete reaction of 5.05 grams of zinc with excess $HCl(aq)$?

    $Zn(s) + 2\ HCl(aq) \longrightarrow ZnCl_2(aq) + H_2(g)$

    (Note: R = 0.0821 L·atm/mol·K
       atomic mass of Zn = 65.4)

    (A) $\left(\dfrac{5.05}{65.4}\right)\left(\dfrac{760}{763}\right)(0.0821)(313)$
    (B) $\left(\dfrac{5.05}{65.4}\right)\left(\dfrac{763}{760}\right)(0.0821)(40)$
    (C) $\left(\dfrac{5.05}{65.4}\right)\left(\dfrac{760}{763}\right)(0.0821)(40)$
    (D) $\left(\dfrac{5.05}{65.4}\right)\left(\dfrac{763}{760}\right)(0.0821)(313)$

11. If one isotope of an element has a mass number of 208 and an atomic number of 82, then another isotope of this element could have

    (A) 124 neutrons.
    (B) 126 neutrons.
    (C) a mass number of 208.
    (D) an atomic number of 80.

12. A sample of a pure compound is analyzed and found to contain 0.537 moles of N, 1.074 moles of H, and 0.537 moles of Cl. What is the empirical formula of this compound?

    (A) NH_4Cl
    (B) NH_2Cl
    (C) $NHCl_2$
    (D) $N_2H_2Cl_2$

13. Given the reactions and thermodynamic data below, calculate the enthalpy of formation for C_6H_5OH in kcal/mol.

reaction	$\Delta H°$ (kcal)
$C_6H_5OH + 7\ O_2 \rightarrow 6\ CO_2 + 3\ H_2O$	729.8
$C + O_2 \rightarrow CO_2$	94.4
$2\ H_2 + O_2 \rightarrow 2\ H_2O$	136.8

    (A) −247.0
    (B) −41.7
    (C) 41.7
    (D) 247.0

14. What is the percent yield if 78 g of C_6H_6 reacts and 82 g of $C_6H_5NO_2$ is formed according to the reaction below?

    $C_6H_6 + HNO_3 \rightarrow C_6H_5NO_2 + H_2O$

    (Molecular weights: $C_6H_6 = 78$, $C_6H_5NO_2 = 123$)

    (A) 33%
    (B) 50%
    (C) 67%
    (D) 100%

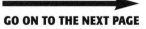

GO ON TO THE NEXT PAGE

15. Hydrogen fluoride, HF, is a gas at room temperature, while water, H_2O, is a liquid. Which is the best explanation for this observed difference in physical properties?

    (A) The difference in molecular weights indirectly accounts for the difference in boiling points because of van der Waals forces.

    (B) The O-H bond dipoles of water are greater than the F-H bond dipoles of HF and account for the greater dipole-dipole interactions between water molecules.

    (C) Hydrogen bonding between water molecules is significantly greater than that between HF molecules.

    (D) Dispersion forces are significant between HF molecules but not between water molecules.

16. When 100 g of an unknown compound is dissolved in water to produce 1.00 liter of solution, the pH of the resulting solution is measured as 4.56. Which of the following statements is most likely TRUE of the unknown compound?

    (A) It is a strong base with a formula weight of less than 50 g/mol.

    (B) It is a weak base with a pK_b of less than 5.

    (C) It is a strong acid with a formula weight of less than 50 g/mol.

    (D) It is a weak acid with a pK_a of more than 0.

17. Thirty-five mL of 0.10 M KOH is required to neutralize 50 mL of a monoprotic acid solution. The molarity of the acid solution is

    (A) $(35)(50)(0.10)$.

    (B) $(35/0.10)(50)$.

    (C) $(50/35)(0.10)$.

    (D) $(35/50)(0.10)$.

18. When 22.2 g of a soluble ionic compound (formula weight =111 g/mol) are added to 1.0 kg of water ($K_f = 1.86°C/m$), the freezing point of the resulting solution is $-1.12°C$. Which of the following could be the general formula of the ionic compound?

    (A) MX

    (B) MX_2

    (C) MX_3

    (D) M_2X_3

19. Compute the sum of the $X_1 + X_2 + X_3 + X_4 + X_5$ in the following nuclear equation (atomic numbers: Mg = 12, He = 2):

    $$^{26}_{X_1}Mg + ^{X_2}_{0}n \rightarrow ^{X_3}_{X_4}He + ^{X_5}_{10}Ne$$

    (A) 40

    (B) 41

    (C) 42

    (D) 43

20. The balanced equation below is for a spontaneous oxidation-reduction reaction.

    $$8\,Al(s) + 3\,NO_3^-(aq) + 5\,OH^-(aq) + 18\,H_2O(l) \rightarrow$$
    $$8\,Al(OH)_4^-(aq) + 3\,NH_3(g)$$

    Which of the following is the best oxidizing agent?

    (A) $Al(s)$

    (B) $NO_3^-(aq)$

    (C) $NH_3(g)$

    (D) $Al(OH)_4^-(aq)$

21. What is the pH of a saturated aqueous solution of $Ca(OH)_2$? The K_{sp} of $Ca(OH)_2$ is 8.0×10^{-6}.

    (A) 12.4

    (B) 7.0

    (C) 1.6

    (D) 1.0

GO ON TO THE NEXT PAGE

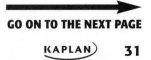

22. Which of the following transformations could occur at the anode of an electrochemical cell?

    (A) $Cr_2O_7^{2-} \rightarrow CrO_4^{2-}$
    (B) $Cr^{2+} \rightarrow CrO_4^{2-}$
    (C) $Cr_2O_7^{2-} \rightarrow Cr^{2+}$
    (D) $CrO_4^{2-} \rightarrow Cr^{3+}$

23. A portion of an organic molecule is pictured below, though not necessarily with accurate geometry. What are the approximate degree measures of angles a, b, and c, respectively?

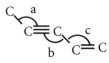

    (A) 109.5°, 120°, and 109.5°
    (B) 120°, 120°, and 120°
    (C) 120°, 180°, and 120°
    (D) 180°, 180°, and 120°

24. The diagram below indicates a pair of *p* orbitals. What kind of bond is formed by overlapping *p* orbitals within a molecule?

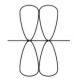

    (A) σ bonds found in single, double, and triple bonds
    (B) π bonds found in triple but not in double bonds
    (C) π bonds found in double but not in triple bonds
    (D) π bonds found in double and triple bonds

25. Which of the following is NOT true of acetylene (ethyne, C_2H_2)?

    (A) It does not have a permanent dipole moment.
    (B) The carbon atoms are sp^2 hybridized.
    (C) It has two π bonds.
    (D) It is a linear molecule.

STOP

READING COMPREHENSION
Questions: 20
Time: 25 minutes

Directions: Each of the following sets of questions is preceded by descriptive material. After reading the material, select the best answer to each question.

Attempts to find a medication that can halt the progression of cocaine addiction have centered on drugs that influence dopaminergic function in the brain, since the rewarding and habit-forming effects of cocaine have been shown to be due to cocaine's action at dopaminergic neural synapses. Normally in the dopaminergic synapse, vesicles in the presynaptic cell release dopamine into the synapse, where the dopamine binds to postsynaptic receptors and transmits a signal to the postsynaptic cell. Subsequently, the dopamine is taken back up into the presynaptic cell and either repackaged into storage vesicles for another release or broken down via monoamine oxidase (MAO) and other enzymes to its metabolites, dihydroxyphenylacetic acid (DOPAC) and homovanillic acid (HVA). Cocaine, however, blocks the reuptake of dopamine into the presynaptic cell, leaving the neurotransmitter in the synapse to have prolonged interaction with its receptors. This acute activation of dopaminergic neurotransmission produces cocaine's rewarding effects, such as euphoria.

Conversely, cocaine craving, which plays a central role in the development of addiction, is thought to be produced by the opposite phenomenon: decreased levels of dopamine in the synapse and the accompanying deactivation of dopaminergic neurotransmission. By blocking reuptake from the synapse, cocaine prevents the presynaptic cell from "recycling" dopamine for release, as normally takes place. Simultaneously, the dopamine in the synapse remains there so long that it becomes vulnerable to synaptic enzymes such as catechol-O-methyltransferase (COMT). The post-cocaine result is dopamine depletion, an imbalance that leads to craving for more of the drug.

Investigators turned to the dopamine agonist bromocriptine as a potential treatment to counteract cocaine craving. Bromocriptine, like cocaine, increases dopaminergic neurotransmission, although by a different mechanism; it stimulates dopamine receptors on the postsynaptic cell. As a result, in small quantities it

can temporarily correct the dopamine imbalance caused by cocaine abuse and thereby reduce the abuser's craving. However, bromocriptine has adverse side effects, which prevent it from being used compulsively or in large amounts. Bromocriptine has been shown to be useful as a short-term treatment for cocaine abusers, but it has not fulfilled researchers' hopes of being effective in eliminating cocaine addiction.

1. Which of the following is MOST likely to happen as a result of cocaine administration?

    (A) The level of HVA in the presynaptic cell rises.

    (B) The level of HVA in the presynaptic cell falls.

    (C) The level of DOPAC in the presynaptic cell rises.

    (D) The level of HVA and DOPAC in the presynaptic cell both rise.

2. According to the passage, the euphoria produced by cocaine is due to the fact that cocaine causes

    (A) released dopamine to be active for a longer time.

    (B) released dopamine to be turned over more rapidly.

    (C) more dopamine receptors to become available.

    (D) more dopamine to be released into the synapse.

3. It can be inferred that cocaine has which of the following effects on the presynaptic cell?

    (A) It depletes the cell's store of MAO.

    (B) It shunts dopamine away from storage to metabolism.

    (C) It lowers the amount of dopamine stored in presynaptic vesicles.

    (D) It causes the cell to become dormant.

GO ON TO THE NEXT PAGE

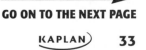

4. Which of the following does NOT take place in normal dopaminergic neurotransmission?

   (A) Uptake of dopamine into the presynaptic cell
   (B) Breakdown of dopamine by COMT
   (C) Recycling of dopamine by the presynaptic cell
   (D) Breakdown of dopamine by MAO

5. Bromocriptine can be used to counteract cocaine craving because it

   (A) replaces dopamine as a receptor agonist.
   (B) allows dopamine to stay in the synapse for extended periods.
   (C) mimics the action of cocaine in the synapse.
   (D) replenishes depleted vesicles in the presynaptic cell.

6. Which of the following effects do cocaine and bromocriptine share?

   (A) Dopamine depletion
   (B) Aversive side effects
   (C) Dopaminergic activation
   (D) Habit-forming rewards

7. It can be inferred that bromocriptine will cause the level of dopamine in the presynaptic cell to

   (A) rise gradually.
   (B) stay the same.
   (C) be temporarily elevated.
   (D) plummet immediately.

GO ON TO THE NEXT PAGE

Although we know more about so-called Neanderthal men than about any other early population, their exact relation to present-day human beings remains unclear. Long considered subhuman, Neanderthals are now known to have been fully human. They walked erect, used fire, and made a variety of tools. They lived partly in the open and partly in caves. The Neanderthals are even thought to have been the first humans to bury their dead, a practice which has been interpreted as demonstrating the capacity for religious and abstract thought.

The first monograph on Neanderthal anatomy, published by Marcellin Boule in 1913, presented a somewhat misleading picture. Boule took the Neanderthals's low-vaulted cranium and prominent brow ridges, their heavy musculature, and the apparent overdevelopment of certain joints as evidence of a prehuman physical appearance. In postulating for the Neanderthal such "primitive" characteristics as a stooping, bent-kneed posture, a rolling gait, and a forward-hanging head, Boule was a victim of the rudimentary state of anatomical science. Modern anthropologists recognize the Neanderthal bone structure as that of a creature whose bodily orientation and capacities were very similar to those of present-day human beings. The differences in the size and shape of the limbs, shoulder blades, and other parts are simply adaptations that were necessary to handle the Neanderthal's far more massive musculature. Current taxonomy considers the Neanderthals to have been fully human and thus designates them not as a separate species, *Homo neanderthalensis*, but as a subspecies of *Homo sapiens*: *Homo sapiens neanderthalensis*.

The rise of the Neanderthals occurred over some 100,000 years—a sufficient period to account for evolution of the specifically Neanderthal characteristics through free interbreeding over a broad geographical range. Fossil evidence suggests that the Neanderthals inhabited a vast area from Europe through the Middle East and into Central Asia from approximately 100,000 years ago until 35,000 years ago. Then, within a brief period of 5,000–10,000 years, they disappeared. Modern humans, not found in Europe prior to about 33,000 years ago, thenceforth became the sole inhabitants of the region. Anthropologists do not believe that the Neanderthals evolved into modern human beings. Despite the similarities between Neanderthal and modern human anatomy, the differences are major

enough that, among a population as broad ranging as the Neanderthals, such an evolution could not have taken place in a period of only 10,000 years. Furthermore, no fossils of types intermediate between Neanderthals and moderns have been found.

A major alternative hypothesis, advanced by E. Trinkaus and W.W. Howells, is that of localized evolution. Within a geographically concentrated population, free interbreeding could have produced far more pronounced genetic effects within a shorter time. Thus, modern humans could have evolved relatively quickly, either from Neanderthals or from some other ancestral type in isolation from the main Neanderthal population. These humans may have migrated throughout the Neanderthal areas, where they displaced or absorbed the original inhabitants. One hypothesis suggests that these "modern" humans immigrated to Europe from the Middle East.

No satisfactory explanation of why modern human beings replaced the Neanderthals has yet been found. Some have speculated that the modern humans wiped out the Neanderthals in warfare; however, there exists no archeological evidence of a hostile encounter. It has also been suggested that the Neanderthals failed to adapt to the onset of the last Ice Age; yet their thick bodies should have been heat conserving and thus well adapted to extreme cold. Finally, it is possible that the improved tools and hunting implements of the late Neanderthal period made the powerful Neanderthal physique less of an advantage than it had been previously. At the same time, the Neanderthals's need for a heavy diet to sustain this physique put them at a disadvantage compared to the less massive moderns. If this was the case, then it was improvements in human culture—including some introduced by the Neanderthals themselves—that made the Neanderthal obsolete.

8. Boule considered all of the following as evidence that Neanderthals were subhuman EXCEPT

   (A) posture.
   (B) bone structure.
   (C) cranial structure.
   (D) ability to use tools.

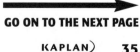

GO ON TO THE NEXT PAGE

9. The passage BEST supports which of the following conclusions?

   (A) Neanderthals were less intelligent than early modern humans.
   (B) Neanderthals were poorly adapted for survival.
   (C) There was probably no contact between Neanderthals and early modern humans.
   (D) Neanderthals may have had a capacity for religious and abstract thought.

10. According to the passage, the latest that any Neanderthal might have existed was

    (A) 100,000 years ago.
    (B) 35,000 years ago.
    (C) 33,000 years ago.
    (D) 25,000 years ago.

11. By inference from the passage, the most important evidence that Neanderthals did NOT evolve into modern humans is the

    (A) major anatomical differences between Neanderthals and modern humans.
    (B) brief time in which Neanderthals disappeared.
    (C) difference in the geographical ranges of Neanderthals and modern humans.
    (D) gap of many thousands of years between the latest Neanderthal fossils and the earliest modern human fossils.

12. All of the following are hypotheses about the disappearance of the Neanderthals EXCEPT

    (A) the Neanderthal physique became a handicap instead of an advantage.
    (B) the Neanderthals failed to adapt to climatic changes.
    (C) the Neanderthals evolved into modern humans.
    (D) modern humans exterminated the Neanderthals.

13. It can be inferred from the passage that the rate of evolution is directly related to the

    (A) concentration of the species population.
    (B) anatomical features of the species.
    (C) rate of environmental change.
    (D) adaptive capabilities of the species.

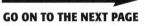

GO ON TO THE NEXT PAGE

The population of the United States is growing older and will continue to do so until well into the next century. For the first time in American history, elders outnumber teenagers. The U.S. Census Bureau projects that 39 million Americans will be 65 or older by the year 2010, 51 million by 2020, and 65 million by 2030. This demographic trend is due mainly to two factors: increased life expectancy, and the occurrence of a "baby boom" in the generation born immediately after World War II. People are living well beyond the average life expectancy in greater numbers than ever before, too. In fact, the number of U.S. citizens 85 years old and older is growing six times as fast as the rest of the population.

The "graying" of the United States is due in large measure to the aging of the generation born after World War II, the "baby boomers." The baby boom peaked in 1957, with over 4.3 million births that year. More than 75 million Americans were born between 1946 and 1964, the largest generation in U.S. history. Today, millions of "boomers" are already moving into middle age; in less than two decades, they will join the ranks of America's elderly.

What will be the social, economic, and political consequences of the aging of America? One likely development will involve a gradual restructuring of the family unit, moving away from the traditional nuclear family and towards an extended, multigenerational family dominated by elders, not by their adult children.

The aging of the U.S. population is also likely to have far-reaching effects on the nation's workforce. In 1989, there were approximately 3.5 workers for every person 65 and older; by the year 2030, there'll only be 2 workers for every person 65 and older. As the number of available younger workers shrinks, elderly people will become more attractive as prospective employees. Many will simply retain their existing jobs beyond the now-mandatory retirement age of 65. In fact, the phenomenon of early retirement, which has transformed the U.S. workforce over the past four decades, will probably become a thing of the past. In 1950, about 50 percent of all 65-year old men still worked; today, only 15 percent of them do. The median retirement age is currently 61. Yet recent surveys show that almost half of today's retirees would prefer to be working, and in decades to come, their counterparts will be doing just that.

Finally, the great proportional increase in the number of older Americans will have significant effects on the nation's economy in the areas of Social Security and health care. A recent government survey showed that 77 percent of elderly Americans have annual incomes of less than $20,000; only 3 percent earn more than $50,000. As their earning power declines and their need for health care increases, most elderly Americans come to depend heavily on federal and state subsidies. With the advent of Social Security in 1935 and Medicaid/Medicare in 1965, the size of those subsidies has grown steadily until by 1990, spending on the elderly accounted for 30 percent of the annual federal budget.

Considering these figures, and the fact that the elderly population will double within the next 40 years, it's clear that major government policy decisions lie ahead. In the first 50 years of its existence, for example, the Social Security fund has received $55 billion more in employee/employer contributions than it has paid out in benefits to the elderly. Yet time and again the federal government has "borrowed" this surplus without repaying it to pay interest on the national debt.

Similarly, the Medicaid/Medicare system is threatened by the continuous upward spiral of medical costs. The cost of caring for disabled elderly Americans is expected to double in the next decade alone. And millions of Americans of all ages are currently unable to afford private health insurance. In fact, the United States is practically unique among developed nations in lacking a national health care system. Its advocates say such a system would be far less expensive than the present state of affairs, but the medical establishment and various special interest groups have so far blocked legislation aimed at creating it. Nonetheless, within the next few decades, an aging U.S. population may well demand that such a program be implemented.

14. Based on the information contained in the passage, which of the following statements about the U.S. elderly population is TRUE?

(A) It is largely responsible for the nation's current housing shortage.

(B) It is expected to double within the next 40 years.

(C) It is the wealthiest segment of the U.S. population.

(D) It represents almost 30 percent of the U.S. population.

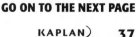

GO ON TO THE NEXT PAGE

15. According to the passage, the majority of elderly people in the United States

    (A) currently earn less than $20,000 per year.
    (B) will suffer some sort of disability between the ages of 65 and 75.
    (C) have been unable to purchase their own homes.
    (D) continue to work at least 20 hours per week.

16. The fact that health care costs for disabled elderly Americans are expected to double in the next 10 years indicates which of the following statements?

    (A) The federal government will be unable to finance a national health care system.
    (B) The Medicaid/Medicare system will probably become even more expensive in the future.
    (C) Money will have to be borrowed from the Social Security fund to finance the Medicaid/Medicare system.
    (D) "Baby boomers" will be unable to receive federal health benefits as they grow older.

17. According to the U.S. Census Bureau, today's elderly population is

    (A) larger than the current population of teenagers.
    (B) larger than the current population of "boomers."
    (C) smaller than the number of elderly people in 1950.
    (D) smaller than the number of elderly people in 1970.

18. The author speculates that, in future decades, the typical U.S. family will probably be

    (A) youth oriented.
    (B) subsidized by Social Security.
    (C) multigenerational.
    (D) wealthier than today's family.

19. The author suggests that, over the past three decades, many of today's elderly people

    (A) supplemented their incomes by working past the age of retirement.
    (B) lost their Social Security benefits.
    (C) have experienced a doubling in their cost of living.
    (D) have come to depend heavily on government subsidies.

20. According to the author, the federal government has not yet instituted a program mandating health care for all U.S. citizens because

    (A) the federal deficit must first be eliminated.
    (B) such a program would be too expensive.
    (C) legislative lobbies have prevented it.
    (D) Medicaid and Medicare have made it unnecessary.

STOP

QUANTITATIVE ABILITY
Questions: 24
Time: 20 minutes

Directions: Choose the **best** answer to each of the following questions.

1. Which of the following is equal to $\dfrac{12 \times 10^5}{16 \times 10^9}$?
   (A) 7.5×10^{-6}
   (B) 7.5×10^{-5}
   (C) 7.5×10^{-4}
   (D) 7.5×10^4

2. Which of the following is equal to $\sqrt{0.000004}$?
   (A) 0.2
   (B) 0.02
   (C) 0.002
   (D) 0.0002

3. Which of the following is equal to the value of 7% of 3% of 4?
   (A) 0.00084
   (B) 0.0084
   (C) 0.084
   (D) 0.84

4. Which of the following is equal to $\dfrac{1}{5 + \dfrac{1}{5 + \dfrac{2}{3}}}$?
   (A) $\dfrac{5}{26}$
   (B) $\dfrac{17}{88}$
   (C) $\dfrac{15}{68}$
   (D) $\dfrac{10}{51}$

5. Which of the following is equal to $\dfrac{2}{3} + \dfrac{5}{6} - \dfrac{7}{12} - \dfrac{1}{24}$?
   (A) $\dfrac{2}{3}$
   (B) $\dfrac{3}{4}$
   (C) $\dfrac{7}{8}$
   (D) $\dfrac{23}{24}$

6. Line ℓ is perpendicular to the line with the equation $y = -\dfrac{1}{5}x$, and the point $(3, -10)$ is on line ℓ. Which of the following is an equation of line ℓ ?
   (A) $y = -\dfrac{1}{5}x - \dfrac{47}{5}$
   (B) $y = 5x - 25$
   (C) $y = 5x$
   (D) $y = 5x - 5$

7. When Allen was at the department store, he spent 10 percent of the money he originally had with him on tennis equipment and 55 percent of the money he originally had with him on golf equipment. After these purchases, he had $210 left. How much money did Allen have originally?
   (A) $350
   (B) $490
   (C) $540
   (D) $600

8. There are five purple marbles and six yellow marbles in a bag. If two balls are drawn at random (one after the other without replacement), what is the probability of selecting two purple marbles?
   (A) $\dfrac{20}{121}$
   (B) $\dfrac{25}{121}$
   (C) $\dfrac{2}{11}$
   (D) $\dfrac{5}{11}$

GO ON TO THE NEXT PAGE

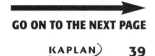

9. What is the value of x if $\sqrt{x-16} = 26 - 21$?

   (A) 41
   (B) 37
   (C) 27
   (D) 21

10. Elaine had an average (arithmetic mean) score of 76 on the first three exams she took and a score of 84 on her fourth exam. What was her average (arithmetic mean) score on all four exams?

   (A) 77
   (B) 78
   (C) 79
   (D) 80

11. At a certain company, the ratio of the number of clerical employees to the number of nonclerical employees is 5 to 2. If there is a total of 630 employees working at this company, how many employees working at this company are clerical employees?

   (A) 180
   (B) 350
   (C) 441
   (D) 450

12. A train traveled from Xaviertown to Youngstown. It traveled the first half of the distance at an average speed of 60 miles per hour, and it traveled the second half of the distance at an average speed of 100 miles per hour. What was the average speed of the train, in miles per hour, for the entire distance traveled?

   (A) 68
   (B) 75
   (C) 80
   (D) 84

13. What is the value of $a \div \dfrac{1}{b^2}$ when $a = \dfrac{18}{48}$ and $b = \dfrac{1}{3}$?

   (A) $\dfrac{1}{24}$
   (B) $\dfrac{1}{8}$
   (C) $\dfrac{3}{4}$
   (D) $\dfrac{27}{8}$

14. Which of the following is equal to $(3x - 7y)^2$?

   (A) $9x^2 + 49x^2$
   (B) $9x^2 + 21xy + 49y^2$
   (C) $9x^2 - 21xy + 49y^2$
   (D) $9x^2 - 42xy + 49y^2$

15. What is the value of x if $\sqrt{2x - 3} = 7$?

   (A) 14
   (B) 20
   (C) 26
   (D) 29

16. What is the value of x if $\dfrac{3}{5} + \dfrac{7}{x - 4} = 3$?

   (A) $\dfrac{107}{8}$
   (B) $\dfrac{19}{3}$
   (C) $\dfrac{95}{12}$
   (D) $\dfrac{83}{12}$

17. If $y = \dfrac{5x + 2}{x - 6}$ for all $x \neq 6$, then which of the following gives x in terms of y for all values of y where the expression for x in terms of y is defined?

   (A) $x = \dfrac{2 + 6y}{5 - y}$
   (B) $x = \dfrac{2 + 6y}{y + 5}$
   (C) $x = \dfrac{2 + 6y}{y - 5}$
   (D) $x = \dfrac{2 - 6y}{y - 5}$

18. If 16 ounces equal 1 pound and a ton equals 2,000 pounds, then how many ounces are there in 3 tons?

   (A) 6,000
   (B) 24,000
   (C) 32,000
   (D) 96,000

GO ON TO THE NEXT PAGE

 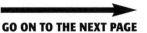

19. What is the value of x if $5x - y = 3$ and $2x + 7y = 4$?

    (A) $\dfrac{33}{37}$

    (B) $\dfrac{25}{37}$

    (C) $\dfrac{14}{37}$

    (D) $-\dfrac{17}{37}$

20. Which of the following is the equation of a line that is perpendicular to the y-axis?

    (A) $x = 0$
    (B) $x = 3$
    (C) $y = 3$
    (D) $y = -2x$

21. How many different pairs of people can be selected from a group of seven people?

    (A) 14
    (B) 21
    (C) 28
    (D) 35

22. James has packed 10 white socks in a suitcase. He wants to add enough black socks so that the probability of randomly selecting a white sock from the suitcase is 1/5. How many black socks should he add to the suitcase?

    (A) 30
    (B) 35
    (C) 40
    (D) 45

23. Below is the graph of the function $y = f(x)$, line l passing through the points $(a, f(a))$ and $(b, f(b))$ on the graph of f, and line m, which is tangent to the graph of f at $(a, f(a))$.

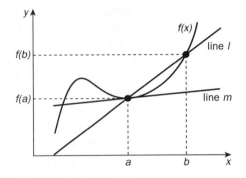

    Which of the following statements are TRUE?

    I. Line m is the derivative of f at $x = a$.

    II. The slope of line l is the average rate of change of f from a to b.

    III. The slope of line is given by
    $$\lim_{\Delta x \to 0} \frac{f(a + \Delta x) - f(a)}{\Delta x}.$$

    (A) Only I
    (B) Only III
    (C) Both I and III
    (D) Both II and III

24. $4! =$

    (A) 4
    (B) 16
    (C) 20
    (D) 24

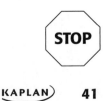

STOP

Answers and Explanations

VERBAL ABILITY

1. **B**   For the first blank, look for a word that describes a desert and explains why the mummies are still intact. After the comma, there is an important context clue. The word *whereas* signifies contrast. It indicates that the Egyptian conditions are different from those described in the second half of the sentence, which is where the conditions found in tropical rain forests are explained. So the context clue *whereas* indicates that the first blank will be the opposite of humid. Likewise, the second blank tells about Aztec mummies, which you know will be the opposite of what is true of Egyptian mummies. If the Egyptian mummies are still intact, then Aztec mummies must not have survived.

    A good prediction for this sentence is: "The dryness of the desert explains why Egyptian mummies are still around, whereas the humidity in tropical rain forests explains why so few Aztec mummies have survived."

    Predictions for both blanks are pretty precise, so start with either one. Looking for a word that means "dryness" for the first blank directs you to (B) and (C). Both *aridity* and *dehydration* mean "lacking in moisture," but the second word in (C), *decayed*, is the opposite of what you're looking for. You need a word that means "survived." (B), *endured*, is perfect. Hold onto (B) and check the others. The first word in (A) and (D) eliminates these answers. All of these words may be true of the desert, but none of them means "dry."

2. **C**   In this sentence, you learn that they did something until only one option remained open to them—a desperate, last-minute solution. They must have waited or put off their work until they had no recourse.

    A good prediction for this sentence is: "They delayed until there was no choice but a last-minute solution to solve the problem."

    Starting with the first blank because the prediction is pretty definite, (B) and (C) look good. Eliminate (B) because the second word, *envision*, that is, "predict or foresee," does not convey the meaning of a solution. The second word in (C), *implement*, means "execute or achieve," so (C) works well for both blanks. Based on the first word, (A) and (D) can be eliminated. Of these only (A), *filibustered*, suggests delaying, but it has a more specific meaning that is not applicable here. To filibuster is to interrupt or delay something from occurring by engaging in activities such as long speeches and discourse.

3. **D**   This is a fairly long sentence whose blanks occur toward the end. Take the sentence apart, paraphrasing what each phrase means, and pay close attention to the first few lines, which will tell you how to fill in the blanks. The context clue *but because* after the first comma is critical in directing you to the right answer. *But* indicates that a contrast is coming, and the word *because* tells you that an explanation will be given. The second part of the sentence will contrast with the first and will tell you why it is so. In the first part, you learn that the engine was a *marvel* that reduced pollution. However, it was not *fuel-efficient*. The word *because* tells you that the lack of fuel efficiency led to something, unlike the fact that the engine was so marvelous. The fact that it reduced pollution must not have been important anymore, since there was a *panic over fuel shortages*.

    A good prediction for this sentence is: "The engine was rejected or modified in the 1970s, when concerns about pollution gave way to panic over fuel shortages."

    Working with the first blank, (C) and (D) look good. While *modified* in the first blank of (C) makes sense, the second phrase, *opinion on*, is too broad. You're not told if it was a positive or negative opinion that gave way or what direction it gave way to. This answer, then, is not precise enough and would not warrant modifying the engine. In (D), if a *preoccupation with* pollution gave way to panic over fuel shortages, that would explain why the engine was no longer valued. This is a much stronger phrase than *opinion on*. This looks like the best answer, but check the others to be sure. Eliminate (A) and (B) based on the first word in each, since neither of them suggests that the engine was rejected or changed in anyway.

4. **C** The semicolon between these two clauses is a context clue. It tells you that the second thought will be a continuation of, or will support, the first thought. The basic meaning of the first half of the sentence is that friendship has its limits no matter what. The first blank must be filled with something that reinforces the notion of having limits in all cases. The second half of the sentence says that advice that is thrust upon someone cannot be considered an act of friendship. The second blank will be filled with a word that describes advice that is *thrust insistently* on someone—advice that is not asked for.

A prediction for this sentence is: "All friendship, no matter how close, has boundaries; unwanted advice, when thrust upon someone, is rarely a sign of friendship."

Choice (C) looks good right away because the first word, *intimate*, matches your prediction of *close*, and the second word, *unsolicited*, is perfect, too. Choice (A) and (D) can be eliminated because the first word in each is the opposite of *close*. The first word in (B) might be all right if nothing else were better, but can be eliminated on the basis of the second word. *Obverse* means "inside out or upside down," which doesn't make sense in this context.

5. **A** The word *despite* is a context clue that tells you that there is a change or contrast later in the sentence. Despite something from the critics, the poet's work sold steadily.
The critics must not have favored the poetry, which would explain why it would be surprising that the work still sold well. For the first blank, look for a word that suggests the critics' disapproval. The second blank is harder to figure out. You know the word will describe the critics, but many words, both positive and negative, could work here. Evaluate the meaning of each of the choices to narrow it down.

A good prediction, for the first blank at least, is: "Despite negative responses from (some type) of critics, the poetry sold well."

Starting with the first blank since it is more precise, (A) seems to be just right. *Vitriol* means severe criticism, which would work in the first blank, and *influential* in the second blank explains why it's surprising that these type of critics' responses did not negatively impact the sales of the book. Run through the other answers quickly. Choice (C) does not fit well in the first blank because *tedium* may be defined as boredom. Receiving boring responses from the critics does not mean that the responses were negative. (B) and (D) can be eliminated because of the second word in each. It is not logical that the response of obscure or ineffectual critics would explain the contrast suggested by the word *despite*. If the critics have no influence, it would not be surprising that the books sold well. Look for a word that would justify the context clue *despite*.

6. **A** The commas after the first blank are important clues that tell you what type of word you are looking for. Because it is set off with commas, the phrase *from production to projection* simply renames the word in the preceding blank. This phrase describes every aspect of the film industry, so the correct word will, too. Since all of these components were *held by one company*, it makes sense that a monopoly would eventually arise. In the second blank, you're looking for something that expresses the fact that monopolies were bound to arise.

A good prediction for this answer is: "Because the different components were arranged so that all aspects of the business were held by one company, monopolistic practices were bound to arise."

Predictions for both of these blanks are pretty definite, but the second is a little more precise, so start there. Choice (A) looks good right away because *inevitable* means that it was bound to happen, which was your prediction for the second blank. *Opportunities for control* works well in the first blank, too. This one looks good. Hold onto it and check the others. Choice (C) can be eliminated because the second word does not convey the meaning that something would have to happen. Choices (B) and (D) can be eliminated because the words for the first blank, *burdens of business* and *means of solicitation*, are not logical in context. Having control of all of the components of the film industry would certainly not be burdens, nor would all of them act as a means of soliciting.

7. **D** The first blank describes something that the peasants tried to conceal as they knelt before the body of the dictator's son. This doesn't sound like a very positive situation. They are kneeling and we know that they live under a dictatorship, so it is likely that the peasants are being required to do this. The second part of the sentence supports this theory. You learn that *far from affection*, something else motivates them. Consequently, you're looking for a negative word in both blanks.

Many words would work in these blanks, so evaluate each choice carefully, looking for two negative words that fit in this context.

Starting with the second blank since you have a little more information to work with there, (D) looks like the best answer. It makes sense that *fear* would bring them to the wake of the dictator's son. The first word, *trepidation*, also fits the sentence, since it means "apprehension." Choice (A) can be eliminated because there is no indication in the sentence that the peasants are concealing *sarcasm*, and they would not show this if they felt something as extreme as *hatred*. Likewise, the second word in (B), *violence*, is not suggested from the clues. (C), *adulation*, is positive.

8. **C** The context clue *despite* at the beginning of this sentence helps you figure this one out. Because *despite* indicates that the two parts of the sentence are contrasting with each other, you know that despite the increased attention on this issue, something has happened. You would expect that with increased attention, there would be fewer crimes committed by this group. However, the word *despite* indicates that what you might expect does not prove to be true. You're looking for the opposite of what you would normally expect given these circumstances.

A good prediction for this one is: "Despite increased attention on juvenile delinquency, there's been an increase in crimes."

Working with the second blank since it is more specific, (B) and (C) look good. After considering the first blank, though, only (C) makes sense. The first words in (B), *offered to*, are not strong enough. Simply offering attention to this issue does not tell you whether or not attention was actually given. You need something more definitive in the first blank to indicate that the expected cause and effect was not realized. Hold onto (C) and check the remaining two. (A) and (D) are inappropriate, since the second word in each doesn't have a contrasting meaning to the first clause. You must have a contrast because of the word *despite* in the first clause.

9. **D**   The context clue *contradicted* tells you that the blank will be opposite in meaning to *cynicism*—something like innocence.

A good prediction: "The Beatles's music was characterized by a superficial innocence subtly contradicted by an inherent, deeper cynicism."

Choice (D) looks good right away because *naiveté* means "innocence." None of the other choices comes close to being opposite in meaning to *cynicism*.

10. **C**   The key word in this sentence is *ambivalent*. An ambivalent attitude is one that contains both positive and negative feelings. You know that the negative side of Jung's attitude is that he attacked Freud. However, even as he attacked Freud, Jung did something that must have been positive in order to have shown ambivalence.

Many positive words would work here, so it would be hard to predict an answer. Instead, go directly to the choices and evaluate each one carefully in the context of the sentence.

Choice (C) looks good since *revered* is a very positive word. Choices (B) and (D) can be eliminated because they are negative. Choice (A) is out because it doesn't make sense in the context of the sentence. If Jung *enlightened* Freud, it might have a positive effect on Freud, but it is impossible to say whether this would have a positive or negative impact on Jung.

Analogies

11. **D** A DRAKE is a male DUCK. Likewise, a BULL is a male OX. The terms for the male of the species in (A) and (B) are *ram* and *rooster*.

12. **D** A PREAMBLE is the formal introduction to a DOCUMENT. Similarly, a PROLOGUE is a speech introducing a PLAY. An interlude (A) is an entertainment or episode that comes in the middle of a play. A letter (B) begins with a salutation or an address, such as "Dear John...."

13. **B** The word *sartorial* refers to clothing; you go to a TAILOR to take care of your SARTORIAL needs. The word *tonsorial* refers to barbers and haircutting; you go to a BARBER to take care of your TONSORIAL needs. Choice (C) wants you to confuse *tonsorial* with *tonsils*.

14. **B** To RUMINATE is to meditate or REFLECT; these words are practically synonyms. Thus, you're looking for a synonym of BROOD; it's WORRY (B). *Ponder* (C) is a synonym of *ruminate* and *reflect*; it lacks the element of anxiety shared by *brood* and *worry*.

15. **B** A PAEAN is a fervent expression of joy or PRAISE. Likewise, a DIRGE is a fervent expression of MOURNING. None of the other choices necessarily involves the feelings of great sadness or loss that would require a dirge.

16. **C** A RECTORY is the house where a CLERIC lives. In the same way, a PALACE is the house where a monarch or POTENTATE lives. A soldier (A) lives in a barracks, a mendicant (B) or beggar may live in the street, and a monk's (D) dwelling place is called a monastery.

17. **D** To perform a PEREGRINATION is to TRAVEL. Similarly, to perform a GYRATION is to circle or REVOLVE. (A) and (B) use "same-field foolers"—words that involve motion but bear no relationship to *gyration*.

18. **D** An ABSTRACT is a summary of the important points of an ARTICLE. Similarly, a SYNOPSIS is a summary of the important points of a story, or NARRATIVE. A statement (A) and a rule (B) might each consist of a single sentence and not require a synopsis. *Summary* (C) is synonymous with *synopsis*.

19. **B** An ABSTEMIOUS person eats and drinks in moderation and does not BINGE. Likewise, a FRUGAL person spends money very carefully and does not SPLURGE. No other choice concerns acting in moderation.

20. **A** By definition, a majestic or AUGUST person behaves with splendor, or GRANDEUR. Also by definition, a CRASS person is gross or coarse and behaves with INDELICACY. Certitude (C) is a defining characteristic of arrogance but not of crassness. Nor is crassness the sole property of youth (D).

21 **C** WATER that's safe to drink is POTABLE. In the same way, FOOD that is safe to eat is EDIBLE. *Palatable* (A) runs a close second here, but it really means "acceptable to the taste," which is not as strong. Food that's poisonous (B) is not safe to consume, and audible (D) means "capable of being heard."

22. **C** Something PICAYUNE is trivial, not worthy of ATTENTION. Likewise, someone laughable or LUDICROUS is unworthy of RESPECT. Choice (B) may have been tempting because one associates authority with respect, but it fits awkwardly with our bridge. (D) is too extreme: just because someone is laughable doesn't mean they're unworthy of compassion.

23. **D** Something IMMUTABLE is incapable of CHANGE. Similarly, something IMMOBILE is incapable of MOVEMENT. *Stasis* (A) is a state of motionlessness; this is the opposite of what we want. *Mutation* (C) is a synonym for change, not movement.

24. **B** A MAELSTROM is a raging, spinning funnel of WATER. Likewise, a TORNADO is a raging, spinning funnel of AIR.

BIOLOGY

1. **B** The hypothalamus is responsible for regulating homeostatic functions such as hunger, thirst, sex drive, water balance, blood pressure, and temperature regulation. Thus, if the hypothalamus were damaged, appetite would be most affected.

    The other answer choices are incorrect because they refer to functions that are not controlled by the hypothalamus; injury to the hypothalamus would not affect them. Choice (A) is incorrect because respiration is controlled by the medulla. Choice (C) is incorrect because motor coordination is controlled by the cerebellum. Choice (D) is incorrect because memory is a function of the cerebral cortex.

2. **D** The lymphatic system is a secondary circulatory system that is distinct from cardiovascular circulation. The vessels of the lymphatic system transport excess interstitial fluid, called lymph, to the cardiovascular system, thereby keeping fluid levels in the body constant. Swellings along lymph vessels, known as lymph nodes, contain phagocytic cells that remove and destroy foreign particles in the lymph. Thus, choice (D) is correct.

    Choice (A) is incorrect because cardiovascular circulation is responsible for the transport of oxygen to the body tissues. Choice (B) is incorrect because the capillaries of the cardiovascular system, not the lacteals of the lymphatic system, are responsible for absorbing carbohydrates from the gastrointestinal tract. Lacteals are responsible for the absorption of fats from the gastrointestinal tract. Choice (C) is incorrect because cerebrospinal fluid is reabsorbed by the cardiovascular system via a sinus in the cranial meninges.

3. **A** The liver is responsible for the processing of nitrogenous wastes. Excess amino acids are absorbed in the small intestine and transported to the liver via the hepatic portal vein. There, the amino acids undergo deamination, in which the amino group is removed from the amino acids and converted into ammonia. In a complex biochemical process, the liver combines ammonia with carbon dioxide to form urea, which is released into the blood and eventually excreted by the kidneys. Thus, (A) is correct.

    (B) is incorrect because the lacteals in the gastrointestinal tract are responsible for the absorption of fat. (C) is incorrect because the storage of protein is not a function of the liver, or any other organ of the body for that matter. Excess protein is broken down into amino acids, which are converted to urea and excreted. (D) is incorrect because the red bone marrow is responsible for the production of red blood cells.

4. **D** tRNA (transfer RNA) carries amino acids to the ribosomes during protein synthesis. (A) is incorrect because hnRNA (heterogeneous nuclear RNA) is a large ribonucleoprotein complex that is a precursor of mRNA (messenger RNA). (B) is incorrect because mRNA carries the complement of a DNA sequence and transports it from the nucleus to the ribosomes. (C) is incorrect because rRNA (ribosomal RNA) is a structural component of ribosomes.

5. **C** Only animal cells contain centrioles, so (C) is correct. Both fungal cells and animal cells are eukaryotic. Eukaryotic cells contain membrane-bound organelles, such as mitochondria and a nucleus, so (A) and (D) are incorrect. Both fungal cells and animal cells contain ribosomes, so (B) is incorrect.

6. **C** Glucagon, which is a pancreatic hormone, increases the blood glucose level by stimulating the conversion of glycogen to glucose.

    (A) is incorrect because insulin's action is antagonistic to that of glucagon; insulin lowers blood glucose level by stimulating the storage of glucose as glycogen in muscle and liver cells. (B) is incorrect because parathyroid hormone raises blood calcium levels and is not involved with glucose regulation. (D) is incorrect because cortisone reduces the body's inflammatory responses. Cortisone, like glucagon, is also responsible for increasing blood glucose levels, but it accomplishes this by increasing protein degradation and promoting gluconeogenesis, not by converting glycogen to glucose.

7. **A** Piloerection is when hair on the skin is raised by tiny, involuntary muscles. In an animal with body hair, piloerection traps air near the skin, which creates an insulatory effect. As humans, we experience piloerection as the "goose pimples" we observe on ourselves when we are cold.

    Choices (B) and (D) are incorrect because perspiration and subcutaneous blood vessel dilation are mechanisms of heat loss. (C) is incorrect because aldosterone secretion is not related to heat conservation; rather, aldosterone is responsible for the reabsorption of sodium from the kidney, so it plays a part in salt and water regulation.

8. **D** During the first stage of mitosis (prophase), chromosomes condense, shorten, and coil. During the second stage of mitosis (metaphase), the chromosomes align at the equatorial plane of the cell. Thus, (B) is incorrect. During the third stage of mitosis (anaphase), the sister chromatids separate. Thus, (C) is incorrect. During the final stage of mitosis (telophase), new nuclear membranes form and cytokinesis occurs. Thus, (A) is incorrect.

9. **B** The basis for the pairing of the two strands of DNA in the double helix is hydrogen bonding. This is because complementary base pairs form hydrogen bonds with each other. T always forms two hydrogen bonds with A, and G always forms three hydrogen bonds with C. This base-pairing forms "rungs" on the interior of the double helix and links the two polynucleotide strands together.

    Choices (A), (C), and (D) are incorrect because they do not correctly identify the type of chemical bond that pairs the two strands of DNA together. Covalent bonding arises from the sharing of electrons between atoms and in biochemistry and is generally responsible for the linking together of monomer units to form polymers: peptide bonds, which link amino acids together, and phosphodiester bonds, which link nucleotides together, are covalent bonds. Hydrophobic interactions are responsible for the tertiary structure of protein molecules in aqueous environments; for example, nonpolar side chains cluster together in the interior of the protein molecule. Ionic bonding arises between charged particles.

10. **D** Vacuoles are membrane-bound sacs that store materials that are ingested, secreted, processed, or digested by the cell.

    Choice (A) is incorrect because mitochondria are the sites of aerobic respiration within the cell and hence the suppliers of energy. (B) is incorrect because the ribosomes are the sites of protein synthesis within the cell. (C) is incorrect because the centrioles are involved in spindle organization during cell division.

11. **C** The concentrations of enzyme and substrate during the course of a reaction greatly affect the reaction rate. When the concentrations of both enzyme and substrate are low, many of the active sites are unoccupied, and the reaction rate is low. Initial increases in the substrate concentration, at constant enzyme concentration, lead to proportional increases in the rate of the reaction because unoccupied active sites on the enzyme readily bind to the additional substrate. However, once most of the active sites are occupied, the reaction rate levels off, regardless of further increases in substrate concentration. Thus, (C) is correct.

12. **A** Retroviruses are a class of viruses that contain RNA as their genetic material; thus (A) is the correct answer. Since eukaryotes do not have the ability to transcribe DNA from RNA, retroviruses must bring the enzyme reverse transcriptase, which transcribes DNA from RNA, with them when they infect a host cell. Yeast cells, muscle cells, and neurons are all eukaryotic cells and contain DNA as their genetic material, so (B), (C), and (D) are incorrect.

13. **A** ACTH (adrenocorticotropic hormone) stimulates the adrenal cortex to synthesize and secrete glucocorticoids such as cortisone.

    (B) is incorrect: ACTH stimulates the adrenal cortex to release cortisone, not norepinephrine. (C) is incorrect as well. Although it is true that the adrenal medulla secretes epinephrine, ACTH stimulates the adrenal cortex, not the adrenal medulla. Similarly, (D) is also incorrect because although ACTH stimulates the adrenal medulla, it is the adrenal cortex, not the adrenal medulla, that secretes cortisone.

14. **A** Amylase is responsible for hydrolyzing starch, a polysaccharide, to maltose, a disaccharide. Amylase is secreted by the salivary glands in the mouth and by the pancreas.

    (B) is incorrect because maltase hydrolyzes maltose, a disaccharide, to two monosaccharide glucose molecules. (C) is incorrect because lipase hydrolyzes lipids. (D) is incorrect because carboxypeptidase hydrolyzes the terminal peptide bond at the carboxyl end of proteins.

15. **A** In transformation, DNA enters the cell from the environment, so (A) is the correct answer. In conjugation (B), genetic material is passed from one cell to another via a conjugation bridge. In transduction (C), bacterial DNA is transferred from one cell to another via a bacteriophage. Binary fission (D) is the process of cell division in prokaryotes.

16. **B** The normal site of fertilization in humans is the fallopian tube, also known as the oviduct.

    (A) is incorrect because normal fertilization does not occur in the ovary. The ovaries are the female gonads; their function is to produce eggs and secrete the hormones estrogen and progesterone. (C) is incorrect because the uterus is the site of implantation for the fertilized egg. (D) is incorrect because the vagina is the site of sperm deposition during intercourse and is also the birth canal.

17. **C**   Muscle contraction results from myosin and actin filaments sliding over each other. During muscle contraction, calcium ions are released into the cytoplasm of a muscle cell in response to an action potential in the motor neuron innervating the muscle. The ions bind to troponin molecules, causing the tropomyosin strands to shift, thereby exposing myosin-binding sites on the actin filaments. The free globular heads of the myosin molecules move toward and then bind to the exposed binding sites on the actin molecules, forming actin-myosin cross-bridges. In creating these cross-bridges, the myosin pulls on the actin molecules, drawing the thin filaments towards the center of the H zone and shortening the sarcomere. The hydrolysis of ATP in the myosin head provides the energy for the powerstroke that results in the dissociation of the myosin head from the actin. The myosin returns to its original position and is now free to bind to another actin molecule and repeat the process, thus further pulling the thin filaments towards the center of the H zone.

   An important principle to remember about muscle contraction is that the thick and thin filaments in the sarcomere never expand, contract, or change their length. Rather, contraction of the sarcomere is accomplished by this pulling and sliding action. Thus, choices (A), (B), and (D) are all incorrect.

18. **B**   The three primary germ layers (ectoderm, endoderm, and mesoderm) are responsible for the differential development of the tissues, organs, and systems of the body at later stages of growth. The musculoskeletal system, circulatory system, excretory system, reproductive system, and the connective tissues, including blood, are all derived from the mesoderm. Thus, the kidney arises from the mesoderm, so (B) is indeed correct.

   (C) is incorrect. Endoderm derivatives include the lining of the digestive system and the associated glands and organs, including the pancreas and liver. The lungs are also derived from the endoderm. (A) is incorrect. The ectoderm gives rise to the epidermis and nervous system.

19. **B** NAD^+ is reduced to NADH during glycolysis.

   (A) is incorrect because $FADH_2$ is produced during the Krebs cycle, not during glycolysis. During glycolysis, one molecule of glucose is converted into two molecules of pyruvate—not one molecule of pyruvate, as (C) incorrectly states. (D) is incorrect because pyruvate, the end product of glycolysis, only goes on to form acetyl CoA during aerobic respiration. During anaerobic respiration, pyruvate is reduced to ethanol or lactic acid.

20. **D**   Your are told that aerobic prokaryotes were engulfed by larger host prokaryotes. This indicates that the inner mitochondrial membrane most likely evolved from the aerobic prokaryotic membrane, while the outer membrane evolved from an invagination of the large host prokaryote's membrane. Thus, the inner membrane enzymes most likely originated from the aerobic prokaryotic symbiont cell's membrane. (D) is the correct answer. (A) and (B) are correct because the enzymes are membrane bound. Cytoplasmic enzymes would most likely remain in the cytoplasm of evolved eukaryotes. (C) is incorrect because enzymes on the plasma membrane of the host cell would most likely appear in the outer membrane of the mitochondria.

21. **C**   Commensalism is the symbiotic interspecific interaction in which one organism is benefited by the association while the other is not affected. An example of commensalism is the relationship between birds and trees. Birds benefit by nesting in trees, while the trees are not affected.

(A) is incorrect because predation is an interaction in which one organism feeds on another. (B) is incorrect because mutualism is a symbiotic relationship from which both organisms derive some benefit. (D), parasitism, is an interaction in which one organism benefits at the expense of another.

22. **D** During inhalation, the diaphragm and the external intercostal muscles contract, pushing the rib cage and chest wall up and out. This causes the thoracic cavity to increase in volume. This volume increase, in turn, reduces the intrapleural pressure, causing the lungs to expand and fill with air.

    (A) is incorrect because oxygen and carbon dioxide are exchanged at the alveoli via passive diffusion. (B) is incorrect because hemoglobin is capable of binding CO_2. In fact, hemoglobin is responsible for transporting carbon dioxide from the tissues to the lungs. (C) is incorrect because gas exchange occurs across the walls of the alveoli, not in the trachea.

23. **D** The light cycle of photosynthesis is initiated by exposure to photons; thus, it can only occur in the presence of light.

    (A) is incorrect because sugar is produced during the dark cycle, not the light cycle. (B) is incorrect because the dark cycle does not need a photon input, so it can proceed in both the presence and the absence of light. (C) is incorrect because ATP is produced during the light cycle, not the dark cycle.

24. **A** The best way to deal with this problem is to construct a Punnett square. We are given the information that the allele for black hair (B) is dominant to the allele for brown hair (b). Thus, the heterozygote parent must have genotype Bb. The parent with brown hair must possess two recessive alleles, and a genotype of bb. Thus, the Punnett square looks like this:

	B	b
b	Bb	bb
b	Bb	bb

We see that half the offspring will have the genotype Bb (and have the phenotype of black hair) and half the offspring will have the genotype bb (and have the phenotype of brown hair). Thus, the phenotypic ratio of the offspring will be 1 black hair: 1 brown hair, or (A).

CHEMISTRY

1. **D** Phosphorus has five valence electrons. It thus needs three more to complete its octet. It can do this by forming three covalent bonds: two to hydrogen and one to chlorine. The Lewis structure is as follows:

The Lewis structure, however, does not necessarily give an accurate representation of the three-dimensional appearance of the molecule. For that we have to use VSEPR theory. There are four regions of electron density around the central P atom—three bonding electron pairs and one nonbonding pair. These will want to be as far apart as possible, resulting in a tetrahedral electronic geometry. In describing the actual molecular geometry, however, we ignore the nonbonding pair and would thus describe the molecule as trigonal pyramidal. It is similar to the structure of NH_3:

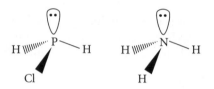

2. **D** Virtually no calculation is needed for this question. The pressure has slightly less than doubled when going from 1.00 atm to 1.80 atm. Because temperature and volume are not changing, the number of moles of gas needs to increase proportionally; i.e., it needs to increase to slightly less than the double, 6.00 moles. The only choice that fits this requirement is (D): an extra 2.4 moles would bring the total number of moles of gas to 5.4 moles.

For completeness, the setup is as follows. From rearranging the ideal gas law:

$$\frac{P1}{n1} = \frac{P2}{n2} = \frac{RT}{V} = \text{constant}$$

$$n2 = \frac{n1}{P1} \times P2 = \frac{3.00}{1.00} \times 1.80 = 5.40 \text{ moles}$$

The extra number of moles needed is therefore 5.4 − 3.0 = 2.4.

(A sidenote: Be careful when applying this approach to questions dealing with changes in temperature. Make sure you are using absolute temperature, in Kelvin. An increase from 20°C to 40°C is NOT a doubling of temperature!)

3. **A** First we must determine the order of the reaction. On going from experiment 1 to experiment 2, the concentration of [B] has increased, but the rate of reaction remains the same. The reaction therefore appears to be independent on the concentration of [B], or in other words, it is zero order with respect to [B]. Comparing experiments 1 and 3, we see that the concentration of [A] has tripled, whereas the rate of reaction has increased by about a factor of nine. The reaction is second order in [A]. We can therefore write:

$$\text{rate} = k[A]^2$$

To determine the rate constant, we need only to arrange the above equation and substitute in values for [A] and the rate for any one experiment:

$$k = \frac{\text{rate}}{[A]2} = \frac{1.87}{(0.181)^2}$$

Note that the rate constant will have units (of M–1s–1 for second-order reactions), but we are ignoring that in this particular question.

4. **D** The spontaneity of a reaction is determined by the free energy change, ΔG. A reaction goes from being spontaneous to nonspontaneous (or vice versa) when the value of ΔG crosses the value of 0. Since $\Delta G = \Delta H - T\Delta S$, and we are told to assume that the values of ΔH and ΔS are not sensitive to changes in temperature, we can solve for the temperature at which the value of ΔG becomes zero. The tricky part is that ΔH and ΔS are reported in different units, and we must be careful to be consistent. We change the value of ΔH from 131 kJ/mol to 131,000 J/mol:

$$0 = 131,000 - T(134)$$
$$T = \frac{131,000}{134}$$

which is slightly less than 1,000 K. (Remember, we always use the absolute temperature in cases like this!) To convert from Kelvin to degrees Celsius, we need to subtract about 300. This brings the value to about 700, which is (D).

The ΔH and ΔS values are reported in different energy units not just to trap you. The magnitude of the enthalpy change is usually much greater than the magnitude of the entropy change for a given reaction, and so expressing one with kJ and the other with J (or kcal and cal) is a common practice.

5. **A** A mole of ideal gas, regardless of the species, occupies 22.4 L at STP, which corresponds to 1 atm pressure and 0°C (or 273 K). The conditions specified in the question stem are thus STP conditions. The mixture occupies a volume of 44.8 L, which means there are two moles of gas present. If the mixture contains 1.5 moles of argon, then there must be $2 - 1.5 = 0.5$ mol of Ne present.

6. **D** The percentage of oxygen by mass is the mass of oxygen divided by the total mass of the compound, multiplied by 100 percent. Even though we are told that the sample weighs 200 g, we actually don't need this to get the answer. Any sample of $CuSO_4 \cdot 5H_2O$, regardless of its weight, will have the same percentage of O by mass because this is dictated by the stoichiometric relationships in the chemical formula.

We can work with the convenient quantity of 1 mole. The weight of a 1-mole sample is just the molecular weight of the compound: $63.5 + 32 + 4 \times 16 + 5 \times (2 \times 1 + 16) = 63.5 + 32 + 64 + 90 = 250$ g. The mass of oxygen in this 1-mole sample is $4 \times 16 + 5 \times 16 = 144$, where the first four come from the sulfate and the other five come from the five water molecules hydrated to the compound. The percentage by mass of oxygen is therefore:

$$\frac{144}{250} \times 100\%$$

Because 144 is more than half of 250, the percentage is more than 50 percent, making (D) the correct choice.

Note again that nowhere did we use the fact that the sample weighs 200 g.

7. **C** Nonmetallic elements are found in the right of the periodic table, and, if neutral, will always have valence electrons in the *p* subshell, which can hold a maximum of six electrons. (If it is not neutral, there is a possibility that electrons have been added or removed so that there are only *s* valence electrons.) The requirement that it be in its ground state means that the orbitals are filled in accordance with the Aufbau principle. Only (C) satisfies these criteria.

(A) is incorrect because its valence electrons are in the *s* subshell. If it is a neutral species, this would be Mg, which is a metal. If it is a nonmetal, it must have had electrons removed or added, making it not neutral (e.g., Al+). (B) is incorrect because the 4*s* orbital should not have filled before the 3*p* orbitals: it does not represent a ground state species. (D) is incorrect because the *p* subshell, with three orbitals, can only have a maximum of six electrons.

8. **D** This rather tricky question on concentration units and solution stoichiometry requires that you apply the definition of molality, or moles of solute per kilogram solvent, although a glance at the answer choices indicates that full calculation is unnecessary. We can calculate the formula weight of aluminum sulfate as 342 g/mol ($2 \times 27 + 3 \times 32 + 12 \times 16$, or $54 + 3 \times 96$). In a 0.3-m solution, there are 3 moles of aluminum sulfate for every kilogram of solvent. So $0.3 \text{ mol/kg} \times 342 \text{ g/mol} = 102.6 \text{ g/kg}$ of solvent. The total mass of a solution produced by dissolving 102.6 g of aluminum sulfate in one kilogram (i.e., 1,000 g) of solvent will then be $102.6 + 1,000 = 1,102.6$ grams. We can set up and rearrange a ratio now to find the quantity of $Al_2(SO_4)_3$ required for the 87.5 g of solution given in the question:

$$\frac{102.6 \text{ g of solute}}{1,102.6 \text{ g of solution}} = \frac{X \text{ g of solute}}{87.5 \text{ g of solution}}$$

$$X = \frac{87.5 \times 102.6}{1,102.6}$$

9. **D** For a molecule to be polar, it must contain polar bonds (bonds formed between elements of different electronegativity in which electron density is not shared equally), and the dipole moments carried by these polar bonds must not cancel vectorially. (A), (B), and (C) are incorrect because even though they all contain polar bonds, these bonds are arranged spatially so that they cancel one another:

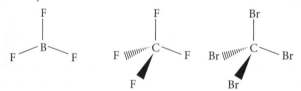

BF_3 has a trigonal planar geometry, and the dipole moments of the polar B–F bonds, when added together vectorially, yield no net dipole moment. Similarly, for the tetrahedral CF_4 and CBr_4.

(D) is correct because the two polar C–Cl bonds do not completely cancel each other.

10. **A** This question tests our knowledge of both stoichiometry and gas laws. First, we need to determine how many moles of hydrogen gas are generated from the reaction and then calculate the volume of the gas under the conditions described. For the first part, the dimensional setup is as follows:

number of moles of H2 produced = $5.05 \text{ g Zn} \times \dfrac{1 \text{ mol Zn}}{65.4 \text{ g}} \times \dfrac{1 \text{ mol hydrogen}}{1 \text{ mol Zn}} = \dfrac{5.05}{65.4}$,

where the atomic weight of Zn of 65.4 g/mol is given and the stoichiometric relationship between Zn and H2 is read from the balanced equation given in the question stem. (For every mole of Zn consumed, one mole of hydrogen gas is produced.) For the second part of calculating the volume, we need to use the ideal gas law. We need to be careful about units because we are using the value of R as given in the question stem to determine the volume in liters, but that means that we need our temperature to be in Kelvin and our pressure to be in atmospheres. $40°C = 313$ K, and because 1 atm = 760 torr, 763 torr = $\frac{763}{760}$ atm.

$$PV = nRT$$

$$V = nRTP \qquad = \text{number of moles of H2} \times \frac{(0.0821 \text{ L·atm/mol·K})(313 \text{ K})}{763/760 \text{ atm}}$$

$$= \text{number of moles of H2} \times \frac{760}{763} \times 0.0821 \times 313$$

$$= \frac{5.05}{65.4} \times \frac{760}{763} \times 0.0821 \times 313$$

which is choice (A).

11. **A**   Isotopes of an element have the same atomic number but different mass numbers. The atomic number is the same as the number of protons, and the mass number is the sum of protons and neutrons. The isotope given in the question has a mass number of 208 and an atomic number of 82; therefore, it has 82 protons and $208 - 82 = 126$ neutrons. Another isotope of the same element hence must also have 82 protons (an atomic number of 82) but a different number of neutrons.

   (B) and (C) are incorrect because each would imply that the two isotopes are the same.

   (D) is incorrect because isotopes of the same element must have the same atomic number (same number of protons), in this case 82.

12. **B**   The empirical formula gives the simplest whole number ratio of the different elements in a compound. Because in this question, the number of moles of each element in the compound has been given to us already, all we need to do is to find the simplest whole number ratio among them; 1.074 is twice the value of 0.537, so N:H:Cl = 0.537:1.074:0.537 = 1:2:1. The empirical formula is thus NH_2Cl.

   (Note that in most questions involving empirical formulas, we would probably just be given the mass of each element in the sample, and we would then first have to determine the number of moles of each by dividing by the atomic mass of the elements.)

13. **C**   Hess's law tells us that the standard change in enthalpy of a reaction, $\Delta H°$, is equal to the sum of the standard enthalpies of formation of the products minus the sum of the standard enthalpies of formation of the reactants. Therefore, for the first reaction in the table, we can write:

   $\Delta H° = 729.8 \text{ kcal} = 6 \times \Delta H°f (CO_2) + 3 \times \Delta H°f (H_2O) - \Delta H°f (C_6H_5OH) - 7 \times \Delta H°f (O_2)$

   O_2 is already in its standard state, and so its enthalpy of formation is zero. The last term in the equation thus vanishes. The enthalpy of formation of carbon dioxide is the enthalpy change of the second reaction in the table (i.e., 94.4 kcal/mol). The enthalpy of formation of one mole of H_2O is one-half the enthalpy change of the third reaction (i.e., 68.4 kcal/mol). (The reaction leads to the formation of two moles of H_2O.) We can now substitute in these values and solve for the unknown, the enthalpy of formation of C_6H_5OH:

   $$729.8 = 6 \times 94.4 + 3 \times 136.8/2 - \Delta H°f (C_6H_5OH)$$

   $$\Delta H°f (C_6H_5OH) = 6 \times 94.4 + 3 \times 68.4 - 729.8 = 600 + 210 - 730$$

   With this approximation, we can see that only (C) is close enough to be correct.

14. **C** The percent yield is the actual yield divided by the theoretical yield multiplied by 100 percent. The theoretical yield is the amount of product expected based purely on stoichiometry. In this question, the theoretical yield is determined as follows:

$$\text{amount of } C_6H_5NO_2 \text{ expected} = \frac{78 \text{ g } C_6H_6}{78 \text{ g/mol } C_6H_6} \times \frac{1 \text{ mol } C_6H_5NO_2}{1 \text{ mol } C_6H_6} \times 123 \text{ g/mol}$$

$$C_6H_5NO_2 = 123 \text{ g } C_6H_5NO_2$$

The actual yield is 82 g. The percent yield is therefore $\frac{82}{123} \times 100\%$. Without actually performing the division, we note that 82 is more than half of 123, so the percentage is greater than 50 percent. Because we get less than the theoretical 123 g that is possible, the yield is not 100 percent. Choice (C) is the only possible response.

15. **C** Hydrogen bonds are a specific type of dipole-dipole interaction. When hydrogen is bonded to a highly electronegative atom, such as oxygen, nitrogen, or fluorine, the hydrogen atom carries little of the electron density of the covalent bond. This partially positively charged hydrogen atom interacts with the partial negative charge located on the electronegative atoms of nearby molecules. Water has two hydrogen atoms per molecule, whereas HF has only one. Water can therefore engage in more hydrogen bond per molecule:

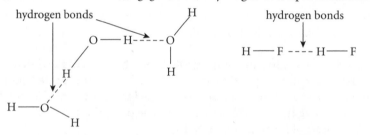

(Note that in the diagram above, we have only indicated the hydrogen bonding for the hydrogen atom(s) of one molecule. Obviously, the electronegative atom can also engage in hydrogen bonding with a hydrogen atom from another molecule.)

(A) is incorrect because H_2O and HF only differ by 2 amu; this difference is insignificant relative to boiling point determination. Besides, HF has the higher molecular weight, so based on this factor alone, we would have expected HF to have a higher boiling point, which contradicts what we are told in the question stem.

(B) is incorrect because the H–F bond is more polar than the H–O bond (fluorine is more electronegative than oxygen), so the H–F dipole-dipole attraction is stronger than that of O–H.

(D) is incorrect because dispersion forces dominate only between nonpolar atoms or molecules. So the dispersion forces between H–F and H–O are insignificant.

16. **D** The easiest way to answer to this question is by eliminating wrong answer choices.

(A) and (B) can be eliminated because the unknown compound resulted in an acidic solution, so it cannot be a base.

We can eliminate (C) as follows. We are given a pH of 4.56. Because $pH = -\log[H^+]$, then the $[H^+] = 1 \times 10^{-pH}$. The $[H^+]$ must then be between 1×10^{-5} M and 1×10^{-4} M. Because the volume is 1 L, then there are between 1×10^{-5} M and 1×10^{-4} mol H+. Looking at (C), if the acid had a formula weight of $50 \frac{g}{mol}$, and 100 g was added to the water, then 2 mol of H+ would form if it were a strong acid. From the previous calculation we know that is impossible. The unknown must be a weak acid.

We can confirm (D) as the correct answer as follows. The formula for K_a is $\frac{[H+][A-]}{[HA]}$. Because the unknown compound must be a weak acid, there will be more undissociated acid in solution than dissociated, making the $[HA] > [H^+][A^-]$, so then $K_a < 1$. If the $K_a < 1$, then the $pK_a > 0$.

17. **D** The molarity of the acid solution can be calculated using the neutralization formula: $M_A V_A = M_B V_B$. Solving for the acid molarity and plugging in we get: $M_A = \frac{M_B V_B}{V_A} = \frac{(.1)(35)}{50}$; or (D).

Note that in this case, the molarity of the solutions is the same as their normality because KOH is monobasic and the acid is monoprotic. Also, even though technically we need to express the volume in L for most calculations (since 1 M = 1 mol/L), we do not need to do the conversion here because all we are interested in is the ratio of the two volumes: $\frac{35 \text{ mL}}{50 \text{ mL}} = \frac{0.035 \text{ L}}{0.050 \text{ L}} = 0.70$.

18. **B** Freezing-point depression is a colligative property—one that depends only on the amount of the substance present. Because the compound in the question is ionic, the formula for the freezing-point depression has to be multiplied by the number of particles formed upon dissolving. The formula for freezing-point depression is $DT_f = K_f m$, where m is the molality of solute particles. In this case, for the molality of solute particles, we need to multiply the molality of the compound by the number of particles formed as the compound dissociates. First, however, let us find out how much the freezing point would change if the compound does not dissociate:

$$DT_f = K_f \frac{\text{moles of compound}}{\text{weight of solvent}} = K_f \frac{\text{mass of compound/formula weight}}{\text{weight of solvent}} = 1.86 \frac{22.2/111}{1}$$
$$= 2(0.2) = 0.4°C$$

The observed freezing point is $-1.12∞C$, which is about three times as much as the calculated value. The unknown ionic compound must therefore dissociate into three particles, making (B) the correct choice.

19. **C** This question on nuclear chemistry requires you to correctly determine the upper and lower numbers on the nuclide symbols. The sum of the nuclear charge (lower) numbers on the right side of the reaction must equal the sum of the charge numbers on the left, but each of these lower numbers corresponds to the atomic number of the associated element. Thus, $X_1 = 12$ and $X_4 = 2$, as given in the question stem. Now, since the mass (upper) numbers on the reactant side must sum to the same value as the mass numbers on the

product side, and since a neutron has a mass number of 1 (i.e., $X_2 = 1$), we can set up an algebraic expression to solve for the desired sum:

$$26 + X_2 = X_3 + X_5$$

$$X_3 + X_5 = 27$$

$$X_1 + X_2 + X_3 + X_4 + X_5 = X_1 + X_2 + X_4 + (X_3 + X_5) = 12 + 1 + 2 + (27) = 42$$

20. B The best oxidizing agent is the species getting reduced. The nitrogen atom goes from an oxidation state of $+5$ in NO_3- to -3 in NH_3, getting reduced and serving as an oxidizing agent.

(A) is wrong because aluminum goes from 0 in $Al(s)$ to $+3$ in $Al(OH)4-$. It is therefore oxidized and acts as a reducing agent.

(C) and (D) are wrong because they represent products of the reaction. If either one of them were a stronger oxidizing agent than NO_3-, the reaction as given would not be spontaneous.

21. A This question requires no calculation. Because we are dealing with a base, (B), (C), and (D) can all be eliminated.

If we had wanted to proceed with a full calculation, we would have proceeded as follows. Calcium hydroxide dissociates to yield one calcium ion and two hydroxide ions, and so if $\times$ M calcium hydroxide dissociates, we would have $\times M$ of Ca^2+ and $2x\ M\ OH^-$. When the solution is saturated, the concentrations of these ions satisfy the following condition:

$$[Ca^2+][OH-]^2 = Ksp = 8.0 \times 10^{-6}$$

where the square is needed for the hydroxide ion concentration because the dissociation reaction is of the form:

$$Ca(OH)_2 \rightarrow Ca^2+ + 2OH-$$

Recall that for an equilibrium expression, the concentration of the species is raised to its stoichiometric coefficient. Proceeding with our calculation, we substitute in the expressions for the concentrations of the ions:

$$Ca^2+][OH^-]^2 = (x)(2x)^2 = 4x^3 = 8.0 \times 10^{-6}$$

$$x^3 = 2.0 \times 10^{-6}$$

$$x = (2.0 \times 10^{-6})^{1/3}$$

$$= (2.0)^{1/3} \times 10^{-2}$$

But again because of the stoichiometry of the dissociation reaction, the hydroxide ion concentration is 2x, or $2 \times (2.0)^{1/3} \times 10^{-2}$. The pOH of the solution is the negative log of this number, which is about 2, since $\log (10^{-2}) = -2$ and so $-\log (10^{-2}) = 2$. The pH of the solution is $14 - pOH$, or about 12.

22. **B** Oxidation occurs at the anode and reduction at the cathode (mnemonic: An Ox – Red Cat). Only in the reaction shown in (B) is chromium being oxidized. Assignations of oxidation numbers are as follows:

(A) $2x - 14 = -2$
$\uparrow \quad \uparrow$
$x \quad -2$
$Cr_2O_7^{2-} \longrightarrow$
$Cr = +6$

$x - 8 = -2$
$\uparrow \quad \uparrow$
$x \quad -2$
$CrO_4^{2-} \longrightarrow$
$Cr = +6$

(C) $2x - 14 = -2$
$\uparrow \quad \uparrow$
$x \quad -2$
$Cr_2O_7^{2-} \longrightarrow$
$Cr = +6$

Cr_2
$Cr2$

(B)

$x - 8 = -2$
$\uparrow \quad \uparrow$
$-2 \quad x$
$CrO_4^{2-} \longrightarrow$
$Cr = +6$

(D) $x - 8 = -2$
$\uparrow \quad \uparrow$
$-2 \quad x$
$CrO_4^{2-} \longrightarrow \quad Cr^{3+}$
$Cr = +6$

$Cr^{2+} \longrightarrow$
$Cr = +6$

23. **D** Numbering the carbon atoms from left to right, we notice that carbon 2 and carbon 3 form a triple bond and a single bond each. They are thus both *sp* hybridized, and the bond angles a and b must be 180° (i.e., carbons 1–4 are linear). Carbon 4 forms a double bond and a single bond (with presumably another single bond, not shown, to a hydrogen atom or something else). It is thus *sp2* hybridized with a bond angle of 120°. A more accurate representation of the structure of the molecule may be as follows:

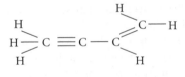

24. **D** Overlapping orbitals that are perpendicular to the axis of the bond are features of π bonds. Because the overlap is not cylindrically symmetric, rotation about the interatomic axis would break such bonds. A double bond consists of one *s* and one π bond, whereas a triple bond consists of one *s* and two π bonds. Choice (A) is incorrect because *s* bonds, found in single bonds, are formed when the overlap is along the axis joining the atoms. (B) and (C) are incorrect because double and triple bonds differ only in the number of π bonds, not in the nature of the π bonds.

25. **B** Because each carbon of acetylene has two bonding partners (one carbon and one hydrogen), it is *sp* hybridized. The rest of the choices are all true and therefore incorrect. Acetylene, or ethyne, is a linear molecule with a triple bond (one *s* and two π bonds). Because it is also symmetric, the (already weak) polarity of the C–H bonds cancel each other vectorially, and the molecule does not have a net dipole moment, making it nonpolar: it is only slightly soluble in water. The statements in (A), (C), and (D) are all true.

READING COMPREHENSION

1. **B** Paragraph 1 states that, normally, "dopamine is taken back up into the presynaptic cell" and broken down into metabolites like DOPAC and HVA. But cocaine "blocks the reuptake of dopamine into the presynaptic cell." We can therefore infer that, with less dopamine to process, there will be a corresponding DECREASE in the level of metabolites like HVA, and (B) is correct. If (B) is true, (A) must be false. (C) is wrong because levels of DOPAC, like those of HVA, should fall, not rise. (D) combines the mistakes of choices (A) and (C).

2. **A** A tricky one. According to the last two sentences of paragraph 1, when cocaine blocks the reuptake of dopamine in the presynaptic cell, this exposes the postsynaptic neurotransmitter to "prolonged" and "acute" dopaminergic neurotransmission, resulting in euphoria. The key word here is *prolonged*: cocaine causes released dopamine to be active for a longer time (A). (B), (C), and (D) subtly distort the author's point: it's not that dopamine "turns over" more rapidly, that more dopamine receptors become available, or that more dopamine is released into the synapse. The euphoria occurs because the released dopamine is active for a longer duration than normal.

3. **C** As with question 1, the correct answer here can be inferred from paragraph 1's description of what happens to the presynaptic cell under normal circumstances. Normally, "dopamine is taken back up into the presynaptic cell and either repackaged into storage vesicles, etc..." If cocaine "blocks the reuptake of dopamine into the presynaptic cell," then it follows that those storage vesicles will have lower-than-normal amounts of dopamine, (C). (A) is wrong because dopamine is "broken down via MAO"—in other words, less dopamine doesn't necessarily mean less MAO. (B) distorts the same sentence: in reality, storage and metabolism are both shortchanged when dopamine reuptake is blocked by cocaine. Dormant cells (D) are never mentioned in the passage.

4. **B** According to paragraph 1, incorrect choices (A), (C), and (D) all take place in normal dopaminergic neurotransmission. The end of paragraph 2 says that (B), the breakdown of dopamine by COMT, is what causes cocaine craving. This breakdown does not occur in normal dopaminergic neurotransmission.

5. **A** According to the first two sentences of paragraph 3, bromocriptine is a "dopamine agonist" that "stimulates dopamine receptors," a fact restated in (A). Contrary to choices (B) and (C), neither cocaine nor bromocriptine works in the synapse but in the presynaptic and postsynaptic cells, respectively. Because bromocriptine doesn't work on the presynaptic cell, (D) is also wrong.

6. **C** The second sentence of paragraph 3 says that "bromocriptine, like cocaine, increases dopaminergic neurotransmission." (C) correctly restates this fact. (A) is wrong because, unlike cocaine, bromocriptine doesn't cause dopamine depletion. (B) is tempting because cocaine addiction and craving are obviously both problematic, but they aren't side effects, technically speaking. At any rate, the author asserts that, of the two drugs, only bromocriptine has "adverse side effects." Neither drug is said to have "habit-forming rewards" (D).

7. **B** Paragraph 3 says that bromocriptine works on the postsynaptic cell, not the presynaptic cell. The safest inference here, then, is that bromocriptine will not affect the level of dopamine in the presynaptic cell, which will stay the same (B).

8. **D** Whereas paragraph 1 tells us that Neanderthal man used tools (D), Boule was an anatomist who concerned himself only with the Neanderthal physique. The second and third sentences of paragraph 2 say that Boule considered Neanderthals "primitive" because of such characteristics as their "stooping, bent-kneed posture" (A), prominent brows and overdeveloped joints (i.e., bone structure) (B), and their "low-vaulted cranium" (C).

9. **D** The "best supported" point is usually a direct restatement of material in the passage. The author argues at the end of paragraph 1 that Neanderthals showed "the capacity for religious and abstract thought," so (D) is best. This point also contradicts (A)'s notion that Neanderthals were less intelligent than early modern humans. (B) is considered and rejected in the third sentence of the final paragraph. Paragraphs 3 and 4 suggest that, contrary to (C), there probably WAS contact between Neanderthals and early modern humans.

10. **D** This detail question requires a careful reading of paragraph 3. The author says that Neanderthals "inhabited a vast area...until 35,000 years ago...then, within a brief period of 5,000–10,000 years, they disappeared." Therefore, the latest that any Neanderthal might have existed is not 35,000 years ago but 10,000 years later, or 25,000 years ago.

11. **A** (A) can be inferred from the second-to-last sentence of paragraph 3: despite their anatomical similarities, "the [anatomical] differences are major enough" that early humans did not evolve from Neanderthals. Neanderthals did disappear quickly (B), but the author doesn't suggest that this is why humans couldn't have evolved from Neanderthals. (C) distorts a point in paragraph 4, the theory of localized evolution, which posits a way that humans COULD HAVE evolved from Neanderthals. (D) is contradicted by paragraph 3, which suggests that there is an overlap, not a gap, between the dates of the latest Neanderthal and earliest modern human fossils.

12. **C** Each incorrect choice is discussed in the final paragraph, which offers various explanations for the disappearance of the Neanderthals. The Neanderthals's "need for a heavy diet to sustain" their physique eliminates (A). Some people think "the Neanderthals failed to adapt to the onset of the last Ice Age" (B), and some think that "modern humans wiped out the Neanderthals in warfare (D). (C) is correct: whereas paragraph 4's theory of localized evolution suggests that modern humans may have evolved from Neanderthals, it doesn't explain why the Neanderthals themselves disappeared.

13. **A** The key word in this question stem is *evolution*, which directs you to paragraph 4's discussion of localized evolution. If interbreeding "within a geographically concentrated population" could have produced "far more pronounced genetic effects within a shorter time," then you can infer that the rate of evolution is directly related to the concentration of species population, (A). Choices (B), (C), and (D) raise issues that the passage suggests may have factored into the extinction of the Neanderthal subspecies but not into the evolution of a species.

14. **B** The first sentence of paragraph 6 states that "the elderly population will double within the next 40 years," so (B) is correct. The passage never mentions a housing shortage (A). (C) contradicts paragraph 5, which states that "77 percent of elderly Americans have annual incomes of less than $20,000." As for (D), the author never specifies what percentage of the total population is elderly.

15. **A** The second sentence of paragraph 5 says that 77 percent of elders, a solid majority, earn less than $20,000 per year (A). (B) thoroughly distorts the second sentence of the final paragraph. The inability of elders to purchase their own homes (C) is never mentioned in the passage, and whereas paragraph 4 discusses elderly Americans in the workforce, it doesn't say how many hours a week they work (D).

16. **B** In the final paragraph, the author says that "the Medicaid/Medicare system is threatened by the continuous upward spiral of medical costs." If health care expenses for "disabled elderly Americans"—a subset of those people covered by Medicaid/Medicare—is likely to double within 10 years, then the threat is real: Medicaid/Medicare will indeed probably become more expensive in the future (B). The obstacle to a federally funded national health care system is not monetary (A) but rather opposition from "the medical establishment and various special interest groups." (C) distorts paragraph 6, which says that the federal government has borrowed from Social Security to "pay interest on the national debt," not health care expenses. Finally, (D) overreaches: the author doesn't suggest that rising health care costs for the disabled elderly will actually prevent baby boomers from receiving health benefits, only that such rising costs will place increasing strain on the federal health benefit system.

17. **A** A relatively easy detail question, (A) restates the second sentence of the passage. (B) distorts information in paragraph 2, which says that the "graying" of the "baby boomers" will contribute to the future rise of the elderly population. (C) and (D) are completely unsubstantiated in the passage.

18. **C** Paragraph 3 asserts that, in the future, the typical U.S. family will be restructured "towards an extended, multigenerational family" (C). Because such a family will be "dominated by elders," it will not be youth oriented (A). Contrary to (B), the author suggests that the Social Security system will be unable to subsidize adequately the greatly enlarged elderly population. (D) runs counter to the thrust of paragraphs 5, 6, and 7; indeed, paragraph 5 notes that, as people grow older, "their earning power decreases and their need for health care increases."

19. **D** Paragraph 5 states that, especially since the advent of Medicaid/Medicare in 1965, "most elderly Americans [have] come to depend heavily on federal and state subsidies;" thus, (D) is correct. (A) contradicts paragraph 4, which says that whereas 50 percent of 65-year old men worked in 1950, only 15 percent do today. (B) is a distortion of paragraph 6: whereas the federal government has often borrowed from the Social Security fund to pay interest on the national debt, the author never suggests that this caused many elderly Americans to lose their Social Security benefits. The cost of living (D) is never discussed in the passage.

20. **C** We end with a fairly straightforward detail question. In the final paragraph, the author states that we don't yet have a national health care system because "the medical establishment and various special interest groups have so far blocked legislation aimed at creating it"; thus, (C) is correct. The obstacles in choices (A) and (B) are never suggested, and (D) contradicts the author, who obviously feels that a national health care system is necessary.

QUANTITATIVE ABILITY

1. **B** First group the integers 12 and 16 together and group the powers 10^5 and 10^9 together.

    Then $\dfrac{12 \times 10^5}{16 \times 10^9} = \left(\dfrac{12}{16}\right) \times \left(\dfrac{10^5}{10^9}\right)$. Now $\dfrac{12}{16} = \dfrac{3}{4} = 0.75$. To work with $\dfrac{10^5}{10^9}$, you need to know a law of exponents. The law you need to know is that whenever you divide powers with the same base, you subtract the exponents and keep the same base. Algebraically, $\dfrac{b^x}{b^y}$
    $= b^{x-y}$. So $\dfrac{10^5}{10^9} = 10^{5-9} = 10^{-4}$. Now $\dfrac{12 \times 10^5}{16 \times 10^9} = 0.75 \times 10^{-4}$. None of the answer choices is 0.75×10^{-4}. However, each answer choice is 7.5 times something. Let's multiply the 0.75 in $\times 10^{-4}$ by 10 to obtain 7.5. However, we must keep the value of 0.75×10^{-4} the same. To adjust for the fact that we multiplied 0.75 by 10, let's divide 10^{-4} by 10. Then

    $$0.75 \times 10^{-4} = (0.75 \times 10) \times \left(\frac{10^{-4}}{10}\right)$$
    $$= (0.75 \times 10) \times \frac{10^{-4}}{10^1}$$
    $$= 7.5 \times 10^{-4-1}$$
    $$= 7.5 \times 10^{-5}$$

2. **C** Remember the convention that the radical symbol always means the nonnegative square root of the (nonnegative) number. For example, 64 has two square roots, 8 and –8, while $\sqrt{64} = 8$.

    Since 4 is a perfect square, $4 = 2^2$. Let's reexpress the quantity under the radical sign, 0.000004, as the product of two factors, where one factor is 4 and the other factor is 10 raised to an exponent. (Hopefully this exponent will be even—it will certainly be negative—so that when we take half of it we will get an integer.) Then we'll use the law of radicals, which says that the (nonnegative) square root of a product is equal to the product of the (nonnegative) square roots. Algebraically, if $a \geq 0$ and $b \geq 0$, then $\sqrt{ab} = \sqrt{a}\sqrt{b}$.

    Now $0.000004 = 4 \times 10^{-6}$. The exponent –6 is indeed even. So

    $$\sqrt{0.000004} = \sqrt{4 \times 10^{-6}}$$
    $$= \sqrt{4} \times \sqrt{10^{-6}}$$
    $$= 2 \times 10^{-3}$$
    $$= 0.002$$

3. B Convert the percents to decimals and then do the multiplication. Whenever you convert a percent to a decimal (and also whenever you convert a percent to a fraction), you divide the percent by 100%, thus having the percent symbols drop out. First, let's convert 7% and 3% to decimals. $7\% = \dfrac{7\%}{100\%} = \dfrac{7}{100} = 0.07$ and, similarly, $3\% = 0.03$. So 7% of 3% of 4 is equal to $0.07 \times 0.03 \times 4$. Now just find the value of $0.07 \times 0.03 \times 4$. Working this out, we have that $0.07 \times 0.03 \times 4 = 0.0021 \times 4 = 0.0084$, and choice (B) is correct.

4. B
$$\cfrac{1}{5 + \cfrac{1}{5 + \cfrac{2}{3}}} = \cfrac{1}{5 + \cfrac{1}{\frac{15}{3} + \frac{2}{3}}} = \cfrac{1}{5 + \cfrac{1}{\left(\frac{17}{3}\right)}} = \cfrac{1}{5 + \frac{3}{17}} = \cfrac{1}{\frac{85}{17} + \frac{3}{17}} = \cfrac{1}{\left(\frac{88}{17}\right)} = \frac{17}{88}$$

5. C To add the fractions, find a common denominator for the fractions. The largest denominator, 24, is a multiple of the denominator 3 ($24 = 8 \times 3$), the denominator 6 ($24 = 4 \times 6$), and the denominator 12 ($24 = 2 \times 12$). So 24 can be used as a common denominator. Actually, 24 is also the least common denominator. Then

$$\frac{2}{3} + \frac{5}{6} - \frac{7}{12} - \frac{1}{24} = \frac{2}{3} \times \frac{8}{8} + \frac{5}{6} \times \frac{4}{4} - \frac{7}{12} \times \frac{2}{2} - \frac{1}{24}$$
$$= \frac{16}{24} + \frac{20}{24} - \frac{14}{24} - \frac{1}{24}$$
$$= \frac{16 + 20 - 14 - 1}{24}$$
$$= \frac{21}{24}$$
$$= \frac{7}{8}$$

6. B The graph of a line has to satisfy the equation $y = mx + b$, where m is the slope and b is the y-intercept. If two lines are perpendicular to each other, then the slope of one line is the negative inverse of the other. We are told that line ℓ is perpendicular to the line $y = -\frac{1}{5}x$, so the slope of ℓ must equal 5. In the $y = mx + b$, we know that m must equal 5. To find b, we substitute the point (3, −10) into the equation. We are given that the point (3, −10) is on the line, so $x = 3$ and $y = -10$ must satisfy the equation $y = 5x + b$. By substituting $x = 3$ and $y = -10$, we get

$$y = mx + b$$
$$y = 5x + b$$
$$-10 = 5(3) + b$$
$$-10 = 15 + b$$
$$-10 - 15 = b$$
$$-25 = b$$

Now we know that m = 5 and b = −25, so our equation is y = 5x − 25, which is choice (B).

7. **D** Since Allen spent 10% of the money he originally had on tennis equipment and 55% of the money he originally had on golf equipment, he spent a total of 10% + 55%, or 65% of the money he originally had with him at the store. We were able to add these two percents because they are percents of the same whole. Since he spent 65% of the original amount of money, he had 100% − 65% or 35% of the original amount left. He had $210 left. If we call T the number of dollars of the original amount, then 35% of T is 210. Now find the value of T. The word *of* means "times" in this instance, so $35\% \times T = 210$. Now convert 35% to a fraction. Whenever you convert a percent to a fraction (and also whenever you convert a percent to a decimal), you divide the percent by 100%, thus having the percent symbols drop out. So $\frac{35\%}{100\%} = \frac{35}{100} = \frac{7}{20}$. So $\frac{7}{20} \times T = 210$, and $T = 210 \times \frac{20}{7} = 30 \times 20 = 600$.

8. **C** The probability of two independent events occurring together is the product of their individual probabilities. The probability of selecting the first marble is $\frac{5}{11}$ and the probability of selecting the second marble is $\frac{4}{10}$. (Don't forget to subtract 1 since you are not putting the second one back!) The probability of drawing two purple marbles is then $\frac{5}{11} \times \frac{4}{10} = \frac{20}{110} = \frac{2}{11}$.

9. **A** Solve the equation $\sqrt{x - 16} = 26 - 21$ for x.

$$\sqrt{x - 16} = 26 - 21$$

Simplify the right side: $\sqrt{x - 16} = 5$

Square both sides: $(\sqrt{x - 16})^2 = 5^2$

Simplify each side: $x - 16 = 25$

Add 16 to both sides: $x = 41$

10. **B** You need to know the average formula: average $= \frac{\text{sum of the terms}}{\text{number of terms}}$. In this question, it is also important to be familiar with the average formula in the rearranged form: sum of the terms = average × number of terms. Elaine's average score on all 4 exams was $\frac{\text{sum of the four scores}}{4}$. So the sum of all 4 scores must first be found. Elaine's average on the first 3 exams was 76, so the sum of her scores on the first 3 exams was 76 × 3, or 228. The sum of her scores on all 4 exams is equal to the sum of her scores on the first 3 exams plus her score on the fourth exam, or 228 + 84, which is 312. Her average on all 4 exams was $\frac{312}{4}$, which is 78. Choice (B) is correct.

11. **D** The ratio of 5 to 2 tells us that for every five clerical employees, there are two nonclerical employees. It also tells us that there are a total of $5 + 2 = 7$ equal parts. These 7 equal parts make up the total of 630 employees. So each of these equal parts is $\frac{630}{7} = 90$ employees. The clerical employees consist of 5 of these equal parts, so there are 5×90, or 450 clerical employees.

12. **B** In distance, rate (or speed), and time problems, we use the formula: distance = rate × time. It will be convenient to work with this formula in the forms

$$\text{rate} = \frac{\text{distance}}{\text{time}} \quad \text{and time} = \frac{\text{distance}}{\text{rate}}$$

when solving this problem.

It's important to keep in mind that the average speed for an entire trip is always the total distance divided by the total time. Never take the average of speeds. In this question, a greater amount of time was spent traveling the first half of the distance at an average speed of 60 miles per hour than was spent traveling the second half of the distance at the greater average speed of 100 miles per hour, so the average speed (in miles per hour) must be closer to 60 than to 100. Just realizing this enables you to eliminate choices (C) and (D).

One way to solve this question is to pick a value for the distance between Xaviertown and Youngstown. Always pick a number that is easy to work with. Here, we should pick a number that is a multiple of the numbers 100 and 60. Let's use 600 for the distance between the towns. Let's now state the total distance traveled: the 600 miles we have selected as the distance between the towns. Now let's find the total time traveled. We know that 300 miles were traveled from Xaviertown to the midpoint and 300 miles were traveled from the midpoint to Youngstown. The time taken to travel from Xaviertown to the midpoint was $\frac{300 \text{ miles}}{60 \text{ miles per hour}}$, which is $\frac{300}{60}$ hours, or 5 hours. The time taken to travel from the midpoint to Youngstown was $\frac{300}{100}$ hours, or 3 hours. The total time traveled was $5 + 3$ hours, which is 8 hours. The total distance traveled was 600 miles, and the total time traveled was 8 hours. So the average speed for the trip was $\frac{600}{8}$ miles per hour, or 75 miles per hour.

13. **D** $a = \dfrac{18}{48}$

$b = \dfrac{1}{3}$

$\dfrac{a}{\left(\dfrac{1}{b^2}\right)} = a \times b^2 = \dfrac{(18 \times 9)}{48} = \dfrac{(18 \times 3)}{16} = \dfrac{(9 \times 3)}{8} = \dfrac{27}{8}$

14. **D** The expression $(3x - 7y)^2$ is of the form $(c - d)^2$. We have that $(c - d)^2 = c^2 - 2cd + d^2$. Now replace c by $3x$ and d by $7y$. Then

$(3x - 7y)^2 = (3x)^2 - 2(3x)(7y)^2$

$\qquad\qquad = 9x^2 - 42xy + 49y^2$

If you did not remember that $(c - d)^2 = c^2 - 2cd + d^2$, you can multiply out $(3x - 7y)^2$ directly using the FOIL rule. Thus,

$(3x - 7y)^2 = (3x - 7y)(3x - 7y)$

$\qquad\qquad = (3x)(3x) - (3x)(7y) - (7y)(3x) + (7y)(7y)$

$\qquad\qquad = 9x^2 - 21xy - 21xy + 49y^2$

$\qquad\qquad = 9x^2 - 42xy + 49y^2$

15. **C** Solve the equation $\sqrt{2x - 3} = 7$ for x.

$$\sqrt{2x - 3} = 7$$

Square both sides: $\quad (\sqrt{2x - 3})^2 = 7^2$

Simplify each side: $\quad \sqrt{2x - 3} = 49$

Add 3 both sides: $\qquad\qquad 2x = 52$

Divide both sides by 2: $\qquad x = \dfrac{52}{2} = 26$

16. **D** Solve the equation $\dfrac{3}{5} + \dfrac{7}{x - 4} = 3$ for x.

$$\dfrac{3}{5} + \dfrac{7}{x - 4} = 3$$

Subtract $\dfrac{3}{5}$ from both sides: $\quad \dfrac{7}{x - 4} = 3 - \dfrac{3}{5}$

Simplify the right side: $\quad \dfrac{7}{x - 4} = \dfrac{15}{5} - \dfrac{3}{5}$

$$\dfrac{7}{x - 4} = \dfrac{12}{5}$$

Cross multiply: $\qquad\qquad 7(5) = 12(x - 4)$

Multiply out each side: $\qquad 35 = 12x - 48$

Add 48 to both sides: $\qquad 83 = 12x$

Divide both sides by 12: $\qquad x = \dfrac{83}{12}$

17. **C** Solve the equation $y = \dfrac{5x + 2}{x - 6}$ for x in terms of y.

$$y = \frac{5x + 2}{x - 6}$$

Multiply both sides by $x - 6$:	$(x - 6)y = 5x + 2$
Multiply out the left side:	$xy - 6y = 5x + 2$
Subtract $5x$ from both sides:	$xy - 6y - 5x = 2$
Add $6y$ to each side:	$xy - 5x = 2 + 6y$
Factor out an x from the left side:	$x(y - 5) = 2 + 6y$
Divide both sides by 12:	$x = \dfrac{2 + 6y}{y - 5}$

18. **D** First find the number of ounces in 1 ton. Then, to find the number of ounces in 3 tons, multiply the number of ounces in 1 ton by 3. Since a ton is 2,000 pounds and a pound is 16 ounces, the number of ounces in 1 ton is $2,000 \times 16$, or $32,000$. Since there are 32,000 ounces in one ton, the number of ounces in 3 tons is $32,000 \times 3$, which is 96,000.

19. **B** Notice that this question requires you to find the value of x. So make sure that you indicate the value of x for the answer, not the value of y. Let's try to multiply both sides of the equation $5x - y = 3$ by an appropriate number, so that when we add the corresponding sides of the equation that results (from multiplying both sides of the equation $5x - y = 3$ by an appropriate number) and the equation $2x + 7y = 4$, the y-terms will cancel out. The coefficient of y in the first equation, $5x - y = 3$, is -1, and the coefficient of y in the second equation, $2x + 7y = 4$, is 7. If we multiply both sides of the first equation by 7 and keep the second equation the same, we will get two equations where there is a $-7y$ in one equation and a $7y$ in the other equation. Then if we add the corresponding sides of these two equations, the y-terms will cancel out, since $-7y$ and $7y$ added together equal 0. Then we will be left with an equation with just the variable x, which we can solve for x.

Multiplying both sides of the equation $5x - y = 3$ by 7, we have $7(5x - y) = 7(3)$, and multiplying out each side gives $35x - 7y = 21$.

Now add the corresponding sides of the equations $35x - 7y = 21$ and $2x + 7y = 4$. The y-terms will cancel out.

$$\begin{array}{r} 35x - 7y = 21 \\ +(2x + 7y = 4) \\ \hline 37x \qquad = 25 \end{array}$$

Dividing both sides of the equation $37x = 25$ by 37, we have that $x = \dfrac{25}{37}$.

Incorrect choice (C) is the value of y. Always be careful to answer what the question requires.

20. **C** The y-axis is a vertical line, so a line perpendicular to that will be a horizontal line. A horizontal line has a constant y-value. Therefore choice (C) is correct.

Choice (A) is $x = 0$. Each point on the line with this equation has an x-coordinate of 0. This line is vertical. This line is the y-axis itself. So the line $x = 0$ is certainly not perpendicular to the y-axis.

Choice (B) is $x = 3$. Each point on the line with this equation has an x-coordinate of 3 and this line is vertical. So the line $x = 3$ is parallel to the y-axis, not perpendicular to the y-axis.

Choice (D) is $y = -2x$. This is the equation of a line with a negative slope. This line is not parallel to either axis, and therefore it is not perpendicular to either axis. The y-values of this line decrease with movement from left to right.

21. **B** There are 7 different people that can be chosen first. For each of these 7 people chosen first, there are 6 people that can be chosen second. So there is a total of 7×6, or 42 *ordered* pairs of people that can be chosen. However, the order in which two people are chosen does not matter. Thus, choosing *A* first and then *B* is the same as choosing *B* first and then *A*. So to find the number of different pairs of people that can be chosen, the number of ordered pairs, 42, must be divided by 2. So the number of different pairs of people that can be chosen is $\frac{42}{2}$, or 21, and choice (B) is correct.

22. **C** Use the three-part probability formula: probability $= \frac{(\#\text{desired outcomes})}{(\#\text{ of possible outcomes})}$. Solving this formula for the number of possible outcomes gives # of possible outcomes $= \frac{(\#\text{ of desired outcomes})}{\text{Probability}}$. Given that your probability is $\frac{1}{5}$ and the number of desired outcomes, pulling out a white sock, is 10, plug these in and solve for the number of possible outcomes. # of possible outcomes $= \frac{10}{(\frac{1}{5})} = 50$. If the number of possible outcomes is 50 and the number of desired outcomes is 10, then the number of undesired outcomes, black socks, must be the difference between the two, or 40. So he must add 40 black socks to the suitcase. The answer is (C).

23. **D** Statement (II) is true, because the average rate of change between two points is given by the slope of the secant line between them. Statement (I) is false because the derivative is the *slope* of the tangent line, not the line itself. Statement (III) is true because the slope of the tangent line is the limit of the difference quotient giving the slope of the secant line between point a and a point very close to a (i.e. $a + \Delta x$).

Let's pause here to talk about test strategy. Say that the first thing you do is determine that statement (I) is incorrect, because you've drilled into your brain that the derivative is the slope of the tangent line. The very next thing you should do is cross off answer choices (A) and (C). Even if you have no idea whether statements (II) and (III) are correct, you can guess between the two remaining answer choices, (B) and (D), and you have a 50 percent chance of guessing correctly. Those are pretty good odds for guessing on a test.

24. **D** The factorial of a positive whole number n is defined as:
$n! = (n)(n-1)(n-2)\dots(2)(1)$
Using this definition, we can see that $4! = 4 \cdot 3 \cdot 2 \cdot 1 = 24$.

CHAPTER FIVE

The Importance of Vocabulary

INTRODUCTION

The broader your vocabulary, the better you are likely to do on the PCAT Verbal Ability section. PCAT does not test whether you know exactly what a particular word means. It tests if you have a broad and diverse understanding of vocabulary. Here is a bit of comforting information: if you have only an idea of what a word means, you have as good a chance of correctly answering a question as you would if you knew the precise dictionary definition.

Here is some more good news: one of the most difficult aspects of vocabulary use isn't tested on the exam. You won't have to distinguish between words with very similar meanings or between words that differ only in nuance. For example, you won't have to master the subtle differences between loquacious, verbose, and garrulous. If you see any of those words, you will simply need to know that they have to do with being wordy or talkative. The test format will provide context clues to make your job easier.

This chapter will help you increase your verbal ability by arming you with common strategies for broadening your vocabulary. It will also help you discern the meaning of an unfamiliar word by identifying the word's root.

TECHNIQUES FOR LEARNING VOCABULARY

Develop a game plan

A great vocabulary can't be built overnight. You can't cram all your study into a week and expect to remember much. You'll only remember the words you learn if you take the time to review them. *Repetition and reinforcement* are critical.

Personalize your study methods

Try several techniques and pick the ones that work best for *you*. If you learn well by seeing, make flash cards of new words (or groups of words), and run through them whenever you have a few spare minutes. If you own a cassette player and you learn better by hearing, make a vocabulary tape.

Be strategic

How *well* you use your time between today and the exam can be just as important as how *much* time you spend.

Remember: The aim is word recognition

You won't have to define words on a blank piece of paper, use them in an essay, or spout them in conversation. Practice the strategies you learn in the lessons and labs that allow you to take advantage of the *context clues* inherent in all verbal formats.

Learn words in groups

Related words are far easier to memorize than words chosen at random from a list. Create your own groups: the very act of categorizing words will help you remember their definitions.

Keep building your vocabulary whenever you read

Whether you're reading for school or for pleasure, jot down unfamiliar words and look them up when you get a chance. Keep a list and review it from time to time.

Supplement your vocabulary study by learning word roots

Each day, familiarize yourself with a few more word roots. Make sure to look up any unfamiliar words

Indulge in dictionary "browsing"

When looking up a new word, check to see whether other words on the same page are related. Don't limit yourself to definitions: take advantage of all the information in a word entry, including the etymology, pronunciation, and so on.

Become an omnivorous reader

Read as much as you can. Make a special habit of reading newspaper editorials, syndicated columns, and news magazines: all are good sources of words.

A FEW WORDS THAT ARE EASY TO REMEMBER

You're more likely to remember a word if you can remember something interesting about it (that's why, when you're learning a foreign language, you always remember the dirty words). Here are some words with interesting stories behind them. Look them up in a dictionary.

cavalier

Originally, a cavalier was a horseman, a knight, or an aristocrat. People like that could afford to be proud or careless.

chimerical

A chimera is a mythical beast with the head of a lion, the body of a goat, and the tail of a snake. It also breathes fire. It's not surprising that chimerical would mean "unreal."

juggernaut

The original Juggernaut was an idol representing the Hindu god Krishna. It was drawn on a huge cart through the streets of Puri, India, in an annual festival, and people were sometimes crushed beneath its wheels. (Some European observers thought that people were deliberately throwing themselves under the wheels, but in fact these deaths were accidental.)

maudlin

This word comes from the name of Mary Magdalene, the penitent prostitute in the New Testament. Some paintings of Mary weeping for her sins are very maudlin indeed.

meretricious

Meretrix is the Latin word for prostitute. Enough said.

ostracism

This word sounds a little like **oyster**, and in fact there is a tenuous connection. In ancient Athens, ostracism was temporary banishment, and it was imposed upon a citizen by popular vote. In those days, the Athenians used potsherds, bits of broken pottery, as ballots. And since potsherds often look somewhat like oyster shells, the Greek word for potsherd (*ostrikon*) derives from the Greek word for oyster (*ostreion*), which is also where the English word **oyster** comes from.

laconic, spartan

These words derive from **Laconia** and **Sparta**, which are two different names for the same place: a city-state in Ancient Greece. The Spartans, or Laconians, were famous for their austere way of life and their curt manner of speech.

sybaritic

The citizens of Sybaris, an ancient Greek city, were just the opposite of the Spartans, or Laconians. The Sybarites were famous for their devotion to luxury and pleasure.

choleric, melancholy, phlegmatic, sanguine

These words derive from the same source: ancient medical theory. Up until approximately the 17th century, it was believed that physical and mental health depended upon the proper balance of four "humors" or bodily fluids. Too much bile, or choler, caused irritability; black bile, or melancholy, caused sadness; too much phlegm caused apathy or sluggishness; too much blood caused excessive cheerfulness. Although this theory was exploded centuries ago, the words remain.

serendipity

Serendip is an old name for Sri Lanka. An 18th-century English writer named Horace Walpole wrote an otherwise forgotten story about three princes of Serendip, who had a knack for making valuable discoveries by accident.

Now look up these words in a dictionary (preferably an unabridged one) and note the derivation of each word as well as its meaning:

apocryphal

behemoth

cherubic

cynic

gargantuan

hackneyed

masochist

pariah

posh

quixotic

seraphic

stoic

utopia

KNOW YOUR ROOTS

You can make the task of learning words more manageable by using word roots. Roots have a "multiplier" effect: memorizing one root can help you understand and remember a number of different words.

Suppose you see the word **circumnavigate** on the test, for example, but you don't know its meaning. If you recognize the root CIRCUM, you'll know that the word has something to do with a circle. If you also know the root NAV, meaning "sailing" (as in **navy**), you can guess that the word means "to sail around something," which is basically correct. Typically, it means to sail around the world.

We use the term *root* loosely here to include both prefixes and actual, etymological roots, often based on Greek or Latin words. Whereas prefixes always introduce words (e.g., ANTE- in **antecedent** and NON- in **nonentity**), roots can be found at the beginning, middle, or end of words (e.g., ANIM in **animate** and **unanimous**).

A few words of warning are in order, though. For one thing, breaking a word down into its roots generally produces only an approximate definition, not a precise definition. Often, over the centuries, a word will have acquired a specific meaning that is not reflected in its etymology.

For example, E means "out of," and GREG means "flock," but something egregious is "out of the flock" in a very specific, figurative way that you would not be able to figure out simply by breaking the word down into its roots. Something egregious stands out by being conspicuously bad.

Similarly, A means "not, without," and GNO means "know," but agnostic denotes a very specific kind of not knowing, as you'll see if you look it up in a dictionary.

You need to use a certain amount of caution when using word roots to figure out unfamiliar words, or the results can be misleading. A word may contain a combination of letters that looks like one of the roots on the root list but really means something different.

What does BELL mean in **belligerent**, **bellicose**, and **antebellum**? Does it mean the same thing in **belladonna**?

Think about what DEM means in **democracy**, **demographics**, and **demagogue**. Does it mean the same thing in **demolition**?

Sometimes two distinctly different roots look exactly the same, usually because they derive from different languages. There's no totally reliable way to tell them apart, although if you can partly understand a word through other word roots, context, or anything else, often common sense will do the rest.

In **antacid** and **antiperspirant**, does ANT mean "against" or "before"? How about in **antiquity** and **anticipate**?

In **homicide**, does HOM mean "human being" or "same"? How about in **homogenize**, **homonym**, or **homosexual**?

What approximately does PER mean in each of the following words: **perfidy**, **perimeter**, **permanent**, **perambulate**?

Finally, here's what is probably the most frequent example. In **inanimate**, **invisible**, and **inadvisable**, does IN mean "in" or "not"? How about in **invade**?

Notice that some roots, especially certain short prefixes, change their forms before certain letters. It's **exit**, but **egregious**; **inexorable**, but **impossible**. This is a common linguistic phenomenon; certain sounds change or drop out before certain other sounds to make the words easier to pronounce.

CHAPTER SIX

Mastering Sentence Completion and Analogies

THE FOUR BASIC PRINCIPLES OF SENTENCE COMPLETIONS

Principle 1. Every clue is right in front of you.

Each sentence contains a few crucial clues that determine the answer. For a sentence to be used on the PCAT, the answer must already be in the sentence. Clues *in the sentence* limit the possible answers, and finding these clues will guide you to the correct answer.

For example, could the following sentence be on the PCAT?

The student thought the test was quite _____ .

(A) long
(B) unpleasant
(C) predictable
(D) ridiculous
(E) indelible

No. Because nothing in the sentence hints at which word to choose, it would be a terrible test question.

Now let's change the sentence to get a question that *could* be answered:

Since the student knew the form and content of the questions in advance, the test was quite _____ for her.

(A) long
(B) unpleasant
(C) predictable
(D) ridiculous
(E) indelible

What are the important clues in this question? Well, the word *since* is a great structural clue. It indicates that the missing word follows logically from part of the sentence. Specifically, the missing word must follow from "knew the form and content ... in advance." That means the test was predictable.

Principle 2. Look for what's directly implied and expect clichés.

We're not dealing with poetry here. These sentences aren't excerpted from the works of Toni Morrison or William Faulkner. The correct answer is the one most directly implied by the meanings of the words in the sentence.

Principle 3. Don't imagine strange scenarios.

Read the sentence literally, not imaginatively. Pay attention to the meaning of the words, not associations or feelings that you have.

Principle 4. Look for structural road signs.

Structural road signs are key words that will point you to the right answer, such as *since*. The missing words in Sentence Completions will usually have a relationship similar or opposite to other words in the sentence. Key words, such as *and* or *but*, will tell you which it is.

A semicolon by itself always connects two closely related clauses. If a semicolon is followed by a structural road sign, then that road sign determines the direction. Just like on the highway, there are road signs in each question that tell you to go ahead or to take a detour.

"Straight-ahead" signs are used to make one part of the sentence support or elaborate another part. They continue the sentence in the same direction. The positive or negative charge of what follows is not changed by these clues. Straight-ahead clues include: *and, similarly, in addition, consequently, since, also, thus, because, ; (semicolon),* and *likewise.*

"Detour" signs change the direction of the sentence. They make one part of the sentence contradict or qualify another part. The positive or negative charge of an answer is changed by these clues. Detour signs include: *but, despite, yet, however, unless, rather, although, while, on the other hand, unfortunately,* and *nonetheless.*

In the following examples, test your knowledge of Sentence Completion road signs by choosing the right answers (in the parentheses):

1. The winning argument was _____ *and* persuasive. (cogent, flawed)

2. The winning argument was _____ *but* persuasive. (cogent, flawed)

3. The play's script lacked depth and maturity; *likewise,* the acting was altogether _____. (sublime, amateurish)

4. The populace _____ the introduction of the new taxes, *since* they had voted for them overwhelmingly. (applauded, despised)

5. *Despite* your impressive qualifications, I am _____ to offer you a position with our firm. (unable, willing)

6. Scientists have claimed that the dinosaurs became extinct in a single, dramatic event, *yet* new evidence suggests a _____ decline. (headlong, gradual)

7. The first wave of avant-gardists elicited _____ from the general population, *while* the second was completely ignored. (indifference, shock)

By concentrating on the road signs, it's easier to find your way through each question and arrive at the right answers (1. cogent, 2. flawed, 3. amateurish, 4. applauded, 5. unable, 6. gradual, 7. shock). Now that you understand road signs, let's look at Kaplan's Method for Sentence Completions and try it out on some practice questions.

Kaplan Strategy

Kaplan's basic principles for success on Sentence Completions are:
- Look for clues in the sentence.
- Focus on what's directly implied.
- Pay attention to the meanings of the words.
- Keep an eye out for structural road signs.

Kaplan's Four-Step Method for Sentence Completions

Step 1. Read the sentence, looking for structural road signs and other clues to where the sentence is heading.

Step 2. In your own words, predict the answer.

Step 3. Select the choice that most closely matches your prediction.

Step 4. Read your choice back into the sentence to make sure it fits.

Kaplan's Four-Step Method for Two-blank Sentence Completions

Step 1. Read the sentence, looking for structural road signs and other clues to where the sentence is heading.

Step 2. Decide which blank is easier to predict and make a prediction for that blank.

Step 3. Eliminate choices that don't match your prediction for that blank.

Step 4. Read the remaining choices into your sentence and select the choice that works for both blanks.

THE FOUR BASIC PRINCIPLES OF ANALOGIES

Principle 1: Every analogy consists of two words, called the stem pair, that provide a clue to completing the second pairing.

In each PCAT analogy question, a stem pair of words is separated by a colon. This stem pair is followed by a single word, for which you must determine the appropriate pairing from the designated answer choices, based on the relationship of the stem pair. Following is an example of a PCAT analogy question:

AIRPLANE : HANGAR :: BOAT:

(A) Depot
(B) Sail
(C) Dock
(D) Station

Can you identify a relationship between the stem pair?

Principle 2: There will always be a direct and necessary relationship between the words in the stem pair.

The first step to solving an analogy question is to look for clues in the stem pair. How do the two words that make up the stem pair relate to each other? Are they opposites? Do they depend on each other in some specific way? Is one word specific to the other in some way?

Let's take a look at another example:

BOLOGNA: COLD CUT :: PARFAIT:

(A) Banana
(B) Dessert
(C) Pastrami
(D) Entreé

What is the relationship between BOLOGNA and COLD CUT? BOLOGNA *is a type of* COLD CUT. Likewise, you can apply this relationship to the single word PARFAIT to find the answer: PARFAIT *is a type of* DESSERT. This short sentence that expresses the relationship is called a *bridge*.

Principle 3: Applying the bridge to the incomplete pair can help identify the correct answer.

Here are some keys to building good bridges:
 • Build a sentence that makes the relationship between the two words clear.
 • Make sure the bridge expresses a direct and necessary relationship.
 • Keep the sentence short and to the point.
 • Avoid qualifying phrases such as *could, sometimes, may* or *may not*, etc.

A good bridge should help you predict the word that could plausibly complete the analogy. Build your bridge before looking at the answer choices – this will help you avoid answer traps or trick answers.

Practice building bridges for the following stem pairs:

PLATITUDE : TRITE

AIRPLANE : HANGAR

LUCIDITY : OBSCURITY

LETHARGY : ENERGY

FOAL : HORSE

Take a look at the following answers. Note that there are no qualifying words and that the bridges establish a definitive relationship. Yours may be slightly different but should express the direct and clear relationship between the two words.

PLATITUDE is always TRITE.

AIRPLANES are found within a HANGAR.

LUCIDITY is a lack of OBSCURITY.

LETHARGY is a lack of ENERGY.

FOAL is a young HORSE.

Principle 4: Working backwards can help when all else fails.

What if you can't build a bridge between the stem words? Or you don't know some of the stem words? Or you know you understand one half of the analogy, but you don't know how to complete it?

When the going gets tough, the tough work backwards.

Let's see how this is done.

The first thing to remember when you encounter a hard question is to skip it until you've answered all the questions that don't give you trouble. If you do have the time to go back to it, here are our tips for working backwards:

1. If you can't build a bridge, pay attention to the parts of speech of the stem words. Consider different ways to build a bridge.
2. Look for trap answer choices and eliminate them.
3. Try out the remaining answer choices and see if one of them makes sense.
4. If you're stuck, guess.

Let's take a look at each of these strategies.

Pay Attention to Parts of Speech

If an analogy confuses you, you should take a look at the **parts of speech** in the question—that is, whether the words are **nouns**, **verbs**, **adjectives**, etc. With very few exceptions, parts of speech are always consistent within an analogy. In other words, if the first word of one word pair is an adjective and the second word a noun, then the same is true for the other word pair.

Eliminate Trap Answer Choices

The right answer to an Analogy question will create the same strong bridge as between the stem pair. Wrong answer choices, on the other hand, come in two principal varieties: the first variety is exemplified by a weak bridge; the second by a strong, but wrong, bridge that has no relationship to the stem pair.

Take a look at the example we used earlier:

AIRPLANE : HANGAR :: BOAT

(A) Sail
(B) Station
(C) Dock
(D) Depot

Which answer choices can you eliminate? Without even referring to the stem pair, it is easy to see that there is no plausible bridge connection between BOAT and choices B and D, so these can be eliminated immediately. A strong bridge could be created between BOAT and SAIL, but this would be the wrong bridge. The right answer, choice C, is obvious if you know the relationship between the stem pair. If you don't know the stem pair relationship, then you have increased your chances of guessing correctly by 50% by simply eliminating the two most unlikely answers.

Kaplan's Strategy

Kaplan's basic principles for success on Analogies are:

- There will always be a direct and necessary relationship between the words in the stem pair; the single word will share this relationship with the correct answer choice.
- Practice creating and identifying strong bridges.
- Recognize answer traps to save time and increase your chances of guessing correctly.

Kaplan's Four-Step Method for Analogies

Step 1. Find a strong bridge between the stem words. Be flexible: sometimes it's easier to use the second word first.

Step 2. Plug the answer choices into the bridge. Make sure to keep the same word order that you used with the stem pair.

Step 3. Adjust the bridge as necessary. You want your bridge to be simple and somewhat general, but if more than one answer choice fits into your bridge, it is too general. Make it a little more specific and try the answer choices again.

Step 4. If you are stuck, eliminate all answer choices with weak bridges. If two choices have the same bridge when paired with a single word, eliminate them both; there can only be one correct pairing. Work backwards from the remaining choices to the stem pair and make your best guess.

REVIEW PROBLEMS

Try the following Sentence Completion and Analogy questions using Kaplan's Four-Step Method. They are more difficult than the ones you have encountered up to this point, but you should be able to handle them. Time yourself; you only have about 30 seconds to complete each question.

1. The yearly financial statement of a large corporation may seem _____ at first, but the persistent reader soon finds its pages of facts and figures easy to decipher.

    (A) bewildering

    (B) surprising

    (C) inviting

    (D) misguided

    (E) uncoordinated

2. The giant squid's massive body, adapted for deep-sea life, breaks apart in the reduced pressures of higher ocean elevations, making the search for an intact specimen one of the most _____ quests in all of marine biology.

    (A) controversial

    (B) meaningful

    (C) elusive

    (D) popular

    (E) expensive

3. Organic farming is more labor intensive and thus initially more _____, but its long-term costs may be less than those of conventional farming.

    (A) uncommon

    (B) stylish

    (C) restrained

    (D) expensive

    (E) difficult

4. Unfortunately, there are some among us who equate tolerance with immorality; they feel that the _____ of moral values in a permissive society is not only likely but _____.

    (A) decline … possible

    (B) upsurge … predictable

    (C) disappearance … desirable

    (D) improvement … commendable

    (E) deterioration … inevitable

5. CITIZENSHIP : PASSPORT :: PURCHASE :

    (A) Receipt

    (B) Product

    (C) Ticket

    (D) Visa

6. DRAWL : SPEAK :: LOPE :
   (A) Throw
   (B) Aim
   (C) Run
   (D) Slice

7. INVIDIOUS : OFFEND :: EVANESCENT :
   (A) Shock
   (B) Disappear
   (C) Grow
   (D) Rubbish

8. PANEGYRIC : CRITICAL :: POLEMIC :
   (A) Succinct
   (B) Impartial
   (C) Verbose
   (D) Direct

SOLUTIONS TO REVIEW PROBLEMS

1. **A** If you use the Four-Step Method, you will first look for road signs in the sentence. You should recognize the key word *but*, which indicates that the correct answer will mean the opposite of how the financial statement is described at the conclusion of the sentence, "easy to decipher." In your own words, that opposite may be "difficult to understand." Choice (A), *bewildering*, is your answer. None of the other choices is an opposite of "easy to decipher" and can be eliminated.

2. **B** This is a pretty straightforward Sentence Completion. The key here is the word *intact*, which means that, although specimens have been collected, they have often (if not always) not been intact when recovered. You can fairly assert that recovering an intact specimen is difficult. When you look for a synonym for *difficult* in the answer choices, you should recognize *elusive* (C) as your answer.

3. **D** The key word in this sentence is, again, *but*. You also get a big clue with the phrase "long-term costs" in the second half of the sentence. Your answer, expensive (D), is the only answer that has anything to do with costs.

4. **E** Use the Four-Step Method for Two-Blank Sentence Completions. Your road signs in this one are *unfortunately* in the first half of the sentence and *not only* in the second. *Unfortunately* tells you that the answer will be words containing a negative charge. *Not only* tells us that both words will fit that charge.

5. **A** A passport is a proof of citizenship, and a receipt is a proof of purchase.

6. **C** To drawl is to speak in a slow, drawn-out manner, and to lope is to run in a slow, drawn-out manner.

7. **B** Someone who is invidious is likely to offend; something that is evanescent is likely to disappear.

8. **B** Being critical is the opposite of being panegyric, or praising, and being impartial is the opposite of being polemic, or argumentative.

CHAPTER SEVEN

The Basis of Life

LIFE ACTIVITIES

Animals use energy obtained from the digestion of food to maintain their internal environment and regulate the basic activities of life. The following terms are used to describe the acquisition, conversion, and some of the uses of energy by a living organism:

- **Metabolism**–The sum of all chemical reactions that occur in the body. Metabolism can be divided into **catabolic reactions**, which break down large chemicals and release energy, and **anabolic reactions**, which build up large chemicals and require energy.
- **Ingestion**–The acquisition of food and other raw materials
- **Digestion**–The process of converting food into a usable soluble form so that it can pass through membranes in the digestive tract and enter the body
- **Absorption**–The passage of nutrient molecules through the lining of the digestive tract into the body proper. Absorbed molecules pass through cells lining the digestive tract by diffusion or active transport.
- **Transport**–The circulation of essential compounds required to nourish the tissues and the removal of waste products from the tissues
- **Assimilation**–The building up of new tissues from digested food materials
- **Respiration**–The consumption of oxygen by the body. Cells use oxygen to convert glucose into ATP, a ready source of energy for cellular activities.
- **Excretion**–The removal of waste products (such as carbon dioxide, water, and urea) produced during metabolic processes like respiration and assimilation
- **Synthesis**–The creation of complex molecules from simple ones (anabolism)
- **Regulation**–The control of physiological activities. The body's metabolism functions to maintain its internal environment in a changing external environment. This is known as **homeostasis** and includes regulation by hormones and the nervous system. **Irritability** is the ability to respond to a stimulus and is part of regulation.
- **Growth**–An increase in size caused by a synthesis of new materials
- **Photosynthesis**–The process by which plants convert CO_2 and H_2O into carbohydrates. Sunlight is harnessed by chlorophyll to drive this reaction.
- **Reproduction**–The generation of additional individuals of a species

BIOCHEMISTRY

All living things are composed primarily of the elements carbon, hydrogen, oxygen, nitrogen, sulfur, and phosphorus. Traces of magnesium, iodine, iron, calcium, and other minerals are also components of **protoplasm**, the substance of life.

The unit of an element is the atom. The unit of a compound is the **molecule**. **Atoms** are joined by chemical bonds to form **compounds**. Water (H_2O), carbon dioxide (CO_2), and glucose ($C_6H_{12}O_6$) are some familiar compounds.

The chemical compounds in living matter can be divided into inorganic and organic compounds. **Inorganic compounds** are compounds that do not contain the element carbon, including salts and HCl. **Organic compounds** are made by living systems and contain carbon. They include carbohydrates, lipids, proteins, and nucleic acids.

Carbohydrates

Carbohydrates are composed of the elements carbon, hydrogen, and oxygen in a 1:2:1 ratio, respectively. They are used as storage forms of energy or as structural molecules. For example, glucose and glycogen store energy in animals, whereas starch stores energy in plants. You may be required to recognize the following types of carbohydrates, but you do not need to memorize their structure.

Monosaccharide

Monosaccharides like glucose and fructose are single sugar subunits.

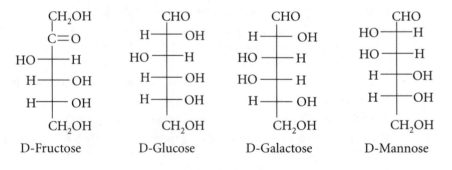

Figure 7.1

Glucose, $C_6H_{12}O_6$, has a hexagonal structure with a six-carbon ring and H and OH bonded to each carbon.

Disaccharide

Disaccharides such as maltose and sucrose are composed of two monosaccharide subunits joined by **dehydration synthesis,** which involves loss of a water molecule.

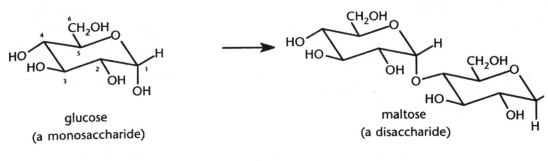

glucose
(a monosaccharide)

maltose
(a disaccharide)

Figure 7.2

Polysaccharide

Polysaccharides are **polymers** or chains of repeating monosaccharide subunits. Glycogen and starch are polysaccharides. Cellulose is a polysaccharide that serves a structural role in plants. These polysaccharides are insoluble in water.

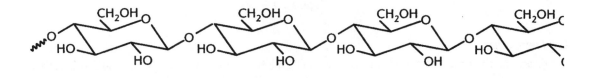

Cellulose, a 1,4´-β-D-Glucose polymer

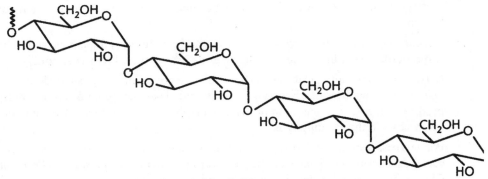

Starch, a 1,4´α -D-Glucose polymer

Figure 7.3

Polysaccharides are formed by removing water (**dehydration**). By adding water, large polymers can be broken down into smaller subunits in a process called **hydrolysis**.

Lipids (Fats and Oils)

Like carbohydrates, lipids are also composed of C, H, and O, but their H:O ratio is much greater than 2:1 because they have much more H than O. A lipid consists of 3 **fatty acid** molecules bonded to a single **glycerol** backbone. Fatty acids have long carbon chains that give them their hydrophobic (fatty) character and carboxylic acid groups that make them acidic. Three dehydration reactions are needed to form one fat molecule. Lipids do not form polymers.

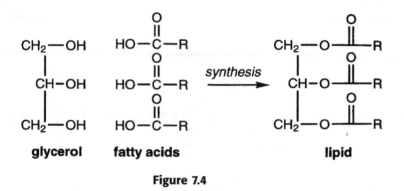

glycerol   **fatty acids**   **lipid**

Figure 7.4

Lipid derivatives

Lipids are the chief means of food storage in animals. They release more energy per gram weight than any other class of biological compounds. They also provide insulation and protection against injury because they are a major component of fatty (**adipose**) tissue. Some lipid derivatives are as follows:

- **Phospholipids** contain glycerol, two fatty acids, a phosphate group, and nitrogen-containing alcohol; e.g., lecithin (a major constituent of cell membranes) and cephalin (found in brain, nerves, and neural tissue).

- **Waxes** are esters of fatty acids and monohydroxylic alcohols. They are found as protective coatings on skin, fur, leaves of higher plants, and on the exoskeleton of many insects; e.g., lanolin.

- **Steroids** have three fused cyclochexane rings and one fused cyclopentane ring. They include **cholesterol**, the **sex hormones** testosterone and estrogen, and **corticosteroids**.

- **Carotenoids** are fatty, acid-like carbon chains containing conjugated double bonds and carrying six-membered carbon rings at each end. These compounds are the **pigments** that produce red, yellow, orange, and brown colors in plants and animals. Two subgroups are the **carotenes** and the **xanthophylls**.

- **Porphyrins**, also called tetrapyrroles, contain four joined **pyrrole** rings. They are often complexed with a metal. For example, the porphyrin **heme** complexes with Fe in hemoglobin. Chlorophyll is complexed with Mg.

Proteins

Proteins are composed primarily of the elements C, H, O, and N but may also contain phosphorus (P) and sulfur (S). They are polymers of **amino acids**.

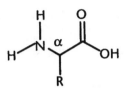

Figure 7.5

Amino acids are joined by **peptide bonds** through dehydration reactions. Chains of such bonds produce a polymer called a **polypeptide**, or simply peptide. This is another term for protein. The sequence of amino acids in a protein is referred to as the 1° (primary) structure. Proteins can also coil or fold to form helices and β-pleated sheets. These are considered part of the protein's 2° (secondary) structure.

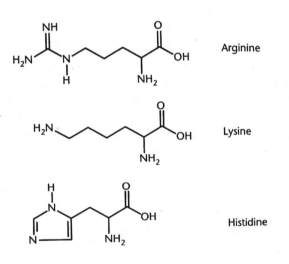

Arginine

Lysine

Histidine

Figure 7.6

Protein structure

- **Primary structure**—Sequence of amino acids
- **Secondary structure**—Based on hydrogen bonding between adjacent amino acids and results in β-pleated sheets or α helices.
- **Tertiary Structure**—Three-dimensional structure that is based on R-group interactions between adjacent amino acids. Results in globular or fibrous proteins. The hydrophobic amino acids are crowded in the center with hydrophilic amino acids at the outer edge and periphery.
- **Quaternary Structure**—The interaction and joining of two or more independent polypeptide chains.

Proteins can be classified on the basis of structure:

- **Simple proteins**—These are composed entirely of amino acids.
- **Albumins and globulins**—These are primarily globular in nature. They are functional proteins that act as carriers or enzymes.
- **Scleroproteins**—These are fibrous in nature and act as structural proteins. Collagen is a scleroprotein.
- **Conjugated proteins**—These contain a simple protein portion plus at least one nonprotein fraction.
- **Lipoproteins**—Proteins bound to **lipid**
- **Mucoproteins**—Proteins bound to **carbohydrate**
- **Chromoproteins**—Proteins bound to pigmented molecules
- **Metalloproteins**—Proteins complexed around a **metal ion**
- **Nucleoproteins**—Proteins containing histone or protamine (nuclear protein) bound to **nucleic acids**

Protein function

- **Hormones**—These are proteins that function as chemical messengers secreted into the circulation. Insulin and ACTH are protein hormones.
- **Enzymes**—These are biological catalysts that act by increasing the rate of chemical reactions important for biological functions (e.g., amylase, lipase, and ATPase).
- **Structural proteins**—These contribute to the physical support of a cell or tissue. They may be extracellular (e.g., collagen in cartilage, bone, and tendons) or intracellular (e.g., proteins in cell membranes).
- **Transport proteins**—These are carriers of important materials. For example, hemoglobin carries oxygen in the circulation, and the cytochromes carry electrons during cellular respiration.
- **Antibodies**—These bind to foreign particles (antigens), including disease-causing organisms, that have entered the body.

Enzymes

Enzymes are organic catalysts. A catalyst is any substance that affects the rate of a chemical reaction without itself being changed. Enzymes are crucial to living things because all living systems must have **continuous-controlled** chemical activity. Enzymes regulate metabolism by speeding up or slowing down certain chemical reactions. They affect the reaction rate by decreasing the activation energy.

Enzymes are **proteins**, and thus, thousands of different enzymes can conceivably be formed. Many enzymes are conjugated proteins and have a nonprotein **coenzyme**. In these cases, both components must be present for the enzyme to function.

Enzymes are very selective; they may catalyze only one reaction or one specific class of closely related reactions. The molecule upon which an enzyme acts is called the **substrate**. There is an area on each enzyme to which the substrate binds called the **active site**. The two models that follow describe the binding of the enzyme to the substrate.

1. Enzymes do NOT alter the equilibrium constant.
2. Enzymes are NOT consumed in the reaction. This means that they will appear in both the reactants and the products.
3. Enzymes are pH and temperature sensitive, with optimal activity at specific pH ranges and temperatures.

Lock and key theory

This theory holds that the spatial structure of an enzyme's active site is exactly complementary to the spatial structure of its substrate. The two fit together like a lock and key. In other words, receptors are large proteins that contain a recognition site (lock) that is directly linked to transduction systems. When a drug or endogenous substance (key) binds to the receptor, a sequence of events is started. Although this theory has been largely discounted, it is still frequently used as a teaching tool in Pharmacy schools when explaining drug interactions with receptors and enzymes.

Induced fit theory

This more widely accepted theory describes the active site as having flexibility of shape. When the appropriate substrate comes in contact with the active site, the conformation of the active site changes to fit the substrate.

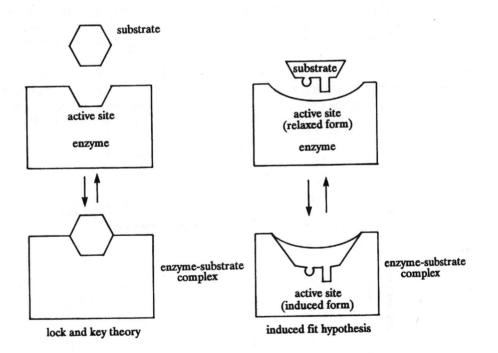

Figure 7.7

Most enzyme reactions are reversible. The product synthesized by an enzyme can be decomposed by the same enzyme. An enzyme that synthesizes maltose from glucose can also hydrolyze maltose back to glucose.

Enzyme action and the reaction rate depend on several environmental factors including temperature, pH, and the concentration of enzyme and substrate.

In general, as the temperature increases, the rate of enzyme action increases, until an optimum temperature is reached (usually around 40°C). Beyond optimal temperature, heat alters the shape of the active site of the enzyme molecule and deactivates it, leading to a rapid drop in rate.

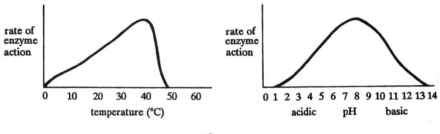

Figure 7.8

For each enzyme there is an optimal pH; above and below that, enzymatic activity declines. Maximal activity of many human enzymes occurs around pH 7.2, which is the pH of most body fluids. Exceptions include **pepsin**, which works best in the highly acidic conditions of the stomach (pH = 2), and pancreatic enzymes, which work optimally in the alkaline conditions of the small intestine (pH = 8.5). In most cases, the optimal pH matches the conditions under which the enzyme operates.

The concentrations of substrate and enzyme greatly affect the reaction rate. When the concentrations of both enzyme and substrate are low, many of the active sites on the enzyme are unoccupied, and the reaction rate is low. Increasing the substrate concentration will increase the reaction rate until all of the active sites are occupied. After this point, further increase in substrate concentration will not increase the reaction rate.

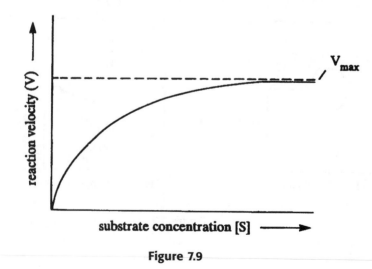

Figure 7.9

Competitive inhibition

The active site of an enzyme is specific for a particular substrate or class of substrates. However, it is possible for molecules that are similar to the substrate to bind to the active site of the enzyme. If a similar molecule is present in a concentration comparable to the concentration of the substrate, it will compete with the substrate for bonding sites on the enzyme and interfere with enzyme activity. This is known as competitive inhibition because the enzyme is inhibited by the inactive substrate, or competitor.

Noncompetitive inhibition

A noncompetitive inhibitor is a substance that forms strong covalent bonds with an enzyme and consequently may not be displaced by the addition of excess substrate. Therefore, noncompetitive inhibition is irreversible. A noncompetitive inhibitor may be bonded at, near, or remote from the active site. When the inhibition takes place at a site other then the active site, this is called **allosteric inhibition**. (*Allosteric* means "other site" or "other structure.") The interaction of an inhibitor at an allosteric site changes the structure of the enzyme so that the active site is also changed.

Examples of enzyme activity

Every reaction in the body is regulated by enzymes. Some of the basic reaction types are listed below.

Hydrolysis reactions function to digest large molecules into smaller components. **Lactase** hydrolyzes lactose to the monosaccharides glucose and galactose. **Proteases** degrade proteins to amino acids, and **lipases** break down lipids to fatty acids and glycerol.

In multicellular organisms, digestion can begin outside of the cells in the gut. Other hydrolytic reactions occur within cells.

Synthesis reactions (including dehydrations) can be catalyzed by the same enzymes as hydrolysis reactions, but the directions of the reactions are reversed.

These reactions occur in different parts of the cell. For example, protein synthesis occurs in the ribosomes and involves dehydration synthesis between amino acids.

Synthesis is required for growth, repair, regulation, protection, and production of food reserves such as fat and glycogen by the cell. The survival of an organism depends on its ability to ingest substances that it needs but cannot synthesize. Once ingested, these substances are converted into useful products.

Certain vitamin cofactors and essential amino acids cannot be synthesized by humans. If they are not available in the diet, deficiency diseases will occur.

Many enzymes require the incorporation of a nonprotein molecule to become active. These molecules, called **cofactors**, can be metal cations such as Zn^{2+} or Fe^{2+} or small organic groups called coenzymes. Most coenzymes cannot be synthesized by the body and are obtained from the diet as vitamin derivatives. Cofactors that bind to the enzyme by strong covalent bonds are called **prosthetic groups**.

CELL BIOLOGY

The cell is the fundamental unit of all living things. Every function in biology involves a process that occurs within cells or at the interface between cells. Therefore, to understand biology, you need to appreciate the structure and function of different parts of the cell.

Cell Theory

The cell was not discovered or studied in detail until the development of the microscope in the 17th century. Since then, much more has been learned, and a unifying theory known as the Cell Theory has been proposed.

The Cell Theory may be summarized as follows:
- All living things are composed of cells.
- The cell is the basic functional unit of life.
- The chemical reactions of life take place inside the cell.
- Cells arise only from pre-existing cells.
- Cells carry genetic information in the form of **DNA**. This genetic material is passed from parent cell to daughter cell.

Cell Structure

The components of the cell are specialized in their structure and function. These organelles include the nucleus, ribosomes, endoplasmic reticulum, golgi apparatus, vesicles, vacuoles, lysosomes, mitochondria, chloroplasts, and centrioles.

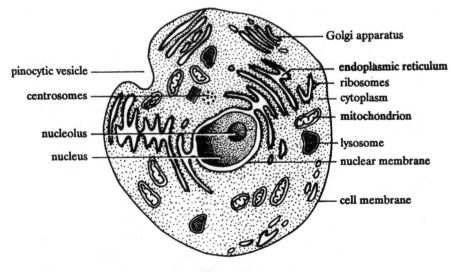

Figure 7.10

There are millions of species of "living things" that can be divided into five kingdoms: monerans, protists, fungi, plants, and animals. Within these five kingdoms are two major types of cells: prokaryotes and eukaryotes. The word *prokaryote* means "before nucleus," and prokaryotic cells lack a nucleus.

Cell Membrane

The cell membrane (plasma membrane) encloses the cell and exhibits selective permeability; it regulates the passage of materials into and out of the cell. According to the generally accepted **fluid mosaic model**, the cell membrane consists of a phospholipid bilayer with proteins embedded throughout. The lipids and many of the proteins can move freely within the membrane.

The phospholipid bilayer has a specific structure that forms spontaneously. Phospholipid molecules are arranged such the long, nonpolar, hydrophobic, "fatty" chains of carbon and hydrogen face each other, with the phosphorus-containing, polar, hydrophilic heads facing outward. The hydrophobic heads face the watery regions inside and outside the cell, while the hydrophobic tails face each other in a water-free region.

As a result of its lipid bilayer structure, a plasma membrane is readily permeable to both small, nonpolar hydrophobic molecules, such as oxygen, and small polar molecules, such as water. Small charged particles are usually able to cross the membrane through protein channels. However, charged ions and larger charged molecules cross the membrane with the assistance of **carrier proteins**.

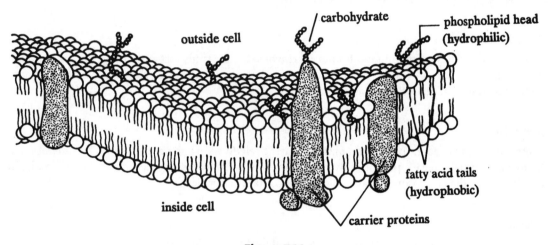

Figure 7.11

Nucleus

The nucleus controls the activities of the cell, including cell division. It is surrounded by a nuclear membrane. The nucleus contains the DNA, which is complexed with structural proteins called **histones** to form **chromosomes**. The **nucleolus** is a dense structure in the nucleus where **ribosomal RNA** (rRNA) synthesis occurs.

Ribosome

Ribosomes are the sites of protein production and are synthesized by the nucleolus. Free ribosomes are found in the cytoplasm, whereas bound ribosomes line the outer membrane of the endoplasmic reticulum.

Endoplasmic Reticulum

The endoplasmic reticulum (ER) is a network of membrane-enclosed spaces involved in the transport of materials throughout the cell, particularly those materials destined to be secreted by the cell.

Golgi Apparatus

The Golgi apparatus receives vesicles and their contents from the smooth ER, modifies them (e.g, glycosylation), repackages them into vesicles, and distributes them to the cell surface by exocytosis.

Mitochondria

Mitochondria are the sites of aerobic respiration within the cell and hence the suppliers of energy. Each mitochondria is bounded by an outer and inner phospholipid bilayer.

Cytoplasm

Most of the cell's metabolic activity occurs in the cytoplasm. Transport within the cytoplasm occurs by **cyclosis** (streaming movement within the cell).

Vacuole/Vesicle

Vacuoles and vesicles are membrane-bound sacs involved in the transport and storage of materials that are ingested, secreted, processed, or digested by the cell. Vacuoles are larger than vesicles and are more likely to be found in plant than in animal cells.

Centrioles

Centrioles are involved in spindle organization during cell division and are not bound by a membrane. Animal cells usually have a pair of centrioles that are oriented at right angles to each other and lie in a region called the centrosome. Plant cells do not contain centrioles.

Lysosome

Lysosomes are membrane-bound vesicles that contain **hydrolytic enzymes** involved in intracellular digestion. Lysosomes break down material ingested by the cell. An injured or dying tissue may "commit suicide" by rupturing the lysosome membrane and releasing its hydrolytic enzymes; this process is called **autolysis**.

Cytoskeleton

The cytoskeleton supports the cell, maintains its shape, and functions in cell motility. It is composed of microtubules, microfilaments, and intermediate filaments.

Microtubules are hollow rods made up of polymerized **tubulin** that radiate throughout the cell and provide it with support. Microtubules provide a framework for organelle movement within the cell. Centrioles, which direct the separation of chromosomes during cell division, are composed of microtubules. **Cilia** and **flagella** are specialized arrangements of microtubules that extend from certain cells and are involved in cell motility and cytoplasmic movement.

Microfilaments are solid rods of **actin**, which are important in cell movement as well as support. Muscle contraction, for example, is based on the interaction of actin with myosin. Microfilaments move materials across the plasma membrane, for instance, in the contraction phase of cell division and in amoeboid movement.

Plant Cells

Plant cells differ from the animal cells described above in the following ways:

- No centrosome
- Presence of cell wall composed of cellulose
- Chloroplasts in many cells of green plants are sites of synthesis of organic compounds
- No lysosomes
- Many vacuoles/mature plant cells usually contain one large vacuole

TRANSPORT ACROSS THE CELL MEMBRANE

Substances can move into and out of cells in various ways. Some methods occur passively, without energy, whereas others are active and require energy expenditure (adenosine triphosphate).

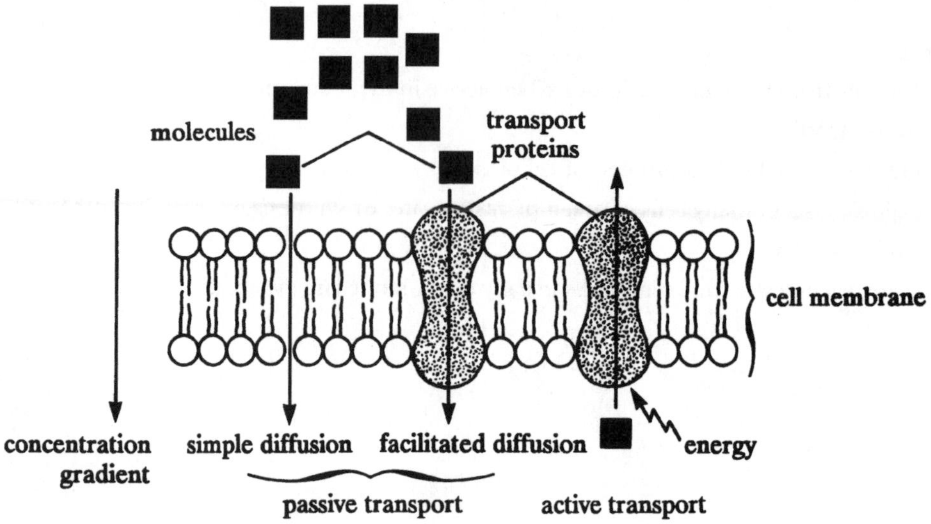

Figure 7.12

Simple Diffusion

Simple diffusion is the net movement of dissolved particles down their concentration gradients—from a region of higher concentration to a region of lower concentration. This is a passive process that requires no external source of energy.

Osmosis

Osmosis is the simple diffusion of water from a region of lower solute concentration to a region of higher solute concentration. When the cytoplasm of a cell has a lower solute concentration than the extracellular medium, the medium is said to be **hypertonic** to the cell, and water will flow out of the cell. This process, also called **plasmolysis**, will cause the cell to shrivel.

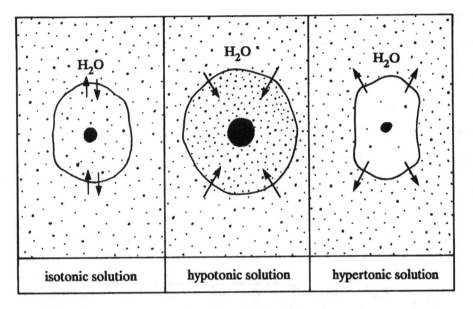

| isotonic solution | hypotonic solution | hypertonic solution |

Figure 7.13

If the extracellular environment is less concentrated than the cytoplasm of the cell, the extracellular medium is said to be **hypotonic**, and water will flow into the cell causing it to swell and **lyse** (burst). For example, red blood cells will burst if placed in distilled water. Fresh water protozoa have contractile vacuoles to pump out excess water and prevent bursting.

Facilitated Diffusion

Facilitated diffusion (passive transport) is the net movement of dissolved particles down their concentration gradient through special channels or carrier proteins in the cell membrane. This process, like simple diffusion, does not require energy.

Active Transport

Active transport is the net movement of dissolved particles against their concentration gradient with the help of transport proteins. Unlike diffusion, active transport requires energy. These carrier molecules aid in the regulation of the cell's internal content of ions and large molecules. The passage of specific ions and molecules is facilitated by these carrier molecules, such as:

- **Energy independent carriers**—facilitate the movement of compounds along a concentration gradient
- **Symporters**—move two or more ions or molecules
- **Antiporters**—exchange one or more ions (or molecules) for another ion or molecule
- **Pumps**—energy-dependent carriers (require ATP); e.g., sodium potassium pump

Endocytosis

Endocytosis is a process in which the cell membrane invaginates, forming a vesicle that contains extracellular medium (see Figure 7.14). **Pinocytosis** is the ingestion of fluids or small particles, and **phagocytosis** is the engulfing of large particles. Particles may bind to receptors on the cell membrane before being engulfed.

Exocytosis

In exocytosis, a vesicle within the cell fuses with the cell membrane and releases its contents to the outside. Fusion of the vesicle with the cell membrane can play an important role in cell growth and intercellular signalling (see Figure 7.14). Note that in both endocytosis and exocytosis, the material never actually crosses through the cell membrane.

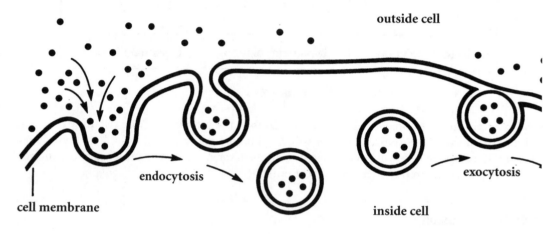

Figure 7.14 Endocytosis and Exocytosis

CIRCULATION

Circulation is the transportation of material within cells and throughout the body of a multicellular organism.

Intracellular Circulation

Materials move about within a cell in a number of ways. Some examples include:

- **Brownian movement**–kinetic energy spreads small suspended particles throughout the cytoplasm of the cell.
- **Cyclosis or streaming**–the circular motion of cytoplasm around the cell transports molecules.
- **Endoplasmic reticulum**–this provides channels throughout the cytoplasm and provides a direct continuous passageway from the plasma membrane to the nuclear membrane.

Extracellular Circulation

A number of systems have been devised to deal with the movement of materials on a larger scale through the body of an organism. Examples include:

Diffusion

If cells are in direct or close contact with the external environment, **diffusion** can serve as a sufficient means of transport for food and oxygen from the environment to the cells. In larger, more complex animals, diffusion is important for the transport of materials between cells and the interstitial fluid that bathes the cells.

Circulatory system

Complex animals, whose cells are too far from the external environment to transport materials by diffusion, require a circulatory system. It generally includes vessels to transport fluid and a pump to drive the circulation.

REVIEW PROBLEMS

1. All of the following are components of the Cell Theory EXCEPT

    (A) all living things are composed of cells.

    (B) all living things contain mitochondria.

    (C) cooperation among cells allows for complex functioning in living things.

    (D) all cells arise from pre-existing cells.

2. A eukaryotic cell contains organelles specialized for various activities. Name the organelles involved and the role they play in the following activities.

    (A) Ingestion

    (B) Digestion

    (C) Transport of proteins

3. Which of the following activities occurs in the Golgi apparatus?

    (A) Synthesis of proteins

    (B) Breakdown of lipids and carbohydrates

    (C) Catalysis of various oxidative reactions

    (D) Modification and packaging of proteins

    (E) Photosynthesis

4. Draw the fluid mosaic model of the cell membrane. How does this model account for the passage of materials across the membrane?

5. Prokaryotes and eukaryotes differ in a number of ways. Compare them in terms of the following characteristics.

    (A) Organization of genetic material

    (B) Site of cellular respiration

    (C) Presence of membrane-bound organelles

6. A researcher treats a solution containing animal cells with ouabain, a substance that interferes with the Na^+/K^+ pump embedded in the cell membrane, and causes the cell to lyse. Which of the following statements best explains ouabain's mechanism of action?

    (A) Treatment with ouabain results in high levels of extracellular Ca^{2+}.

    (B) Treatment with ouabain results in high levels of extracellular K^+ and Na^+.

    (C) Treatment with ouabain increases intracellular concentrations of Na^+.

    (D) Treatment with ouabain decreases intracellular concentrations of Na^+.

7. Prokaryotic cells and eukaryotic animal cells both have
   (A) DNA.
   (B) ribosomes.
   (C) a cell wall.
   (D) A and B.

8. What is the significance of the lysosomal membrane?

9. Describe the kinetic effects of increasing substrate concentration while enzyme concentration remains constant.

10. What determines enzyme specificity?

SOLUTIONS TO REVIEW PROBLEMS

1. **B** Discussed in cell theory section.

2. **A** Cellular ingestion is a function of the cell membrane and vesicles. The cell membrane invaginates around a food particle and pinches off, enclosing the material in a vesicle that can travel freely in the cytoplasm. This is known as endocytosis.

   B The organelles involved in digestion are lysosomes, vesicles, and mitochondria. A lysosome is a membrane-bound sac containing hydrolytic enzymes. It fuses with a vesicle, allowing its enzymes to chemically degrade the ingested material. The products of lysosomal digestion are released into the cytoplasm where they can be used by the cell. Glucose is metabolized in mitochondria via aerobic respiration.

   C The endoplasmic reticulum forms a long, interconnecting series of passageways through which proteins are transported. Smooth ER secretes proteins into cytoplasmic vesicles that are transported to the Golgi apparatus. Microtubules are involved in the transport of proteins in some specialized cells such as neurons.

3. **D** Discussed in cell biology section.

4.   According to the fluid mosaic model in Figure 7.11, the individual molecules of the lipid bilayer are in constant motion within the plane of the membrane. This fluidity allows ions and small molecules to diffuse directly across the cell membrane. However, large molecules cannot cross the membrane without the aid of special carrier protein molecules, which are embedded within the phospholipid bilayer. Some substances cannot cross the membrane at all. This selective permeability allows the cell membrane to control tightly the passage of materials into and out of the cell.

5. **A** In prokaryotes, the genetic material is composed of a single circular molecule of DNA localized in a region of the cell called the nucleoid. Eukaryotes have highly coiled linear strands of DNA organized into chromosomes within a membrane-bound nucleus.

   B In prokaryotes, cellular respiration occurs directly at the cell membrane, whereas in eukaryotes, cellular respiration occurs across the mitochondrial membrane and within the mitochondria itself.

   C Prokaryotes do not contain any membrane-bound organelles, whereas eukaryotes contain a number of membrane-bound organelles, such as the nucleus, lysosomes, vesicles, ER, and mitochondria.

6. **C** This question requires an understanding of osmosis and the action of Na/K (adenosine triphosphatase). When a cell is placed in a hypertonic solution (a solution having a higher solute concentration than the cell), fluid will diffuse out the cell into the solution, resulting in cell shrinkage. When a cell is placed in a hypotonic solution (a solution having a lower solute concentration than the cell), fluid will diffuse from the solution into the cell, causing the cell to expand and possibly lyse. The Na/K ATPase moves three sodium ions out for every two potassium ions it lets into the cell. Therefore, inhibition of the Na/K ATPase by ouabain will cause a net increase in the Na^+ concentration inside the cell, and water will diffuse in down its concentration gradient, causing the cell to swell and then lyse.

7. **D** Discussed in cell biology section.

8. The lysosomal membrane serves an important function. It protects the cell from the hydrolytic actions of the enzymes it contains. If the membrane were to burst, these enzymes would digest cellular components and ultimately kill the cell.

9. When substrate concentration is low, the reaction proceeds slowly. Initial increases in substrate concentration greatly increase the reaction rate because of the binding of substrate to available active sites. Eventually, a point is reached at which all of the active sites are occupied, and the addition of more substrate will not hasten the reaction appreciably. Eventually, at very high levels of substrate, the reaction rate approaches a maximum, V_{max}.

10. Enzyme specificity is determined by the unique 3D spatial structure of the active site. According to the induced fit hypothesis, an enzyme's active site is capable of undergoing a conformational change when the appropriate substrate comes into contact with it, such that the substrate is held in place to form an enzyme-substrate complex.

CHAPTER EIGHT

Reproduction

CELL DIVISION

Cell division is the process by which a cell doubles its organelles and cytoplasm, replicates its DNA, and then divides in two. For **unicellular organisms**, cell division is a means of reproduction, whereas for **multicellular organisms**, it is a method of growth, development, and replacement of worn-out cells. Cell division can follow two different courses, mitosis and meiosis.

Mitosis

Mitosis is the division and distribution of the cell's DNA to its two daughter cells such that each cell receives a complete copy of the original genome. Nuclear division (**karyokinesis**) is followed by cell division (**cytokinesis**). Before the initiation of mitosis, the cell undergoes a period of growth and replication of genetic material called interphase.

Interphase

A cell normally spends at least 90 percent of its life in interphase. During this period, each chromosome is replicated so that during division, a complete copy of the genome can be distributed to both daughter cells. After replication, the chromosomes consist of two identical **sister chromatids** held together at a central region called the **centromere**. During interphase, the individual chromosomes are not visible. The DNA is uncoiled and is called **chromatin**.

In summary, the growth period for the eukaryotic cell is interphase. There are four total parts to interphase, with the last part being mitosis. The four parts are as follows:

1. **G1**–Initiates interphase. Is described as the active growth phase and can vary in length. The cell increases in size and synthesizes proteins. The length of the G1 phase determines the length of the entire cell cycle.
2. **S**–The period of DNA synthesis
3. **G2**–The cell prepares to divide. It grows and synthesizes proteins.
4. **M**–Cell division occurs (mitosis), resulting in two identical daughter cells.

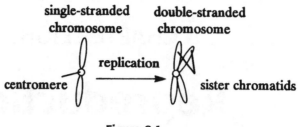

Figure 8.1

Prophase

During prophase, the chromosomes condense, and the centriole pairs (in animals) separate and move towards the opposite poles of the cell. The spindle apparatus forms between them, and the nuclear membrane dissolves, allowing the spindle fibers to interact with the chromosomes.

Metaphase

The centriole pairs are now at opposite poles of the cell. The fibers of the spindle apparatus attach to each chromatid at the centromere to align the chromosomes at the center of the cell (equator), forming the **metaphase plate**.

Anaphase

The centromeres split so that each chromatid has its own distinct centromere, thus allowing sister chromatids to separate. The sister chromatids are pulled toward the opposite poles of the cell by the shortening of the spindle fibers. Spindle fibers are composed of microtubules.

Telophase

The spindle apparatus disappears. A nuclear membrane forms around each set of newly formed chromosomes. Thus, each nucleus contains the same number of chromosomes (the diploid number, 2n) as the original or parent nucleus. The chromosomes uncoil, resuming their interphase form.

Cytokinesis

Near the end of telophase, the cytoplasm divides into two daughter cells, each with a complete nucleus and its own set of organelles. In animal cells, a **cleavage furrow** forms, and the cell membrane indents along the equator of the cell and finally pinches through the cell, separating the two nuclei.

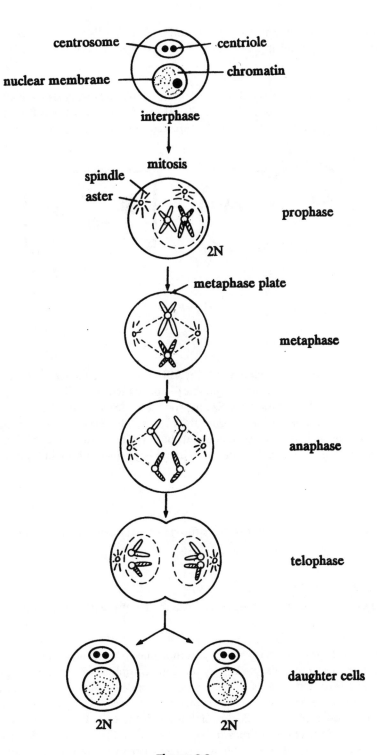

Figure 8.2

Plant cells

There are two major differences between cell division in animal cells and plant cells. One is that plant cells lack centrioles. The spindle apparatus is synthesized by microtubule organizing centers that are not visible.

Also, cytokinesis in animal cells proceeds through production of a cleavage furrow. Plant cells are rigid and cannot form a cleavage furrow. They divide by the formation of a **cell plate**, an expanding partition that grows outward from the interior of the cell until it reaches the cell membrane.

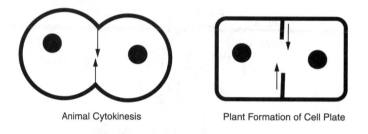

Animal Cytokinesis   Plant Formation of Cell Plate

Figure 8.3

Meiosis

Sexual reproduction differs from asexual reproduction in that there are two parents involved. Sexual reproduction occurs via the fusion of two gametes—specialized sex cells produced by each parent. **Meiosis** is the process by which these sex cells are produced. Meiosis is similar to mitosis in that a cell duplicates its chromosomes before undergoing the process. However, whereas mitosis preserves the diploid number of the cell, meiosis produces the **haploid** (1N) number, halving the number of chromosomes. Meiosis involves two divisions of **primary sex cells** resulting in four haploid cells called **gametes**.

Interphase

As in mitosis, the parent cell's chromosomes are replicated during interphase, resulting in the 2N number of sister chromatids.

First meiotic division

The first division produces two intermediate daughter cells with N chromosomes with sister chromatids.

Prophase I—The chromatin condenses into chromosomes, the spindle apparatus forms, and the nucleoli and nuclear membrane disappear. Homologous chromosomes (chromosomes that code for the same traits, one inherited from each parent) come together and intertwine in a process called **synapsis**. Since at this stage, each chromosome consists of two sister chromatids, each synaptic pair of homologous chromosomes contains four chromatids and is therefore often called a **tetrad**. Sometimes chromatids of homologous chromosomes break at corresponding points and exchange equivalent pieces of DNA; this process is called crossing over. Note that crossing over occurs between homologous chromosomes and not between sister chromatids of the same chromosomes (the latter are identical, so crossing over would not produce any genetic variation). The chromatids involved are left with an altered but complete set of genes. Recombination among chromosomes results in increased genetic diversity within a species. Note that sister chromatids are no longer identical after recombination has occurred.

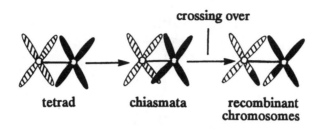

Figure 8.4

Metaphase I—Homologous pairs (tetrads) align at the equatorial plane, and each pair attaches to a separate spindle fiber by its kinetochore.

Anaphase I—The homologous pairs separate and are pulled to opposite poles of the cell. This process is called **disjunction**, and it accounts for a fundamental Mendelian law. During disjunction, each chromosome of paternal origin separates (or disjoins) from its homologue of maternal origin, and either chromosome can end up in either daughter cell. Thus, the distribution of homologous chromosomes to the two intermediate daughter cells is random with respect to parental origin. Each daughter cell will have a unique pool of genes from a random mixture of maternal and paternal origin.

Telophase I—A nuclear membrane forms around each new nucleus. At this point, each chromosome still consists of sister chromatids joined at the centromere.

Second meiotic division

This second division is very similar to mitosis, except that meiosis II is not preceded by chromosomal replication. The chromosomes align at the equator, separate and move to opposite poles, and are surrounded by a reformed nuclear membrane. The new cells have the haploid number of chromosomes. Note that in women, only one of these daughter cells becomes a functional gamete.

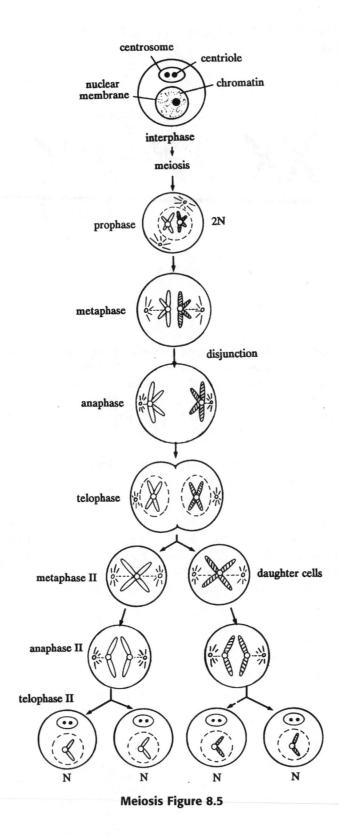

Meiosis Figure 8.5

ASEXUAL REPRODUCTIVE MECHANISMS

Asexual reproduction is the production of offspring without **fertilization**. New organisms are formed by division of a single parent cell. Offspring are essentially genetic carbon copies of their parent cells. Thus, except for random mutations, the offspring are genetically identical to the parent cells. The different types of asexual reproduction are fission, budding, regeneration, and parthenogenesis. Prokaryotes reproduce asexually. Among animals, asexual reproduction is more prevalent in invertebrates than vertebrates. All **plants**, simple and complex, use asexual reproduction in some form.

Fission

Binary fission is a simple form of asexual reproduction seen in prokaryotic organisms. The DNA replicates, and a new plasma membrane and cell wall grow inward along the midline of the cell, dividing it into two equally sized cells with equal amounts of cytoplasm, each containing a duplicate of the parent chromosome. A very similar process occurs in some primitive eukaryotic cells. Fission occurs in one-celled organisms such as amoebae, paramecia, algae, and bacteria. In summary, in binary fission, each of the daughter cells must receive an identical set of genetic information.

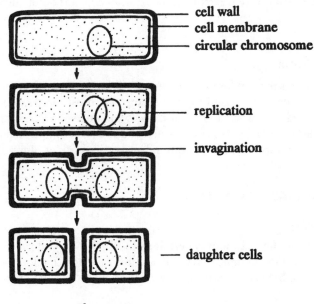

Figure 8.6

Budding

Budding is the replication of the nucleus followed by unequal cytokinesis. The cell membrane pinches inward to form a new cell that is smaller in size but genetically identical to the parent cell. The new cell subsequently grows to adult size. The new cell may separate immediately from the parent, or it may remain attached to it, develop as an outgrowth, and separate at a later stage. Budding occurs in hydra and yeast.

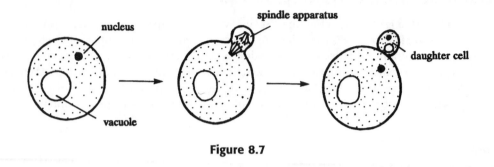

Figure 8.7

Regeneration

Regeneration is the regrowth of a lost or injured body part. Replacement of cells occurs by mitosis. Some lower animals such as hydra and starfish have extensive regenerative capabilities. If a starfish loses an arm, it can regenerate a new one; the severed arm may even be able to regenerate an entire body, as long as the arm contains a piece of an area called the central disk. Salamanders and tadpoles can generate new limbs (the extent of regeneration depends on the nerve damage to the severed body part).

Parthenogenesis

Parthenogenesis is the development of an unfertilized egg into an adult organism. This process occurs naturally in certain lower organisms. For example, in most species of bees and ants, the males develop from unfertilized eggs, whereas the worker bees and queen bees develop from fertilized eggs. Artificial parthenogenesis can be performed in some animals. For example, the eggs of rabbit and frogs can be stimulated to develop without fertilization by electric shock or pinprick.

Asexual Reproduction in Plants

Spore formation

All plants exhibit **alternation of generations** in which a diploid generation is succeeded by a haploid generation. The diploid **sporophyte** generation produces haploid spores, which develop into the haploid **gametophyte** generation. Spores are specialized cells with hard coverings that prevent loss of water.

Vegetative propagation

Undifferentiated tissues in plants, called **meristems**, provide a source of cells that can develop into an adult plant. Vegetative propagation can occur naturally or through human intervention. Propagation is advantageous because it introduces no genetic variation and is a rapid form of reproduction.

Natural vegetative propagation—Vegetative propagation can occur as a natural means of plant reproduction:

- **Bulbs** split to form several bulbs. This occurs in tulips and daffodils.
- **Tubers** are underground stems with buds, like the eyes of potatoes, that can develop into adult plants.

- **Runners** are stems running above and along the ground, extending from the main stem. Runners can produce new roots and upright stems as they do in strawberry and lawn grasses.
- **Rhizomes** (stolons) are woody, underground stems. They can develop new upright stems as they do in ferns and iris plants.

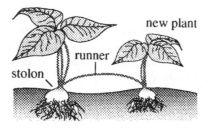

Figure 8.8

Artificial Vegetative Propagation—Humans may use vegetative propagation in agriculture:

- A **cut** piece of stem can develop new roots in water or moist ground. This can be used to grow geranium and willow. Synthetic plant hormones called **auxins** can be used to accelerate root formation.
- Stems of certain plants, like blackberry and raspberry, will take root when bent to the ground and covered with soil. This process is called **layering**.
- The stem of one plant, called the **scion**, can be attached to the rooted stem of another closely related plant called the **stock**. The **cambium** tissue of both stems must be in contact.

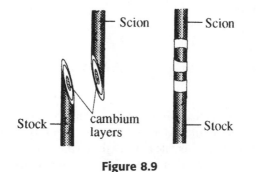

Figure 8.9

SEXUAL REPRODUCTIVE MECHANISMS

Sexual reproduction differs from asexual reproduction in that there are two parents involved and the end result is a genetically unique offspring. Sexual reproduction occurs via the fusion of two gametes—specialized sex cells produced by each parent. Sexual reproduction requires the following:

- The production of **functional sex cells** or **gametes** by adult organisms
- The union of these cells (**fertilization** or **conjugation**) to form a zygote
- The development of the zygote into another adult, completing the cycle

Sexual Reproduction in Animals

Sexual reproduction in animals is a complex process involving the formation and fertilization of gametes and regulation of these processes by both parents.

Gonads

The gametes are produced in specialized organs called the **gonads**. The male gonads, called **testes**, produce sperm in the tightly coiled seminiferous tubules. The female gonads, called **ovaries**, produce **oocytes** (eggs). Some species are **hermaphrodites**, which have both functional male and female gonads. These include the hydra and the earthworm.

Spermatogenesis

Spermatogenesis, or sperm production, occurs in the seminiferous tubules. Diploid cells called spermatogonia undergo meiosis to produce four haploid sperm of equal size. The mature sperm is an elongated cell with a head, tail, neck, and body. The **head** consists almost entirely of the nucleus, which contains the paternal genome. The tail (**flagellum**) propels the sperm, whereas mitochondria in the neck and body provide energy for locomotion.

Oogenesis

Oogenesis, the production of female gametes, occurs in the ovaries. One diploid primary female sex cell undergoes meiosis in the ovaries to produce a **single mature egg**. Each meiotic division produces a **polar body**, a small cell that contains little more than the nucleus. The mature ovum is a large cell containing most of the cytoplasm, RNA, organelles, and nutrients needed by a developing embryo. The polar bodies rapidly degenerate.

Fertilization

Fertilization is the union of the egg and sperm nuclei to form a zygote with a diploid number of chromosomes.

External fertilization—External fertilization occurs in vertebrates that reproduce in water (fish and amphibians). The female lays eggs in the water, and the male deposits sperm in the vicinity. The lack of direct passage of sperm from male to female reduces the chances of fertilization considerably. Many eggs must be laid to ensure some fertilization success. The sperm have flagella, enabling them to swim through the water to the eggs.

Internal fertilization—Internal fertilization is practiced by terrestrial vertebrates and provides a direct route for sperm to reach the egg cell. This increases the chance for fertilization success, and females produce fewer eggs. The number of eggs produced is affected by other factors as well. If the early development of the offspring occurs outside of the mother's body, more eggs will be laid to increase the chances of offspring survival. The amount of parental care after birth is also related to the number of eggs produced. Species that care for their young produce fewer eggs.

Human Reproduction

Male reproductive physiology

The **testes** are located in an external pouch called the **scrotum** that maintains the testes' temperature at 2°C–4°C lower than body temperature, a condition essential for sperm survival. Sperm pass from the testes through the **vas deferens** to the **ejaculatory duct** and then to the **urethra**. The urethra passes through the penis and opens to the outside at its tip. In males, the urethra is a common passageway for both the reproductive and excretory systems. The testes are also the sites of production of testosterone. **Testosterone** regulates secondary male sex characteristics including facial and pubic hair and voice changes.

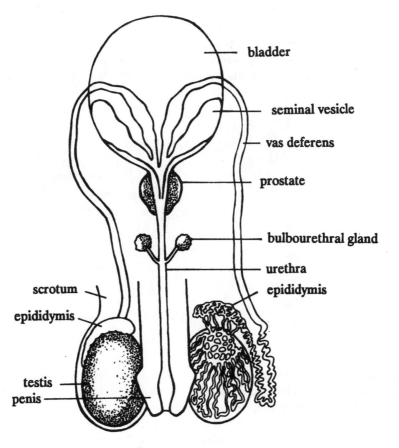

Figure 8.10

Spermatogenesis

Spermatogenesis, or sperm production, occurs in the seminiferous tubules. Diploid cells called **spermatogonia** differentiate into diploid cells called **primary spermatocytes**, which undergo the first meiotic division to yield two haploid **secondary spermatocytes** of equal size; the second meiotic division produces four haploid **spermatids** of equal size. After meiosis, the spermatids undergo a series of changes leading to the production of mature sperm, or **spermatozoa**, which are specialized for transporting the sperm nucleus to the egg, or **ovum**. The mature sperm is an elongated cell with a head, neck, body, and tail. The head consists almost entirely of the nucleus. The tail (flagellum) propels the sperm, while mitochondria in the neck and body provide energy for locomotion. A caplike structure called the **acrosome**, derived from the Golgi apparatus, develops over the anterior half of the head. The acrosome contains enzymes needed to penetrate the tough outer covering of the ovum. After a male has reached sexual maturity, approximately 3 million primary spermatocytes begin to undergo spermatogenesis per day, the maturation process taking a total of 65–75 days.

Female reproductive anatomy

The **ovaries** are found in the abdominal cavity, below the digestive system. The ovaries consist of thousands of follicles; a **follicle** is a multilayered sac of cells that contains, nourishes, and protects an immature ovum. It is actually the follicle cells that produce estrogen. Once a month, an immature ovum is released from the ovary into the abdominal cavity and drawn into the nearby **oviduct**. The oviducts are also known as ovanan or fallopian tubes. Each fallopian tube opens into the upper end of a muscular chamber called the **uterus**, which is the site of fetal development. The lower, narrow end of the uterus is called the **cervix**. The cervix connects with the vaginal canal, which is the site of sperm deposition during intercourse and is also the passageway through which a baby is expelled during childbirth. At birth, all the eggs that a female will ovulate during her lifetime are already present in the ovaries.

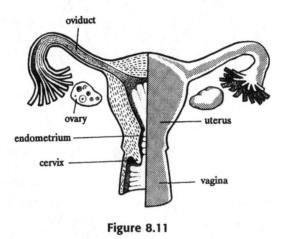

Figure 8.11

Oogenesis

Oogenesis, which is the production of female gametes, occurs in the ovarian follicles. At birth, all of the immature ova, known as **primary oocytes,** that a female will produce during her lifetime are already in her ovaries. Primary oocytes are diploid cells that form by mitosis in the ovary. After menarche (the first time a female gets her period), one primary oocyte per month completes meiosis I, yielding two daughter cells of unequal size—a **secondary oocyte** and a small cell known as a **polar body**. The secondary oocyte is expelled from the follicle during ovulation. Meiosis II does not occur until fertilization. The oocyte cell membrane is surrounded by two layers of cells; the inner layer is the **zona pellucida**, and the outer layer is the **corona radiata**. Meiosis II is triggered when these layers are penetrated by a sperm cell, yielding two haploid cells—a mature ovum and another polar body. (The first polar body may also undergo meiosis II; eventually, the polar bodies die.) The mature ovum is a large cell containing a lot of cytoplasm, RNA, organelles, and nutrients needed by a developing embryo.

Female sex hormones

The ovaries synthesize and secrete the female sex hormones including estrogens and progesterone. The secretion of both estrogens and progesterone is regulated by LH and FSH, which, in turn, are regulated by GnRH.

Estrogens—Estrogens are steroid hormones necessary for normal female maturation. They stimulate the development of the female reproductive tract and contribute to the development of secondary sexual characteristics and sex drive. Estrogens are also responsible for the thickening of the endometrium (uterine wall). Estrogens are secreted by the ovarian follicles and the corpus luteum.

Progesterone—Progesterone is a steroid hormone secreted by the corpus luteum during the luteal phase of the menstrual cycle. Progesterone stimulates the development and maintenance of the endometrial walls in preparation for implantation.

The menstrual cycle

The hormonal secretions of the ovaries, the hypothalamus, and the anterior pituitary play important roles in the female reproductive cycle. From puberty through menopause, interactions between these hormones result in a monthly cyclical pattern known as the menstrual cycle. The menstrual cycle may be divided into the follicular phase, ovulation, the luteal phase, and menstruation.

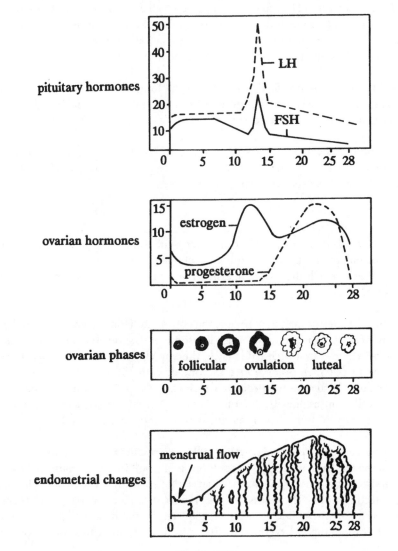

Figure 8.12

Follicular phase—The follicular phase begins with the cessation of the menstrual flow from the previous cycle. During this phase, **FSH** (Follicle Stimulating Hormone) from the anterior pituitary promotes the development of the follicle, which grows and begins secreting estrogen.

Ovulation—Midway through the cycle, ovulation occurs—a mature ovarian follicle bursts and releases an ovum. Ovulation is caused by a surge in **LH** (Luteinizing Hormone) that is preceded, and in part caused, by a peak in estrogen levels.

Women ovulate approximately once every four weeks (except during pregnancy and, usually, lactation) until menopause, which typically occurs between the ages of 45 and 50. During menopause, the ovaries become less sensitive to the hormones that stimulate follicle development (FSH and LH), and eventually they atrophy. The remaining follicles disappear, estrogen and progesterone levels greatly decline, and ovulation stops. The profound changes in hormone levels are often accompanied by physiological and psychological changes that persist until a new balance is reached.

Luteal phase—After ovulation, LH induces the ruptured follicle to develop into the **corpus luteum**, which secretes estrogen and progesterone. **Progesterone** causes the glands of the endometrium to mature and produce secretions that prepare it for the implantation of an embryo. Progesterone and estrogen are essential for the maintenance of the endometrium.

Menstruation—If the ovum is not fertilized, the corpus luteum atrophies. The resulting drop in progesterone and estrogen levels causes the endometrium (with its superficial blood vessels) to slough off, giving rise to the menstrual flow (**menses**).

If fertilization occurs, the developing placenta produces **hCG** (human Chorionic Gonadotrophin), maintaining the corpus luteum and, thus, the supply of estrogen and progesterone that maintains the uterus, until the placenta takes over production of these hormones.

Fertilization

An egg can be fertilized during the 12–24 hours after ovulation. Fertilization occurs in the lateral, widest portion of the fallopian tube. Sperm must travel through the vaginal canal, cervix, uterus, and into the fallopian tubes to reach the ovum. Sperm remain viable and capable of fertilization for 1–2 days after intercourse.

The first barrier that the sperm must penetrate is the corona radiata. Enzymes secreted by the sperm aid in penetration of the corona radiata. The acrosome is responsible for penetrating the zona pellucida; it releases enzymes that digest this layer, thereby allowing the sperm to come into direct contact with the ovum cell membrane. Once in contact with the membrane, the sperm forms a tubelike structure called the **acrosomal process,** which extends to the cell membrane and penetrates it, fusing the sperm cell membrane with that of the ovum. The sperm nucleus now enters the ovum's cytoplasm. It is at this stage of fertilization that the ovum completes meiosis II.

The acrosomal reaction triggers a **cortical reaction** in the ovum, causing calcium ions to be released into the cytoplasm; this, in turn, initiates a series of reactions that result in the formation of the **fertilization membrane.** The fertilization membrane is a hard layer that surrounds the ovum cell membrane and prevents multiple fertilizations. The release of $Ca2+$ also stimulates metabolic changes within the ovum, greatly increasing its metabolic rate. This is followed by the fusion of the sperm nucleus with the ovum nucleus to form a diploid zygote. The first mitotic division of the zygote soon follows.

Multiple births

Monozygotic (identical) twins—Monozygotic twins result when a single zygote splits into two embryos. If the splitting occurs at the two-cell stage of development, the embryos will have separate chorions and separate placentas; if it occurs at the blastula stage, then the embryos will have only one chorionic sac and will therefore share a placenta and possibly an amnion. Occasionally the division is incomplete, resulting in the birth of "Siamese" twins, which are attached at some point on the body, often sharing limbs or organs. Monozygotic twins are genetically identical because they develop from the same zygote. Monozygotic twins are therefore of the same sex, blood type, and so on.

Dizygotic (fraternal) twins—Dizygotic twins result when two ova are released in one ovarian cycle and are fertilized by two different sperm. The two embryos implant in the uterine wall individually, and each develops its own placenta, amnion, and chorion (although the placentas may fuse if the embryos implant very close to each other). Fraternal twins share no more characteristics than any other siblings because they develop from two distinct zygotes.

Sexual Reproduction in Plants

The life cycles of plants are characterized by an alternation of the diploid **sporophyte** generation and the haploid gametophyte generation. The relative lengths of the two stages vary with the plant type. In general, the evolutionary trend has been towards increased dominance of the sporophyte generation.

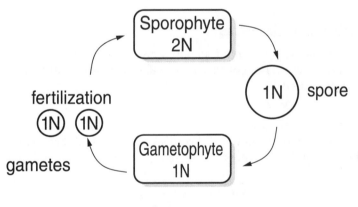

Figure 8.13

Gametophyte generation

The haploid gametophyte generation produces **gametes** by mitosis. Union of the male and female gametes at fertilization restores the diploid sporophyte generation. Thus, the gametophytes reproduce sexually, whereas the sporophyte generation reproduces asexually.

Mosses—In mosses, the gametophyte is the dominant generation. The sporophyte is a smaller, short-lived organism that depends on the gametophyte for energy and nutrients. The sporophytes grow on top of the gametophytes and produce spores that develop into gametophytes.

Sporophyte generation

The diploid sporophyte generation produces a haploid (monoploid) **spore** by meiosis. The spores divide by mitosis to produce the haploid, or gametophyte, generation.

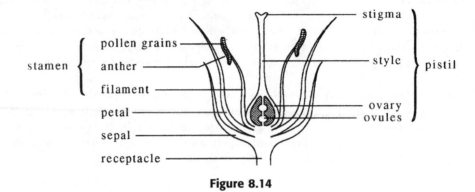

Figure 8.14

Ferns—In ferns, the **sporophyte** generation is the dominant, familiar form. The sporophyte releases spores from the undersides of its leaves that develop into small heart-shaped gametophytes.

Angiosperms—Flowering plants or angiosperms have gametophytes consisting of a few cells that exist for a very short time. The woody plant that is seen (maple, rose, etc.) is the sporophyte stage.

Sexual Reproduction in Angiosperms

The **flower** is the reproductive structure of angiosperms. Some species of plants have flowers that contain only stamens (male plants) and other flowers that contain only pistils (female plants). Flowers have the following distinct parts:

Stamen

The stamen is the male organ of the flower and consists of a thin, stalk-like **filament** with a terminal sac called the **anther**. The anther produces monoploid spores that develop into pollen grains.

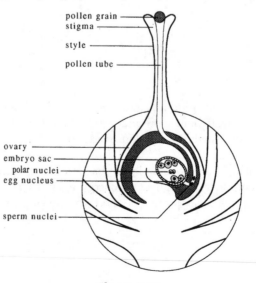

Figure 8.15

Seed formation

The zygote divides mitotically to form the cells of the mass of cells called the embryo. The embryo consists of the following parts:

- **Epicotyl**–This is the precursor of the upper stem and leaves.
- **Cotyledons**–These are the seed leaves. Dicots have two seed leaves, whereas monocots have only one.
- **Hypocotyl**–This develops into the lower stem and root.
- **Endosperm**–The endosperm grows and feeds the embryo. In dicots, the cotyledon absorbs the endosperm.
- **Seed coat**–Develops from the outer covering of the ovule. The embryo and its seed coat together comprise the seed.

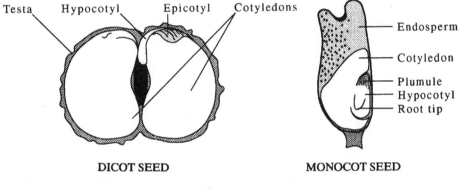

Figure 8.16

Seed Dispersal

The fruit, in which most seeds develop, is formed from the ovary walls, the base of the flower, and other consolidated flower pistil components. The fruit may be fleshy like a tomato or dry like a nut. It serves as a means of seed dispersal. The fruit enables the seed to be carried more frequently or effectively by air, water, or animals (ingestion and subsequent elimination). The seed is released from the ovary and will germinate under proper conditions of temperature, moisture, and oxygen.

Plant Development

Growth in higher plants is restricted to the embryonic (undifferentiated) cells called **meristem** cells. These tissues undergo active cell reproduction. Gradually, the cells elongate and differentiate into cell types characteristic of the species.

Apical meristem

The apical meristem is found in the tips of roots and stems. Growth in length occurs only at these points.

Lateral meristem

The lateral meristem or **cambium** is located between the xylem and phloem. This tissue permits growth in diameter and can differentiate into new xylem and phloem cells. It is not an active tissue in monocots (grasses) or herbaceous dicots (alfalfa) but is predominant in woody dicots like oaks.

REVIEW PROBLEMS

1. What roles do microtubules and microfilaments play in cell division?

2. If the haploid number of an organism is 13, what is its diploid number?

3. What distinguishes binary fission from budding?

4. Fill in the blanks with the name of the appropriate stage of mitosis.

    (A) During _____, the chromosomes separate and move to opposite poles of the cell.
    (B) The nuclear membrane begins to dissolve during _____.
    (C) The centromeres of the replicated chromosomes have completely split by _____.
    (D) During _____, nucleoli disappear.
    (E) Chromosomes condense, shorten, and coil during _____.
    (F) Centromeres line up at the equatorial plate during _____.
    (G) During _____, a cleavage furrow is formed.

5. Upon ovulation, the oocyte is released into the

    (A) fallopian tube.
    (B) ovary.
    (C) follicle.
    (D) abdominal cavity.
    (E) uterus.

6. Describe three ways in which sexual reproduction promotes genetic variability. How does genetic variability benefit a species?

7. How do metaphase and anaphase of mitosis differ from metaphase I and anaphase I of meiosis?

8. The chromosome number of offspring produced via parthenogenesis is

    (A) diploid.
    (B) haploid.
    (C) 2N.
    (D) both A and C.

9. Name two ways in which mitosis in plant cells differs from mitosis in animal cells.

10. Which of the following is true about the alternation of generations in plants?

    (A) The haploid gametophyte generation reproduces sexually.
    (B) The diploid gametophyte generation reproduces asexually.
    (C) The diploid sporophyte generation reproduces sexually.
    (D) The haploid sporophyte generation reproduces sexually.

SOLUTIONS TO REVIEW PROBLEMS

1. Microtubules and microfilaments play important roles in cell division. Microtubules form the mitotic spindle, which is responsible for separating sister chromatids. During prophase, a radial array of microtubules forms around the centrioles. The microtubules "push" the centrioles to opposite poles of the cell, forming the bipolar spindle apparatus. When the chromosomes align at the metaphase plate, these spindle fibers attach to the centromeres. During anaphase, the fibers shorten and pull on the centromeres, separating the sister chromatids and moving them towards opposite poles of the cell.

   After anaphase, microfilaments (actin filaments) and myosin filaments under the cell membrane contract, leading to the indentation of the membrane at the metaphase plate and the subsequent division of the parent cell into two daughter cells.

2. Gametes are produced by meiosis, a process in which the chromosome number of the parent cell is reduced by one half. Thus, if the haploid number (N) of a particular organism is 13, then the diploid number (2N) must be 26.

3. Although both are forms of asexual reproduction, binary fission results in the formation of two equally sized cells, whereas budding results in the formation of two asymmetric cells because of unequal division of cytoplasm (cytokinesis) after mitosis. Binary fission occurs in bacteria and blue-green algae, whereas budding is characteristic of hydra and yeast.

4. **A** anaphase

   B prophase

   C anaphase

   D prophase

   E prophase

   F metaphase

   G telophase

5. **D** This subtle point about ovulation eludes most people and remains hard to believe until the organs are examined in anatomy class in medical school. The ruptured ovarian follicle releases an oocyte into the abdominal cavity, close to the entrance of the fallopian tube. With the aid of beating cilia, the oocyte is drawn into the fallopian tube, through which it travels until it reaches the uterus. If it is fertilized (in the fallopian tube), it will implant in the uterine wall; if it is not fertilized, it will be expelled along with the uterine lining during menstruation.

6. Sexual reproduction promotes genetic variability through the independent assortment of homologous chromosomes, the crossing over between homologous chromosomes during meiosis, and the random fertilization of a sperm and an egg.

   The independent assortment of chromosomes during gametogenesis allows for tremendous genetic variability by creating numerous possible combinations of chromosomes in a given gamete. During metaphase I, homologous chromosomes pair and randomly align at the metaphase plate. The random positioning of the homologous pairs determines which chromosomes are pulled toward each pole of the cell during anaphase. Thus, each resultant daughter cell has a random assortment of chromosomes, some of maternal origin and some of paternal origin.

In addition to independent assortment, a random exchange of genes between chromosomes can occur via recombination. This allows for greater genetic variability by creating new combinations of genes on each chromosome. Recombination occurs during prophase I of meiosis, when homologous pairs of chromosomes align themselves side by side and exchange genetic information in a process called crossing over .

Genetic variability is further enhanced by fertilization. An egg cell containing one of the millions of possible gene combinations fuses with a sperm cell containing another of the millions of possible combinations of different genes to create a zygote with a unique assortment of maternal and paternal genes.

Genetic variability benefits a species because it increases the chances that the offspring will be able to adapt to a myriad of potential environmental stresses and conditions.

7. In metaphase of mitosis, replicated chromosomes line up in single file; during anaphase, sister chromatids separate and move to opposite poles of the cell. In metaphase I of meiosis, homologous pairs of replicated chromosomes line up; during anaphase I, the homologous chromosomes separate, but sister chromatids remain attached.

8. **B** Discussed in section on parthenogenesis under asexual reproduction.

9. Plant cells lack centrioles. During cell division, plant cells form a cell plate, whereas animal cells divide by cytokinesis.

10. **A** The sporophyte generation is the dominant generation in angiosperms, flowering plants. It is diploid and produces haploid spores by meiosis, thus reproducing asexually. The spores develop into the haploid gametophyte generation, which reproduces sexually. Gametophytes produce gametes that join through fertilization to give the diploid sporophyte.

CHAPTER NINE

Genetics

Genetics is the study of how traits are inherited from one generation to the next. The basic unit of heredity is the **gene**. Genes are composed of DNA and are located on **chromosomes**. When a gene exists in more than one form, the alternative forms are called **alleles**. The genetic makeup of an individual is the individual's **genotype**; the physical manifestation of the genetic makeup is the individual's **phenotype**. Some phenotypes correspond to a single genotype, whereas other phenotypes correspond to several different genotypes. Knowledge of genetics will help reveal the concepts of evolution by the process of natural selection.

MENDELIAN GENETICS

In the 1860s, Gregor Mendel developed the basic principles of genetics through his experiments with the **garden pea**. Mendel studied the inheritance of individual pea traits by performing genetic **crosses**: he took true-breeding individuals (which, if self-crossed, produce progeny only with the parental phenotype) with different traits, mated them, and statistically analyzed the inheritance of the traits in the progeny.

Mendel's First Law: Law of Segregation

Mendel postulated four principles of inheritance:

1. Genes exist in alternative forms (now referred to as **alleles**). A gene controls a specific trait in an organism.

2. An organism has **two alleles** for each inherited trait, one inherited from each parent.

3. The two alleles **segregate** during meiosis, resulting in gametes that carry only one allele for any given inherited trait.

4. If two alleles in an individual organism are different, only one will be fully expressed, and the other will be silent. The expressed allele is said to be **dominant**, the silent allele, **recessive**. In genetics problems, dominant alleles are typically assigned capital letters, and recessive alleles are assigned lowercase letters. Organisms that contain two copies of the same allele are **homozygous** for that trait; organisms that carry two different alleles are **heterozygous**. The dominant allele is expressed in the phenotype. This is known as **Mendel's Law of Dominance**. In the cross shown on the next page, Yy will appear as yellow as YY.

Genes	Genotype	Phenotype
YY	Homozygous	Yellow
Yy	Heterozygous	Yellow
yy	Homozygous	Green

Monohybrid cross

The principles of Mendelian inheritance can be illustrated in a cross between two true-breeding pea plants, one with purple flowers and the other with white flowers. Because only one trait is being studied in this particular mating, it is referred to as a **monohybrid cross**. The individuals being crossed are the **Parental** or **P generation**; the progeny generations are the **Filial** or **F generations**, with each generation numbered sequentially (e.g., F1, F2, etc.).

The purple flower parent has the genotype PP (i.e., it has two P alleles) and is homozygous dominant. The white flower parent has the genotype pp and is homozygous recessive. When these individuals are crossed, they produce F1 plants that are 100 percent heterozygous (genotype = Pp). Because purple is dominant to white, all the F1 progeny have the purple flower phenotype.

Punnett square

One way of predicting the genotypes expected from a cross is by drawing a **Punnett square diagram**. The parental genotypes are arranged around a grid. Because the genotype of each progeny will be the sum of the alleles donated by the parental gametes, their genotypes can be determined by looking at the intersections on the grid. A Punnett square indicates all the potential progeny genotypes, and the relative frequencies of the different genotypes and phenotypes can be easily calculated.

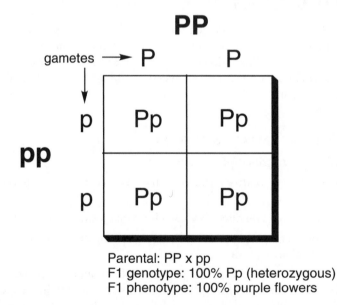

Parental: PP x pp
F1 genotype: 100% Pp (heterozygous)
F1 phenotype: 100% purple flowers

Figure 9.1

When the F1 generation from our monohybrid cross is self-crossed (i.e., Pp × Pp), the F2 progeny are more genotypically and phenotypically diverse than their parents. Because the F1 plants are heterozygous, they will donate a P allele to half of their descendants and a p allele to the other half. One-fourth of the F2 plants will have the genotype PP, 50 percent will have the genotype Pp, and 25 percent will have the genotype pp. Because the homozygous dominant and heterozygous genotypes both produce the dominant phenotype purple flowers, 75 percent of the F2 plants will have purple flowers, and 25 percent will have white flowers.

This is a standard pattern of Mendelian inheritance. Its hallmarks are the disappearance of the silent (recessive) phenotype in the F1 generation and its subsequent reappearance in 25 percent of the individuals in the F2 generation. If we were to take a closer look at the physical characteristics of the plants themselves, we would find that the 1:2:1 genotypic ratio produces a 3:1 phenotypic ratio.

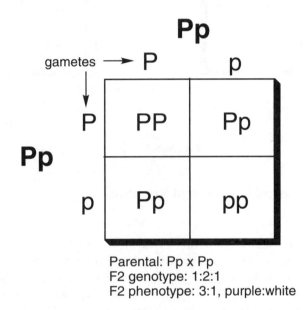

Parental: Pp x Pp
F2 genotype: 1:2:1
F2 phenotype: 3:1, purple:white

Figure 9.2

Testcross

Mendel also developed the testcross, which is a diagnostic tool to determine the genotype of an organism. Only with a recessive phenotype can genotype be predicted with 100 percent accuracy. If the dominant phenotype is expressed, the genotype can be either homozygous dominant or heterozygous. Thus, homozygous recessive organisms always breed true. This fact can be used to determine the unknown genotype of an organism with a dominant phenotype. In a procedure known as a testcross, or **backcross**, an organism with a dominant phenotype of unknown genotype (Ax) is crossed with a phenotypically recessive organism (genotype aa). Since the recessive parent is homozygous, it can donate only the recessive allele, a, to the progeny. If the dominant parent's genotype is AA, all of its gametes will carry an A, and all of the progeny will have genotype Aa. If the dominant parent's genotype is Aa, half of the progeny will be Aa and express the dominant phenotype, and half will be aa and express the recessive phenotype. In a testcross, the appearance of the recessive phenotype in the progeny indicates that the phenotypically dominant parent is genotypically heterozygous.

Testcross: aa x A?

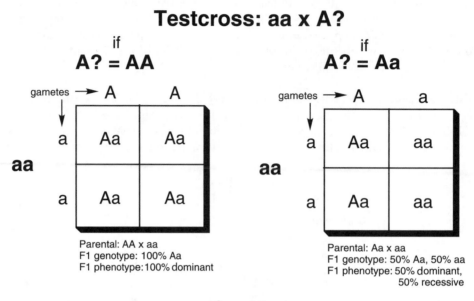

Figure 9.3

Mendel's Second Law: Law of Independent Assortment

Dihybrid cross

The segregation principle provides a satisfactory explanation for the inheritance of a single gene; however, if one wants to follow more than one gene pair, the dihybrid cross, also developed by Mendel, can be used. The principles of the monohybrid cross can be extended to a dihybrid cross in which the parents differ in **two traits**, as long as the genes are on separate chromosomes and assort independently during meiosis. Genes on the same chromosome will stay together unless **crossing over** occurs. Crossing over exchanges information between chromosomes and may break the linkage of certain patterns. For example, red hair is usually linked with freckles, but some blondes and brunettes have freckles as well.

This is known as **Mendel's Law of Independent Assortment**.

In the following example, a purple-flowered tall pea plant is crossed with a white-flowered dwarf pea plant; both plants are doubly homozygous (tall is dominant to dwarf, T = tall allele, t = dwarf allele; purple is dominant to white, P = purple allele, p = white allele). The purple parent's genotype is TTPP, and it thus produces only TP gametes; the white parent's genotype is ttpp and produces only tp gametes. The F1 progeny will all have the genotype TtPp and will be phenotypically dominant for both traits.

When the F1 generation is self-crossed (TtPp × TtPp), it produces four different phenotypes: tall purple, tall white, dwarf purple, and dwarf white, in the ratio 9:3:3:1, respectively. This is the typical pattern for Mendelian inheritance in a dihybrid cross between heterozygotes with independently assorting traits.

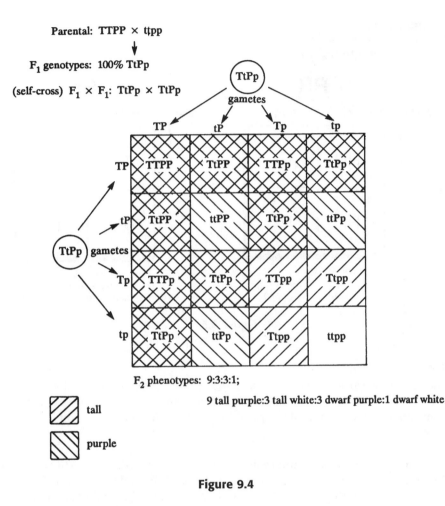

Figure 9.4

Non-Mendelian Inheritance Patterns

In real life, inheritance patterns are often more complicated than Mendel would have hoped. One major source of complications is in the relationship between **phenotype** and **genotype**. In theory, 100 percent of individuals with the recessive phenotype have a homozygous recessive genotype, and 100 percent of individuals with the dominant phenotype have either homozygous or heterozygous genotypes. Such clean concordance between genotype and phenotype is not always the case.

Incomplete dominance

Some progeny phenotypes are apparently **blends** of the parental phenotypes. The classic example is flower color in snapdragons: homozygous dominant red snapdragons, when crossed with homozygous recessive white snapdragons, produce 100 percent pink progeny in the F1 generation. When F1 progeny are self-crossed, they produce red, pink, and white progeny in the ratio of 1:2:1, respectively. The pink color is the result of the combined effects of the red and white genes in heterozygotes. An allele is incompletely dominant if the phenotype of the heterozygote is an intermediate of the phenotypes of the homozygotes.

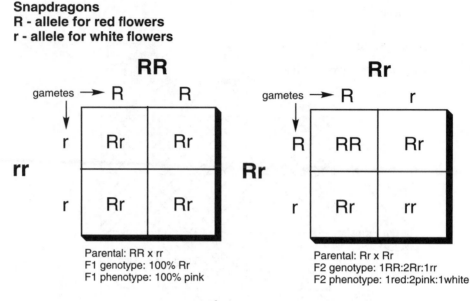

Snapdragons
R - allele for red flowers
r - allele for white flowers

Figure 9.5

Codominance

Codominance occurs when **multiple** alleles exist for a given gene and more than one of them is **dominant**. Each dominant allele is fully dominant when combined with a recessive allele, but when two dominant alleles are present, the phenotype is the result of the expression of both dominant alleles simultaneously.

The classic example of codominance and multiple alleles is the inheritance of **ABO blood groups** in humans. Blood type is determined by three different alleles: I^A, I^B, and i. Only two alleles are present in any single individual, but the population contains all three alleles. I^A and I^B are both dominant to i. Individuals who are homozygous I^A or heterozygous I^Ai have blood type A; individuals who are homozygous I^B or heterozygous I^Bi have blood type B; and individuals who are homozygous ii have blood type O. However, I^A and I^B are codominant; individuals who are heterozygous $I^A I^B$ have a distinct blood type, AB, which combines characteristics of both the A and B blood groups.

Sex Determination

The two members of each of the chromosome pairs are identical in shape except for one pair: the sex chromosomes. As you all know, different species vary in their systems of sex determination. In sexually differentiated species, most chromosomes exist as pairs of homologues called **autosomes**, but sex is determined by a pair of sex chromosomes. All humans have 22 pairs of autosomes; additionally, women have a pair of homologous X chromosomes, and men have a pair of heterologous chromosomes, an X and a Y chromosome. The sex chromosomes pair during meiosis and segregate during the first meiotic division. Since females can produce only gametes containing the X chromosome, the gender of a zygote is determined by the genetic contribution of the male gamete. If the sperm carries a Y chromosome, the zygote will be male; if it carries an X chromosome, the zygote will be female. For every mating, there is a 50 percent chance that the zygote will be male and a 50 percent chance that it will be female.

Genes that are located on the X or Y chromosome are called **sex linked**. In humans, most sex-linked genes are located on the X chromosome, although some Y-linked traits have been found (e.g., hair on the outer ears).

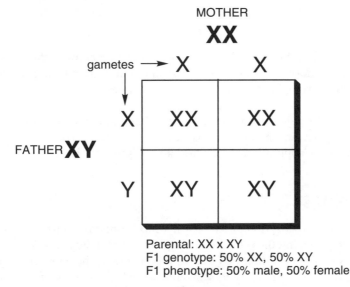

Parental: XX x XY
F1 genotype: 50% XX, 50% XY
F1 phenotype: 50% male, 50% female

Figure 9.6

Sex Linkage

In humans, women have two X chromosomes, and men have only one. As a result, recessive genes that are carried on the X chromosome will produce the recessive phenotypes whenever they occur in men because no dominant allele is present to mask them. The recessive phenotype will thus be much more frequently found in men. Examples of sex-linked recessives in humans are the genes for **hemophilia** and for **color-blindness**.

The pattern of inheritance for a sex-linked recessive is somewhat complicated. Because the gene is carried on the X chromosome, and men pass the X chromosome only to their daughters, affected men cannot pass the trait to their male offspring. Affected men will pass the gene to all of their daughters. However, unless the daughter also receives the gene from her mother, she will be a phenotypically normal carrier of the trait. Because all of the daughter's male children will receive their only X chromosome from her, half of her sons will receive the recessive sex-linked allele. Thus, sex-linked recessives generally affect only men; they cannot be passed from father to son, but they can be passed from father to grandson via a daughter who is a carrier, thereby skipping a generation.

Drosophila Melanogaster

Modern work with the fruit fly (*Drosophila melanogaster*) helped to provide explanations for Mendelian genetic patterns. The fruit fly provides several advantages for genetic research:

- It reproduces often (short life cycle).
- It reproduces in large numbers (large sample size).
- Its chromosomes (especially in the salivary gland) are large and easily recognizable in size and shape.
- Its chromosomes are few (4 pairs, $2n = 8$).
- Mutations occur relatively frequently.

Through genetic and mutational analyses of *D. melanogaster*, scientists have elucidated the patterns of embryological development, discovering how genes expressed early in development can affect the adult organism.

Environmental Factors

The environment can often affect the expression of a gene. Interaction between the environment and the genotype produces the phenotype. For example, Drosophila with a given set of genes have crooked wings at low temperatures but straight wings at higher temperatures.

Temperature also influences the hair color of the **Himalayan hare**. The same genes for color result in white hair on the warmer parts of the body and black hair on colder parts. If the naturally warm portions are cooled (e.g., by the application of ice), the hair will grow in black.

MOLECULAR GENETICS

Genes are composed of **DNA** (deoxyribonucleic acid), which contains information **coded** in the sequence of its base pairs, providing the cell with a blueprint for protein synthesis. (The process of protein synthesis involves RNA and is discussed later in this chapter.) These proteins regulate all life functions. Furthermore, DNA has the ability to **self-replicate**, which is crucial for cell division and hence for organismal reproduction. DNA is the basis of **heredity**; self-replication ensures that its coded sequence will be passed on to successive generations. This is the central dogma of molecular genetics. DNA is **mutable** and can be altered under certain conditions, altering the corresponding characteristics in the organism. Changes in DNA are stable and can be passed from generation to generation, providing the basis for evolution.

Central Dogma of Molecular Genetics

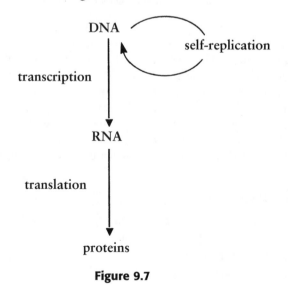

Figure 9.7

STRUCTURE OF DNA

The basic unit of DNA is the **nucleotide**, which is composed of **deoxyribose** (a sugar) bonded to both a phosphate group and a nitrogenous base. There are two types of bases: **purines** and **pyrimidines**. The purines in DNA are **adenine** (A) and **guanine** (G), and the pyrimidines are **cytosine** (C) and **thymine** (T). The phosphate and sugar form a chain with the bases arranged as side groups off the chain.

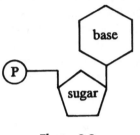

Figure 9.8

A DNA molecule is a **double-stranded helix** with the sugar-phosphate chains on the outside of the helix and the bases on the inside. T always forms two hydrogen bonds with A, and G always forms three hydrogen bonds with C. This base-pairing forms "rungs" on the interior of the double helix that link the two polynucleotide chains together. This is known as the **Watson-Crick DNA Model**.

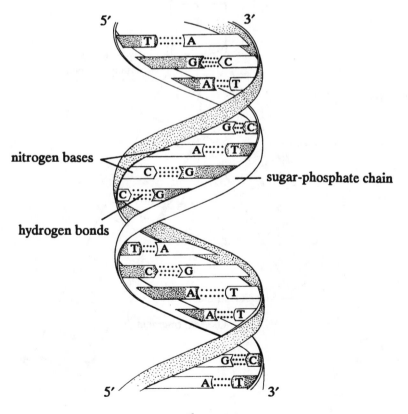

Figure 9.9

FUNCTION OF DNA

DNA Replication

The double-stranded DNA molecule unwinds and separates into two single strands. Each strand acts as a template for **complementary base-pairing** in the synthesis of two new daughter helices. Each new daughter helix contains an intact strand from the parent helix and a newly synthesized strand; thus, DNA replication is **semiconservative**. The daughter DNA helices are identical in composition to each other and to the parent DNA. One daughter strand is the **leading strand**, and the other daughter strand is the **lagging strand**. The leading strand is continuously synthesized by DNA polymerase in the 5′ → 3′ direction. The lagging strand is synthesized discontinuously in the 5′→ 3′ direction (since DNA polymerase synthesizes only in that direction) as a series of short segments known as **Okazaki fragments**; however, overall growth of the lagging strand occurs in the 3′ → 5′ direction (see Figure 9.9).

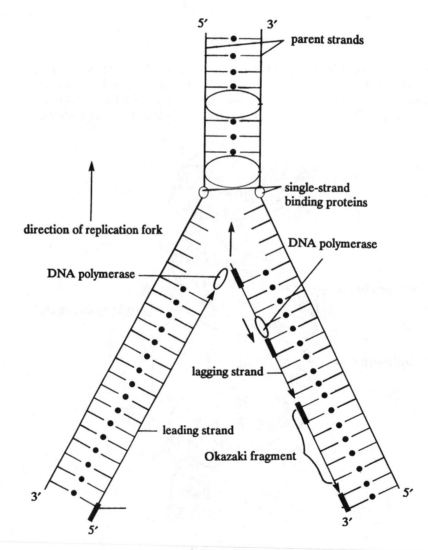

Figure 9.10

The Genetic Code

The language of DNA consists of four "letters": **A**, **T**, **C**, and **G**. The language of **proteins** consists of 20 "words": the **20 amino acids**. The DNA language must be translated by mRNA in such a way as to produce the 20 words in the amino acid language; hence, the **triplet** code. The base sequence of mRNA is translated as a series of triplets, otherwise known as **codons**. A sequence of three consecutive bases codes for a particular amino acid; e.g., the codon GGC specifies glycine, and the codon GUG specifies valine. The genetic code is **universal** for almost all organisms.

Given that 64 different codons are possible based on the triplet code, and only 20 amino acids need to be coded, the code must contain **synonyms**. Most amino acids have more than one codon specifying them. This property is referred to as the **degeneracy** or **redundancy** of the genetic code.

Second Base

First Base (5′)	U	C	A	G	Third Base (3′)
U	UUU UUC } Phe UUA UUG } Leu	UCU UCC UCA UCG } Ser	UAU UAC } Tyr UAA UAG } *Stop*	UGU UGC } Cys UGA } *Stop* UGG } Trp	U C A G
C	CUU CUC CUA CUG } Leu	CCU CCC CCA CCG } Pro	CAU CAC } His CAA CAG } Gln	CGU CGC CGA CGG } Arg	U C A G
A	AUU AUC } Ile AUA AUG } *Start* or Met	ACU ACC ACA ACG } Thr	AAU AAC } Asn AAA AAG } Lys	AGU AGC } Ser AGA AGG } Arg	U C A G
G	GUU GUC GUA GUG } Val	GCU GCC GCA GCG } Ala	GAU GAC } Asp GAA GAG } Glu	GGU GGC GGA GGG } Gly	U C A G

Figure 9.11

RNA

The Structure of RNA

RNA, ribonucleic acid, is a polynucleotide structurally similar to DNA except that its sugar is **ribose**, it contains **uracil** (U) instead of thymine, and it is usually **single-stranded**. RNA can be found in both the nucleus and the cytoplasm. There are several types of RNA, all of which are involved in some aspect of protein synthesis: mRNA, tRNA, and rRNA.

Messenger mRNA (mRNA)

mRNA carries the complement of a DNA sequence and transports it from the **nucleus** to the **ribosomes**, where protein synthesis occurs. mRNA is assembled from ribonucleotides that are **complementary** to the "sense" strand of the DNA. The mRNA has the "inverted" complementary or negative codes of the original master on DNA. For example, because the DNA code for the amino acid valine is AAC, the mRNA is the complementary UUG. mRNA is **monocistronic**; i.e., one mRNA strand codes for one polypeptide.

Transfer RNA (tRNA)

tRNA is a small RNA found in the cytoplasm that aids in the translation of mRNA's nucleotide code into a sequence of amino acids. tRNA brings amino acids to the ribosomes during protein synthesis. There is at least 1 type of tRNA for each amino acid; there are approximately 40 known types of tRNA.

Ribosomal RNA (rRNA)

rRNA is a structural component of ribosomes and is the most abundant of all RNA types. rRNA is synthesized in the **nucleolus**.

PROTEIN SYNTHESIS

Transcription

Transcription is the process whereby information coded in the base sequence of DNA is transcribed into a strand of mRNA that leaves the nucleus through nuclear pores. The remaining events of protein synthesis occur in the cytoplasm.

Translation

Translation is the process whereby mRNA codons are translated into a sequence of amino acids. Translation occurs in the cytoplasm and involves tRNA, ribosomes, mRNA, amino acids, enzymes, and other proteins.

tRNA

tRNA brings amino acids to the **ribosomes** in the correct sequence for polypeptide synthesis; tRNA "recognizes" both the amino acid and the mRNA codon. This dual function is reflected in its three-dimensional structure: one end contains a three-nucleotide sequence, the **anticodon**, which is complementary to one of the mRNA codons; the other end is the site of amino acid attachment. Each amino acid has its own **aminoacyl-tRNA synthetase**, which has an active site that binds to both the amino acid and its corresponding tRNA, catalyzing their attachment to form an aminoacyl-tRNA complex.

Ribosomes

Ribosomes are composed of two subunits (consisting of proteins and rRNA), one large and one small, that bind together only during protein synthesis. Ribosomes have three binding sites: one for mRNA and two for tRNA—the P site (peptidyl-tRNA binding site) and the A site (aminoacyl-tRNA complex binding site). The P site binds to the tRNA attached to the growing polypeptide chain, whereas the A site binds to the incoming aminoacyl-tRNA complex.

Polypeptide synthesis

Polypeptide synthesis can be divided into three distinct stages: initiation, elongation, and termination. Synthesis begins when the ribosome binds to the mRNA near its 5' end. The ribosome scans the mRNA until it binds to a **start codon** (AUG). The initiator aminoacyl-tRNA complex, methionine-tRNA (with the anticodon 3'-UAC-5'), base pairs with the start codon. In **elongation**, hydrogen bonds form between the mRNA codon in the A site and its complementary anticodon on the incoming aminoacyl-tRNA complex. A peptide bond is formed between the amino acid attached to the tRNA in the A site and the fmet attached to the tRNA in the P site. After peptide bond formation, a ribosome carries uncharged tRNA in the P site and peptidyl-tRNA in the A site. The cycle is completed by **translocation**, in which the ribosome advances three nucleotides along the mRNA in the 5' to 3' direction. In a concurrent action, the uncharged tRNA from the P site is expelled, and the peptidyl-tRNA from the A site moves into the P site. The ribosome then has an empty A site ready for entry of the aminoacyl-tRNA corresponding to the next codon.

Polypeptide synthesis **terminates** when one of three special mRNA **termination codons** (UAA, UAG, or UGA) arrives in the A site. These codons signal the ribosome to terminate translation; they do not code for amino acids. Frequently, many ribosomes simultaneously translate a single mRNA molecule, forming a structure known as a **polyribosome**.

After the release of the protein from the ribosome, the protein immediately assumes the characteristic native conformation. This conformation is determined by the **primary** sequence of amino acids. Furthermore, the polypeptide chains can form intramolecular and intermolecular cross-bridges with **disulfide bonds**. The result is a complex, intertwined functional protein.

GENETIC PROBLEMS

Although genetic replication is very accurate, chromosome number and structure can be altered by abnormal cell division during meiosis or by mutagenic agents. This can result in the appearance of abnormal characteristics of the offspring in question.

Nondisjunction

Nondisjunction is either the failure of homologous chromosomes to separate properly during meiosis I or the failure of sister chromatids to separate properly during meiosis II. The resulting **zygote** might either have three copies of that chromosome, called **trisomy** (somatic cells will have 2N + 1 chromosomes), or might have a single copy of that chromosome, called **monosomy** (somatic cells will have 2N − 1 chromosomes). A classic case of trisomy is the birth defect **Down's syndrome**, which is caused by trisomy of **chromosome 21**. Most monosomies and trisomies are lethal, causing the embryo to spontaneously abort early in the pregnancy.

Nondisjunction of the sex chromosomes may also occur, resulting in individuals with extra or missing copies of the X or Y chromosomes.

Chromosomal Breakage

Chromosomal breakage may occur spontaneously or be induced by environmental factors, such as mutagenic agents and X rays. The chromosome that loses a fragment is said to have a deficiency.

Mutations

Mutations are changes in the genetic information of a cell coded in the DNA. Mutations that occur in **somatic** cells can lead to tumors in the individual. Mutations that occur in the sex cells (**gametes**) will be transmitted to the offspring. Most mutations occur in regions of DNA that do not code for proteins and are silent (not expressed in the phenotype). Mutations that do change the sequence of amino acids in proteins are most often recessive and deleterious.

Mutagenic agents

Mutagenic agents induce mutations. These include cosmic rays, X rays, ultraviolet rays, and radioactivity, as well as chemical compounds such as **colchicine** (which inhibits spindle formation, thereby causing polyploidy) or **mustard gas**. Mutagenic agents are sometimes also **carcinogenic**.

Mutation types

In a gene mutation, nitrogen bases are **added**, **deleted**, or **substituted**, thus creating different genes; inappropriate amino acids may be inserted into polypeptide chains, and a mutated protein may be produced. Therefore, a mutation is a genetic "error" with the "wrong" base or no base on the DNA at the particular position.

In a **point mutation**, a nucleic acid is replaced by another nucleic acid. The number of nucleic acids substituted may vary, but generally point mutations involve between one and three nucleotides. There are three possible effects on the **codon**, the sequence of three nucleotides that determines the identity of the amino acid. First, the new codon may code for the same amino acid (a **silent mutation**). Second, the new codon may code for a different amino acid (a **missense mutation**). Finally, the new codon may be a stop codon (a **nonsense mutation**). Point mutations may not be lethal if they code for the same amino acid or if the amino acid is not crucial to the functioning of the protein. The length of the genome does not change.

In a **frameshift mutation**, nucleic acids are deleted or inserted into the genome sequence. This frequently is lethal. The insertion or deletion of nucleic acids throws off the entire sequence of codons from that point on because the genome is "read" in groups of three nucleic acids. Since nucleic acids are inserted or deleted, the length of the genome changes.

Examples of genetic disorders

- **Phenylketonuria** (PKU) is a molecular disease caused by the inability to produce the proper enzyme for the metabolism of **phenylalanine**. A degradation product (phenylpyruvic acid) accumulates. Therefore, these individuals are unable to consume diet products containing aspartame. The administration of any product that contains phenylalanine, such as aspartame, to an individual with any of the hyperphenylaninemia conditions could be detrimental to their general health. Hyperphenylaninemia may result from an impaired conversion of phenylalanine to tyrosine. The most common and clinically important impairment is phenylketonuria, which is characterized by an increased concentration of phenylalanine in blood, increased concentration of phenylalanine and its by-products (such as phenylpyruvate, phenylacetate, and phenyllactate) in urine, and mental retardation. Phenylketonuria is a condition caused by a deficiency of phenylalanine hydrolase. It is important to note that although this is a rare condition, the Food and Drug Administration requires that the following warning be placed on all food products that contain aspartame: Caution phenylketonurics—contains phenylalanine.

- **Sickle-cell anemia** is a disease in which red blood cells become crescent-shaped because they contain defective **hemoglobin**. The sickle-cell hemoglobin carries less oxygen. This disease is caused by a substitution of valine (GUA or GUG) for glutamic acid (GAA or GAG) because of a single base-pair substitution in the gene coding for hemoglobin.

CYTOPLASMIC INHERITANCE

Heredity systems exist outside the nucleus. For example, **DNA** is found in **chloroplasts** and **mitochondria** and other cytoplasmic bodies. These cytoplasmic genes may interact with nuclear genes and are important in determining the characteristics of their organelles. Drug resistance in many microorganisms is regulated by cytoplasmic DNA, known as **plasmids**, that contain one or more genes.

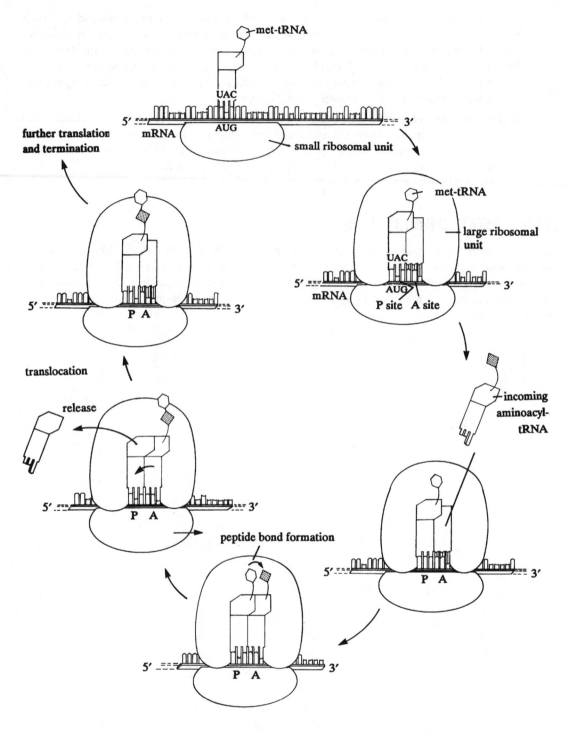

Figure 9.12

BACTERIAL GENETICS

Bacterial Genome

The bacterial genome consists of a single circular chromosome located in the **nucleoid** region of the cell. Many bacteria also contain smaller circular rings of DNA called **plasmids**, which contain accessory genes. **Episomes** are plasmids that are capable of integration into the bacterial genome.

Replication

Replication of the bacterial chromosome begins at a unique origin of replication and proceeds in both directions simultaneously. DNA is synthesized in the 5' to 3' direction.

Genetic Variance

Bacterial cells reproduce by **binary fission** and proliferate very rapidly under favorable conditions. Although binary fission is an **asexual** process, bacteria have three mechanisms for increasing the genetic variance of a population: **transformation**, **conjugation**, and **transduction**.

Transformation

Transformation is the process by which a foreign chromosome fragment (**plasmid**) is incorporated into the bacterial chromosome via recombination, creating new inheritable genetic combinations.

Conjugation

Conjugation can be described as **sexual mating** in bacteria; it is the transfer of genetic material between two bacteria that are temporarily joined. A cytoplasmic conjugation bridge is formed between the two cells, and genetic material is transferred from the donor male (+) type to the recipient female (−) type. Only bacteria containing plasmids called sex factors are capable of conjugating. The best studied sex factor is the **F factor** in *E. coli*. Bacteria possessing this plasmid are termed F+ cells; those without it are called F− cells. During conjugation between an F+ and an F− cell, the F+ cell replicates its F factor and donates the copy to the recipient, converting it to an F+ cell. Genes that code for other characteristics, such as **antibody resistance**, may be found on the plasmids and transferred into recipient cells along with these factors.

Sometimes the sex factor becomes integrated into the bacterial genome. During conjugation, the entire bacterial chromosome replicates and begins to move from the donor cell into the recipient cell. The conjugation bridge usually breaks before the entire chromosome is transferred, but the bacterial genes that enter the recipient cell can easily recombine with the bacterial genes already present to form novel genetic combinations. These bacteria are called **Hfr** cells, meaning that they have a **high frequency of recombination**.

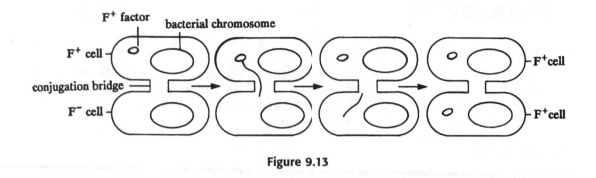

Figure 9.13

Transduction

Transduction occurs when fragments of the bacterial chromosome accidentally become packaged into viral progeny produced during a viral infection. These **virions** may infect other bacteria and introduce new genetic arrangements through recombination with the new host cell's DNA. The closer two genes are to one another on a chromosome, the more likely they will be to transduce together. This fact allows geneticists to map genes to a high degree of precision.

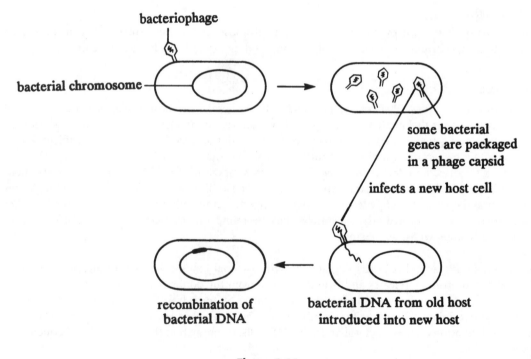

Figure 9.14

Recombination

Recombination occurs when linked genes are separated. It occurs by breakage and rearrangements of adjacent regions of DNA when organisms carrying different genes or alleles for the same traits are crossed.

Gene Regulation

The regulation of gene expression (**transcription**) enables prokaryotes to control their metabolism. Regulation of transcription is based on the accessibility of **RNA polymerase** to the genes being transcribed and is directed by an **operon**, which consists of **structural** genes, an **operator** gene, and a **promoter** gene. Structural genes contain sequences of DNA that code for **proteins**. The operator gene is the sequence of **nontranscribable** DNA that is the **repressor** binding site. The **promoter** gene is the noncoding sequence of DNA that serves as the initial binding site for RNA polymerase. There is also a **regulator** gene, which codes for the synthesis of a repressor molecule that binds to the operator and blocks RNA polymerase from transcribing the structural genes.

RNA polymerase must also move past the operator gene to transcribe the structural genes. Regulatory systems function by preventing or permitting the RNA polymerase to pass on to the structural genes. Regulation may be via **inducible systems** or **repressible systems**. Inducible systems are those that require the presence of a substance, called an **inducer**, for transcription to occur. Repressible systems are in a constant state of transcription unless a **corepressor** is present to inhibit transcription.

Inducible systems

In an inducible system, the repressor binds to the operator, forming a barrier that prevents RNA polymerase from transcribing the structural genes. For transcription to occur, an inducer must bind to the repressor, forming an **inducer-repressor complex**. This complex cannot bind to the operator, thus permitting transcription. The proteins synthesized are thus said to be inducible. The structural genes typically code for an enzyme, and the inducer is usually the substrate, or a derivative of the substrate, upon which the enzyme normally acts. When the substrate (inducer) is present, enzymes are synthesized; when it is absent, enzyme synthesis is negligible. In this manner, enzymes are transcribed only when they are actually needed.

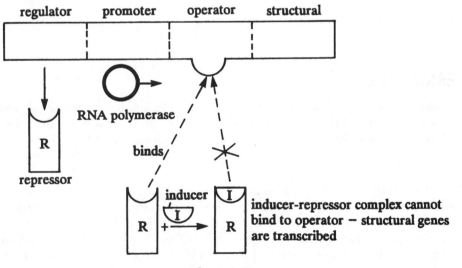

Figure 9.15

Repressible systems

In a repressible system, the repressor is inactive until it combines with the corepressor. The repressor can bind to the operator and prevent transcription only when it has formed a repressor-corepressor complex. Corepressors are often the **end-products** of the biosynthetic pathways they control. The proteins produced (usually enzymes) are said to be repressible because they are normally being synthesized; transcription and translation occur until the corepressor is synthesized. Operons containing mutations such as deletions or whose regulator genes code for defective repressors are incapable of being turned off; their enzymes, which are always being synthesized, are referred to as **constitutive**.

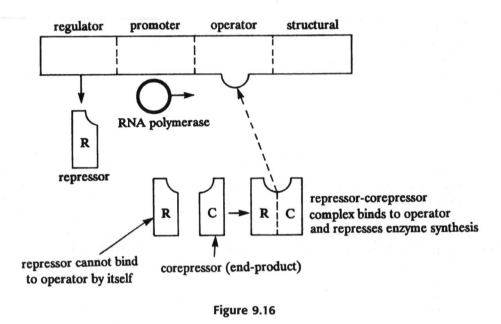

Figure 9.16

BACTERIOPHAGE

A bacteriophage is a virus that infects its host bacterium by attaching to it, boring a hole through the bacterial cell wall, and injecting its DNA while its protein coat remains attached to the cell wall. Once inside its host, the bacteriophage enters either a lytic cycle or a lysogenic cycle.

Lytic Cycle

The phage DNA takes control of the bacterium's genetic machinery and manufactures numerous progeny. The bacterial cell then bursts (**lyses**), releasing new virions, each capable of infecting other bacteria. Bacteriophages that replicate by the lytic cycle, killing their host cells, are called **virulent**. If the initial infection takes place on a bacterial **lawn** (a plated culture), then very shortly a **plaque** or clearing in the lawn occurs, corresponding to the area of lysed bacteria. The physical characteristics of a plaque are useful in identifying mutant phage strains that may arise.

Lysogenic Cycle

If the bacteriophage does not lyse its host cell, it becomes **integrated** into the bacterial genome in a harmless form (**provirus**), lying dormant for one or more generations. The virus may stay integrated indefinitely, replicating along with the bacterial genome. However, either spontaneously or as a result of environmental circumstances (e.g., radiation, ultraviolet light, or chemicals), the provirus can reemerge and enter a lytic cycle. Bacteria containing proviruses are normally resistant to further infection (**superinfection**) by similar phages.

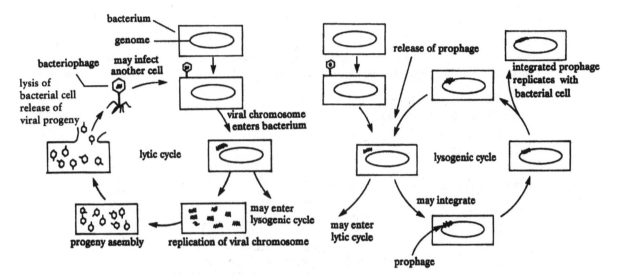

Figure 9.17 Bacteriophage Lifecycle

REVIEW PROBLEMS

1. A woman with blood genotype $I^A i$ and a man with blood genotype $I^B i$ have two children, both type AB. What is the probability that a third child will be blood type AB?

    (A) 25%
    (B) 33%
    (C) 50%
    (D) 66%

2. In humans, the allele for black hair (B) is dominant to the allele to brown hair (b), and the allele for curly hair (C) is dominant to the allele for straight hair (c). When a person of unknown genotype is crossed against a straight- and brown-haired individual, the phenotypic ratio is

    25% curly black hair
    25% straight black hair
    25% curly brown hair
    25% straight brown hair

    What is the genotype of the unknown parent?

    (A) BBCC
    (B) BbCC
    (C) Bbcc
    (D) bbCc
    (E) BbCc

3. Which of the following is TRUE concerning a sex-linked recessive disorder that is lethal in infancy?

    (A) Females are unable to carry the gene.
    (B) It will cause death in both males and females.
    (C) Male children of male carriers will be carriers.
    (D) It will cause death only in males.
    (E) It will serve to increase the potential son/daughter ratio in a cross between a female carrier and a normal male.

4. Assuming classical Mendelian inheritance, how can one differentiate between a homozygous dominant individual and one who is heterozygous for the dominant trait?

    (A) By crossing the individuals in question
    (B) By crossing each individual with a known homozygous recessive and examining the offspring
    (C) By crossing each individual with a known heterozygote and examining the offspring
    (D) By crossing each individual with a known homozygous dominant and examining the offspring
    (E) Both B and C

5. If a male hemophiliac (XhY) is crossed with a female carrier of both color blindness and hemophilia (XcXh), what is the probability that a female child will be phenotypically normal?

   (A) 0%
   (B) 25%
   (C) 50%
   (D) Same as for a male child
   (E) Not enough information given

6. Explain the concept of Mendel's law of segregation.

7. Why are lethal dominant alleles much less common than lethal recessive alleles?

8. In the DNA of a fruit fly (*Drosophila melanogaster*), 20 percent of the bases are cytosines. What percent are adenines?

9. Nucleotides are linked by

   (A) hydrogen bonds.
   (B) phosphodiester bonds.
   (C) covalent bonds.
   (D) van der Waals bonds.

10. Many point mutations do not have any effect on the gene product. What are two possible explanations for this observation?

11. You have just sequenced a piece of DNA that reads: 5' TCTTTGAGACATCC 3'

    a. What would be the base sequence in the mRNA transcribed from this DNA?
    b. Using the chart of the genetic code, establish the amino acid sequence of the protein coded for by this DNA.

12. What are three differences between DNA and RNA?

SOLUTIONS TO REVIEW PROBLEMS

1. **A** This is a cross between two heterozygotes for a trait that has codominant alleles. The inheritance pattern for human blood groups is not a simple dominant/recessive pattern because the A and B alleles are both phenotypically expressed when the genotype is AB.

   This is a cross between a woman heterozygous for blood type A and a man heterozygous for blood type B: $I^A i \times I^B i$.

F1 genotypes:	25% $I^A I^B$	phenotypes:	25% type AB
	25% $I^B i$		25% type B
	25% $I^A i$		25% type A
	25% ii		25% type O

   The birth of each child is an independent event. Hence, the fact the first two children this couple had were type AB has no influence whatsoever on the probability that a third child will be AB. So there is a 25 percent chance that any child, not just the third, will be type AB.

2. **E** In this dihybrid problem, a doubly recessive individual is crossed with an individual of unknown genotype—this is known as a testcross. The straight- and brown-haired individual has the genotype bbcc and can thus produce gametes of only one class, bc. Looking at the F1 offspring, there is a 1:1:1:1 phenotypic ratio. The fact that both the recessive and dominant traits are present in the offspring means that the unknown parental genotype must contain both recessive alleles (b and c). The unknown parental genotype must therefore be BbCc. If you want to double-check the answer, you can work out the Punnett square for the cross BbCc × bbcc: BbCc can produce four different types of gametes, BC, Bc, bC, and bc, whereas bbcc can produce only bc gametes, as previously mentioned.

   So the unknown parental genotype is BbCc, choice (E).

3. **D** A sex-linked recessive gene is one that is carried on the X chromosome and can be passed from fathers to daughters only and from mothers to both sons and daughters. An early-acting lethal sex-linked recessive will kill all males in infancy because men are XY and lack a dominant allele to mask the effects of the recessive lethal. Men cannot be carriers of the lethal gene, as there will be no men of reproductive age with this gene to pass it on to offspring. Therefore, the gene will be inherited only from female carriers, who will pass the lethal gene to 50 percent of their offspring (all of their sons will die in infancy). A female can never be homozygous, because that would mean that she inherited one of the lethal alleles from her father—but that is impossible because all afflicted males die in infancy. Hence, there will be no female deaths as a result of the lethal allele. Thus, choices A, B, and C can be ruled out. A cross between a female carrier and a normal man will produce 25 percent carrier daughters, 25 percent normal daughters, 25 percent homozygous sons (who will die in infancy), and 25 percent normal sons. Because 50 percent of all sons will die, the potential son/daughter ratio will decrease, and thus, choice (E) is wrong. So the correct answer is (D), ALL males with the early-acting, sex-linked lethal recessive allele will die.

4. **E** To differentiate between a homozygous dominant and a heterozygous dominant for a trait that exhibits classic dominant/recessive Mendelian inheritance, one must perform a cross that results in offspring that reveal the unknown parental genotype; this is known as a testcross. If we cross the homozygous dominant with a homozygous recessive, we will get 100 percent phenotypically dominant offspring; if we cross the heterozygous dominant

with the homozygous recessive, we will get 50 percent phenotypically dominant and 50 percent phenotypically recessive offspring. Thus, using a homozygous recessive as a testcrosser will allow us to distinguish between the two. We can also use a known heterozygote as the testcrosser because when this is crossed with the homozygous dominant, 100 percent phenotypically dominant offspring are produced, and when it is crossed with the heterozygote, the phenotypic ratio of the offspring is 3:1 dominant:recessive. Hence, the correct answer is (E), because both (B) and (C) are viable options. Crossing both dominants with a known homozygous dominant, as in (D), will produce 100 percent phenotypically dominant offspring for both crosses, not allowing us to distinguish between the homozygote and the heterozygote. Crossing the individuals in question, as in (A), will also result in 100 percent phenotypically dominant offspring and hence will be useless to us.

5. C   In this problem, we are told that the female in this cross is a carrier of two sex-linked traits: color blindness and hemophilia. We are also told that the genes for these traits are not found on the same X chromosome, as indicated by her genotype, XcXh. So of the female offspring, half, or 50 percent, will be phenotypically normal.

6. The chromosomal basis for Mendel's law of segregation is as follows: for any given trait, all individuals have two alleles located on separate, but homologous, chromosomes, one inherited from each parent. During meiosis, or gamete formation, these homologous chromosomes pair and line up along the equatorial plate. As meiosis proceeds, the spindle fibers attached to the homologues move them towards opposite poles of the cell. Because the alleles are on different chromosomes, they segregate and wind up in different gametes. The paired condition of the alleles is restored with the fusion of egg and sperm during fertilization.

7. Lethal dominant alleles are much less common than lethal recessive alleles because a lethal dominant allele kills both heterozygotes and homozygotes, preventing the transmission of the allele to offspring (unless the gene is late acting). Dominant lethals usually appear in an individual as a result of spontaneous mutations and die with that individual. Thus, the frequency with which dominant lethals appear in the gene pool always remains very low. Lethal recessive alleles also kill homozygotes; however, heterozygotes are phenotypically normal and will not die as a result of their single copy of the lethal recessive. Hence, heterozygotes are able to pass on the lethal allele to offspring and thus maintain the frequency of the allele in the gene pool.

8. If 20 percent of the bases are cytosines, then 20 percent of the bases must also be guanines (because they base-pair). The remaining 60 percent (100 − 20 − 20 = 60) of bases are adenines and thymines. Again, because of complementary base-pairing, 30 percent are adenines and 30 percent are thymines. So 30 percent of the bases are adenines.

9. A   Nucleotides are linked by hydrogen bonds. A always binds to T with two hydrogen bonds, whereas C and G bind with three hydrogen bonds. Note that phosphodiester bonds are covalent bonds.

10. A point mutation causes the substitution of one base pair for another. Sometimes, as in the case of sickle-cell anemia, it may have a very profound effect on the gene product (hemoglobin) because it changes the message carried by the gene. In some cases, however, a mutated gene codes for the same product. This can be explained by the redundancy of the genetic code. Most amino acids have more than one triplet coding for them. The substitution of the third cytosine in the triplet CCC (proline) for any of the remaining bases (G, A, or U) will not change the amino acid sequence because the codons CCG, CCA, and CCU code for proline as well. In eukaryotes, a point mutation may occur in an intron and thus will not affect the gene product because noncoding regions are excised after transcription.

11. a. The mRNA will be: 5' GGAUGUCUCAAAGA 3' (Remember that mRNA is antiparallel to DNA!).

    b. The code is as follows: GG AUG UCU CAA AGA, which codes for Met-Ser-Gln-Arg.

12. 1) DNA is double-stranded; RNA is single-stranded; 2) DNA has the nitrogen base thymine; RNA has uracil; and 3) the sugar in DNA is deoxyribose; the sugar in RNA is ribose.

CHAPTER TEN

Vertebrate Embryology

Embryology is the study of the development of a unicellular zygote into a complete, multicellular organism. In the course of nine months, a unicellular human zygote undergoes cell division, cellular differentiation, and morphogenesis in preparation for life outside the uterus. Much of what is known about mammalian development stems from the study of less complex organisms such as sea urchins and frogs.

EARLY DEVELOPMENTAL STAGES

Fertilization

An egg can be fertilized within 12–24 hours after ovulation. Fertilization occurs in the lateral, widest portion of the oviduct when sperm traveling from the vagina encounter an egg. If more than one egg is fertilized, **fraternal twins** may be conceived.

Cleavage

Early embryonic development is characterized by a series of rapid mitotic divisions known as cleavage. These divisions lead to an increase in cell number without a corresponding growth in cell protoplasm (i.e., the total volume of cytoplasm remains constant). Thus, cleavage results in progressively smaller cells, with an increasing ratio of nuclear-to-cytoplasmic material. Cleavage also increases the surface-to-volume ratio of each cell, thereby improving gas and nutrient exchange. This early developmental process consists of a series of very rapid, synchronous mitotic divisions that converts the zygote's single large cell into a solid ball of cells, known as the merula, then into the blastula.

The first complete cleavage of the zygote occurs approximately 32 hours after fertilization. The second cleavage occurs after 60 hours, and the third cleavage after approximately 72 hours, at which point the eight-celled embryo reaches the uterus. As cell division continues, a solid ball of embryonic cells, known as the **morula**, is formed. **Blastulation** begins when the morula develops a fluid-filled cavity called the **blastocoel**, which by the fourth day becomes a hollow sphere of cells called the **blastula**. The blastula is the stage of the embryo that implants in the uterus.

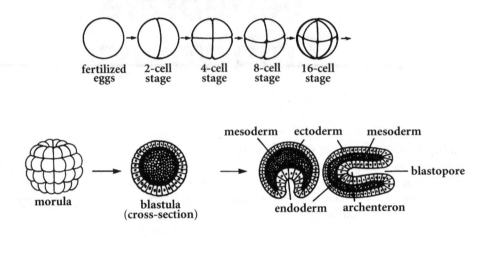

Figure 10.1

Gastrulation

Once implanted in the uterus, cell migrations transform the single-cell layer of the blastula into a three-layered structure called a gastrula. These three primary germ layers are responsible for the differential development of the tissues, organs, and systems of the body at later stages of growth:

1. **Ectoderm**—Integument (including the epidermis, hair, nails, and epithelium of the nose, mouth, and anal canal), the lens of the eye, the retina, and the nervous system

2. **Endoderm**—Epithelial linings of the digestive and respiratory tracts (including the lungs) and parts of the liver, pancreas, thyroid, and bladder lining

3. **Mesoderm**—Musculoskeletal system, circulatory system, excretory system, gonads, connective tissue throughout the body, and portions of digestive and respiratory organs

Neurulation

By the end of gastrulation, regions of the germ layers begin to develop into a rudimentary nervous system; this process is known as **neurulation**. A rod of mesodermal cells, called the **notochord**, develops along the longitudinal axis just under the dorsal layer of ectoderm. The notochord has an inductive effect on the overlying ectoderm, causing it to bend inward and form a groove along the dorsal surface of the embryo. The dorsal ectoderm folds on either side of the groove; these neural folds grow upward and finally fuse, forming a closed tube. This is the neural tube, which gives rise to the brain and spinal cord (central nervous system). Once the neural tube is formed, it detaches from the surface ectoderm. The cells at the tip of each neural fold are called the **neural crest cells**. These cells migrate laterally and give rise to many components of the peripheral nervous system, including the **sensory ganglia**, **autonomic ganglia**, **adrenal medulla**, and **Schwann cells**.

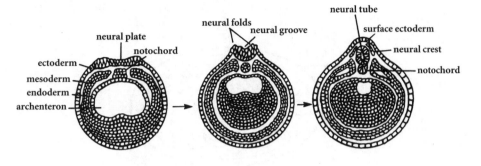

Figure 10.2. Amphilian Neurulation

Development

The developmental process can be divided into internal and external development.

Internal development

- Follows the neurulation process.
- Includes organogenesis, growth, and gametogenesis:

    Organogenesis: The body organs begin to form. In this process, the cells interact, differentiate, change physical shape, proliferate, and migrate.

    Growth: The organs increase in size, which is a continual process from infancy to childhood to adulthood.

    Gametogenesis: Eggs develop in women and sperm develop in men, which results in the possibility of reproduction occurring.

- The fertilization cycle continues, and then cleavage begins.

External development

The early development of many animals occurs outside of the mother's body, on land or in the water. Fish and amphibians lay eggs that are fertilized externally in the water. The embryo develops within the egg, feeding on nutrients stored in the yolk. Reptiles, birds, and some mammals (like the duck-billed platypus) develop externally on land. Fertilization occurs internally, and the fertilized egg is then laid. Eggs provide protection for the developing embryo. The eggs also include the following embryonic membranes:

- **Chorion**—The chorion lines the inside of the shell. It is a moist membrane that permits gas exchange.
- **Allantois**—This sac-like structure is involved in respiration and excretion and contains numerous blood vessels to transport O_2, CO_2, water, salt, and nitrogenous wastes.
- **Amnion**—This membrane encloses the amniotic fluid. Amniotic fluid provides an aqueous environment that protects the developing embryo from shock.
- **Yolk sac**—The yolk sac encloses the yolk. Blood vessels in the yolk sac transfer food to the developing embryo.

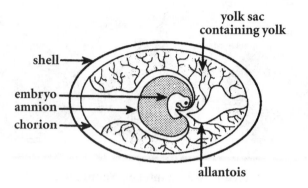

Figure 10.3

Nonplacental internal development

Early development within the body of the mother protects the young. Certain animals, including **marsupials** and some tropical fish, develop in the mother **without** a placenta. Without a placenta, exchange of food and oxygen between the young and the mother is limited. The young may be born very early in development.

Placental internal development

The growing fetus receives oxygen directly from its mother through a specialized circulatory system. This system not only supplies oxygen and nutrients to the fetus but removes carbon dioxide and metabolic wastes as well. The two components of this system are the **placenta** and the **umbilical cord**, which both develop in the first few weeks after fertilization.

The placenta and the umbilical cord are outgrowths of the four extra-embryonic membranes formed during development: the **amnion**, **chorion**, **allantois**, and **yolk sac**. The **amnion** is a thin, tough membrane containing a watery fluid called amniotic fluid. Amniotic fluid acts as a shock absorber of external pressure and localized pressure from uterine contractions during labor. Placenta formation begins with the **chorion**, a membrane that completely surrounds the amnion. A third membrane, the **allantois**, develops as an outpocketing of the gut. The blood vessels of the allantoic wall enlarge and become the umbilical vessels, which will connect the fetus to the developing placenta. The **yolk sac**, the site of early development of blood vessels, becomes associated with the umbilical vessels.

GESTATION

Human pregnancy, or gestation, is approximately nine months (266 days) and can be subdivided into three **trimesters**. The primary developments that occur during each trimester are described below.

First trimester

During the first weeks, the major organs begin to develop. The heart begins to beat at approximately 22 days, and soon afterward, the eyes, gonads, limbs, and liver start to form. By five weeks' the embryo is 10 mm in length; by six weeks' the embryo has grown to 15 mm. The cartilaginous skeleton begins to turn into bone by the seventh week. By the end of eight weeks, most of the organs have formed, the brain is fairly developed, and the embryo is referred to as a fetus. At the end of the third month, the fetus is about 9 cm long.

Second trimester

During the second trimester, the fetus does a tremendous amount of growing. It begins to move around in the amniotic fluid, its face appears human, and its toes and fingers elongate. By the end of the sixth month, the fetus is 30–36 cm long.

Third trimester

The seventh and eighth months are characterized by continued rapid growth and further brain development. During the ninth month, antibodies are transported by highly selective active transport from the mother to the fetus for protection against foreign matter. The growth rate slows and the fetus becomes less active, as it has less room to move about.

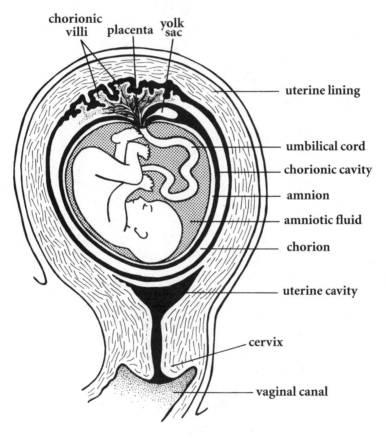

Figure 10.4

Birth and maturation

Childbirth is accomplished by labor, a series of strong uterine contractions. Labor can be divided into three distinct stages. In the first stage, the **cervix** thins out and dilates, and the amniotic sac ruptures, releasing its fluids. During this time, contractions are relatively mild. The second stage is characterized by rapid contractions, resulting in the birth of the baby, followed by the cutting of the umbilical cord. During the final stage, the uterus contracts, expelling the placenta and the umbilical cord.

The embryo develops into the adult through the process of maturation, which involves cell division, growth, and differentiation. In some animals, maturation is suspended in a temporary state. For example, arthropods have a pupal stage. Mammals develop uninterrupted. Differentiation of cells is complete when all organs reach adult form.

REVIEW PROBLEMS

1. Which of the following developmental stages has the greatest nuclear-to-cytoplasmic material ratio?

   (A) Four-celled zygote
   (B) Eight-celled zygote
   (C) Morula
   (D) Blastula

2. Name the three embryonic germ layers. Identify the embryological origin of the following structures: nails, thyroid, lens, testes, aorta, peripheral nerves, and lung epithelium.

3. Describe the structure of a blastula.

4. What is a determinate cleavage? When does the embryo first differentiate into germ layers?

5. What is an ectopic pregnancy?

6. How do marsupials differ from other mammals?

SOLUTIONS TO REVIEW PROBLEMS

1. **D** Discussed in early development section.

2. The three embryonic germ layers are the endoderm, the mesoderm, and the ectoderm. The thyroid and lung epithelium are of endodermal origin. The testes and the aorta are of mesodermal origin. The nails, lens, and peripheral nerves are of ectodermal origin.

3. The name *blastula* refers to an early stage of development in which the embryo consists of a hollow ball of cells surrounding a cavity called the blastocoel.

4. A determinate cleavage results in cells whose differentiation pathways are clearly defined; these cells are incapable of individually developing into complete organisms. The appearance of the three primary germ layers—the endoderm, mesoderm, and ectoderm—occurs during gastrulation.

5. In a normal pregnancy, the blastula implants in the uterus. In an ectopic pregnancy, the embryo implants outside the uterus; for example, in the fallopian tube. An embryo cannot be maintained for long outside of the uterus; it will abort spontaneously, and hemorrhaging will follow.

6. Marsupials are nonplacental mammals. The offspring are born early and move to a pouch for the rest of their development.

CHAPTER ELEVEN

Vascular Systems in Animals and Plants

CIRCULATION IN INVERTEBRATES

Protozoans

The protozoans are heterotrophic cells that generally consume other cells or food particles. The word *protozoa* means "first animal." With respect to the vascular system, the movement of gases and nutrients is accomplished by simple diffusion within the cell.

Cnidarians

Hydras and other cnidarians have body walls that are two cells thick. All cells are in direct contact with either the internal or external environments so there is no need for a specialized circulatory system.

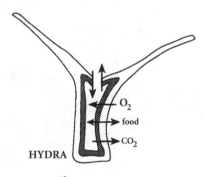

Figure 11.1

Arthropods

Arthropods have **open circulatory systems** in which blood (interstitial fluid) is in direct contact with the body tissues. The blood is circulated primarily by body movements. Blood flows through a **dorsal vessel** and into spaces called **sinuses** where exchange occurs.

Annelids

The earthworm (annelida) uses a **closed circulatory system** to deliver materials to cells that are not in direct contact with the external environment. In a closed circulatory system, blood is confined to blood vessels. Blood moves towards the head in the **dorsal vessel**, which functions as the main heart by coordinated contractions. Five pairs of vessels called **aortic loops** connect the dorsal vessel to the **ventral vessel** and function as additional pumps. Earthworm blood lacks any red blood cells. A hemoglobin-like pigment is dissolved in the aqueous solution.

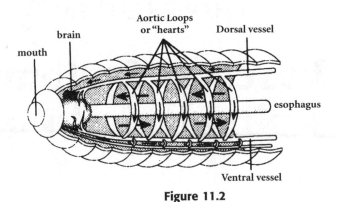

Figure 11.2

CIRCULATION IN HUMANS

The human cardiovascular system is composed of a muscular, four-chambered heart, a network of blood vessels, and the blood itself. Blood is pumped into the **aorta**, which branches into a series of **arteries**. The arteries branch into **arterioles** and then into microscopic **capillaries**. Exchange of gases, nutrients, and cellular waste products occurs via diffusion across capillary walls. The capillaries then converge into **venules** and eventually into **veins**, leading deoxygenated blood back toward the heart.

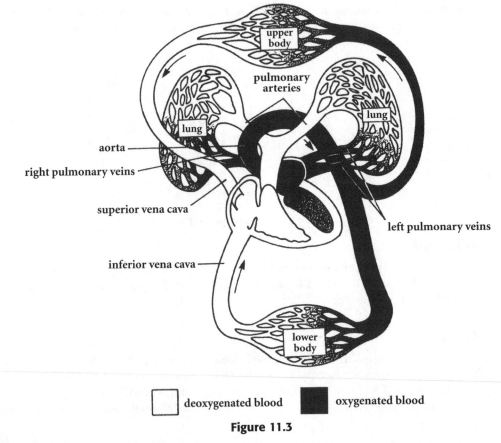

Figure 11.3

The Heart

The heart is the driving force of the circulatory system. The right and left halves can be viewed as two separate pumps: the right side of the heart pumps **deoxygenated** blood into **pulmonary** circulation (toward the lungs), whereas the left side pumps **oxygenated** blood into **systemic** circulation (throughout the body). The two upper chambers are called atria, and the two lower chambers are called ventricles. The **atria** are thin-walled, whereas the **ventricles** are extremely muscular. The left ventricle is more muscular than the right ventricle because it is responsible for generating the force that propels systemic circulation and because it pumps against a higher resistance.

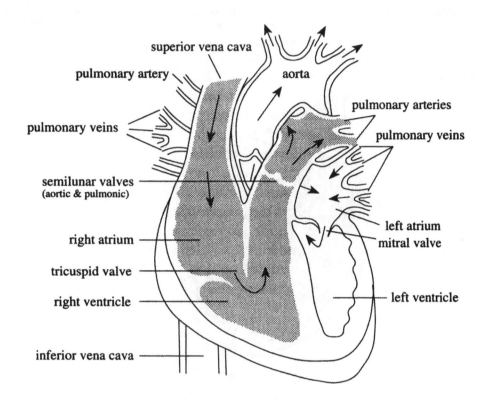

Figure 11.4. Human Heart

Valves

The **atrioventricular valves**, located between the atria and ventricles on both sides of the heart, prevent backflow of blood into the atria. The valve on the right side of the heart has three cusps and is called the **tricuspid valve**. The valve on the left side of the heart has two cusps and is called the **mitral valve**. The **semilunar valves** have three cusps and are located between the left ventricle and the aorta (the aortic valve) and between the right ventricle and the pulmonary artery (the pulmonic valve).

Contraction

Phases–The heart's pumping cycle is divided into two alternating phases, **systole** and **diastole,** which together make up the **heartbeat.** Systole is the period during which the ventricles contract. Diastole is the period of cardiac muscle relaxation during which blood drains into all four chambers. **Cardiac**

output is defined as the total volume of blood the left ventricle pumps out per minute. Cardiac output = **heart rate** (number of beats per minute) × **stroke volume** (volume of blood pumped out of the left ventricle per contraction).

Mechanism and control–Cardiac muscle contracts rhythmically without stimulation from the nervous system, producing impulses that spread through its internal conducting system. An ordinary cardiac contraction originates in, and is regulated by, the **sinoatrial (SA) node** (the **pacemaker**), a small mass of specialized tissue located in the wall of the right atrium. The SA node spreads impulses through both atria, stimulating them to contract simultaneously. The impulse arrives at the **atrioventricular (AV) node**, which conducts slowly, allowing enough time for atrial contraction and for the ventricles to fill with blood. The impulse is then carried by the **bundle of His (AV bundle)**, which branches into the right and left bundle branches, and through the **Purkinje fibers** in the walls of both ventricles, generating a strong contraction.

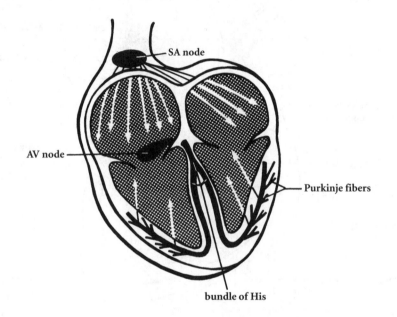

Figure 11.5. Contraction

The **autonomic nervous system** modifies the rate of heart contraction. The parasympathetic system innervates the heart via the **vagus nerve** and causes a decrease in the heart rate. The sympathetic system innervates the heart via the cervical and upper thoracic ganglia and causes an increase in the heart rate. The adrenal medulla exerts hormonal control via epinephrine (adrenaline) secretion, which causes an increase in heart rate.

Blood Vessels

The three types of blood vessels are arteries, veins, and capillaries. **Arteries** are thick-walled, muscular, elastic vessels that transport oxygenated blood away from the heart—except for the **pulmonary arteries,** which transport deoxygenated blood from the heart to the lungs. **Veins** are relatively thinly walled, inelastic vessels that conduct deoxygenated blood towards the heart—except for the **pulmonary veins,** which carry oxygenated blood from the lungs to the heart. Much of the blood flow in veins depends on their compression by skeletal muscles during movement, rather than on the pumping of the heart. Venous circulation is often at odds with gravity; thus, larger veins, especially those in the legs, have valves that prevent backflow. Capillaries have very thin walls composed of a single layer of endothelial cells, across which respiratory gases, nutrients, enzymes, hormones, and wastes can readily diffuse. **Capillaries** have the smallest diameter of all three types of vessels; red blood cells must often travel through them single file.

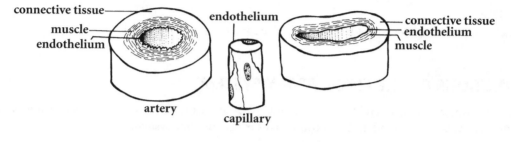

Figure 11.6

Lymph Vessels

The lymphatic system is a secondary circulatory system distinct from the cardiovascular circulation. Its vessels transport excess **interstitial fluid**, called **lymph**, to the cardiovascular system, thereby keeping **fluid** levels in the body constant. **Lymph** nodes are swellings along lymph vessels containing phagocytic cells (**leukocytes**) that filter the lymph, removing and destroying foreign particles and pathogens.

Blood

On the average, the human body contains four to six liters of blood. Blood has both liquid (55 percent) and cellular components (45 percent). **Plasma** is the liquid portion of the blood. It is an aqueous mixture of nutrients, salts, respiratory gases, wastes, hormones, and blood proteins (e.g., immunoglobulins, albumin, and fibrinogen). The cellular components of the blood are erythrocytes, leukocytes, and platelets.

Erythrocytes (red blood cells, RBCs)

Erythrocytes are the oxygen-carrying components of blood. An erythrocyte contains approximately 250 million molecules of hemoglobin, each of which can bind up to four molecules of oxygen. When hemoglobin binds oxygen, it is called **oxyhemoglobin**. This is the primary form of oxygen transport in the blood. Erythrocytes have a distinct biconcave, disklike shape, which gives them both increased surface area for gas exchange and greater flexibility for movement through those tiny capillaries. **Erythrocytes** are formed from stem cells in the **bone marrow** where they lose their nuclei, mitochondria, and membranous organelles. Once mature, RBCs circulate in the blood for about 120 days, after which they are phagocytized by special cells in the spleen and liver.

Leukocytes

Leukocytes are larger than erythrocytes and serve protective functions. Some white blood cells (WBCs) phagocytize foreign matter and organisms such as bacteria. Others migrate from the blood to tissue, where they mature into stationary cells called **macrophages**. Other WBCs, called **lymphocytes**, are involved in immune response and the production of antibodies (B cells) or cytolysis of infected cells (T cells).

Platelets

Platelets are cell **fragments** that lack nuclei and are involved in clot formation.

FUNCTIONS OF THE CIRCULATORY SYSTEM

Blood transports nutrients and O_2 to tissue and wastes and CO_2 from tissue. Platelets are involved in injury repair. Leukocytes are the main component of the immune system.

Transport of Gases

Erythrocytes transport O_2 throughout the circulatory system. Actually, the hemoglobin molecules in erythrocytes bind to O_2. Each hemoglobin molecule is capable of binding to four molecules of O_2. Hemoglobin also binds to **CO_2**.

Transport of Nutrients and Waste

Amino acids and **simple sugars** are absorbed into the bloodstream at the intestinal capillaries and, after processing, are transported throughout the body. Throughout the body, metabolic **waste products** (e.g., water, urea, and carbon dioxide) diffuse into capillaries from surrounding cells; these wastes are then delivered to the appropriate excretory organs.

Clotting

When platelets come into contact with the exposed collagen of a damaged vessel, they release a chemical that causes neighboring platelets to adhere to one another, forming a **platelet plug**. Subsequently, both the platelets and the damaged tissue release the clotting factor thromboplastin. **Thromboplastin**, with the aid of its cofactors calcium and vitamin K, converts the inactive plasma protein **prothrombin** to its active form, **thrombin**. Thrombin then converts **fibrinogen** (another plasma protein) into fibrin. Threads of **fibrin** coat the damaged area and trap blood cells to form a clot. Clots prevent extensive blood loss while the damaged vessel heals itself. The fluid left after blood clotting is called **serum**.

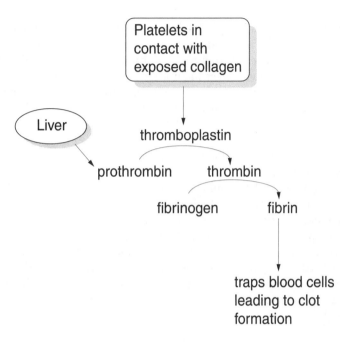

Figure 11.7

The Human Immune System

The body has the ability to distinguish between "self" and "nonself" and to "remember" nonself entities (**antigens**) that it has previously encountered. These defense mechanisms are an integral part of the immune system. The immune system is composed of nonspecific and specific defense mechanisms. The specific immune system comprises **humoral** immunity, which involves the production of antibodies, and **cell-mediated** immunity, which involves cells that combat fungal and viral infection. **Lymphocytes** are responsible for both of these immune mechanisms. The body also has a number of nonspecific defense mechanisms.

Nonspecific defense mechanisms

The body uses a number of nonspecific defenses against foreign material: (1) **Skin** is a physical barrier against bacterial invasion. In addition, pores on the skin's surface secrete sweat, which contains an enzyme that attacks bacterial cell walls. (2) Passages (e.g., the respiratory tract) are lined with ciliated **mucous-coated epithelia**, which filter and trap foreign particles. (3) **Macrophages** engulf and destroy foreign particles. (4) The **inflammatory** response is initiated by the body in response to physical damage: injured cells release **histamine**, which causes blood vessels to dilate, thereby increasing blood flow to the damaged region. **Granulocytes** attracted to the injury site phagocytize antigenic material. An inflammatory response is often accompanied by a **fever**. (5) Proteins called interferons are produced by cells under viral attack. **Interferons** diffuse to other cells, where they help prevent the spread of the virus.

Inappropriate response to certain foods and pollen can cause the body to form antibodies and release histamine. These responses are called **allergic** reactions.

Humoral immunity

One of the body's defense mechanisms is the production of **antibodies**. These responses are very specific to the antigen involved. Humoral immunity is responsible for the proliferation of antibodies after exposure to antigens. Antibodies, also called **immunoglobulins** (Igs), are complex proteins that recognize and bind to specific antigens and trigger the immune system to remove them. Antibodies either attract other cells (such as leukocytes) to phagocytize the antigen or cause the antigens to clump together (**agglutinate**) and form large insoluble complexes, facilitating their removal by phagocytic cells.

Active immunity refers to the production of antibodies during an immune response. Active immunity can be conferred by **vaccination**; an individual is injected with a weakened, inactive, or related form of a particular antigen, which stimulates the immune system to produce specific antibodies against it. Active immunity may require weeks to build up. Passive immunity involves the transfer of antibodies produced by another individual or organism. Passive immunity is acquired either passively or by injection. For example, during pregnancy, some maternal antibodies cross the placenta and enter fetal circulation, conferring passive immunity upon the fetus. Although passive immunity is acquired immediately, it is very short-lived, lasting only as long as the antibodies circulate in the blood system. **Passive immunity** is usually not very specific. **Gamma globulin**, the fraction of the blood containing a wide variety of antibodies, can be used to confer temporary protection against hepatitis and other diseases by passive immunity.

Rejection of transplants

Transplanted tissues or organs are detected as foreign bodies by the recipient's immune system. The resulting immune response can cause the transplant to be **rejected**. Immunosuppressing drugs can be used to lower the immune response to transplants and decrease the likelihood of rejection.

ABO blood types

Erythrocytes have characteristic cell-surface proteins (**antigens**). Antigens are macromolecules that are foreign to the host organism and trigger an immune response. The two major groups of red blood cell antigens are the **ABO group** and the **Rh factor**.

Blood Type	Antigen	Antibody	Can Donate To	Can Receive From
A	A	anti-B	A and AB	A and O
B	B	anti-A	B and AB	B and O
AB	A and B	none	AB only	universal acceptor
O	none	anti-A and anti-B	all (universal donor)	O only

Type A blood has the A antigen present. It is extremely important during blood transfusions that **donor** and **recipient** blood types be appropriately matched. The aim is to avoid transfusion of red blood cells that will be clumped ("rejected") by antibodies (proteins in the immune system that bind specifically to antigens) present in the recipient's plasma. The rule of blood matching is as follows: if the donor's antigens are already in the recipient's blood, no clumping occurs. **Type AB** blood is termed the "**universal recipient**," as it has neither anti-A nor anti-B antibodies. **Type O** blood is considered to be the "**universal donor**"; it will not elicit a response from the recipient's immune system because it does not possess any surface antigens.

Rh factor

The Rh factor is another antigen that may be present on the surface of red blood cells. Individuals may be Rh+, possessing the Rh antigen, or Rh–, lacking the Rh antigen. Consideration of the Rh factor is particularly important during **pregnancy**. An Rh– woman can be sensitized by an **Rh+ fetus** if fetal red blood cells (which will have the Rh factor) enter maternal circulation during birth. If this woman subsequently carries another Rh+ fetus, the anti-Rh antibodies she produced when sensitized by the first birth may cross the placenta and destroy fetal red blood cells. This results in a severe anemia for the fetus, known as **erythroblastosis fetalis**. Erythroblastosis is not caused by ABO blood-type mismatches between mother and fetus because anti-A and anti-B antibodies cannot cross the placenta.

TRANSPORT SYSTEMS IN PLANTS

Transport systems in plants must supply plant cells with nutrients and remove waste products. In plants, circulation is called **translocation**. The plant **stem** is the primary organ of transport in the plant. **Vascular bundles** run up and down the stem. The vascular bundle at the center of the stem contains xylem, phloem, and cambium cells.

Xylem

Xylem cells are **thick-walled**, often hollow cells located on the **inside** of the vascular bundle (towards the center of the stem). They carry water and minerals up the plant, and their thick walls give the plant its rigid support. Older xylem cells die and form the heartwood used for lumber. The outer layer of xylem is alive and is called the **sapwood**. Two types of xylem cells have been differentiated: **vessel cells** and **tracheids**. The rise of water in the xylem is explained by the following:

- **Transpiration pull**—As water evaporates from the leaves of plants, a vacuum is created that pulls water up the stem.
- **Capillary action**—Any liquid in a thin tube will rise because of the surface tension of the liquid and interactions between the liquid and the tube.
- **Root pressure**—Water entering the root hairs exerts a pressure that pushes water up the stem.

Phloem

Phloem cells are **thin-walled** cells on the **outside** of the vascular bundle. They usually transport nutrients (especially carbohydrates produced in the leaves) down the stem. The phloem cells are living and include **sieve tube cells** and **companion cells**. If a tree is girdled by removing a strip of bark around the trunk, the phloem connections are severed, and the tree will die.

Cambium

Cambium cells (two layers thick) are the actively dividing, undifferentiated cells that give rise to xylem and phloem. They are found between the xylem and phloem cell layers; as they divide, the cells near the phloem differentiate into phloem cells, and the cells near the xylem differentiate into xylem cells.

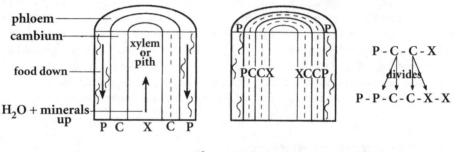

Figure 11.8

Gross structure of a woody stem

Proceeding from the outside inwards, the following layers occur: epidermis (outer-bark), cortex, phloem, cambium, xylem, and pith (tissue involved in storage of nutrients and plant support). The phloem, cambium, and xylem layers are known as the **fibrovascular bundle**.

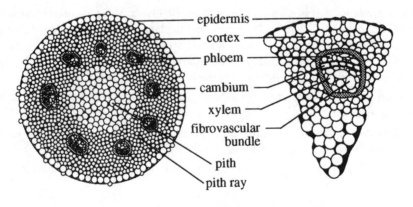

Figure 11.9

Root

The root functions to **absorb** materials through the root hairs and anchor the plant. Some roots provide storage for energy reserves (such as turnips and carrots). **Root hairs** are specialized cells of the root epidermis with thin-walled projections. They increase the surface area for absorption of water and minerals from the soil. Like the stem, the root has the following layers: epidermis, cortex, phloem, xylem, and cambium. The epidermis contains the root hair cells.

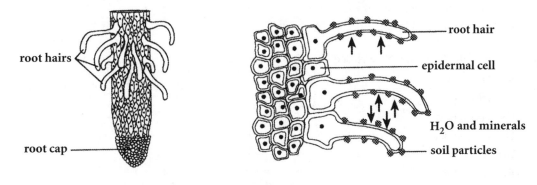

Figure 11.10

Regions of growth in the plant

Meristem refers to the actively dividing, undifferentiated cells of a plant. **Cambium,** lying between the phloem and xylem, is a type of meristem called lateral meristem. It provides for lateral growth of the stem by adding to the phloem or xylem (i.e., growth in diameter). **Apical meristem** is also located at the tips of roots and stems where division leads to increase in length. After actively dividing, the new cells elongate (zone of elongation) and finally differentiate into one of the many specialized cells of the plants.

REVIEW PROBLEMS

1. Erythrocytes are anaerobic. Why is this advantageous for the organism?

2. The lymphatic system
   (A) transports hormones throughout the body.
   (B) transports absorbed chylomicrons to the circulatory system.
   (C) filters the blood.
   (D) does both A and B.

3. Which of the following have closed circulatory systems?
   (A) Humans
   (B) Jellyfish
   (C) Lobsters
   (D) Earthworms
   (E) A and B
   (F) A and D

4. How does water travel upwards in the xylem of plants?

5. Draw the reactions of the clotting process. Include all of the proteins and cofactors involved.

6. What type of cells is responsible for antibody production? How do antibodies combat antigens?

7. What role do the surface proteins on erythrocytes play in blood transfusions?

SOLUTIONS TO REVIEW PROBLEMS

1. If erythrocytes were aerobic, they would use some of the O_2 that they carry for their own energy requirements, thus decreasing the amount of O_2 transported to the rest of the body. Because they are anaerobic, they do not have any O_2 requirements of their own and can deliver all the O_2 they carry to other cells.

2. **B** The main function of the lymphatic system is to collect excess interstitial fluid and return it to the circulatory system, maintaining the balance of body fluids. However, this is not one of the answer choices. A second function of the lymphatic system is to absorb chylomicrons from the small intestine and deliver them to cardiovascular circulation; this is choice (B). Transport of hormones and filtration of blood are not functions of the lymphatic system, so choices (A), (C), and (D) are incorrect.

3. **F** All organisms that have bodies where all cells are not in contact with the external environment require an effective circulatory system. Annelids are the simplest organisms with closed circulatory systems, and all more advanced organisms have closed systems. Arthropods have open circulatory systems in which the blood is not differentiated from the interstitial fluid.

4. There are three explanations for the movement of water against the pull of gravity in the xylem of plants. Transpiration pull occurs when water evaporates from the leaves of plants. Capillary action pulls any liquid up a thin tube. Root pressure is caused by water entering the root hairs and pushing water up the stem.

5. See Figure 11.7

6. Antibodies are produced by plasma cells derived from B lymphocytes. Antibodies recognize and bind to specific antigens, tagging them so that they are easily recognized by phagocytic cells. Antibodies can also cause the antigens to agglutinate and form insoluble complexes, which facilitate their removal.

7. In a blood transfusion, the donor blood must be carefully matched with the blood of the recipient. If the erythrocytes in the donor blood have a different class of surface proteins (antigens) than the recipient's erythrocytes, the recipient's immune system might "attack" the surface protein of the donor, thus rejecting the donor blood. For example, if the donor blood is type A and the recipient blood is type B, the recipient's anti-A antibodies would attack the donor's erythrocytes, because type A blood has type A antigens.

CHAPTER TWELVE

Endocrinology

CHEMICAL REGULATION IN ANIMALS

The endocrine system acts as a means of internal communication, coordinating the activities of the organ systems. Endocrine glands synthesize and secrete chemical substances called **hormones** directly into the circulatory system. (In contrast, **exocrine glands**, such as the gall bladder, secrete substances that are transported by ducts.)

Glands that synthesize or secrete hormones include the pituitary, hypothalamus, thyroid, parathyroids, adrenals, pancreas, testes, ovaries, pineal, kidneys, gastrointestinal glands, heart, and thymus. Some hormones regulate a single type of cell or organ, whereas others have more widespread actions. The specificity of hormonal action is usually determined by the presence of specific receptors on or in the target cells.

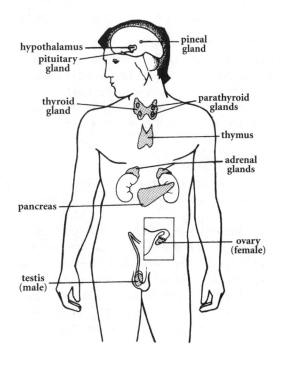

Figure 12.1

Adrenal Glands

The adrenal glands are situated on top of the kidneys and consist of the adrenal cortex and the adrenal medulla.

Adrenal cortex

In response to stress, the adrenocorticotropic hormone (ACTH) which is produced by the anterior pituitary, stimulates the adrenal cortex to produce more than two dozen different steroid hormones, collectively known as **adrenocortical steroids**, or simply corticosteroids. In the blood stream, these corticosteroids are bound to transport proteins called **transcortins**. Corticosteroids exert their mechanism of action by determining which genes are transcribed in the nuclei of their target cells and at what particular rate. The subsequent changes in the nature and given concentration of the enzymes will affect cellular metabolism.

- **Glucocorticoids**

  Glucocorticoids, such as **cortisol** and **cortisone**, are involved in glucose regulation and protein metabolism. Glucocorticoids raise blood glucose levels by promoting protein breakdown and **gluconeogenesis** and decreasing protein synthesis. Glucocorticoids increase the plasma glucose levels and are antagonistic to the effects of insulin. As a whole, the glucocorticoids release amino acids from skeletal muscle as well as lipids from adipose tissue. They also promote peripheral use of lipids and have antiinflammatory effects.

- **Mineralocorticoids**

  Mineralocorticoids, particularly **aldosterone**, regulate plasma levels of sodium and potassium and, consequently, the total extracellular water volume. Aldosterone causes active reabsorption of sodium and passive reabsorption of water in the **nephron**. This results in an increase in both blood volume and blood pressure. Excess production of aldosterone results in excess retention of water with resulting hypertension (high blood pressure). The mineralocorticoids are stimulated by angiotensin II and inhibited by ANP.

- **Cortical sex hormones**

  The adrenal cortex secretes small quantities of **androgens** (male sex hormones) like androstenedione and dehydroepiandrosterone in both men and women. Because in men, most of the androgens are produced by the **testes**, the physiologic effect of the adrenal androgens is quite small. In women, however, overproduction of the adrenal androgens may have masculinizing effects, such as excessive facial hair.

Adrenal medulla

The adrenal medulla produces **epinephrine** (adrenaline) and **norepinephrine** (noradrenaline), both of which belong to a class of amino acid-derived compounds called **catecholamines**.

Epinephrine increases the conversion of glycogen to glucose in liver and muscle tissue, causing an increase in blood glucose levels and an increase in the basal metabolic rate. Both epinephrine and norepinephrine increase the rate and strength of the heartbeat and dilate and constrict blood vessels in such a way as to increase the blood supply to skeletal muscles, the heart, and the brain, while decreasing the blood supply to the kidneys, skin, and digestive tract. Both epinephrine and norepinephrine will also promote the release of lipids by adipose tissue. These effects are known as the "fight or flight response" and are elicited by sympathetic nervous stimulation in response to stress.

Epinephrine will inhibit certain vegetative functions, such as digestion, which are not immediately important for survival. Both of these hormones are also **neurotransmitters**. The release of these hormones is stimulated during sympathetic activation by sympathetic preganglionic fibers.

Pituitary Gland

The pituitary (**hypophysis**) is a small, trilobed gland lying at the base of the brain. The two main lobes, anterior and posterior, are functionally distinct. (In humans, the third lobe, the intermediate lobe, is rudimentary.) Specifically, the pituitary gland hangs below the hypothalamus and is connected by a slender cord known as the **infundibulum**.

Anterior pituitary

The anterior pituitary synthesizes both direct hormones, which directly stimulate their target organs, and tropic hormones, which stimulate other endocrine glands to release hormones. The hormonal secretions of the anterior pituitary are regulated by hypothalamic secretions called releasing/inhibiting hormones or factors.

Direct hormones

- **Growth hormone (GH, somatotropin)**

  GH promotes bone and muscle growth. GH also promotes protein synthesis and lipid mobilization and catabolism. In children, a GH deficiency can lead to stunted growth (**dwarfism**), while overproduction of GH results in **gigantism**. Overproduction of GH in adults causes **acromegaly**, a disorder characterized by a disproportionate overgrowth of bone, localized especially in the skull, jaw, feet, and hands.

- **Prolactin**

  Prolactin stimulates milk production and secretion in female mammary glands.

Tropic hormones

- **Adrenocorticotropic hormone (ACTH)**

  ACTH stimulates the adrenal cortex to synthesize and secrete glucocorticoids and is regulated by the releasing hormone corticotrophin-releasing factor (CRF).

- **Thyroid-stimulating hormone (TSH)**

  TSH stimulates the thyroid gland to synthesize and release thyroid hormones, including thyroxin.

- **Luteinizing hormone (LH)**

  In women, LH stimulates ovulation and formation of the **corpus luteum**. LH is also responsible for regulating progesterone secretion in women. In men, LH stimulates the interstitial cells of the testes to synthesize testosterone.

- **Follicle-stimulating hormone (FSH)**

  In women, FSH causes maturation of ovarian follicles that begin secreting estrogen; in men, FSH stimulates maturation of the seminiferous tubules and sperm production.

- **Melanocyte-stimulating hormone (MSH)**

  MSH is secreted by the intermediate lobe of the pituitary. In mammals, the function of MSH is unclear, but in frogs, MSH causes darkening of the skin via induced dispersion of molecules of pigment in melanophore cells.

- **Endorphins**

  These are neurotransmitters that have pain-relieving properties.

Posterior pituitary

The posterior pituitary (**neurohypophysis**) does not synthesize hormones; it stores and releases the peptide hormones **oxytocin** and **ADH**, which are produced by the neurosecretory cells of the hypothalamus. Hormone secretion is stimulated by action potentials descending from the hypothalamus.

- **Oxytocin**

  Oxytocin, which is secreted during childbirth, increases the strength and frequency of uterine muscle contractions. Oxytocin secretion is also induced by suckling; oxytocin stimulates milk secretion in the mammary glands.

- **Antidiuretic hormone (ADH; vasopressin)**

  ADH increases the permeability of the nephron's **collecting duct** to water, thereby promoting water reabsorption and increasing blood volume, which subsequently increases blood pressure. ADH is secreted when plasma osmolarity increases, as sensed by osmoreceptors in the hypothalamus, or when blood volume decreases, as sensed by baroreceptors in the circulatory system.

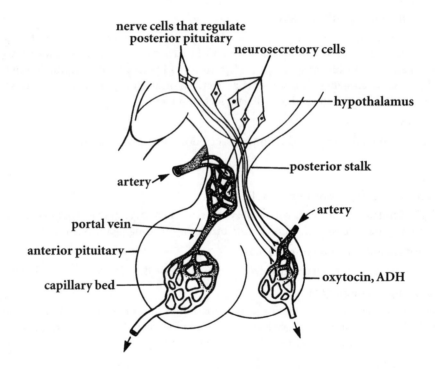

Figure 12.2

Hypothalamus

The hypothalamus is part of the forebrain and is located directly above the pituitary gland. The hypothalamus receives neural transmissions from other parts of the brain and from peripheral nerves that trigger specific responses from its **neurosecretory cells**. The neurosecretory cells regulate pituitary gland secretions via negative feedback mechanisms and through the actions of inhibiting and releasing hormones.

Interactions with anterior pituitary

Hypothalamic-releasing hormones stimulate or inhibit the secretions of the anterior pituitary. For example, GnRH stimulates the anterior pituitary to secrete FSH and LH. Releasing hormones are secreted into the hypothalamic-hypophyseal portal system. In this circulatory pathway, blood from the capillary bed in the hypothalamus flows through a portal vein into the anterior pituitary, where it diverges into a second capillary network. In this way, releasing hormones can immediately reach the anterior pituitary.

A complicated feedback system regulates the secretions of the endocrine system. For example, when the plasma levels of adrenal cortical hormones drop, hypothalamic cells (via a negative feedback mechanism) release ACTH-releasing factor (ACTH-RF) into the portal system. When the plasma concentration of corticosteroids exceeds the normal plasma level, the steroids themselves exert an inhibitory effect on the hypothalamus.

Interactions with the posterior pituitary

Neurosecretory cells in the hypothalamus synthesize both oxytocin and ADH and transport them via their axons into the posterior pituitary for storage and secretion.

Thyroid

Thyroid hormones affect the function of nearly every organ system in the body. In children, thyroid hormones are essential for growth and development; in adults, thyroid hormones are essential for maintenance of metabolic stability. The thyroid hormones, **thyroxine (T4)** and **triiodothyronine (T3)** are formed on the glycoprotein **thyroglobulin**, which is synthesized in the thyroid cell. Because of the specific tertiary structure of this glycoprotein, iodinated tyrosine residues present in thyroglobulin are able to bind together to form active thyroid hormones. With respect to thyroid hormone characteristics, the following principles apply:

- T3 is five times more potent that T4.
- T4 and T3 are transported in the blood by the proteins TBG, TBPA, and albumin. Approximately 99.5 percent of these hormones are bound to these proteins. Note: Only an unbound hormone is able to enter a cell and elicit a cellular response.
- All of the T4 in the body is formed and secreted by the thyroid gland; however, only 20 percent of T3 is produced by the thyroid gland.
- The majority of T3 is produced by the conversion of T4 to T3 by the enzyme 5'—monodeiodase found primarily in the peripheral tissues.

Thyroid hormones (thyroxine and triiodothyronine)

Thyroxine (T_4) and triiodothyronine (T_3) are derived from the iodination of the amino acid **tyrosine**. Thyroid hormones are necessary for growth and neurological development in children. They increase the rate of metabolism throughout the body.

In **hypothyroidism**, thyroid hormones are undersecreted or not secreted at all. Common symptoms of hypothyroidism include a slowed heart rate and respiratory rate, fatigue, cold intolerance, and weight gain. Hypothyroidism in newborn infants, called **cretinism**, is characterized by mental retardation and short stature. In **hyperthyroidism**, the thyroid is overstimulated, resulting in the oversecretion of thyroid hormones. Symptoms often include increased metabolic rate, feelings of excessive warmth, profuse sweating, palpitations, weight loss, and protruding eyes. In both disorders, the thyroid often enlarges, forming a bulge in the neck called a goiter.

Calcitonin

Calcitonin decreases plasma Ca^{2+} concentration by inhibiting the release of Ca^{2+} from bone. Calcitonin secretion is regulated by plasma Ca^{2+} levels. Calcitonin is antagonistic to the parathyroid hormone.

Pancreas

The pancreas is both an **exocrine** organ and an **endocrine** organ. The exocrine function is performed by the cells that secrete digestive enzymes into the small intestine via a series of ducts. The endocrine function is performed by small glandular structures called the **islets of Langerhans**, which are composed of alpha and beta cells. Alpha cells produce and secrete glucagon; beta cells produce and secrete insulin.

- **Glucagon** stimulates protein and fat degradation, the conversion of glycogen to glucose, and gluconeogenesis, all of which serve to increase blood glucose levels. Glucagon's actions are largely antagonistic to those of insulin.

- **Insulin** is a protein hormone secreted in response to a high blood glucose concentration. It stimulates the uptake of glucose by muscle and adipose cells and the storage of glucose as glycogen in muscle and liver cells, thus lowering blood glucose levels. It also stimulates the synthesis of fats from glucose and the uptake of amino acids. Insulin's actions are antagonistic to those of **glucagon** and the **glucocorticoids**. Underproduction of insulin, or an insensitivity to insulin, leads to **diabetes mellitus**, which is characterized by hyperglycemia (high blood glucose levels). Diabetes is the most common endocrine disorder and is characterized by long-term complications involving the eyes, nerves, kidneys, and blood vessels. On the next page is a table differentiating between Type I and Type II diabetes.

Distinguishing Characteristics	Type I	Type II
% Diabetics	10	90
Age onset	Usually <30	Usually >30
Pathogenesis	Presence of islet cell antibodies	
	Autoimmune	Resistance to insulin
	Decreased insulin secretion	Hepatic glucose production
Plasma insulin	Usually none	Low, normal, or high: etiology dependent
Family history	Usually none	Strong
Obesity	Uncommon	Common

Parathyroid Glands

The parathyroid glands are four small, pea-shaped structures embedded in the posterior surface of the thyroid. These glands synthesize and secrete **parathyroid hormone (PTH)**, which regulates plasma Ca^{2+} concentration. PTH raises the Ca^{2+} concentration in the blood by stimulating Ca^{2+} release from the bone and decreasing Ca^{2+} excretion in the kidneys. Calcium in bone is bonded to phosphate, and breakdown of the bone releases phosphate as well as calcium. Parathyroid hormone compensates for this by stimulating excretion of phosphate by the kidneys.

Kidneys

When blood volume falls, the kidneys produce **renin**—an enzyme that converts the plasma protein angiotensinogen to angiotensin I. Angiotensin I is converted to angiotensin II, which stimulates the adrenal cortex to secrete **aldosterone**. Aldosterone helps to restore blood volume by increasing sodium reabsorption at the kidney, leading to an increase in water. This removes the initial stimulus for renin production. The kidneys also produce **erythropoietin (EPO)**. EPO is a glycoprotein that stimulates red blood cell production; it is normally produced in the kidneys. This hormone causes the following:

- Stimulation of the stem cells to differentiate into rubriblasts (least mature erythrocyte)
- Increased rate of mitosis
- Increased release of reticulocytes from the bone marrow
- Increased hemoglobin (HgB) formation, which allows the critical HgB concentration necessary for maturity to be reached at a more rapid rate

Gastrointestinal Hormones

Ingested food stimulates the stomach to release the hormone gastrin. **Gastrin** is carried to the gastric glands and stimulates the glands to secrete HCl in response to food in the stomach. Secretion of pancreatic juice, or the exocrine secretion of the pancreas, is also under hormonal control; the hormone **secretin** is released by the small intestine when acidic food material enters from the stomach. Secretin stimulates the secretion of an alkaline bicarbonate solution from the pancreas that neutralizes the acidity of the **chyme** (partially digested food coming from the stomach). The hormone **cholecystokinin** is released from the small intestine in response to the presence of fats and causes the contraction of the gallbladder and release of bile into the small intestine. **Bile** is involved in the digestion of fats.

Pineal Gland

The pineal gland is a tiny structure at the base of the brain that secretes the hormone **melatonin**. The role of melatonin in humans is unclear, but it is believed to play a role in the regulation of **circadian rhythms**—physiological cycles lasting 24 hours. Melatonin secretion is regulated by light and dark cycles in the environment. In primitive vertebrates, melatonin lightens the skin by concentrating pigment granules in melanophores. (Melatonin is an antagonist to MSH.)

MECHANISM OF HORMONE ACTION

Hormones are classified on the basis of their chemical structure into two major groups: peptide hormones and steroid hormones. There are two ways in which hormones affect the activities of their target cells: via extracellular receptors or intracellular receptors.

Peptides

Peptide hormones range from simple short peptides (amino acid chains), such as ADH, to complex polypeptides, such as insulin. Peptide hormones act as first messengers. Their binding to **specific receptors** on the surface of their target cells triggers a series of enzymatic reactions within each cell, the first of which may be the conversion of ATP to cyclic adenosine monophosphate (cAMP); this reaction is catalyzed by the membrane-bound enzyme adenylate cyclase. **Cyclic AMP** acts as a **second messenger,** relaying messages from the extracellular peptide hormone to cytoplasmic enzymes and initiating a series of successive reactions in the cell. This is an example of a **cascade effect**; with each step, the hormone's effects are amplified. Cyclic AMP activity is inactivated by the cytoplasmic enzyme phosphodiesterase.

Steroids

Steroid hormones, such as estrogen and aldosterone, belong to a class of lipid-derived molecules with a characteristic ring structure. They are produced by the testes, ovaries, placenta, and adrenal cortex. Because they are lipid soluble, steroid hormones enter their target cells directly and bind to specific receptor proteins in the cytoplasm. This receptor-hormone complex enters the nucleus and directly activates the expression of specific genes by binding to receptors on the chromatin. This induces a change in mRNA transcription and protein synthesis.

REGULATION IN PLANTS

Plant hormones are primarily involved in the regulation of growth. They are produced by actively growing parts of the plant, such as the **meristematic tissues** in the apical region (apical meristem) of shoots and roots. They are also produced in young, growing leaves and developing seeds.

Auxins

Auxins are an important class of plant hormones associated with several types of growth patterns.

Auxins are responsible for **phototropism**, which is the tendency of the shoots of plants to bend towards light sources (particularly the sun). When light strikes the tip of a plant from one side, the auxin supply on that side is **reduced**. Thus, the illuminated side of the plant grows more slowly than the shaded side. This asymmetrical growth in the cells of the stem causes the plant to bend towards the light side. **Indole-acetic** acid is one of the auxins associated with phototropism.

Geotropism is the growth of portions of plants toward or away from gravity.

- **Negative geotropism** causes shoots to grow upward, away from the acceleration of gravity. If a plant is turned on its side (horizontally), the shoot will eventually turn upward again. Gravity increases the concentration of auxin on the lower side of the horizontally placed plant, whereas the concentration on the upper side decreases. This unequal distribution of auxins stimulates cells on the lower side to elongate faster than cells on the upper side, causing the plant to grow vertically.
- **Positive geotropism** causes roots to grow towards the pull of gravity. Horizontally placed roots have the same auxin distribution as horizontally placed stems, but the effect on the root cells is opposite. Cells exposed to a higher concentration of auxin are inhibited from growing, whereas the cells on the upper side continue to grow. This causes the root to turn downwards.

Auxins produced in the terminal bud of a plant's growing tip move downward in the shoot and inhibit development of lateral buds. Auxins also initiate the formation of lateral roots, while they inhibit root elongation.

Gibberellins

Gibberellins stimulate rapid stem elongation, particularly in plants that normally do not grow tall (e.g., dwarf plants). They inhibit the formation of new roots and stimulate the production of new phloem cells by the cambium (whereas auxins stimulate the production of new xylem cells). Gibberellins also terminate the dormancy of seeds and buds. They induce some biennial plants to flower during their first year of growth.

Kinins

Kinins also promote cell division. Kinetin is an important type of cytokinin. The ratio of kinetin to auxin is of particular importance in the determination of the timing of the differentiation of new cells. The action of kinetin is enhanced when auxin is present.

Ethylene

Ethylene stimulates fruit ripening. Ethylene also induces senescence or aging.

Inhibitors

Inhibitors block cell division and serve an important role in growth regulation. They are particularly important to the maintenance of dormancy in the lateral buds and seeds of plants during autumn and winter. Inhibitors break down gradually with time (and in some cases are destroyed by cold) so buds and seeds can become active in the next growing season. Abscisic acid is one of the most important inhibitors.

Antiauxins

Antiauxins regulate the activity of auxins. For example, indoleacetic acid oxidase regulates the concentration of indoleacetic acid. An increase in the concentration of indoleacetic acid increases the amount of indoleacetic acid oxidase produced.

REVIEW PROBLEMS

1. Name the different parts of the adrenal gland and the hormones secreted from each.

2. Discuss the relationship between the hypothalamus and the pituitary gland.

3. Increased activity of the parathyroid gland leads to
   - **(A)** a decrease in blood glucose levels.
   - **(B)** an increase in metabolic rate.
   - **(C)** a decrease in body temperature.
   - **(D)** a decrease in the rate of bone resorption.
   - **(E)** an increase in blood Ca^{2+} concentrations.

4. Which of the following statements concerning growth hormone is NOT true?
   - **(A)** Overproduction of growth hormone in children results in gigantism.
   - **(B)** Overproduction of growth hormone in adults results in acromegaly.
   - **(C)** A deficiency of growth hormone results in dwarfism.
   - **(D)** It promotes growth of bone and muscle.
   - **(E)** It is secreted by the hypothalamus.

5. Describe the regulation of plasma Ca^{2+} concentration. Include all of the hormones and organs involved.

6. Thyroid hormone deficiency may result in
   - **(A)** acromegaly.
   - **(B)** cretinism.
   - **(C)** gigantism.
   - **(D)** hyperthyroidism.

7. Match the following hormones with their respective functions

    (A) growth hormone   1.   promotes growth of muscle

    (B) ACTH   2.   stimulates the release of glucose into the blood

    (C) oxytocin   3.   prepares the uterus for implantation of a fertilized egg

    (D) progesterone   4.   stimulates the secretion of glucocorticoids

    (E) aldosterone   5.   increases the rate of metabolism

    (F) glucagon   6.   induces water reabsorption in the kidneys

    (G) thyroxine   7.   increases uterine contractions during childbirth

8. What is negative feedback?

9. Why is the level of blood glucose so important? What hormones are involved in the regulation of blood glucose levels?

10. Destruction of all beta cells in the pancreas would cause

    (A) glucagon secretion to stop and a decrease in blood glucose.
    (B) glucagon secretion to stop and an increase in blood glucose.
    (C) insulin secretion to stop and an increase in blood glucose.
    (D) insulin secretion to stop and a decrease in blood glucose.

11. A man trapped for three days underneath the ruins of a collapsed building was rescued and rushed to the nearest hospital. He suffered from internal bleeding and was very dehydrated. Why was a high level of aldosterone found in his blood?

12. Oxytocin and vasopressin are

    (A) produced and released by the hypothalamus.
    (B) produced and released by the pituitary.
    (C) produced by the hypothalamus and released by the pituitary.
    (D) produced by the pituitary and released by the hypothalamus.

13. Explain negative geotropism.

SOLUTIONS TO REVIEW PROBLEMS

1. The adrenal gland is divided into the adrenal cortex and the adrenal medulla. The adrenal cortex secretes steroid hormones called mineralocorticoids (e.g., aldosterone) as well as glucocorticoids (e.g., cortisol). The adrenal medulla secretes the catecholamines norepinephrine and epinephrine, which are amino acid derivatives.

2. The posterior pituitary stores and secretes hormones produced by the neurosecretory cells of the hypothalamus. In contrast, the anterior pituitary produces hormones whose secretions are regulated by hypothalamic releasing hormones. Hypothalamic releasing hormones stimulate the anterior pituitary to secrete a particular hormone, whereas hypothalamic inhibiting hormones inhibit anterior pituitary secretions. The releasing and inhibiting hormones are secreted into a circulatory pathway known as the hypothalamic-hypophyseal portal system.

3. **E** Discussed in section on parathyroid glands.

4. **E** Discussed in section on hormones of the anterior pituitary.

5. Calcium levels in the blood are regulated by two hormones—calcitonin and parathyroid hormone (PTH). Calcitonin is secreted by the thyroid gland when plasma Ca^{2+} levels are high and decreases the plasma Ca^{2+} concentration by inhibiting bone resorption (which releases Ca^{2+} into the blood). When plasma Ca^{2+} levels are low, PTH is secreted by the parathyroid glands. PTH increases plasma Ca2+ concentration by increasing bone resorption, increasing Ca^{2+} reabsorption in the kidney (thus reducing the amount of Ca^{2+} excreted in the urine), and stimulating the conversion of vitamin D into its active form (1,25-dihydroxycholecalciferol), which increases intestinal absorption of Ca^{2+}.

6. **B** Discussed in section on thyroid gland.

7. **A** 1

    B 4

    C 7

    D 3

    E 6

    F 2

    G 5

8. Negative feedback is a means of regulation whereby an end-product inhibits one or more of the earlier steps that lead to its production or secretion. For example, high plasma levels of thyroxine inhibit the pituitary gland from secreting TSH, thus removing the stimulus on the thyroid to secrete more thyroxine. Negative feedback mechanisms are also used by the body to regulate enzyme production and activity.

9. Glucose is the primary source of energy used by cells during aerobic respiration, so blood glucose levels determine the amount of energy available for cellular activity. Many hormones involved in the regulation of blood glucose levels do so by stimulating the liver either to store or release glucose. When glucose levels are low, the adrenal medulla secretes epinephrine, which stimulates the liver to convert glycogen stores into glucose and release it into the blood. Epinephrine also acts on muscles, transforming their glycogen stores into lactic acid, which is transported to the liver and converted to glucose. The pancreas secretes glucagon, which also stimulates the liver to convert glycogen to glucose. When additional glucose is needed, the adrenal cortex secretes glucocorticoids, which stimulate the liver to synthesize glucose from noncarbohydrates in a process called gluconeogenesis. Insulin is antagonistic to glucagon, epinephrine, and glucocorticoids; it lowers blood glucose levels by stimulating the uptake of glucose by adipose and muscle tissue and by promoting the conversion of glucose into glycogen in liver and muscle cells.

10. **C** Discussed in section on endocrine functions of the pancreas.

11. Internal bleeding leads to a decrease in the volume of blood in the circulatory system. Aldosterone causes increased water reabsorption in the nephrons, leading to an increase in blood volume. Thus, the man's body responded to the blood loss by secreting aldosterone.

12. **C** Discussed in section on anterior pituitary.

13. Gravity increases the concentration of auxin on the lower side of a plant. The auxin stimulates the cells on the lower side to elongate faster, causing the plant to grow vertically.

CHAPTER THIRTEEN

Neuroscience

The **nervous system** includes all of the neural tissues in the body. Neural tissue, with supporting blood vessels and connective tissue, are the components of the nervous system, such as the brain, spinal cord, as well as complex sensory organs like the eye and ear. The two major divisions of the nervous system are the central nervous system (CNS) and the peripheral nervous system (PNS). In general, the nervous system enables organisms to receive and respond to **stimuli** from their external and internal environments. **Neurons** are the functional units of the nervous system. A neuron converts stimuli into **electrochemical signals** that are conducted through the nervous system. The nervous system responds to stimuli more rapidly than the endocrine system.

NEURON

Structure

The neuron is an elongated cell consisting of several **dendrites**, a **cell body**, and a single **axon. Dendrites** are cytoplasmic extensions that receive information and transmit it toward the cell body. The cell body (**soma**) contains the nucleus and controls the metabolic activity of the neuron. The **axon** is a long cellular process that transmits impulses away from the cell body. Most mammalian axons are sheathed by an insulating substance known as myelin, which allows axons to conduct impulses faster. Myelin is produced by cells known as glial cells. (**Oligodendrocytes** produce myelin in the central nervous system, and **Schwann cells** produce myelin in the peripheral nervous system.) The gaps between segments of myelin are called **nodes of Ranvier**. The axons end as swellings known as synaptic terminals (sometimes also called synaptic buttons or knobs). **Neurotransmitters** are released from these terminals into the **synapse** (or synaptic cleft), which is the gap between the axon terminals of one cell and the dendrites of the next cell. Axons traveling from the spine to the tip of the foot may be very long.

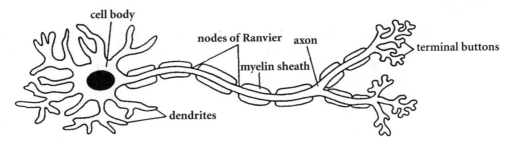

Figure 13.1

There are four major types of cells in the CNS and two major types in the PNS. Here is a summary table of each cell type and function.

Cells in the CNS and PNS	
Cell type	Cell function
CNS	
Astrocytes	Maintain the integrity of the blood brain barrier, regulate nutrient and dissolved gas concentrations, and absorb and recycle neurotransmitters.
Oligodendrocytes	Myelinate CNS axons as well as provide structural framework for the CNS.
Microglia	Remove cellular debris and pathogens.
Ependymal cells	Line the brain ventricles and aid in the production, circulation, and monitoring of cerebral spinal fluid.
PNS	
Satellite cells	Surround the neuron cell bodies in the ganglia.
Schwann cells	Enclose the axons in the PNS and aid in the myelination of some peripheral axons.

Table 13.1

Norepinephrine and **acetylcholine** are two neurotransmitters often found in the nervous system. Here is a summary on the production of these neurotransmitters. When norepinephrine is synthesized, its immediate precursor is dopamine. The synthesis of norepinephrine begins in the axoplasm of the terminal nerve endings of adrenergic fibers. However, its synthesis is completed inside the vesicles of these fibers. The basic steps in the synthesis of norepinephrine are as follows. Tyrosine is converted to DOPA through the process of hydroxylation, and then DOPA undergoes decarboxylation to become dopamine. Dopamine is then transported into the vesicles of the adrenergic fibers where it undergoes hydroxylation to become norepinephrine. In the adrenal medulla, norepinephrine is transformed into epinephrine through the process of methylation. Choline is combined with Acetyl-CoA to become acetylcholine.

Function

Neurons are specialized to receive signals from sensory receptors or from other neurons in the body and transfer this information along the length of the axon. Impulses, known as **action potentials**, travel the length of the axon and invade the nerve terminal, thereby causing the release of neurotransmitter into the synapse. When a neuron is at rest, the potential difference between the extracellular space and the intracellular space is called the resting potential.

Resting potential

Even at rest, a neuron is **polarized**. This potential difference is the result of an unequal distribution of ions between the inside and outside of the cell. A typical resting membrane potential is **–70 millivolts** (mV), which means that the inside of the neuron is more negative than the outside. This difference is caused by selective ionic permeability of the neuronal cell membrane and is maintained by the **active transport** by the Na^+/K^+ pump (also called the Na^+/K^+ ATPase).

The concentration of K^+ is higher inside the neuron than outside; the concentration of Na^+ is higher outside than inside. Additionally, negatively charged proteins are trapped inside of the cell. The resting potential is created because the neuron is **selectively permeable** to K^+, so K^+ diffuses down its concentration gradient, leaving a net negative charge inside. (Neurons are **impermeable** to Na^+, so the cell remains polarized.)

Because the transmission of action potentials lead to the disruption of the ionic gradients, the gradients must be restored by the Na^+/K^+ pump. This pump, using ATP energy, transports 3 Na^+ out for every 2 K^+ it transports into the cell.

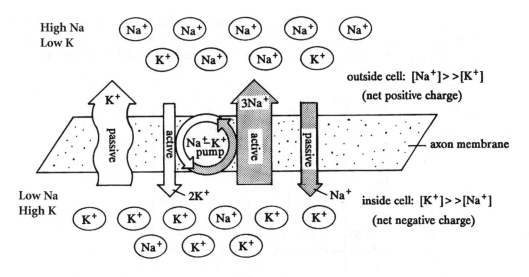

Figure 13.2

Action potential

The nerve cell body receives both excitatory and inhibitory impulses from other cells. If the cell becomes sufficiently excited or depolarized (i.e., the inside of the cell becomes less negative), an **action potential** is generated. The minimum threshold membrane potential (usually around −50 mV) is the level at which an action potential is initiated. Depolarization occurs during phase I, repolarization occurs during phase II, and hyperpolarization occurs during phase III. Figure 13.3 depicts this process.

Ion channels located in the nerve cell membrane open in response to these changes in voltage and are therefore called voltage-gated ion channels. An action potential begins when **voltage-gated Na⁺ channels** open in response to **depolarization**, allowing Na⁺ to rush down its electrochemical gradient into the cell, causing a rapid further depolarization of that segment of the cell. The voltage-gated Na⁺ channels then close, and **voltage-gated K⁺ channels** open, allowing K⁺ to rush out down its electrochemical gradient. This returns the cell to a more negative potential, a process known as **repolarization**. In fact, the neuron may shoot past the resting potential and become even more negative inside than normal; this is called hyperpolarization. Immediately after an action potential, it may be very difficult or impossible to initiate another action potential; this period of time is called the **refractory period**.

The action potential is often described as an **all-or-none response.** This means that whenever the threshold membrane potential is reached, an action potential with a consistent size and duration is produced. The nerve fires maximally, or not at all. Stimulus intensity is coded by the **frequency** of action potentials.

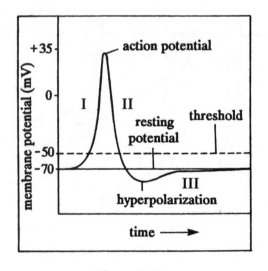

Figure 13.3

Impulse propagation

Although axons can theoretically propagate action potentials bidirectionally, information transfer will occur only in one direction: from dendrite to synaptic terminal. (This is because synapses operate only in one direction and because refractory periods make the backward travel of action potentials impossible.) Different axons can propagate action potentials at **different speeds**. The greater the **diameter** of the axon and the more heavily it is **myelinated**, the faster the impulses will travel. Myelin increases the conduction velocity by insulating segments of the axon, so that the membrane is permeable to ions only in the nodes of Ranvier. In this way, the action potential "jumps" from node to node.

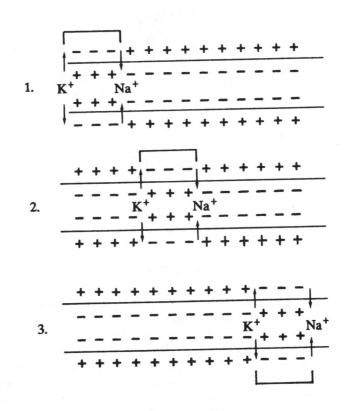

Figure 13.4

Synapse

The synapse is the gap between the **axon terminal** of one neuron (called the presynaptic neuron because it is before the synapse) and the **dendrites** of another neuron (**postsynaptic neuron**). Neurons may also communicate with postsynaptic cells other than neurons, such as cells in muscles or glands; these are called **effector cells**. The nerve terminal contains thousands of membrane-bound vesicles full of chemical messengers known as **neurotransmitters**. When the action potential arrives at the nerve terminal and depolarizes it, the synaptic vesicles fuse with the presynaptic membrane and release neurotransmitter into the synapse. The neurotransmitter **diffuses** across the synapse and acts on receptor proteins embedded in the postsynaptic membrane. The neurotransmitter will lead to depolarization of the post synaptic cell and consequent firing of an action potential. Neurotransmitter is removed from the synapse in a variety of ways: it may be taken back up into the nerve terminal (via a protein known as an uptake carrier) where it may be reused or degraded; it may be degraded by enzymes located in the synapse (e.g., **acetylcholinesterase** inactivates the neurotransmitter **acetylcholine**); it may simply diffuse out of the synapse.

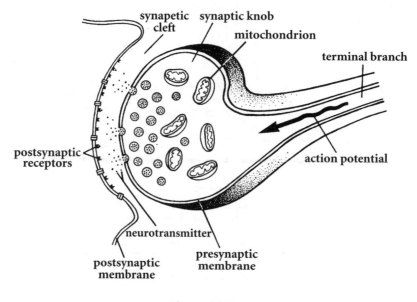

Figure 13.5

When a nerve impulse reaches the neuromuscular junction, several hundred vesicles of acetylcholine are released from the nerve terminal into the synaptic cleft. As the action potential spreads over the nerve terminal, calcium channels open that allows large quantities of calcium to diffuse into the interior of the terminal. These calcium ions exert attractive forces on the acetylcholine vesicles and draw them to the neural membrane. Some of these vesicles will fuse with the neural membrane, emptying their acetylcholine into the synaptic cleft by the process of exocytosis. Sodium is involved in the propagation of the action potential; however, it is not responsible for the release of acetylcholine by the nerve terminal into the synaptic cleft.

Effects of drugs

- **Curare** blocks the postsynaptic acetylcholine receptors so that acetylcholine is unable to interact with the receptor. This leads to paralysis by blocking nerve impulses to muscles.
- **Botulism toxin** prevents the release of acetylcholine from the presynaptic membrane and also results in paralysis.
- **Anticholinesterases** are used as nerve gases and in the insecticide Parathion. As the name implies, these substances inhibit the activity of the **acetylcholinesterase** enzyme. As a result the acetylcholine is not degraded in the synapse and continues to affect the postsynaptic membrane. Therefore, no coordinated muscular contractions can take place.

INVERTEBRATE NERVOUS SYSTEMS

Protozoa

Unicellular organisms possess no organized nervous system. The single-celled organisms may respond to stimuli such as touch, heat, light and chemicals.

Cnidaria

Cnidarians have a simple nervous system called a **nerve net**. This network of nerve cells may have limited centralization. Some jellyfish have clusters of cells and pathways that coordinate the relatively complex movements required for swimming.

Annelida

Earthworms possesses a primitive central nervous system consisting of a defined ventral nerve cord and an anterior "brain" of fused ganglia (i.e., clusters of nerve cell bodies). Definite nerve pathways lead from receptors to effectors.

Arthropoda

Arthropod brains are similar to those of annelids, but more specialized sense organs are present (e.g., compound or simple eyes, tympanum for detecting sound).

VERTEBRATE NERVOUS SYSTEM

There are many different kinds of neurons in the vertebrate nervous system. Neurons that carry **sensory** information about the external or internal environment to the brain or spinal cord are called **afferent neurons**. Neurons that carry motor commands from the brain or spinal cord to various parts of the body (e.g., muscles or glands) are called **efferent neurons**. Some neurons (**interneurons**) participate only in local circuits, linking sensory and motor neurons in the brain and spinal cord; their cell bodies and their nerve terminals are in the same location.

Nerves are essentially **bundles of axons** covered with connective tissue. A network of nerve fibers is called a **plexus**. Neuronal cell bodies often cluster together: such clusters are called **ganglia** in the periphery; in the central nervous system, they are called **nuclei**. The nervous system itself is divided into two major systems: the central nervous system and the peripheral nervous system.

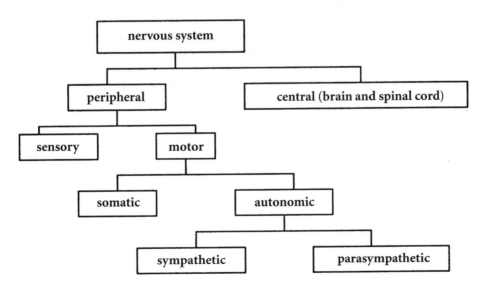

Figure 13.6

Central Nervous System

The CNS consists of the brain and spinal cord.

Brain

The brain is a mass of neurons that resides in the skull. Its functions include interpreting sensory information, forming motor plans, and cognitive function (thinking). The brain consists of an outer portion called the gray matter (cell bodies) and an inner white matter (myelinated axons). The brain can be divided into the forebrain, midbrain, and hindbrain.

Prosencephalon

- The **forebrain** consists of the **telencephalon** and the **diencephalon**. A major component of the telencephalon is the **cerebral cortex**, which is the highly convoluted gray matter that can be seen on the surface of the brain. The cortex processes and integrates sensory input and motor responses and is important for memory and creative thought. The **olfactory bulb** is the center for reception and integration of olfactory input.

  The diencephalon contains the thalamus and hypothalamus. The thalamus is a relay and integration center for the spinal cord and cerebral cortex. The hypothalamus controls visceral functions such as hunger, thirst, sex drive, water balance, blood pressure, and temperature regulation. It also plays an important role in the control of the endocrine system.

Mesencephalon

- The **midbrain** is a relay center for visual and auditory impulses. It also plays an important role in motor control.

Rhombencephalon

- The **hindbrain** is the **posterior** part of the brain and consists of the cerebellum, the pons, and the medulla. The **cerebellum** helps to modulate motor impulses initiated by the cerebral cortex and is important in the maintenance of balance, hand-eye coordination, and the timing of rapid movements. One function of the **pons** is to act as a relay center to allow the cortex to communicate with the cerebellum. The **medulla** (also called the medulla oblongata) controls many vital functions such as breathing, heart rate, and gastrointestinal activity. Together, the midbrain, pons, and medulla constitute the **brainstem**.

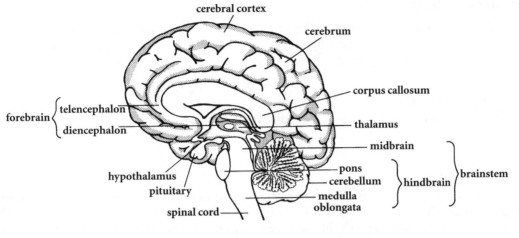

Figure 13.7

Spinal cord

The spinal cord is an elongated extension of the brain which acts as the conduit for sensory information to the brain and motor information from the brain. The spinal cord can also integrate simple motor responses (e.g., **reflexes**) by itself. A cross-section of the spinal cord reveals an outer white matter area containing motor and sensory axons and an inner gray matter area containing nerve cell bodies. Sensory information enters the spinal cord through the **dorsal horn**; the cell bodies of these sensory neurons are located in the dorsal root ganglia. All motor information exits the spinal cord through the **ventral horn**. For simple reflexes like the knee-jerk reflex, sensory fibers (entering through the dorsal root ganglion) synapse directly on ventral horn motor fibers. Other reflexes include interneurons between the sensory and motor fibers that allow for some processing in the spinal cord.

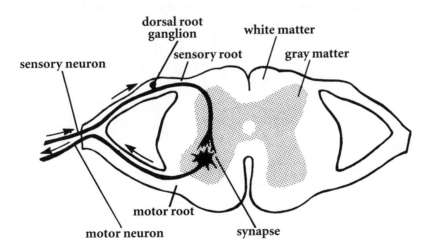

Figure 13.8

Peripheral Nervous Systems

The PNS consists of nerves and ganglia. The sensory nerves that enter the CNS and the motor nerves that leave the CNS are part of the peripheral nervous system. The PNS has two primary divisions: the **somatic** and the **autonomic** nervous systems, each of which has both motor and sensory components.

Somatic nervous system

The somatic nervous system (SNS) innervates skeletal muscles and is responsible for voluntary movement.

Autonomic nervous system

The autonomic nervous system (ANS) is sometimes also called the **involuntary nervous system** because it regulates the body's internal environment without the aid of conscious control. The autonomic innervation of the body includes both sensory and motor fibers. The ANS innervates **cardiac** and **smooth muscle**. Smooth muscle is located in areas such as blood vessels, the digestive tract, the bladder, and bronchi, so it isn't surprising that the ANS is important in blood pressure control, gastrointestinal motility, excretory processes, respiration, and reproductive processes. The ANS is comprised of two subdivisions, the **sympathetic** and the **parasympathetic** nervous systems, which generally act in opposition to one another.

- **Sympathetic nervous system**—The sympathetic division is responsible for the "**flight or fight**" responses that ready the body for action in an emergency situation. It increases blood pressure and heart rate, it increases blood flow to skeletal muscles, and it decreases gut motility. It also dilates the bronchioles to increase gas exchange. The sympathetic nervous system uses **norepinephrine** as its primary neurotransmitter.

- **Parasympathetic nervous system**—The parasympathetic division acts to conserve energy and restore the body to resting activity levels after exertion ("**rest and digest**"). It acts to lower heart rate and to increase gut motility. One very important parasympathetic nerve that innervates many of the thoracic and abdominal viscera is called the **vagus nerve**. It uses **acetylcholine** as its primary neurotransmitter.

Below is a summary table that lists the major functions of the parasympathetic and sympathetic nervous systems.

Comparison of Sympathetic and Parasympathetic Autonomic Functions		
Organ	**Sympathetic effect**	**Parasympathetic effect**
Lens	n/a	Accommodation
Iris	Dilates pupil	Constricts pupil
Salivary glands	Vasoconstriction	Secretion
Sweat glands	Secretion (specific)	Secretion (generalized)
Heart (force and rate)	Increases	Decreases
Peripheral blood vessels	Constriction	Dilation
Visceral blood vessels	Constriction	Dilation
Lungs	Vasodilation, bronchodilation	Bronchoconstriction, secretion
Gastrointestinal tract	Decreases peristalsis and secretion	Increases peristalsis and secretion
Rectum and anus	Inhibits smooth muscle in rectum and constricts sphincter	Increases smooth muscle tone and relaxes sphincter
Adrenal medulla	n/a	secretion
Bladder	Relaxation of the detrusor muscle and constriction of internal sphincter	Contraction of the detrusor muscle and inhibition of internal sphincter
Genitalia	Ejaculation	Penile erection / engorgement of clitoris and labia

SPECIAL SENSES

The body has a number of organs that are specialized receptors, designed to detect stimuli.

The Eye

The eye detects light energy (as **photons**) and transmits information about intensity, color, and shape to the brain. The eyeball is covered by a thick, opaque layer known as the **sclera**, which is also known as the white of the eye. Beneath the sclera is the **choroid** layer, which helps to supply the retina with blood. The choroid is a dark, pigmented area that reduces reflection in the eye. The innermost layer of the eye is the **retina**, which contains the **photoreceptors** that sense light.

The transparent cornea at the front of the eye bends and focuses light rays. The rays then travel through an opening called the **pupil**, whose diameter is controlled by the pigmented, muscular **iris**. The iris responds to the intensity of light in the surroundings (light makes the pupil constrict). The light continues through the lens, which is suspended behind the pupil. The **lens**, the shape and focal length of which is controlled by the **ciliary muscles**, focuses the image onto the retina.

In the retina are **photoreceptors** that transduce light into action potentials. There are two main types of photoreceptors: cones and rods. **Cones** respond to high-intensity illumination and are sensitive to color, whereas rods detect low-intensity illumination and are important in night vision. The cones and **rods** contain various pigments that absorb specific wavelengths of light. The cones contain three different pigments that absorb red, green, and blue wavelengths; the rod pigment, **rhodopsin**, absorbs a single wavelength. The photoreceptor cells synapse onto **bipolar cells,** which in turn synapse onto **ganglion cells**. Axons of the **ganglion cells** bundle to form the optic nerves, which conduct visual information to the brain. The point at which the optic nerve exits the eye is called the **blind spot** because photoreceptors are not present there. There is also a small area of the retina called the **fovea**, which is densely packed with cones and is important for high acuity vision.

The eye contains a jellylike material called **vitreous humor** that helps maintain its shape and optical properties. **Aqueous humor** is formed by the eye and exits through ducts to join the venous blood.

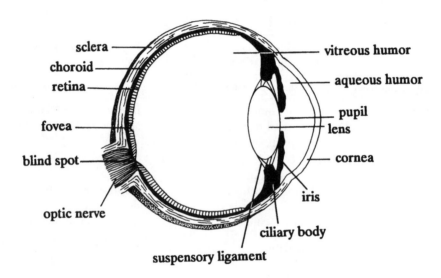

Figure 13.9

Disorders of the eye

- **Myopia (nearsightedness)** occurs when the image is focused in front of the retina.
- **Hyperopia (farsightedness)** occurs when the image is focused behind the retina.
- **Astigmatism** is caused by an irregularly shaped cornea.
- **Cataracts** develop when the lens becomes opaque; light cannot enter the eye, and blindness results.
- **Glaucoma** is an increase of pressure in the eye because of blocking of the outflow of the aqueous humor.

THE EAR

The ear transduces sound energy (**pressure waves**) into impulses perceived by the brain as sound. Sound waves pass through three regions as they enter the ear. First, they enter the **outer ear**, which consists of the **auricle** (external ear) and the **auditory canal**. At the end of the auditory canal is the **tympanic membrane** (eardrum) of the middle ear, which vibrates at the same frequency as the incoming sound. Next, the three bones, or **ossicles** (malleus, incus, and stapes), amplify the stimulus and transmit it through the oval window, which leads to the fluid-filled inner ear. The inner ear consists of the **cochlea** and the **vestibular apparatus**, which is involved in maintaining equilibrium. Vibration of the ossicles exerts pressure on the fluid in the cochlea, stimulating **hair cells** in the **basilar membrane** to transduce the pressure into action potentials, which travel via the auditory (cochlear) nerve to the brain for processing.

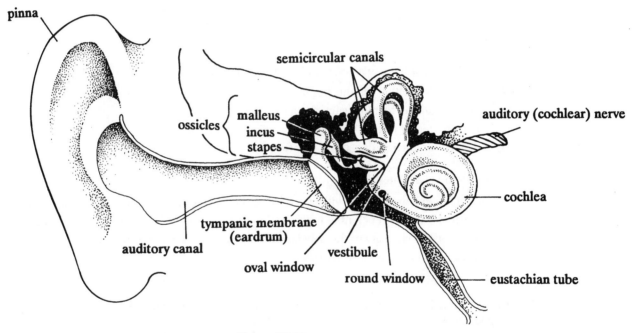

Figure 13.10

REVIEW PROBLEMS

1. Which of the following statements best characterizes an axon?

    (A) It is a long, slender process that fires every time neurotransmitters bind to the postsynaptic membrane.

    (B) It transmits nonelectrical impulses.

    (C) It transmits information from the cell body to the axon terminals.

    (D) None of the above

2. Resting membrane potential depends on

    (A) the differential distribution of ions across the axon membrane.

    (B) active transport.

    (C) selective permeability.

    (D) all of the above.

3. All of the following are associated with the myelin sheath EXCEPT

    (A) faster conduction of nervous impulses.

    (B) nodes of Ranvier forming gaps along the axon.

    (C) increased energy output for nervous impulse conduction.

    (D) saltatory conduction of action potentials.

4. The all-or-none law states that

    (A) all hyperpolarizing stimuli will be carried to the axon terminal without a decrease in size.

    (B) the size of the action potential is proportional to the size of the stimulus that produced it.

    (C) increasing the intensity of the depolarization increases the size of the impulse.

    (D) once an action potential is triggered, an impulse of a given magnitude and speed is produced.

5. Discuss two major differences between the somatic and the autonomic divisions of the peripheral nervous system.

6. By increasing the intensity of the stimulus, the action potential will

    (A) increase in amplitude.

    (B) increase in frequency.

    (C) increase in speed.

    (D) do both B and C.

7. Which of the following pairings is correct?

    (A) sensory nerves–afferent

    (B) motor nerves–afferent

    (C) sensory nerves–efferent

    (D) sensory nerves–ventral

    (E) motor nerves–dorsal

8. When a sensory receptor receives a threshold stimulus, it will do all of the following EXCEPT

   (A) become depolarized.
   (B) transduce the stimulus to an action potential.
   (C) inhibit the spread of the action potential to sensory neurons.
   (D) cause the sensory neuron to send action potentials to the central nervous system.

9. Which of the following structures focuses light on the retina?

   (A) Cornea
   (B) Aqueous humor
   (C) Vitreous humor
   (D) Lens
   (E) Both A and D

10. When the potential across the axon membrane is more negative than the normal resting potential, the neuron is said to be in a state of

    (A) depolarization.
    (B) hyperpolarization.
    (C) repolarization.
    (D) refraction.
    (E) threshold.

11. Chemical X is found to denature all enzymes in the synaptic cleft. What are the effects on acetylcholine if chemical X is added to the cleft and then removed?

    (A) Acetylcholine is not released from the presynaptic membrane.
    (B) Acetylcholine does not bind to the postsynaptic membrane.
    (C) Acetylcholine is not inactivated in the synaptic cleft.
    (D) Acetylcholine is degraded before it acts on the postsynaptic membrane.

12. Which of the following statements concerning the somatic division of the peripheral nervous system is INCORRECT?

    (A) Its pathways innervate skeletal muscles.
    (B) Its pathways are usually voluntary.
    (C) Some of its pathways are referred to as reflex arcs.
    (D) It includes the vagus nerve.

13. In the ear, what structure transduces pressure waves to action potentials?

    (A) Tympanic membrane
    (B) Organ of Corti
    (C) Oval window
    (D) Semicircular canals
    (E) Malleus

SOLUTIONS TO REVIEW PROBLEMS

1. **C** Axons carry information from the cell body of the neuron to the axon terminal by way of action potentials. From there, the impulse is transmitted to another neuron or to an effector. However, the axon does not fire unless the impulse is strong enough to depolarize the axon membrane to the threshold membrane potential.

2. **D** Resting membrane potential is a result of an unequal distribution of ions between the inside and the outside of the cell, and the other facets of cell structure.

3. **C** Discussed in impulse propagation section.

4. **D** Discussed in action potential section.

5. First, the somatic nervous system regulates voluntary actions (except in the cases of monosynaptic and polysynaptic reflexes), whereas the autonomic nervous system regulates involuntary actions. Second, the somatic nervous system innervates skeletal muscle, whereas the autonomic nervous system innervates cardiac and smooth muscle.

6. **B** Discussed in action potential section.

7. **A** Discussed in vertebrate nervous system section.

8. **C** Discussed in vertebrate nervous system section.

9. **E** Discussed in special senses section.

10. **B** When the neuron goes past the resting potential and becomes even more negative inside than normal, this is termed hyperpolarization.

11. **C** Acetylcholine is inactivated in the synaptic cleft by the enzyme acetycholinesterase after it has acted upon the postsynaptic membrane. If chemical X denatures acetylcholinesterase, it will not be able to inactivate acetylcholine and prevent the continuous depolarization of the effector membrane.

12. **D** Discussed in peripheral nervous system section.

13. **B** Discussed in special senses section.

CHAPTER FOURTEEN

Respiration

All living cells need energy for growth, maintenance of homeostasis, defense mechanisms, repair, and reproduction. The cells of the human body and those of other organisms obtain this energy from aerobic respiration (in the presence of oxygen). Respiration refers to the use of **oxygen** by an organism. This process includes the intake of oxygen from the environment, the transport of oxygen in the blood, and the ultimate oxidation of fuel molecules in the cell. **External respiration** refers to the entrance of air into the lungs and the gas exchange between the alveoli and the blood. **Internal respiration** includes the exchange of gas between the blood and the cells and the intracellular processes of respiration.

OVERVIEW OF CELLULAR RESPIRATION

Photosynthesis converts the energy of the sun into the chemical energy of bonds in compounds such as glucose. **Respiration** involves the conversion of the chemical energy in these bonds into the usable energy needed to drive the processes of living cells.

Carbohydrates and fats are the favored **fuel** molecules in living cells. As hydrogen is removed, bond energy is made available. The C-H bond is energy rich; in fact, compared with other bonds, it is capable of releasing the largest amount of energy per mole. In contrast, carbon dioxide contains little usable energy. It is the stable, energy-exhausted end product of respiration.

During respiration, high-energy hydrogen atoms are removed from organic molecules. This is called **dehydrogenation** and is an oxidation reaction. The subsequent acceptance of hydrogen by a hydrogen acceptor (oxygen in the final step) is the reduction component of the redox reaction. Energy released by this reduction is used to form a high-energy phosphate bond in ATP. Although the initial oxidation step requires an energy input, the net result of the redox reaction is energy production. If all of this energy was released in a single step, little could be harnessed. Instead, the reductions occur in a series of steps called the **electron transport chain**.

GLUCOSE CATABOLISM

The degradative oxidation of glucose occurs in two stages: **glycolysis** and **cellular respiration**.

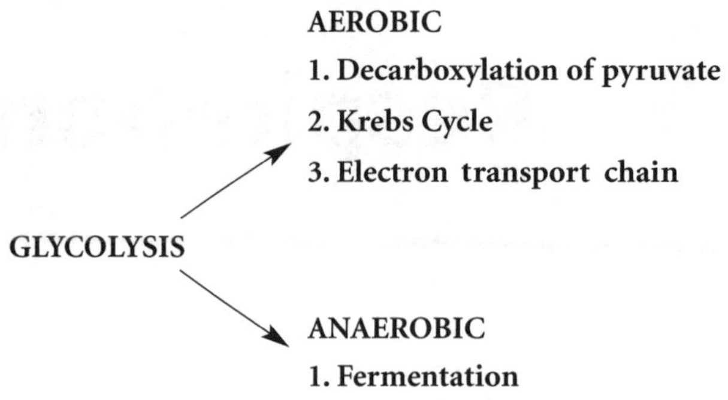

AEROBIC

1. Decarboxylation of pyruvate

2. Krebs Cycle

3. Electron transport chain

GLYCOLYSIS

ANAEROBIC

1. Fermentation

Figure 14.1

Glycolysis

The first stage of glucose catabolism is glycolysis. Glycolysis is a series of reactions that lead to the oxidative breakdown of glucose into two molecules of **pyruvate** (the ionized form of pyruvic acid), the production of ATP, and the reduction of NAD^+ into NADH. All of these reactions occur in the **cytoplasm** and are mediated by specific enzymes. For example, the process of glycolysis is defined as the sequence of reactions that converts glucose into pyruvate with the concomitant production of ATP. The process of glycolysis begins when glucose reacts with hexokinase to form glucose-6-phosphate. When this compound interacts with the enzyme phosphoglucose isomerase, the compound fructose-6-phosphate is formed. After the formation of this compound, it is interacted with the enzyme phosphofructokinase to form the compound fructose 1,6-biphosphate. When interacted with aldolase, glyceraldehyde 3-phosphate is formed. After a number of enzymatic reactions, the compound phosphoenolpyruvate is formed. When acted upon by pyruvate kinase, pyruvate is formed, and the glycolytic pathway is completed.

Glycolytic pathway

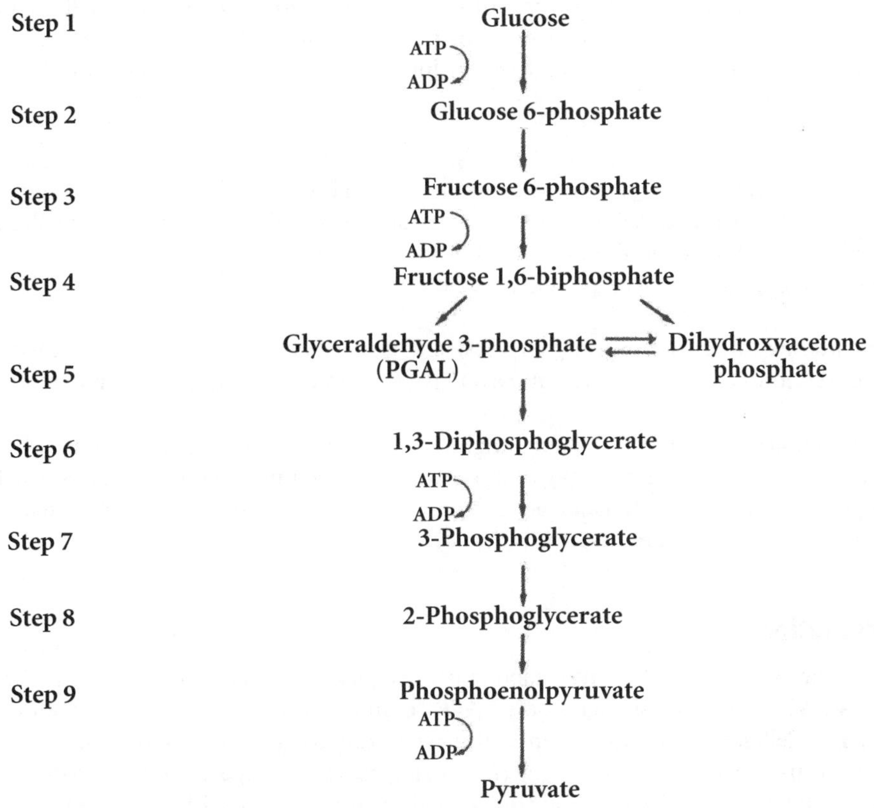

Step 1   **Glucose**

ATP → ADP

Step 2   **Glucose 6-phosphate**

Step 3   **Fructose 6-phosphate**

ATP → ADP

Step 4   **Fructose 1,6-biphosphate**

Glyceraldehyde 3-phosphate ⇌ **Dihydroxyacetone**
(PGAL)   **phosphate**

Step 5

Step 6   **1,3-Diphosphoglycerate**

ATP → ADP

Step 7   **3-Phosphoglycerate**

Step 8   **2-Phosphoglycerate**

Step 9   **Phosphoenolpyruvate**

ATP → ADP

Pyruvate

Figure 14.2

Note that at step 4, fructose 1,6-biphosphate is split into two three-carbon molecules: dihydroxyacetone phosphate and **glyceraldehyde 3-phosphate (PGAL)**. **Dihydroxyacetone phosphate** is isomerized into PGAL so that it can be used in subsequent reactions. Thus, two molecules of PGAL are formed per molecule of glucose, and all of the subsequent steps occur twice for each glucose molecule.

From one molecule of glucose (a six-carbon molecule), two molecules of pyruvate (a three-carbon molecule) are obtained. During this sequence of reactions, two ATP are used (in steps 1 and 3) and four ATP are generated (two in step 6, and two in step 9). Thus, there is a net production of two ATP per glucose molecule. This type of phosphorylation is called **substrate level phosphorylation** because ATP synthesis is directly coupled with the degradation of glucose without the participation of an intermediate molecule such as NAD+. One NADH is produced per PGAL, for a total of two NADH per glucose.

The net reaction for glycolysis is:

$$\text{Glucose} + 2\text{ADP} + 2\text{P}_i + 2\text{NAD}^+ \longrightarrow$$
$$2\text{Pyruvate} + 2\text{ATP} + 2\text{NADH} + 2\text{H}^+ + 2\text{H}_2\text{O}$$

At this stage, much of the initial energy stored in the glucose molecule has not been released and is still present in the chemical bonds of pyruvate. Depending on the capabilities of the organism, pyruvate degradation can proceed in one of two directions. Under **anaerobic** conditions (in the absence of oxygen), pyruvate is reduced during the process of fermentation. Under aerobic conditions (in the presence of oxygen), pyruvate is further oxidized during cell respiration in the mitochondria.

Fermentation

NAD^+ must be regenerated for glycolysis to continue in the absence of O_2. This is accomplished by reducing pyruvate into ethanol or lactic acid. Fermentation refers to all of the reactions involved in this process (i.e., glycolysis and the additional steps leading to the formation of ethanol or lactic acid). Fermentation produces only two ATP per glucose molecule.

Alcohol fermentation often occurs only in yeast and some bacteria. The pyruvate produced in glycolysis is converted to ethanol. In this way, NAD^+ is regenerated and glycolysis can continue.

Lactic acid fermentation occurs in certain fungi and bacteria and in human muscle cells during strenuous activity. When the oxygen supply to muscle cells lags behind the rate of glucose catabolism, the pyruvate generated is reduced to lactic acid. As in alcohol fermentation, the NAD^+ used in step 5 of glycolysis is regenerated when pyruvate is reduced.

Cellular Respiration

Cellular respiration is the most efficient catabolic pathway used by organisms to harvest the energy stored in glucose. Whereas glycolysis yields only **2 ATP** per molecule of glucose, cellular respiration can yield **36–38 ATP**. Cellular respiration is an **aerobic** process; **oxygen** acts as the final acceptor of electrons that are passed from carrier to carrier during the final stage of glucose oxidation. The metabolic reactions of cell respiration occur in the eukaryotic mitochondrion and are catalyzed by reaction-specific enzymes.

Cellular respiration can be divided into three stages: pyruvate decarboxylation, the citric acid cycle, and the electron transport chain.

Pyruvate decarboxylation

The pyruvate formed during glycolysis is transported from the cytoplasm into the mitochondrial matrix where it is decarboxylated (i.e., it loses a CO_2), and the acetyl group that remains is transferred to coenzyme A to form acetyl CoA. In the process, NAD^+ is reduced to NADH.

Citric acid cycle

The citric acid cycle is also known as the **Krebs cycle**. The cycle begins when the two-carbon acetyl group from acetyl CoA combines with oxaloacetate, a four-carbon molecule, to form the six-carbon citrate. Through a complicated series of reactions, two CO_2 are released, and oxaloacetate is regenerated for use in another turn of the cycle.

For each turn of the citric acid cycle one ATP is produced by substrate level phosphorylation via a GTP intermediate. In addition, electrons are transferred to NAD^+ and FAD, generating NADH and $FADH_2$, respectively. These coenzymes then transport the electrons to the electron transport chain, where more ATP is produced via oxidative phosphorylation (see below). Studying the cycle, we can do some bookkeeping; keep in mind that for each molecule of glucose, two pyruvates are decarboxylated and channeled into the citric acid cycle.

$$
\begin{array}{ll}
2 \times 3 \text{ NADH} & 6 \text{ NADH} \\
2 \times 1 \text{ FADH}_2 & 2 \text{ FADH}_2 \\
2 \times 1 \text{ GTP (ATP)} & 2 \text{ ATP}
\end{array}
$$

The net reaction of the citric acid cycle per glucose molecule is:

$$2\text{Acetyl CoA} + 6\text{NAD}^+ + 2\text{FAD} + 2\text{GDP} + 2\text{P}_i + 4\text{H}_2\text{O}$$
$$\longrightarrow 4\text{CO}_2 + 6\text{NADH} + 2\text{FADH}_2 + 2\text{ATP} + 4\text{H}^+ + 2\text{CoA}$$

Electron transport chain

The electron transport chain (ETC) is a complex carrier mechanism located on the inside of the **inner mitochondrial membrane**. During oxidative phosphorylation, ATP is produced when high-energy potential electrons are transferred from NADH and $FADH_2$ to oxygen by a series of carrier molecules located in the inner mitochondrial membrane. As the electrons are transferred from carrier to carrier, free energy is released, which is then used to form ATP. Most of the molecules of the ETC are **cytochromes**, electron carriers that resemble hemoglobin in the structure of their active site. The functional unit contains a central iron atom, which is capable of undergoing a reversible redox reaction (i.e., it can be alternatively reduced and oxidized). Sequential redox reactions continue to occur as the electrons are transferred from one carrier to the next; each carrier is reduced as it accepts an electron and is then oxidized when it passes it on to the next carrier. The last carrier of the ETC passes its electron to the final electron acceptor, O_2. In addition to the electrons, O_2 picks up a pair of hydrogen ions from the surrounding medium, forming water.

$$2\text{H}^+ + 2\text{e}^- + \frac{1}{2}\text{O}_2 \longrightarrow \text{H}_2\text{O}$$

Total Energy Production

To calculate the net amount of ATP produced per molecule of glucose, we need to tally the number of ATP produced by substrate level phosphorylation and the number of ATP produced by oxidative phosphorylation.

Substrate level phosphorylation

Degradation of one glucose molecule yields a net of two ATP from glycolysis and one ATP for each turn of the citric acid cycle. Thus, a total of four ATP are produced by substrate level phosphorylation.

Oxidative phosphorylation

Oxidative phosphorylation is the process that produces more than 90 percent of the ATP used by the cells in our body. The major steps involved in this process occur within the electron transport system (ETS) or respiratory chain of the mitochondria. The steps at the end of the electron transport system where ATP is generated are as follows. Along the ETS, the respiratory enzymes continually pump hydrogen ions from the matrix of the mitochondria to the intermembrane space, which creates a large concentration gradient. At the end of the ETS, hydrogen ions pass through channels in the respiratory enzymes along the concentration gradient. As the hydrogen ions pass through these enzymes, the energy created is used to convert ADP to ATP. Now, specifically looking at the process of oxidative phosphorylation, two pyruvate decarboxylations yield one NADH each for a total of two NADH. Each turn of the citric acid cycle yields three NADH and one $FADH_2$, for a total of six NADH and two $FADH_2$ per glucose molecule. Each $FADH_2$ generates two ATP, as previously discussed. Each NADH generates three ATP except for the two NADH that were reduced during glycolysis; these NADH cannot cross the inner mitochondrial membrane and must transfer their electrons to an intermediate carrier molecule, which delivers the electrons to the second carrier protein complex, Q. Therefore, these NADH generate only two ATP per glucose. So the 2 NADH of glycolysis yield four ATP, the other 8 NADH yield 24 ATP, and the two $FADH_2$ produce 4 ATP, for a total of 32 ATP by oxidative phosphorylation.

The total amount of ATP produced during eukaryotic glucose catabolism is therefore 4 via substrate level phosphorylation plus 32 via oxidative phosphorylation, for a total of 36 ATP. (For prokaryotes, the yield is 38 ATP because the 2 NADH of glycolysis don't have any mitochondrial membranes to cross and therefore don't lose energy.)

Eukaryotic ATP Production per Glucose Molecule

Glycolysis

2 ATP invested (steps 1 and 3)	−	2	ATP
4 ATP generated (steps 6 and 9)	+	4	ATP (substrate)
2 NADH × 2 ATP/NADH (step 5)	+	4	ATP (oxidative)

Pyruvate decarboxylation

2 NADH × 3 ATP/NADH	+	6	ATP (oxidative)

Citric acid cycle

6 NADH × 3 ATP/NADH	+	18	ATP (oxidative)
2 $FADH_2$ × 2 ATP/$FADH_2$	+	4	ATP (oxidative)
2 GTP × 1 ATP/GTP	+	2	ATP (substrate)
Total	+	36	ATP

ALTERNATE ENERGY SOURCES

When glucose supplies run low, the body uses other energy sources. These sources are used by the body in the following preferential order: other carbohydrates, fats, and proteins. These substances are first converted to either glucose or glucose intermediates, which can then be degraded in the glycolytic pathway and the citric acid cycle.

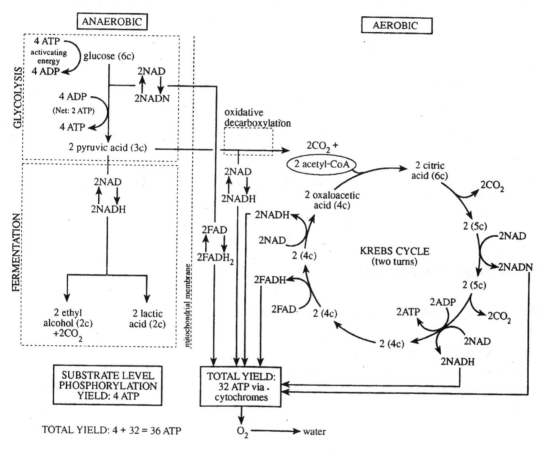

Figure 14.3

Carbohydrates

Disaccharides are hydrolyzed into monosaccharides, most of which can be converted into glucose or glycolytic intermediates. Glycogen stored in the liver can be converted, when needed, into a glycolytic intermediate.

Fats

Fat molecules are stored in adipose tissue in the form of triglyceride. When needed, they are hydrolyzed by **lipases** to **fatty acids** and **glycerol** and are carried by the blood to other tissues for oxidation. Glycerol can be converted into PGAL, a glycolytic intermediate. A fatty acid must first be "activated" in the cytoplasm; this process requires two ATP. Once activated, the fatty acid is transported into the mitochondrion and taken through a series of beta-oxidation cycles that convert it into two-carbon fragments, which are then converted into acetyl CoA. Acetyl CoA then enters the TCA cycle. With each round of b-oxidation of a saturated fatty acid, one NADH and one $FADH_2$ are generated.

Of all the high-energy compounds used in cellular respiration, fats yield the greatest number of ATP per gram. This makes them extremely efficient energy storage molecules. Thus, whereas the amount of glycogen stored in humans is enough to meet the short-term energy needs of about a day, the stored fat reserves can meet the long-term energy needs for about a month.

Proteins

The body degrades proteins only when not enough carbohydrate or fat is available. Most amino acids undergo a **transamination reaction** in which they lose an amino group to form an a-keto acid. The carbon atoms of most amino acids are converted into acetyl CoA, pyruvate, or one of the intermediates of the citric acid cycle. These intermediates enter their respective metabolic pathways, allowing cells to produce fatty acids, glucose, or energy in the form of ATP.

Oxidative deamination removes an ammonia molecule directly from the amino acid. **Ammonia** is a toxic substance in vertebrates. Fish can excrete ammonia, whereas insects and birds convert it to uric acid, and mammals convert it to urea for excretion.

RESPIRATION IN INVERTEBRATES

Unicellular and Simple Multicellular Organisms

Protozoa and Hydra (Phylum: Cnidaria)

In these organisms, every cell is in contact with the external environment (water), and respiratory gases can be exchanged between the cell and the environment by simple diffusion through the cell membrane.

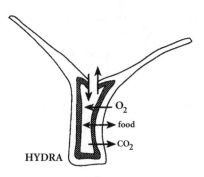

Figure 14.4

Annelids

Mucus secreted by cells on the external surface of the earthworm's body provides a moist surface for gaseous exchange by diffusion. The circulatory system brings O_2 to the cells and waste products such as CO_2 back to the skin for excretion.

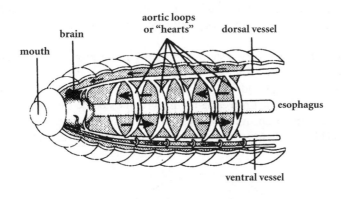

Figure 14.5

Arthropod Phylum

The respiratory system of a grasshopper consists of a series of respiratory tubules called **tracheae** whose branches reach to almost every cell. These tubes open to the surface in openings called **spiracles**. This system thus permits the intake, distribution, and removal of respiratory gases directly between the air and the body cells by diffusion. No carrier of oxygen is needed in this respiratory system, and the efficiency of this system allows insects to have a relatively inefficient open circulatory system.

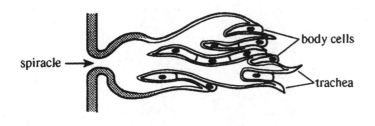

Figure 14.6

RESPIRATION IN HUMANS

In the human respiratory system, air enters the **lungs** after traveling through a series of respiratory **airways**. The air passages consists of the nose, pharynx (throat), larynx, trachea, bronchi, bronchioles, and the alveoli. Gas exchange between the lungs and the circulatory system occurs across the very thin walls of the **alveol**, which are air-filled sacs at the terminals of the airway branches. Three hundred million alveoli provide approximately 100 m^2 of moist respiratory surface for gas exchange. After gas exchange, air rushes back through the respiratory pathway and is exhaled.

The primary functions of the respiratory system in humans are to provide the necessary energy for growth, maintenance of homeostasis, defense mechanisms, repair, and reproduction of cells in the body. The respiratory system also provides a very large area for gas exchange, as well as continually moving oxygenated air over this area, protecting the respiratory surface from infection, dehydration, and temperature changes. It moves air over the vocal cords for the production of sound and assist in the regulation of body pH by regulating the rate of carbon dioxide removal from the blood.

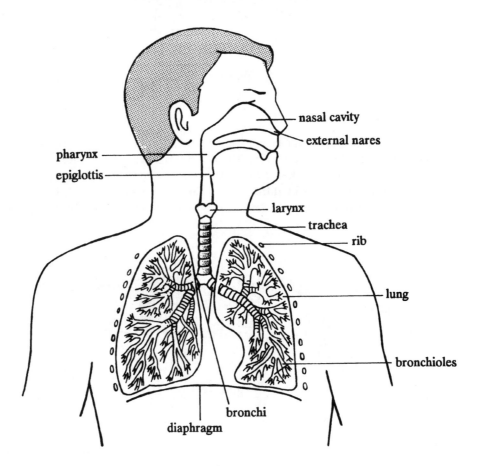

Figure 14.7

Ventilation

Ventilation of the lungs (breathing) is the process by which air is **inhaled** and **exhaled**. The purpose of ventilation is to take in oxygen from the atmosphere and eliminate carbon dioxide from the body.

During **inhalation**, the diaphragm contracts and flattens, and the external intercostal muscles contract, pushing the rib cage and chest wall up and out. This causes the thoracic cavity to increase in **volume**. This volume increase, in turn, reduces the pressure, causing the lungs to expand and fill with air. The phrenic nerve innervates the diaphragm and causes it to contract and flatten. This produces inhalation.

Exhalation is generally a passive process. The lungs and chest wall are highly elastic and tend to recoil to their original positions after inhalation. The diaphragm and external intercostal muscles relax, and the chest wall pushes inward. The consequent decrease in thoracic cavity volume causes the air pressure to increase. This causes the lungs to deflate, forcing air out of the alveoli.

Control of Ventilation

Ventilation is regulated by neurons (referred to as **respiratory centers**) located in the **medulla oblongata**, whose rhythmic discharges stimulate the intercostal muscles or the diaphragm to contract. When the partial pressure of CO_2 rises, the medulla oblongata stimulates an increase in the rate of ventilation.

The primary goal of respiration is to maintain proper concentrations of oxygen, carbon dioxide, and hydrogen ions in tissues. Hence, respiratory activity is highly responsive to changes in the blood levels of these compounds. Excessive carbon dioxide and hydrogen ions are the primary stimulus for respiration. When carbon dioxide and hydrogen ion levels are increased, the respiratory center stimulates both the inspiratory and expiratory muscles of the lungs. Oxygen blood levels do not have a significant effect on the respiratory center. However, oxygen blood levels are monitored by peripheral chemoreceptors, which indirectly stimulate the respiratory center.

Gas Exchange

A dense network of minute blood vessels called the **pulmonary capillaries** surrounds the alveoli. Gas exchange occurs by diffusion across these capillary walls and those of the alveoli; gases move from regions of higher partial pressure to regions of lower partial pressure. Oxygen diffuses from the alveolar air into the blood while carbon dioxide diffuses from the blood into the lungs to be exhaled.

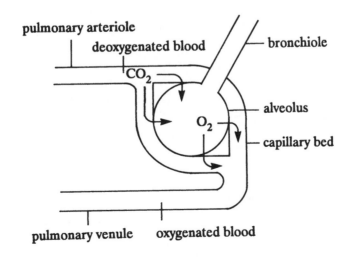

Figure 14.8

RESPIRATION IN PLANTS

In all plants and animals, respiration is continuous, occurring both day and night. However, photosynthesis only takes place during the day. Note that photosynthesis produces glucose and gives off oxygen, whereas respiration requires oxygen to degrade glucose.

Plants undergo aerobic respiration similar to animals. The bonds of glucose are broken in glycolysis to produce two ATP and pyruvic acids. The gases diffuse into the air space entering (or leaving) through the stomatas of the leaf or the lenticels (openings) of woody stems. Thirty-six ATP molecules are produced per molcule of glucose. Anaerobic respiration takes place in simple plants when molecular oxygen is lacking in a manner similar to animals.

REVIEW PROBLEMS

1. What is the net reaction for glycolysis? For the TCA cycle?

2. In glucose degradation
   (A) oxygen is the final electron acceptor.
   (B) oxygen is necessary for ATP synthesis.
   (C) water is the final electron acceptor.
   (D) water is produced.
   (E) both A and D occur.

3. Fatty acids enter the degradative pathway in the form of
   (A) glycerol.
   (B) glucose.
   (C) acetyl CoA.
   (D) brown adipose tissue.
   (E) keto acids.

4. How do ATP, NADH, and $FADH_2$ store energy?

5. How is NAD^+ regenerated, and why is this important?

6. Describe the production of ATP via oxidative phosphorylation.

7. Which of the following is LEAST likely to occur during oxygen debt?
   (A) Buildup of lactic acid
   (B) Buildup of pyruvate
   (C) Decrease in pH
   (D) Fatigue
   (E) Shortage of ATP

8. All of the following facilitate gas exchange in the lungs EXCEPT
   (A) thin alveolar surfaces.
   (B) moist alveolar surfaces.
   (C) differences in the partial pressures of O_2 and CO_2.
   (D) active transport.

9. What muscles play a role in ventilation? Compare the muscular motions involved in inhalation with those involved in exhalation.

10. Which is the correct sequence of the passages air travels through during inhalation?

    (A) pharynx → trachea → bronchioles → bronchi → alveoli

    (B) pharynx → trachea → lungs → bronchi → alveoli

    (C) pharynx → larynx → bronchi → trachea → alveoli

    (D) pharynx → larynx → trachea → bronchi → alveoli

    (E) larynx → pharynx → trachea → bronchi → alveoli

11. Which of the following is generally a passive process?

    (A) Inhalation

    (B) Exhalation

    (C) Gas exchange

    (D) Both A and B

    (E) Both B and C

SOLUTIONS TO REVIEW PROBLEMS

1.   The net reaction for glycolysis is:

Glucose + 2ATP + 4ADP + 2P$_i$ + 2NAD$^+$ →

2 Pyruvate + 2ADP + 4ATP + 2NADH + 2H$^+$ + 2H$_2$O

The net reaction for the TCA cycle is:

2Acetyl CoA + 6NAD+ + 2FAD + 2GDP + 2Pi + 4H2O →

4CO$_2$ + 6NADH + 2FADH$_2$ + 2GTP + 4H+ + 2CoA

2. **E** Discussed in glucose catabolism section.

3. **C** Discussed in alternate energy sources section.

4.   Energy is stored in ATP as high-energy bonds created by the covalent bonding of three phosphates to adenosine. The hydrolysis of ATP to ADP releases inorganic phosphate (P$_i$) and 7 kcal of energy. Hydrolysis of ADP to AMP releases an additional 7 kcal. Alternatively, ATP hydrolysis to AMP + PP$_i$ releases 7 kcal.

NADH and FADH$_2$ are reducing agents that carry chemical energy in the form of high-potential electrons, which can be transferred as hydride ions. In cell respiration, these hydride ions are transferred to the electron transport chain, where energy release is coupled with ATP synthesis during a series of redox reactions.

5.   Step 5 of glycolysis involves the reduction of NAD$^+$ to NADH. Because NAD$^+$ is necessary for glycolysis to continue, it must be regenerated in one of two ways. In the presence of oxygen, oxidative phosphorylation and the ETC can be used to oxidize NADH to NAD$^+$. Alternatively, alcohol or lactic acid fermentation can be used to regenerate NAD$^+$ under anaerobic conditions.

6.   In the electron transport chain, the release of hydrogen ions is coupled with the transfer of electrons. H$^+$ ions accumulate in the mitochondrial matrix and are shuttled across the inner mitochondrial membrane, creating a proton gradient. To cross the inner membrane, the hydrogen ions must pass through ATP synthetases, which catalyze the phosphorylation of ADP into ATP.

7. **B** Discussed in fermentation section.

8. **D** Discussed in gas exchange section.

9. The muscles involved in ventilation are the diaphragm, which separates the thoracic cavity from the abdominal cavity, and the intercostal muscles of the rib cage. During inhalation, the diaphragm contracts and flattens while the external intercostals contract, pushing the rib cage up and out. These actions cause an overall increase in the size of the thoracic cavity. During exhalation, both the diaphragm and the external intercostals relax, causing a decrease in the size of the thoracic cavity. In forced expiration, the internal intercostals contract, pulling the rib cage down.

10. **D** Discussed in vertebrate respiratory system section.

11. **E** Exhalation is generally a passive process involving elastic recoil of the lungs and relaxation of both the diaphragm and the external intercostal muscles. (However, during vigorous exercise, active muscular contraction assists in expiration.) Gas exchange is also a passive process; the gases diffuse down their partial pressure gradients. Inhalation is an active process requiring contraction of the diaphragm and the external intercostals.

CHAPTER FIFTEEN

Autotrophic Nutrition

An **autotroph** is any organism that manufactures its own organic molecules (glucose, amino acids, and fats) from inorganic materials (CO_2, H_2O, and mineral salts). Organic molecules contain potential energy in the form of chemical bonds. Some autotrophs harness the radiant energy of sunlight to form these chemical bonds. This process is called **photosynthesis** and occurs in algae and multicellular green plants. Other simple autotrophic bacteria use chemosynthesis to obtain energy for the manufacture of organic materials.

PHOTOSYNTHESIS

Photosynthesis is a metabolic process where solar energy is trapped, converted to chemical energy, and then subsequently stored in the bonds of plant organic nutrient molecules. All green plants use photosynthesis to convert carbon dioxide and water into **glucose** and oxygen. Glucose can be stored as starch or used as an energy source. In plants, photosynthesis takes place in a specialized organelle called a chloroplast. Photosynthetic bacteria lack chloroplasts but have membranes that function in a similar manner.

Structure of a Chloroplast

In green plants, photosynthesis takes place in the **chloroplast**, a highly organized plastid containing the **chlorophyll** pigment. The chloroplast is bounded by two membranes and contains a network of membranes called **thylakoid membranes**. Chlorophyll resides within the thylakoid membranes. Thylakoid sacs are stacked into columns called **grana** (singular: granum). The fluid matrix of the chloroplast is called the **stroma**. Chlorophyl can best be described as a light-trapping pigment that is the key to the entire process of photosynthesis.

Chlorophyll is a very complex molecule containing over 100 atoms. Chlorophyll is complexed with the metal magnesium. When chlorophyll absorbs photons of light, electrons in the ground state are boosted to an excited state and can be harnessed to drive the reactions of photosynthesis. Chlorophyll absorbs light in the red and blue wavelengths, giving it a green appearance. The principle types are **chlorophyll a** and **chlorophyll b**. These chlorophyll molecules are part of two **photosystems**.

A photosystem is the light-capturing unit of the thylakoid membrane. Each photosystem is composed of a number of chlorophyll molecules. In the center is a single chlorophyll molecule coupled to other proteins that is ultimately excited by the absorbed photon. In **photosystem I**, this **chlorophyll a** molecule is called P700 because it absorbs best at 700 nm. In **photosystem II**, the special chlorophyll a molecule is **P680** because it absorbs best at 680 nm.

Overview of Photosynthesis

Photosynthesis involves the reduction of CO_2 to carbohydrate accompanied by release of oxygen from water. The net reaction is the reverse of respiration—reduction occurs instead of oxidation. This net reaction is shown below:

$$6CO_2 + 12\ H_2O + \text{light energy} \rightarrow C_6H_{12}O_6 + 6O_2 + 6\ H_2O$$

Photosynthesis can be divided into two distinct reactions, the light reactions and the dark reactions. The **light reactions** convert solar energy into chemical energy in the form of **ATP** (by photophosphorylation) and **NADPH**. These reactions must take place in the light. The **dark reactions** are coupled to the light reactions. They incorporate CO_2 into organic molecules in a process called **carbon fixation**. The dark reactions are also called reduction synthesis because carbohydrates are produced by reducing CO_2. Both reactions take place in the chloroplasts.

The Light Reactions

The light reactions, also called photolysis reactions, begin with the absorption of a photon of light by a chlorophyll molecule. When light strikes the special **chlorophyll a P700** molecule in photosystem I, it excites electrons to a higher energy level. These high-energy electrons can flow along two pathways, giving **cyclic electron flow** or **noncyclic electron flow**.

Cyclic electron flow

In cyclic electron flow, the excited electrons of P700 move along a chain of electron carriers. A series of redox reactions ultimately returns the electrons to P700. The reactions are harnessed to produce **ATP** from ADP and Pi in a process called **cyclic photophosphorylation**. The coenzyme carrier **ferrodoxin** is one of the early electron carriers in this electron transport chain.

Noncyclic electron flow

This is the key pathway of the light reactions and involves reactions of both photosystems. Again, photons of light excite electrons in P700 in photosystem I. However, instead of returning to P700 along the carrier chain, the high-energy electrons are transferred to the electron acceptor $NADP^+$. $NADP^+$ is very similar to NAD^+, which functions in cellular respiration. $NADP^+$ accepts the high-energy electrons and forms **NADPH**. P700 is left with electron "holes" and thus is a powerful oxidizing agent.

When light strikes P680 in **photosystem II**, electrons are excited. These electrons travel down the same electron carrier chain used by cyclic electron flow until they reach P700 and fill the electron "holes." This cascade produces ATP by **noncyclic photophosphorylation**.

Now, P680 has electron "holes." P680 is a strong enough oxidizing agent to oxidize water and fill its holes. Water is split into two hydrogen ions and an oxygen atom, and the electrons produced reduce P680. Oxygen atoms combine to form O_2.

The net result of noncyclic electron flow is the production of NADPH and ATP and the photolysis (breakdown) of water.

Chemical Aspects of Photosynthesis

The nature of the photosynthetic reactions was determined using **radioactive isotopes** (tagged atoms) such as **oxygen-18** and **carbon-14**. Using these labeled molecules, it was determined that the O_2 produced in photosynthesis comes from the photolysis of water and not from carbon dioxide. The escape of high-energy electrons from chlorophyll molecules is termed **photoionization**.

The Dark Reactions

The dark reactions use ATP and NADPH produced by the light reactions to reduce CO_2 to carbohydrates, primarily glucose. Although these reactions do not directly require light, they will only occur during the day when the light reactions are replenishing the supply of ATP and NADPH. The dark reactions are also called **carbon-fixation** or **reduction synthesis** reactions.

CO_2 is the source of carbon for carbohydrate production in the **Calvin cycle**. The product of the cycle is the **three-carbon** sugar **phosphoglyceraldehyde (PGAL)**. To produce a three-carbon sugar from CO_2, the cycle must take place three times.

The cycle begins with the addition of CO_2 to **ribulose bisphosphate**, a five-carbon sugar, to produce an unstable six-carbon intermediate that immediately splits to give 2 three-carbon molecules of **3-phosphoglyceric acid**. This acid is phosphorylated by ATP and reduced by NADPH to give **glyceraldehyde-3-phosphate (PGAL)**. Two molecules of PGAL can be converted to glucose, which can then be oxidized to provide usable energy.

The Calvin cycle is similar to the **Krebs cycle** in reverse: (1) carbon dioxide is fed into the cycle; in the Krebs cycle it was produced and released; (2) reducing power is used during the cycle (NADPH); in the Krebs cycle NADH was removed; (3) energy is used in the cycle (conversion of ATP to ADP); in the Krebs cycle, energy was produced when ATP was formed from ADP and inorganic phosphate.

Summary of the Calvin Cycle

Carbon dioxide is fixed to RBP (ribulose bisphosphate), a five-carbon sugar. The resulting unstable six carbon molecule splits to form two molecules of PGA (phosphoglyceric acid). PGA is then phosphorylated and reduced (by ATP and NADPH) to form PGAL. Most of the PGAL is recycled to RBP by a complex series of reactions. In six turns of the Calvin cycle, 12 PGAL are formed from 6 carbon dioxide and 6 RBP. The 12 PGAL recombine to form 6 RBP and 1 molecule of glucose, the net product.

PGAL is generally considered the prime end product of photosynthesis, and it can be used as an immediate food nutrient combined and rearranged to form monosaccharide sugars (e.g., glucose), which can be transported to other cells, or packaged for storage as insoluble polysaccharides such as starch.

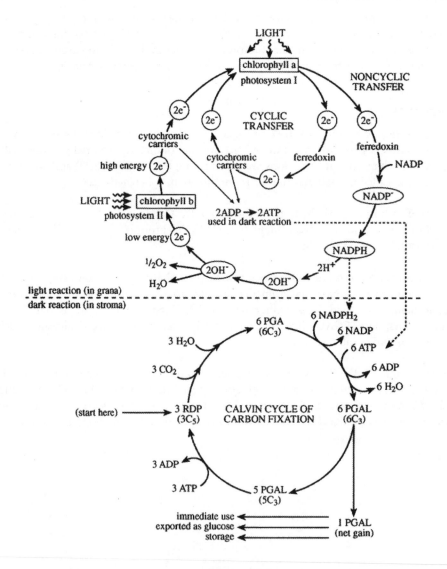

Figure 15.1

PLANT STRUCTURE

The Leaf

The higher multicellular green plants have specialized organs, the **leaves**, which are the principal sites of photosynthesis. The leaves have several adaptations for carrying on photosynthesis:

- **Waxy cuticle** to reduce transpiration and conserve water. Leaves have no openings on their upper surface.

- **Palisade** layer of elongated, chloroplast-containing cells spread over a large surface area. They are directly under the upper epidermis and are well exposed to light.

- **Spongy** layer—The stomata open into air spaces that contact an internal moist surface of loosely packed spongy layer cells. As in animals, the moist surface is necessary for diffusion of gases into and out of cells, for both photosynthesis and respiration. The air spaces also increase the surface area available for gas diffusion by the cells. Spongy cells also contain chloroplasts.

- **Guard** cells surround each of the stomata on the lower surface of the leaves.

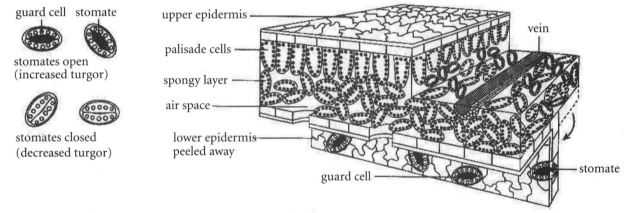

Figure 15.2

Stomata

Stomata are openings in the lower epidermis of a leaf that permit **diffusion** of carbon dioxide, water vapor, and oxygen between the leaf and the atmosphere. The size of the stomata opening is regulated by **guard cells**. The guard cells open stomata during the day to admit CO_2 for photosynthesis and close them at night to limit loss of water vapor (**transpiration**).

During the day, the guard cells, which contain chloroplasts, produce glucose. The presence of a high glucose content in the cells causes them to swell up by osmosis (a condition known as **turgor**). Because the inner wall of the guard cell is thickened, the swelling produces a curvature of the opening between the guard cells, and the stomata opening then increases. At night, photosynthesis ceases, cell turgor decreases, and the stomata closes. During a drought, the stomata will close even during the daytime to prevent loss of water by transpiration. Photosynthesis will cease because of a lack of CO_2.

Vascular bundles

Veins containing **xylem** and **phloem** bring water to the leaf from the roots (xylem) and carry manufactured food out of the leaf (phloem).

The Root

Specialized epidermal cells with thin-walled root hairs are found in the root. They provide an increased surface for **absorption** of water and minerals by **diffusion** and **active transport**.

CHEMOSYNTHESIS

Some bacteria form carbohydrates by use of **chemical energy** rather than by using the radiant energy of the sun. These bacteria oxidize compounds of nitrogen, sulfur, or iron. The small amount of energy released by this oxidation is sufficient for the formation of glucose. The energy produced is sufficient to support the vital functions of these nitrogen, sulfur, and iron bacteria. For example, **nitrifying bacteria** oxidize ammonia and nitrites to nitrates. The plants use these nitrates to make proteins. The bacteria use the energy obtained from this oxidation to make glucose.

REVIEW PROBLEMS

1. The thylakoid membrane sacs are organized into stacks called

   (A) stroma.
   (B) grana.
   (C) chloroplasts.
   (D) none of the above.

2. What are the primary differences between cyclic electron flow and noncyclic electron flow?

3. Which of the following is TRUE of the dark reactions of photosynthesis?

   (A) They occur in the mitochondria.
   (B) They occur at night.
   (C) They do not require light directly but are linked to the light reactions.
   (D) They require light in the UV range.

4. Six turns of the Calvin cycle will produce

   (A) 12 PGAL.
   (B) 6 CO_2.
   (C) 2 glucose.
   (D) 36 ATP.

5. Describe three adaptations of leaves for reduction of water loss.

6. During the day, the environment of the guard cells is

   (A) hypertonic relative to the guard cell cytoplasm.
   (B) hypotonic relative to the guard cell cytoplasm.
   (C) isotonic relative to the guard cell cytoplasm.
   (D) none of the above.

SOLUTIONS TO REVIEW PROBLEMS

1. **B** The thylakoid sacs contain chlorophyll, the photopigment that absorbs light in photosynthesis. They are arranged in columns.

2. Cyclic electron flow involves only photosystem I and leads to the production of ATP by cyclic photophosphorylation. Noncyclic electron flow is the key pathway of photosynthesis. Electrons are excited from P680 in photosystem II to P700 in photosystem I, leading to production of ATP by noncyclic photophosphorylation. Electrons are then removed from water to fill electron "holes" in P680. Water is split and oxygen formed. This process leads to the formation of NADPH, which helps power the dark reactions.

3. **C** The dark reactions do not require light directly because chlorophyll is not involved. However, they depend on the ATP and NADPH, which is generated by the light reactions, and so occur only during the day.

4. **A** In six turns of the Calvin cycle, 12 PGAL are formed from 6 CO_2 and 6 RBP.

5. Leaves have a waxy cuticle that blocks transpiration. The stomata, openings to the environment, are present only on the bottom of leaves and open and close to regulate water conservation. Guard cells surrounding each of the stomata coordinate their opening and closing. Deciduous plants lose their leaves during the winter as an additional means of water conservation.

6. **B** During the day, guard cells fill with glucose, becoming more concentrated than their environment and water flows in. The cells are in a hypotonic environment.

CHAPTER SIXTEEN

Muscles and Locomotion

The musculoskeletal system forms the basic internal framework of the vertebrate body. Muscles and bones work in close coordination to produce voluntary movement. In addition, bone and muscle perform a number of other independent functions. Unicellular organisms may rely on specialized organelles for locomotion. Invertebrates have developed a number of systems for locomotion. Physical support and locomotion are the functions of animal skeletal systems. The muscular system generates force.

UNICELLULAR LOCOMOTION

Protozoans and primitive algae may move by beating **cilia** or **flagella**. The cilia and flagella of all eukaryotic cells possess the same basic structure. Each contains a cylindrical stalk of 11 microtubules—9 paired microtubules arranged in a circle with 2 single microtubules in the center. Flagella achieve movement by means of the power stroke, a thrusting movement generated by the sliding action of microtubules. Return of the cilium or flagellum to its original position is termed the recovery stroke. Amoeba extend **pseudopodia** for locomotion; the advancing cell membrane extends forward, allowing the cell to move.

INVERTEBRATE LOCOMOTION

Hydrostatic Skeleton

Flatworms

The muscles within the body wall of advanced flatworms such as planaria are arranged in two antagonistic layers: longitudinal and circular. The muscles contract against the resistance of the incompressible fluid within the animal's tissues (this fluid is termed the hydrostatic skeleton). Contraction of the circular layer of muscles causes the incompressible interstitial fluid to flow longitudinally, lengthening the animal. Conversely, contraction of the longitudinal layer of muscles shortens the animal. The same type of hydrostatic skeleton assists in the locomotion of annelids, in which each segment of the animal can expand or contract independently.

Segmented worms (annelids)

Earthworms advance principally by the action of muscles on a hydrostatic skeleton. Bristles in the lower part of each segment, called setae, anchor the earthworm temporarily in the earth while muscles push it ahead.

Exoskeleton

An exoskeleton is a hard skeleton that covers all muscles and organs of some invertebrates. Exoskeletons are found principally in arthropods (e.g., insects). Insect exoskeletons are composed of chitin. All exoskeletons are composed of noncellular material secreted by the epidermis. Whereas they offer the animal some protection, exoskeletons impose limitations on growth. Thus, periodic molting and deposition of a new skeleton are necessary to permit body growth.

VERTEBRATE SKELETON

An endoskeleton serves as the framework within all vertebrate organisms. Muscles are attached to the bones, permitting movement. The endoskeleton also provides protection by surrounding delicate vital organs in bone. The rib cage protects the thoracic organs (heart and lungs), whereas the skull and vertebral column protect the brain and spinal cord. The two major components of the skeleton are cartilage and bone.

Structure of the Skeleton

Cartilage

Cartilage is a type of connective tissue that is softer and more flexible than bone. Cartilage is retained in adults in places where firmness and flexibility are needed. For example, in humans, the external ear, the nose, the walls of the larynx and trachea, and the skeletal joints contain cartilage. **Chrondytes** are cells responsible for synthesizing cartillage.

Bone

Bone is a specialized type of mineralized connective tissue that has the ability to withstand physical stress. Ideally designed for body support, bone tissue is hard and strong while, at the same time, somewhat elastic and lightweight. There are two basic types of bone: compact bone and spongy bone.

1. **Compact bone** is dense bone that does not appear to have any cavities when observed with the naked eye. The bony matrix is deposited in structural units called **osteons** (Haversian systems). Each osteon consists of a central microscopic channel called a **Haversian canal**, surrounded by a number of concentric circles of bony matrix (calcium phosphate) called **lamellae**.

2. **Spongy bone** is much less dense and consists of an interconnecting lattice of bony **spicules** (trabeculae); the cavities in between the spicules are filled with yellow or red bone marrow. **Yellow marrow** is inactive and infiltrated by adipose tissue; **red marrow** is involved in blood cell formation.

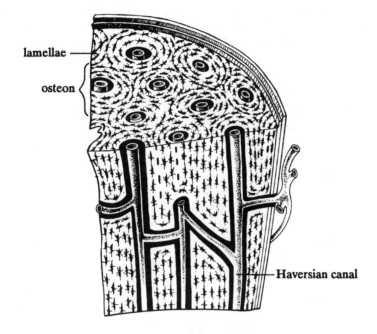

Figure 16.1

Osteocytes

Two other types of cells found in bone tissue are osteoblasts and osteoclasts. **Osteoblasts** synthesize and secrete the organic constituents of the bone matrix; once they have become surrounded by their matrix, they mature into osteocytes. **Osteoclasts** are large, multinucleated cells involved in bone resorption.

Bone formation

Bone formation occurs by either endochondral ossification or by intramembranous ossification. In **endochondral ossification**, existing cartilage is replaced by bone. Long bones arise primarily through endochondral ossification. In **intramembranous ossification**, mesenchymal (embryonic or undifferentiated) connective tissue is transformed into, and replaced by, bone.

Organization of Vertebrate Skeleton

The axial skeleton is the basic framework of the body, consisting of the skull, vertebral column, and the rib cage. It is the point of attachment of the appendicular skeleton, which includes the bones of the appendages and the pectoral and pelvic girdles.

Bones are held together in a number of ways. Sutures or immovable joints hold the bones of the skull together. Bones that move relative to one another are held together by movable joints and are additionally supported and strengthened by ligaments. Ligaments serve as bone-to bone-connectors. Tendons attach skeletal muscle to bones and bend the skeleton at the movable joints.

The point of attachment of a muscle to a stationary bone (the proximal end in limb muscles) is called the **origin**. The point of attachment of a muscle to the bone that moves (distal end in limb muscles) is called the **insertion**. **Extension** indicates a straightening of a joint, whereas **flexion** refers to a bending of a joint.

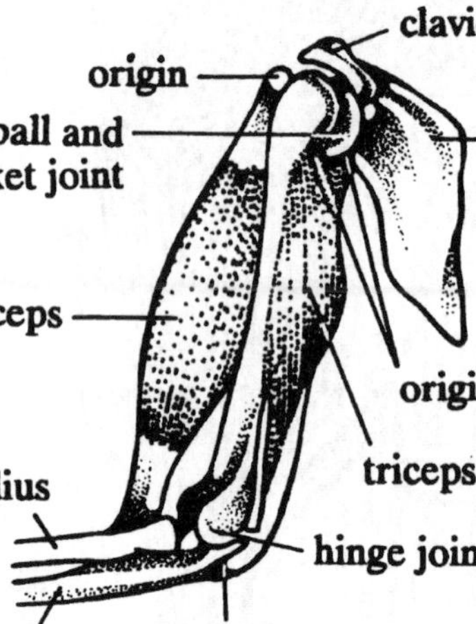

Figure 16.2

MUSCULAR SYSTEM

Muscle tissue consists of bundles of specialized contractile fibers held together by connective tissue. There are three morphologically and functionally distinct types of muscle in mammals: skeletal muscle, smooth muscle, and cardiac muscle.

With respect to the control of the muscular system, the axons of the pyramidal cells of the motor cortex descend to synapse on lower motor neurons in the brain stem and the spinal cord. Because there are no intervening synapses, the **pyramidal system** is able to provide rapid commands to the skeletal muscles and various other organs. Several other centers can issue somatic motor commands as a result of processing performed at the unconscious, involuntary level. These centers and their associated tracts comprise the **extrapyramidal system**. The red nucleus, located in the mesencephalon, is the component of the extrapyramidal system primarily in control of skeletal muscle tone.

SKELETAL MUSCLE

Skeletal muscle is responsible for voluntary movements and is innervated by the somatic nervous system. Each fiber is a multinucleated cell created by the fusion of several mononucleated embryonic cells. Embedded in the fibers are filaments called **myofibrils,** which are further divided into contractile units called **sarcomeres**. The myofibrils are enveloped by a modified endoplasmic reticulum that stores calcium ions and is called the **sarcoplasmic reticulum**. The cytoplasm of a muscle fiber is called sarcoplasm, and the cell membrane is called the sarcolemma. The **sarcolemma** is capable of propagating an action potential and is connected to a system of transverse tubules (T system) oriented perpendicularly to the myofibrils. The **T system** provides channels for ion flow throughout the muscle fibers, and can also propagate an action potential. Because of the high energy requirements of contraction, mitochondria are very abundant in muscle cells, distributed along the myofibrils. Skeletal muscle has striations of light and dark bands and is therefore also referred to as **striated muscle**.

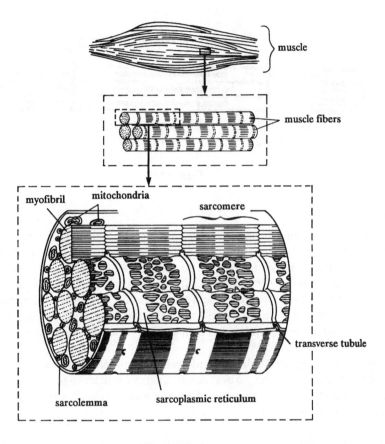

Figure 16.3

The Sarcomere

Structure

The sarcomere is composed of thin and thick filaments. The thin filaments are chains of actin molecules. The thick filaments are composed of organized bundles of myosin molecules.

Electron microscopy reveals that the sarcomere is organized as follows. **Z lines** define the boundaries of a single sarcomere and anchor the thin filaments. The **M line** runs down the center of the sarcomere. The **I band** is the region containing thin filaments only. The **H zone** is the region containing thick filaments only. The **A band** spans the entire length of the thick filaments and any overlapping portions of the thin filaments. Note that during contraction, the A band is not reduced in size, whereas the H zone and I band are.

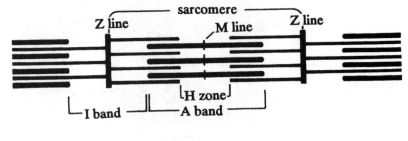

Figure 16.4

Contraction

Muscle contraction is stimulated by a message from the somatic nervous system sent via a motor neuron. The link between the nerve terminal (synaptic bouton) and the sarcolemma of the muscle fiber is called the **neuromuscular junction**. The space between the two is known as the synapse, or synaptic cleft. Depolarization of the motor neuron results in the release of neurotransmitters (e.g., acetylcholine) from the nerve terminal. The neurotransmitter diffuses across the synaptic cleft and binds to special receptor sites on the sarcolemma. If enough of these receptors are stimulated, the permeability of the sarcolemma is altered and an action potential is generated.

Once an action potential is generated, it is conducted along the sarcolemma and the T system and into the interior of the muscle fiber. This causes the sarcoplasmic reticulum to release calcium ions into the sarcoplasm. Calcium ions initiate the contraction of the sarcomere. Actin and myosin slide past each other, and the sarcomere contracts.

An interesting point is that several hours after death, all of the muscles in the body go into a state of **rigor mortis**. In this condition, the muscles contract and become rigid, even without action potentials. The rigidity is caused by an absence of adenosine triphosphate, which is required for the myosin heads to be released from the actin filaments. The muscles typically remain rigid for 12 to 24 hours after death until the muscle proteins are destroyed.

There are five major types of muscle contraction: isotonic, concentric, dynamic, eccentric, and isometric. An **isotonic** contraction occurs when a muscle shortens against a fixed load while the tension on that muscle remains constant. A **concentric** contraction is a type of dynamic contraction where the muscle fibers shorten and the tension on the muscle increases. A **dynamic** contraction includes both concentric and eccentric types of contractions. In general, a dynamic contraction results in the change in length of the muscle with a corresponding change in tension on that muscle. An **eccentric** contraction is a type of dynamic contraction where the muscle fiber lengthens and the tension on the muscle increases. An **isometric** contraction occurs when both ends of the muscle are fixed and no change in length occurs during the contraction, but the tension increases.

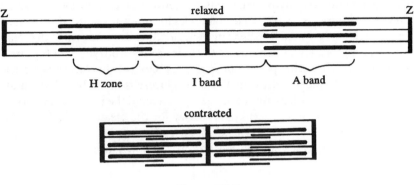

Figure 16.5

Stimulus and muscle response

Individual muscle fibers generally exhibit an all-or-none response; only a stimulus above a minimal value called the threshold value can elicit contraction. The strength of the contraction of a single muscle fiber cannot be increased, regardless of the strength of the stimulus. However, the strength of contraction of the entire muscle can be increased by recruiting more muscle fibers.

- A **simple twitch** is the response of a single muscle fiber to a brief stimulus at or above the threshold stimulus, and consists of a latent period, a contraction period, and a relaxation period. The latent period is the time between stimulation and the onset of contraction. During this time lag, the action potential spreads along the sarcolemma, and Ca^{2+} ions are released. After the contraction period, there is a brief relaxation period in which the muscle is unresponsive to a stimulus; this period is known as the **absolute refractory period**.

- When the fibers of a muscle are exposed to very frequent stimuli, the muscle cannot fully relax. The contractions begin to combine, becoming stronger and more prolonged. This is known as **temporal summation**. The contractions become continuous when the stimuli are so frequent that the muscle cannot relax. This type of contraction is known as **tetanus** and is stronger than a simple twitch of a single fiber. If tetanus is maintained, the muscle will fatigue, and the contraction will weaken.

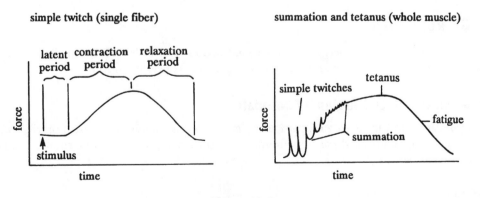

Figure 16.6

- **Tonus** is a state of partial contraction. Muscles are never completely relaxed and maintain a partially contracted state at all times.

During periods of strenuous activity, skeletal muscles convert glucose to pyruvic acid through the process of glycolysis. This process enables skeletal muscles to continue contracting, even in the absence of oxygen. Lactic acid is generated when pyruvic acid is reacted with the enzyme lactate dehydrogenase. This process allows the pyruvate to enter the tricarboxylic acid (or citric acid) cycle. The purpose of the **Cori cycle** during periods of strenuous activity is to convert lactic acid in the liver to glucose for discharge into the bloodstream. Once the glucose is in the blood, the muscles are then able to use the glucose as an immediate source of energy or rebuild their glycogen reserves. Conversion of glucose into pyruvate in the muscle cells is necessary for the creation of ATP during periods of strenuous exercise and does not involve the Cori cycle. During periods of intense exercise, the production of lactic acid is increased, and glycogen is broken down into glucose; however, that is not by means of the Cori cycle.

Smooth Muscle

Smooth muscle is responsible for involuntary actions and is innervated by the autonomic nervous system. Smooth muscle is found in the digestive tract, bladder, uterus, and blood vessel walls, among other places. Smooth muscle cells possess one centrally located nucleus. Smooth muscles lack the striations of skeletal muscle.

Cardiac Muscle

The muscle tissue of the heart is composed of cardiac muscle fibers. These fibers possess characteristics of both skeletal and smooth muscle fibers. As in skeletal muscle, actin and myosin filaments are arranged in sarcomeres, giving cardiac muscle a striated appearance. However, cardiac muscle cells generally have only one or two centrally located nuclei.

Smooth Muscle	Cardiac Muscle	Skeletal Muscle
<ul><li>Nonstriated</li><li>One nucleus per cell</li><li>Involuntary/autonomic nervous system</li><li>Smooth, continuous contractions</li></ul>	<ul><li>Striated</li><li>One to two nuclei per cell</li><li>Involuntary/autonomic nervous system</li><li>Strong, forceful contractions</li></ul>	<ul><li>Striated</li><li>Multinucleated cells</li><li>Voluntary/somatic nervous system</li><li>Strong, forceful contractions</li></ul>

ENERGY RESERVES

ATP is the primary source of energy for muscle contraction. Very little ATP is actually stored in the muscles, so other forms of energy must be stored and rapidly converted to ATP.

Creatine Phosphate and Arginine Phosphate

In vertebrates and some invertebrates, particularly echinoderms, energy can be temporarily stored in a high-energy compound called creatine phosphate. Many invertebrates utilize a similar compound called arginine phosphate.

Myoglobin

Myoglobin is a hemoglobin-like protein found in muscle tissue. Myoglobin has a high oxygen affinity and maintains the oxygen supply in muscles by binding oxygen tightly.

REVIEW PROBLEMS

Questions 1, 2, and 3 are based on the following diagram:

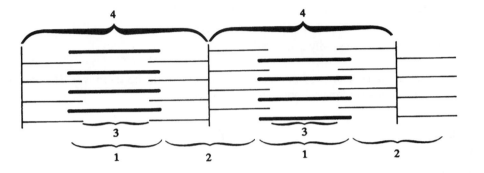

1. During muscle contraction, which of the following regions decrease(s) in length?

    (A) 1 only

    (B) 2 only

    (C) 3 only

    (D) 4 only

    (E) 2, 3, and 4

2. Region 1 refers to

    (A) the thick filaments only.

    (B) the thin filaments only.

    (C) the A band.

    (D) the I band.

    (E) both A and D.

3. Which region represents one sarcomere?

    (A) 1

    (B) 2

    (C) 3

    (D) 4

4. Which of the following cells is correctly coupled with its definition?

    (A) Osteoblasts–bone cells involved in the secretion of bone matrix

    (B) Osteoclasts–immature bone cells

    (C) Osteocytes–multinucleated cells actively involved in bone resorption

    (D) Chondrocytes–undifferentiated bone marrow cells

5. Describe the microscopic structure of compact bone. Include the following terms in your discussion: bone matrix, osteon, Haversian canal, canaliculi, lamellae, lacunae, and osteocyte.

6. When a muscle fiber is subjected to very frequent stimuli
   (A) an oxygen debt is incurred.
   (B) a muscle tonus is generated.
   (C) the threshold value is reached.
   (D) the contractions combine in a process known as summation.
   (E) a simple twitch is repeatedly generated.

7. When a muscle is attached to two bones, usually only one of the bones moves. The part of the muscle attached to the stationary bone is referred to as
   (A) proximal.
   (B) distal.
   (C) origin.
   (D) insertion.
   (E) tetanus.

8. Two processes are involved in bone formation. How do they differ from one another?

   Questions 9–11 refer to the following types of muscle

   I. cardiac muscle

   II. skeletal muscle

   III. smooth muscle

9. Which type of muscle is always multinucleated?
   (A) I only
   (B) II only
   (C) III only
   (D) Both I and II
   (E) Both II and III

10. Which type of muscle has myogenic activity?
    (A) I only
    (B) II only
    (C) III only
    (D) Both I and II
    (E) Both I and III

11. Which type of muscle lacks sarcomeric striations?
    (A) I only
    (B) II only
    (C) III only
    (D) Both II and III

SOLUTIONS TO REVIEW PROBLEMS

1. **E** Discussed in the sarcomere section.

2. **C** Discussed in the sarcomere section.

3. **D** Discussed in the sarcomere section.

4. **A** Discussed in structure of vertebrate skeleton section.

5.   Discussed in structure of vertebrate skeleton section.

6. **D** Discussed in summation section of stimulus and muscle response.

7. **C** Discussed in muscle/bone interactions section.

8.   The processes are called endochondral ossification and intramembranous ossification. In endochrondral ossification, cartilage is replaced with bone. In intramembranous ossification, mesenchyme, or undifferentiated cells, are transformed into bone cells.

9. **B** Discussed in skeletal muscle section.

10. **E** Discussed in smooth muscle and cardiac muscle section.

11. **C** Discussed in smooth muscle section.

CHAPTER SEVENTEEN

Digestion

Animals are **heterotrophic** and thus unable to synthesize their own nutrients. Food provides the raw material for energy, repair, and growth of tissues. The food must first be **ingested**. **Digestion** consists of the degradation of large molecules into smaller molecules that can be **absorbed** into the bloodstream and used directly by cells. **Intracellular** digestion occurs within the cell, usually in membrane-bound vesicles. **Extracellular** digestion refers to a digestive process that occurs outside of the cell, within a lumen or tract.

DIGESTION IN UNICELLULAR ORGANISMS

In unicellular organisms, food capture is effected primarily by **phagocytosis**. Food vacuoles form immediately after ingestion. In the **amoeba**, pseudopods surround and engulf food (phagocytosis) and enclose it in food vacuoles. **Lysosomes** (containing digestive enzymes) fuse with the food vacuole and release their digestive enzymes that act upon the nutrients. The resulting simpler molecules diffuse into the cytoplasm. The unusable end products are eliminated from the vacuole.

In the paramecium, cilia sweep food into the oral groove and **cytopharynx**. A food vacuole forms around food at the lower end of the cytopharynx. Eventually, the vacuole breaks off into the cytoplasm and progresses toward the anterior end of the cell. Enzymes are secreted into the vacuole and the products diffuse into the cytoplasm. Solid wastes are expelled at the anal pore.

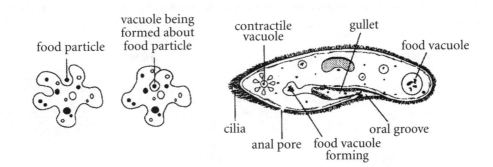

Figure 17.1

DIGESTION IN INVERTEBRATES

Multicellular organisms have developed numerous adaptations for food capture and ingestion, digestion, and absorption. In many animals, the **physical breakdown** of large particles of food into small particles begins by cutting and grinding in the mouth and churning in the digestive tract. The molecular composition is unchanged, but the surface area of the substrates on which the enzymes act is increased. **Chemical breakdown** of molecules is accomplished by enzymatic hydrolysis. The smaller digested nutrients (glucose, amino acids, fatty acids, and glycerol) pass through the semipermeable plasma membrane of the gut cells to be further metabolized or transported.

Cnidarians

The hydra uses intracellular and extracellular digestion. **Tentacles** bring food to the mouth (ingestion) and release the particles into a cup-like sac. The endodermal cells lining this gastrovascular cavity secrete enzymes into the cavity. Thus, digestion principally occurs outside the cells (extracellular). However, once the food is reduced to small fragments the gastrodermal cells engulf the nutrients and digestion is completed intracellularly. Undigested food is expelled through the **mouth**. Every cell is exposed to the external environment, thereby facilitating intracellular digestion.

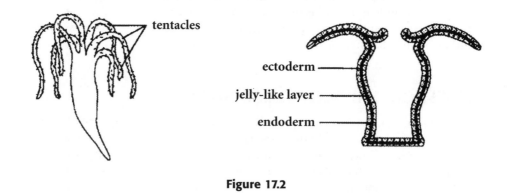

Figure 17.2

Annelids

Like higher animals, **earthworms** have a one-way digestive tract with both a mouth and an anus. This allows **specialization** of different parts of the digestive tract for different functions. These parts include the mouth, pharynx, esophagus, **crop** (to store the food), **gizzard** (to grind the food), **intestine** (which contains a large dorsal fold (**typholosole**) to provide increased surface area for digestion and absorption), and **anus**. Soluble food passes, by diffusion, through the walls of the small intestine into the blood.

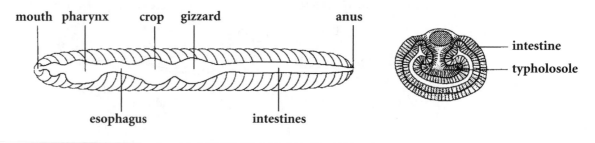

Figure 17.3

Arthropods

Insects have a digestive system similar to that of the earthworm. They also have jaws for chewing and **salivary glands**, which improve food digestion.

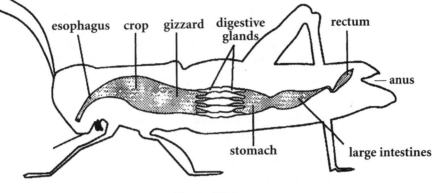

Figure 17.4

DIGESTION IN HUMANS

The human digestive tract begins with the **oral cavity** and continues with the **pharynx**, the **esophagus**, the **stomach**, the **small intestine**, the **large intestine**, and the anus. Accessory organs, such as the salivary glands, the pancreas, the liver, and the gall bladder, also play essential roles in digestion.

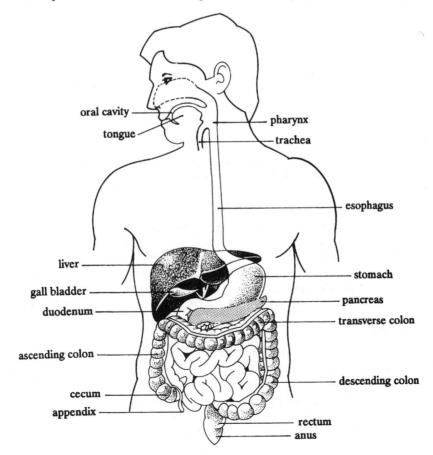

Figure 17.5

The Oral Cavity

The oral cavity (the mouth) is where **mechanical** and **chemical** digestion of food begins. Mechanical digestion is the breakdown of large food particles into smaller particles through the biting and chewing action of teeth (**mastication**). Chemical digestion refers to the enzymatic breakdown of macromolecules into smaller molecules and begins in the mouth when the salivary glands secrete **saliva**. Saliva **lubricates** food to facilitate swallowing and provides a solvent for food particles. Saliva is secreted in response to a nervous reflex triggered by the presence of food in the oral cavity. Saliva contains the enzyme **salivary amylase** (**ptyalin**), which hydrolyzes starch to maltose (a disaccharide).

The Esophagus

The esophagus is the muscular tube leading from the mouth to the stomach. Food is moved down the esophagus by rhythmic waves of involuntary muscular contractions called **peristalsis**.

The body of the esophagus lies within a negative thoracic cavity, and the abdominal cavity has a positive pressure gradient. Therefore, without normal defense mechanisms, the pressure gradients favor a continual reflux of gastric materials into the esophagus. There is a pathological condition known as gastroesophageal reflux disease (GERD). The primary mechanisms by which gastroesophageal reflux may occur are as follows:

- Reflux can occur after spontaneous transient lower esophageal sphincter relaxations not associated with swallowing.
- Resting pressures of the lower esophageal sphincter normally range from 15–35 mmHg above gastric baseline pressure.
- Patients with GERD usually have a decreased lower esophageal reflux pressure (5–10 mmHg above gastric baseline pressure), leading to an increased passage of stomach contents into the esophagus.
- A decreased lower esophageal sphincter pressure is not always associated with the development of GERD; however, the majority of patients with GERD are noted to have a decreased lower esophageal sphincter pressure.

The Stomach

The stomach, a large, muscular organ located in the upper abdomen, stores and partially digests food. The walls of the stomach are lined by the thick gastric mucosa, which contains the glands. These glands secrete **mucus**, which protects the stomach lining from the harshly acidic juices (pH = 2) present in the stomach. They also secrete **pepsin**, protein-hydrolyzing enzyme, and hydrochloric acid (HCl), which kills bacteria, dissolves the intercellular "glue" holding food tissues together, and activates certain proteins. Chief cells synthesize pepsinogen, which is converted to pepsin. Parietal cells synthesize and release HCl and intrinsic factor. The churning of the stomach produces an acidic, semifluid mixture of partially digested food known as **chyme**. The chyme passes into the first segment of the small intestine, the **duodenum**, through the pyloric sphincter.

The Small Intestine

Chemical digestion is completed in the small intestine. The small intestine is divided into three sections: the **duodenum**, the **jejunum**, and the **ileum**. The small intestine is highly **adapted** to **absorption**. To maximize the surface area available for digestion and absorption, the intestine is extremely long (greater than six meters in length) and highly coiled. In addition, numerous finger-like projections called **villi** extend out of the intestinal wall. Villi contain capillaries and lacteals (vessels of the lymphatic system). Amino acids and monosaccharides pass through the villi walls into the capillary system. Large fatty acids and glycerol pass into the lacteals and are then reconverted into fats (fatty acid + glycerol). Note that some nutrients are actively absorbed (i.e., requiring energy), such as glucose and amino acids, whereas others are passively absorbed.

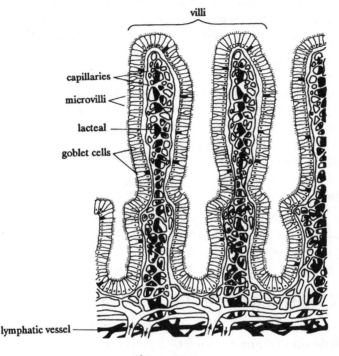

Figure 17.6

Most digestion in the small intestine occurs in the duodenum, where the secretions of the intestinal glands, pancreas, liver, and gall bladder mix together with the acidic chyme entering from the stomach. The intestinal mucosa secretes **lipases** (for fat digestion), **aminopeptidases** (for polypeptide digestion), and **disaccharidases** (digestion of maltose, lactose, sucrose). The disaccharidase **lactase** breaks down lactose (milk sugar). This enzyme is present in infants, but many adults lack the enzyme and are **lactose-intolerant**. Lactose in the small intestine cannot be digested and is metabolized by bacteria, producing intestinal discomfort.

Digestion Enzymes

Here is a summary of some of the most important digestive enzymes. The parietal cell of the stomach secretes two substances: intrinsic factor and hydrochloric acid. **Gastrin**, produced in the G cells of the duodenum, primarily functions to stimulate hydrochloric acid, histamine, and pepsinogen secretion as well as increase gastric blood flow. Gastrin stimulates the parietal cells to produce a substance (**hydrochloric acid**) that denatures proteins and activates digestive enzymes. **Intrinsic factor** is a secretion of the parietal cells that facilitates the absorption of vitamin B_{12} across the intestinal lining. **Cholecystokinin** is produced and stored in the I cells of the duodenal and jejunal mucosa. It is involved in stimulation of pancreatic enzymes and somatostatin secretion as well as gallbladder contraction. **Secretin** is synthesized and stored in the S cells of the upper intestine. It stimulates the secretion of bicarbonate-containing substances from the pancreas and inhibits gastric emptying and gastric acid production.

The Liver

The liver produces **bile** that is stored in the **gall bladder** before release into the small intestine. Bile contains no enzymes; it **emulsifies** fats, breaking down large globules into small droplets. Emulsification of fats exposes a greater surface area of the fat to the action of pancreatic lipase. In the absence of bile, fats cannot be digested. The liver's functions also include storage of glycogen, conversion of ammonia to urea, protein synthesis, detoxification, and cholesterol metabolism.

The Pancreas

The pancreas produces enzymes such as **amylase** for carbohydrate digestion, **trypsin** for protein digestion, and **lipase** for fat digestion. When the pancreas releases chymotrypsin and enterokinase, the enterokinase cleaves trypsinogen to trypsin. Trypsin then cleaves and activates the other zymogens (enzyme precursors). The pancreas secretes a bicarbonate-rich juice that neutralizes the acidic chyme arriving from the stomach. The pancreatic enzymes operate optimally at this higher pH.

The Large Intestine

The large intestine is approximately 1.5 m long and functions in the absorption of salts and the absorption of any water not already absorbed by the small intestine. The **rectum** provides for transient storage of feces before elimination through the anus.

DIGESTION IN PLANTS AND FUNGI

Plants have no digestive system, but intracellular digestive processes similar to those of animals do occur, coordinating the use of nutrients with their production.

Intracellular Digestion

Plants store insoluble polymers, starches, lipids, and proteins in the cells. The principle storage food is starch (a glucose polysaccharide), found in large quantities in seeds, stems, and roots. When nutrients are required, the storage polymers are broken down to simpler molecules (glucose, fatty acids, glycerol, and amino acids) by enzyme **hydrolysis**. The simple products can be used in the storage cell itself or transported by diffusion to other cells.

Extracellular Digestion

Some heterotrophic organisms such as fungi must obtain preformed organic molecules (nutrients) from the environment. Enzymes are secreted, hydrolyzing complex nutrients into simpler molecules, which are then absorbed. Once inside, the simpler molecules can be used for energy or to synthesize larger molecules.

For example, the **rhizoids** of bread mold, a typical saprophyte that lives on dead organic material, secrete enzymes into the external environment (the bread). Digestion produces simple soluble end products (glucose, amino acids, fatty acids, and glycerol), which are absorbed by diffusion into the rhizoid and transported throughout the mold.

In the plant kingdom, the **Venus flytrap** comes the closest to performing actual ingestion. When a fly arrives, certain sensitive tissues entrap the insect. **Enzymes** are secreted to digest the fly and absorb the soluble end products. This is, of course, extracellular digestion. Note that the Venus fly trap is still an autotroph—it photosynthesizes to produce glucose. It uses the insect as a **nitrate** source, as the flytrap grows in nitrogen-poor soils.

REVIEW PROBLEMS

1. Define extracellular digestion. How is the stomach specialized for extracellular digestion?

2. Where are proteins digested?

   (A) Mouth and stomach
   (B) Stomach and large intestine
   (C) Small intestine and large intestine
   (D) Mouth and small intestine
   (E) Stomach and small intestine

3. All of the following processes occur in the mouth EXCEPT

   (A) mechanical digestion.
   (B) moistening of food.
   (C) bolus formation.
   (D) chemical digestion of proteins.
   (E) chemical digestion of starch.

4. The graphs below show the relative activities of pepsin and chymotrypsin in solutions of varying pH. Which graph refers to which enzyme?

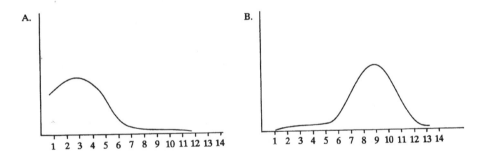

5. Outline the digestion of a piece of bread.

6. Why is pancreatic juice alkaline, and what would happen if its alkaline components were removed?

7. Starch is hydrolyzed into maltose by
    (A) salivary amylase.
    (B) maltase.
    (C) pancreatic amylase.
    (D) both A and C.

8. The intestinal capillaries transport nutrients from the intestines to the
    (A) large intestine.
    (B) liver.
    (C) kidney.
    (D) heart.

9. Describe the digestive system of an earthworm.

SOLUTIONS TO REVIEW PROBLEMS

1. Digestion refers to a mechanical or chemical process whereby macromolecules are converted into smaller molecules that are more readily absorbed and used by cells. Extracellular digestion describes a process in which molecules are broken down outside of the cell. The stomach is a cavity perfectly designed for extracellular digestion. Macromolecules are digested in an environment confined by the lower esophageal and pyloric sphincters. The cells lining the stomach walls are specialized for HCl and pepsinogen secretion by their ability to withstand acidic conditions. Muscular contractions aid in digestion by churning and crushing food. Little absorption occurs in the stomach; chyme is propelled into the small intestine, where further digestion and absorption occur.

2. **E** Protein digestion begins in the stomach with pepsin and continues in the small intestine.

3. **D** Chewing, the mechanical digestion of food, occurs in the mouth, as does moistening of food by saliva and bolus formation. In addition, salivary amylase begins digestion of complex carbohydrates.

4. Graph A refers to pepsin, whereas graph B refers to chymotrypsin. Pepsin is a gastric enzyme; it works best under the highly acidic conditions of the stomach. Chymotrypsin is an enzyme of the small intestine and thus operates optimally in alkaline environments.

5. In the mouth, teeth chew the bread into smaller particles, and salivary amylase digests some of the starch (the major component of bread) into maltose. The bread enters the stomach, where there is no chemical digestion of starch, and then the small intestine. In the small intestine, pancreatic amylase hydrolyzes starch into maltose while maltase, sucrase, and lactase hydrolyze various disaccharides into their respective monosaccharides. Most of the monosaccharides (e.g., glucose, fructose, and galactose) are absorbed into the circulatory system through the intestinal wall.

6. Pancreatic juice is an alkaline fluid that helps neutralize the acidity of the chyme entering the small intestine from the stomach. This is necessary because the small intestine enzymes work optimally at a neutral or alkaline pH. Also, the walls (mucosa) of the small intestine are not specialized for protection against acidic conditions. Therefore, without alkaline pancreatic juice, the intestinal enzymes would not function, and the intestinal walls would be destroyed.

7. **D** Amylase, whether it is produced in the mouth or the pancreas, digests starch into maltose, a disaccharide.

8. **B** Intestinal capillaries transport amino acids and monosaccharides to the liver where initial processing of many nutrients begins.

9. In an earthworm, food is ingested at the mouth and excreted from the anus. The food is ground in the gizzard and absorbed in the intestine, which has a specialized fold to increase the surface area.

CHAPTER EIGHTEEN

Excretion

Excretion refers to the removal of **metabolic wastes** produced in the body. It is distinguished from **elimination**, the removal of indigestible material. Most of the body's activities produce metabolic wastes that must be removed. **Aerobic respiration** leads to the production of **carbon dioxide** and water. **Deamination** of amino acids in the liver leads to the production of **nitrogenous wastes** such as urea and ammonia. All metabolic processes lead to the production of mineral salts, which must be excreted by the kidneys.

EXCRETION IN INVERTEBRATES

Excretion in Protozoans and Cnidarians

In these phyla, all cells are in contact with the external, aqueous environment. Water-soluble wastes, such as **ammonia** and **carbon dioxide**, can exit the cells by simple diffusion through the cell membrane. This type of excretion is **passive**. Some freshwater protozoa, such as the paramecium, possess a contractile **vacuole**—an organelle specialized for water excretion by active transport. Excess water, which continually diffuses into the cell from the hypotonic environment (freshwater), is collected and periodically pumped out of the cell. This permits the cell to maintain its volume and pressure.

Excretion in Annelids

In earthworms, carbon dioxide excretion occurs directly through the moist skin. Two pairs of **nephridia** in each body segment excrete water, mineral salts, and nitrogenous wastes in the form of urea.

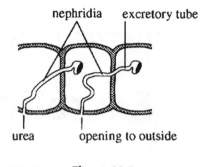

nephridia   excretory tube

urea   opening to outside

Figure 18.1

Excretion in Arthropods

In insects, carbon dioxide is released from the tissues into adjacent tubelike **tracheae**, which are continuous with the external air, through openings called **spiracles**. Nitrogenous wastes are excreted in the form of solid **uric acid** crystals. The use of solid nitrogenous wastes is an adaptation for the conservation of water. Mineral salts and uric acid accumulate in the **Malphigian tubules** and are then transported to the intestine to be expelled with the solid wastes of digestion.

EXCRETION IN HUMANS

The principal organs of excretion in humans are the lungs, liver, skin, and kidneys. In the **lungs**, carbon dioxide and water vapor diffuse from the blood and are continually exhaled. Sweat glands in the **skin** excrete water and dissolved salts (and a small quantity of urea). Perspiration serves to regulate body temperature, since the evaporation of sweat produces cooling. The **liver** processes nitrogenous wastes, blood pigment wastes, and other chemicals for excretion. Urea is produced by the deamination of amino acids in the liver and diffuses into the blood for ultimate excretion in the **kidneys**. Bile salts and red blood pigments are excreted as bile and pass out with the feces. The kidneys function to maintain the osmolarity of the blood; excrete numerous waste products and toxic chemicals; and conserve glucose, salt, and water.

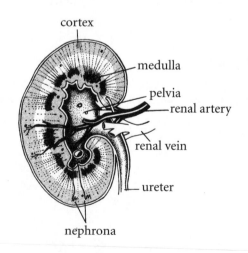

cortex

medulla

pelvia

renal artery

renal vein

ureter

nephrona

Figure 18.2

The Kidneys

The kidneys regulate the concentration of salt and water in the blood through the formation and excretion of urine. The kidneys are bean shaped and are located behind the stomach and liver. Each kidney is composed of approximately one million units called **nephrons**.

Structure

The kidney is divided into three regions: the outer **cortex**, the inner **medulla**, and the renal **pelvis**. A **nephron** consists of a bulb called **Bowman's capsule**, which embraces a special capillary bed called a **glomerulus**. Bowman's capsule leads into a long, coiled tubule that is divided into functionally distinct units: the **proximal convoluted tubule**, the **loop of Henle**, the **distal convoluted tubule**, and the **collecting duct**. The nephron is positioned such that the loop of Henle runs through the medulla, while the convoluted tubules and Bowman's capsule are in the cortex. Concentrated urine in the collecting tubules flows into the pelvis of the kidney, a funnel-like region that opens directly into the **ureter**. The ureters from each kidney empty into the **urinary bladder**, where urine collects until expelled via the **urethra**. Most of the nephron is surrounded by a complex **peritubular capillary** network to facilitate reabsorption of amino acids, glucose, salts, and water.

Urine formation

Filtration, secretion, and reabsorption are the three processes that lead to urine formation.

Filtration—Blood pressure forces 20 percent of the blood plasma entering the glomerulus through the capillary walls and into the surrounding Bowman's capsule. The fluid and small solutes entering the nephron are called the **filtrate**. The filtrate is isotonic with blood plasma. Particles too large to filter through the glomerulus, such as blood cells and albumin, remain in the circulatory system. Filtration is a passive process driven by the hydrostatic pressure of the blood.

Secretion—The nephron secretes substances such as acids, bases, and ions like potassium and phosphate from the interstitial fluid into the filtrate by both **passive** and **active** transport. Materials are secreted from the peritubular capillaries into the nephron tubule.

Body fluid pH remains relatively constant at 7.4; this consistency is attained by the removal of carbon dioxide through lungs or hydrogen ions through the kidneys. Assessment of the pH is measured through the:

- Arterial pH
- Partial pressure of the carbon dioxide (PCO_2)
- Plasma bicarbonate (HCO_3^-)

There are two types of acid-base disorders:

1. **Respiratory**—Affect the blood acidity by causing changes in the PCO_2.
2. **Metabolic**—Affect the blood acidity by causing changes in the HCO_3^-.

Below is a summary of acid-base disorders and compensatory mechanisms by the human body.

Condition	Defect	Blood pH	Compensatory mechanism
Respiratory acidosis	Inc PCO_2	Dec	Inc HCO_3^-
Respiratory alkalosis	Dec PCO_2	Inc	Dec HCO_3^-
Metabolic acidosis	Dec HCO_3^-	Dec	Dec PCO_2
Metabolic alkalosis	Inc HCO_3^-	Inc	Inc PCO_2

Reabsorption—Essential substances (**glucose**, **salts**, and **amino acids**) and water are reabsorbed from the filtrate and returned to the blood. Reabsorption occurs primarily in the proximal convoluted tubule and is an active process. Movement of these molecules is accompanied by the passive movement of water. This results in the formation of **concentrated urine**, which is hypertonic to the blood.

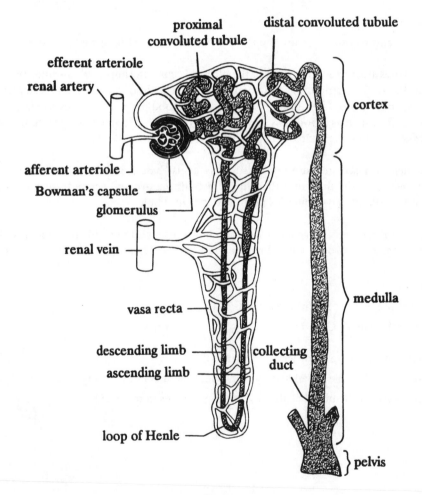

Figure 18.3

Nephron function

Through the **selective permeability** of its walls and the maintenance of an **osmolarity gradient**, the nephron reabsorbs nutrients, salts, and water from the filtrate and returns them to the body, thus maintaining the bloodstream's solute concentration.

The primary function of the nephron is to "clean" the blood plasma of unwanted substances as it passes through the kidney. Because blood plasma contains both wanted and unwanted substances, the nephron will selectively reabsorb wanted substances, at selected portions of the nephron, back into the plasma, while the remaining substances are excreted in the urine. The primary site of nutrient reabsorption in the nephron is the proximal convoluted tubule. The ascending loop of Henle, collecting duct, and descending loop of Henle are the primary sites of regulating water, sodium, and potassium loss in the nephron. The distal convoluted tubule is the primary site for secretion of substances into the filtrate.

Aldosterone, for example, is a hormone that causes an increased exchange transport of sodium and potassium ions along the distal convoluted tubule, the collecting tubule, and the collecting duct, resulting in a decreased excretion of sodium ions in the urine and an increased potassium ion excretion in the urine. Furthermore, it does not affect renal blood flow. The antidiuretic hormone is responsible for the creation of a more concentrated urine or a more dilute urine.

Osmolarity gradient—The selective permeability of the tubules establishes an osmolarity gradient in the surrounding interstitial fluid. By exiting and then reentering at different segments of the nephron, solutes create an osmolarity gradient, with tissue osmolarity increasing from **cortex** to **inner medulla**. The solutes that contribute to the maintenance of the gradient are urea and salt (Na+ and Cl–). The osmolarity of urine (determined by the concentration of dissolved particles) is established in the collecting tubule by means of this **counter-current-multiplier system**: the anatomic arrangement of the loop of Henle within the kidney permits the establishment of the concentration gradient that permits the reabsorption of 99 percent of the filtrate in the collecting tubules. Thus, the production of concentrated urine is possible.

Concentration of urine

The counter-current system causes the medium in the medulla of the kidney to be **hyperosmolar** with respect to the dilute filtrate flowing in the collecting tubule. As the filtrate flowing in the collecting tubules passes through this region of the kidney, on its way to the pelvis and ureter, water flows out of the collecting tubules by **osmosis**. This water is removed by capillaries flowing in the medulla. The reabsorption of water in this zone of the kidney, which permits the concentration of urine, depends on the permeability of the collecting tubules to water. Regulation of the permeability of the collecting tubule to water is accomplished by the hormone **ADH (vasopressin)**. ADH increases the permeability of the collecting duct to water, allowing more water to be absorbed and more concentrated urine to be formed.

EXCRETION IN PLANTS

There is no specific excretory system in plants. Whereas animals excrete the unusable products of metabolism as wastes, plants are able to use many of these "waste" products. These products are used as simple precursors in the synthesis of complex molecules; for example, **carbon dioxide** is used in **photosynthesis**, and **nitrogen** wastes can be reused in the synthesis of **proteins**.

Any excess carbon dioxide, as well as waste oxygen and water vapor, leaves the plant by diffusion through **stomata** (pores in leaves) and **lenticels** (pores in stems). Exit of water vapor through leaf stomates is known as **transpiration**.

REVIEW PROBLEMS

1. Which of the following would most likely filter through the glomerulus into Bowman's capsule?

    (A) Erythrocytes
    (B) Monosaccharides
    (C) Leukocytes
    (D) Platelets
    (E) Proteins

2. Draw a nephron and label all of its segments.

3. Which region of the kidney has the lowest solute concentration?

    (A) Nephron
    (B) Cortex
    (C) Medulla
    (D) Pelvis
    (E) Epithelia

4. In the nephron, amino acids enter the peritubular capillaries via the process of

    (A) filtration.
    (B) secretion.
    (C) excretion.
    (D) reabsorption.
    (E) osmoregulation.

5. The kidneys of desert animals have modified nephrons, which help them survive long periods without water. One would expect such a nephron to

    (A) have a very long loop of Henle.
    (B) have a very short distal tubule.
    (C) have a very short collecting duct.
    (D) be slightly permeable to water.

6. Glucose reabsorption in the nephron occurs in the

    (A) loop of Henle.
    (B) distal tubule.
    (C) proximal tubule.
    (D) collecting duct.

7. Urine is

    (A) hypotonic to the blood.
    (B) hypertonic to the blood.
    (C) hypertonic to the filtrate.
    (D) hypotonic to the vasa recta.
    (E) isotonic to the interstitial fluid in the cortex.

8. Why do protozoans and cnidarians lack an organized excretory system?

SOLUTIONS TO REVIEW PROBLEMS

1. **B** Monosaccharides would most likely filter through the glomerulus. Cells, cell fragments, and proteins remain on the circulatory side.

2. See Figure 18.3.

3. **B** Discussed in nephron function section.

4. **D** Discussed in osmoregulation section.

5. **A** A desert animal must conserve water at all costs. The loop of Henle concentrates sodium in the surrounding interstitial cells to establish a solute gradient for reabsorption of water. The longer the loop of Henle, the greater the distance the filtrate must travel through this gradient. With a greater distance, more water must be reabsorbed and conserved. (B) is incorrect because water is also reabsorbed in the distal tubule. If this section were abnormally short, less water would be conserved. (C) is incorrect by the same line of reasoning. (D) is wrong because if the nephron were less water-permeable, water loss would be greater.

6. **C** Discussed in function of nephron section.

7. **B** Discussed in function of nephron section.

8. Protozoans are single-celled organisms and lack any organs. All exchange of materials occurs through the cell membrane. Cnidarians also exchange materials directly across the cell membrane and get rid of indigested food through their single mouth/anus.

CHAPTER NINETEEN

Animal Behavior

PATTERNS OF ANIMAL BEHAVIOR

Simple Reflexes

Reflexes are simple, automatic responses to simple stimuli. Reflexes can be defined as reliable occurrences of particular behavioral responses after a given environmental stimulus. A **simple reflex** is controlled at the spinal cord. A two-neuron pathway runs from the **receptor** (afferent neuron) to the **motor** or efferent neuron. The efferent nerve innervates the effector (e.g., a muscle or gland). Reflex behavior is important in the behavioral response of lower animals. It is less important in the behavioral repertoire of higher forms of life such as the vertebrates.

Complex Reflexes

More complex reflex patterns involve neural integration at a higher level—the **brainstem** or even the **cerebrum**. For example, the "**startle response**" alerts an animal to a significant stimulus. It can occur in response to potential danger or to hearing one's name called. The startle response involves the interaction of many neurons, a system termed the **reticular activating system**.

Example Reflexes

A reflex is defined as a rapid automatic response to a stimulus. Coughing and sneezing, for example, are **protective reflexes** that operate on the exposure to chemical irritants, toxic vapors, or mechanical stimulation of the respiratory system. Coughing is triggered by irritation of the larynx, and sneezing is triggered by irritation of the wall of the nasal cavity. An **acquired reflex** is another type of reflex that is a complex, learned motor pattern. An example of an acquired reflex would be when an experienced driver steps on the brakes of the car when an animal runs in front of the vehicle. The **baroreceptor reflexes** affect systemic blood pressure and stimulate the respiratory rate when blood pressure declines. The **chemoreceptor reflexes** are stimulated by changes in pH, PCO_2, and PO_2. The **Hering-Breuer reflex** is composed of two different reflexes: the inflation and deflation reflexes. The **inflation reflex** prevents overexpansion of the lungs during forceful breathing, and the **deflation reflex** inhibits the expiratory center and stimulates the inspiratory center when the lungs are in danger of collapsing.

Fixed-Action Patterns

Fixed-action patterns are complex, coordinated, and **innate** behavioral responses to specific patterns of stimulation in the environment. The stimulus that elicits the behavior is referred to as the **releaser**. Because fixed-action patterns are innate, they are relatively unlikely to be modified by learning. An animal has a repertoire of fixed-action patterns and only a limited ability for developing new ones. The particular stimuli that trigger a fixed-action pattern are more readily modified, provided certain cues or elements of the stimuli are maintained.

An example of a fixed-action pattern is the retrieval and maintenance response of many female birds to an egg of their species. Certain kinds of stimuli are more effective than others in triggering a fixed-action pattern. For example, an egg with the characteristics of that species will be more effective than one that only crudely resembles the natural egg. Another type of fixed-action pattern is the characteristic movements made by animals that herd or flock together, such as the swimming actions of fish and the flying actions of locusts.

Behavior Cycles

Daily cycles of behavior are called **circadian rhythms**. Animals with such behavior cycles lose their exact 24-hour periodicity if they are isolated from the natural phases of light and dark. Cyclical behavior, however, will continue with approximate day-to-day phasing. The cycle is thus initiated intrinsically but modified by external factors.

Daily cycles of eating, maintained by most animals, provide a good example of cycles with both **internal** and **external** control. The internal controls are the natural bodily rhythms of eating and satiation. External modulators include the elements of the environment that occur in familiar cyclic patterns, such as dinner bells and clocks.

Sleep and wakefulness are the most obvious examples of cyclic behavior. These behavior patterns have been associated with particular patterns of brain waves.

Environmental Rhythms

In many situations, patterns of behavior are established and maintained mainly by periodic **environmental stimuli**. (A human example of this is the response to traffic lights.) Just as environmental stimuli influence many naturally occurring biological rhythms, biological factors influence behavior governed by periodic environmental stimuli.

LEARNING

Learned behavior involves **adaptive responses** to the environment. Learning is a complex phenomenon that occurs to some extent in all animals. In lower animals, instinctual or innate behaviors are the predominant determinants of behavior patterns, and learning plays a relatively minor role in the modification of these predetermined behaviors. In higher animals, the major share of the response to the environment is learned. The capacity for learning adaptive responses is closely correlated with the degree of **neurologic development** (i.e., the capacity of the nervous system, particularly the cerebral cortex, for flexibility).

Habituation

Habituation is one of the simplest learning patterns. It involves the suppression of the normal startle responses to stimuli. Repeated stimulation will result in decreased responsiveness to that stimulus. The normal autonomic response to that stimulus would serve no useful purpose when the stimulus becomes a part of the background environment, so the response to the stimulus is suppressed. If the stimulus is no longer regularly applied, the response tends to recover over time. This is referred to as **spontaneous recovery**. Recovery of the response can also occur with a modification of the stimulus.

Classical Conditioning

Classical or **Pavlovian** conditioning involves the association of a normally **autonomic** or visceral response with an environmental stimulus. For this reason, the response learned through Pavlovian conditioning is sometimes called a **conditioned reflex**. In Pavlovian conditioning, the normal, innate stimulus for a reflex is replaced by one chosen by the experimenter.

Pavlov's experiments

Pavlov, who won a Nobel prize for his work on digestive physiology, studied the **salivation reflex** in dogs. In 1927 he discovered that if a dog was presented with an **arbitrary stimulus** (e.g., a bell) and then presented with food, the dog would eventually salivate on hearing the bell alone. The food elicited the unconditioned response of salivation. After repeated association of the bell with the food, the bell alone could elicit the salivation reflex. Thus, the innate or unconditioned response would occur with the selected stimulus. Pavlov's terminology, still used today, is described below:

- An established (innate) reflex consists of an **unconditioned stimulus** (US; e.g., food for salivation), and the response that is naturally elicited is termed the **unconditioned response** (UR; e.g., salivation).

- A neutral stimulus is a stimulus that will not by itself elicit the response (before conditioning). During conditioning, the neutral stimulus (the bell) and the unconditioned stimulus (the food) are presented together. Eventually, the neutral stimulus is able to elicit the response in the absence of the unconditioned stimulus, and it is then called the conditioned stimulus (CS). Pavlov's example of a conditioned stimulus is the sound of a bell for salivation.

- The product of the conditioning experience is termed the **conditioned reflex**. The conditioned reflex in Pavlov's experiment was salivation (the conditioned response) following a previously neutral stimulus (now the conditioned stimulus) such as the sound tone.

- Pavlov defined **conditioning** as the establishment of a new reflex (association of stimulus with response) by the addition of a new, previously neutral stimulus to the set of stimuli that are already capable of triggering the response. Thus, Pavlov added a bell tone to the set of stimuli, originally including food, that trigger salivation in the dogs.

Pseudoconditioning

Pseudoconditioning is a phenomenon that can be confused with true classical conditioning. A critical test of conditioning is the determination of whether the conditioning process is actually necessary for the production of a response by a previously "neutral stimulus." In many cases, the so-called "neutral" stimulus is able to elicit the response even before conditioning and hence is not really a neutral stimulus. Pseudoconditioning can be avoided by carefully evaluating all prospective stimuli before conditioning begins.

Operant or Instrumental Conditioning

Operant or instrumental conditioning involves conditioning responses to stimuli with the use of **reward** or **reinforcement**. When the organism exhibits a specific behavioral pattern which the experimenter would like to see repeated, the animal is rewarded. The reinforcement or reward increases the likelihood that the behavior will appear—it has been "reinforced." Although this instrumental conditioning was originally applied to conditioning responses under the voluntary control of the organism, it has been successfully applied more recently to the conditioning of visceral responses such as changes in heartbeat.

Experiments of B.F. Skinner

B.F. Skinner first demonstrated the principles of operant conditioning and reinforcement. In the original operant conditioning experiments, he used the well-known "Skinner box," consisting of a cage with a lever or key and a food dispenser. A food pellet was delivered whenever the animal pressed the lever. Thus, depression of the lever was the operant response under study. In later experiments, Skinner varied the type of reinforcement. Reinforcers fell into two categories:

1. **Positive reinforcement** or **reward** includes providing food, light, or electrical stimulation of the brain's "pleasure centers." After positive reinforcement, the animal was much **more likely** to repeat the desired behavioral response (i.e., to press the bar). In a sense, the animal had developed a positive connection between the action (response) and the reward (stimulus that followed). This type of conditioning is likely to be involved in normal habit formation.

2. **Negative reinforcement** also involves stimulating the brain's pleasure centers. However, in contrast with positive reinforcement, negative reinforcement links the lack of certain behavior with reward (i.e., a bird may learn that it will receive a food pellet if it does not peck on a yellow circle in its cage).

   In this case, the animal has developed a negative connection between action (response) and reward (stimulus that followed). Thus, the animal has developed a *positive* connection between the *lack* of the action and the reward. The animal is **less likely** to repeat the behavioral response.

In addition, **punishment** involves conditioning an organism so that it will stop exhibiting a given behavior pattern. Punishment may involve painfully shocking the organism each time the chosen behavior appears. After punishment, the organism is **less likely** to repeat the behavioral response. The animal develops a negative connection between the stimulus and the response.

A stimulus is usually associated with several possible responses, each response having a different probability of occurrence. These stimulus-behavioral associations are believed to be ordered in a **habit family hierarchy**. For example, a chicken may respond to a light in many ways, but if one particular response is rewarded, it will occur with higher probability in the future. Reward strengthens a specific behavioral response and raises its order in the hierarchy. Punishment weakens a specific behavioral response and lowers its order in the hierarchy.

Modifications of Conditioned Behavior

Extinction

Extinction is the gradual **elimination** of conditioned responses in the absence of reinforcement (i.e., the "unlearning" of the response pattern). In **instrumental and operant conditioning**, the response is diminished and finally eliminated in the absence of reinforcement. The response is not completely unlearned—rather it is inhibited in the absence of reinforcement. It will rapidly reappear if the reinforcement is returned. In **classical conditioning**, extinction occurs when the unconditioned stimulus is removed or was never sufficiently paired with the conditioned stimulus. The conditioned stimulus must be paired with the unconditioned stimulus, at least part of the time, for the maintenance of the conditioned response. When sufficient time elapses after extinction, the conditioned response may again be elicited by the conditioned stimulus. The recovery of the conditioned response after extinction is called **spontaneous recovery**.

Generalization and discrimination

Stimulus generalization is the ability of a conditioned organism to respond to stimuli that are similar, but not identical, to the original conditioned stimulus. The less similar the stimulus is to the original conditioned stimulus, the lesser the response will be. For example, an organism may be conditioned to respond to a stimulus of a 1000-Hz tone, but it may respond to stimuli somewhat higher or lower in pitch. **Stimulus discrimination** involves the ability of the learning organism to respond differentially to slightly different stimuli. For example, if rewards are given for only a very narrow range of sound (such as a tone of 990 to 1010 Hz) but not to stimuli outside this range, the organism will also learn not to respond to stimuli that are very different in tone. A **stimulus generalization gradient** is established after the organism has been conditioned, whereby stimuli further and further away from the original conditioned stimulus elicit responses with decreasing magnitude.

LIMITS OF BEHAVIORAL CHANGE

Imprinting

Imprinting is a process in which environmental patterns or objects presented to a developing organism during a brief **critical period** in early life become accepted permanently as an element of their behavioral environment (i.e., "stamped in") and included in an animal's behavioral response. A **duckling** passes through a critical period in which it learns that the first large moving object it sees is its mother. In the natural environment, this is usually the case. However, other objects can be substituted during this period, and it will follow anything that is substituted for its mother. This phenomenon was first identified by the ethologist **Konrad Lorenz**, who swam in a pond amongst newly hatched ducklings separated from their mother and found that they eventually followed him as if he were their mother.

Critical Period

Critical periods are specific time periods during an animal's early development when it is physiologically able to develop specific behavioral patterns. If the proper environmental pattern is not present during the critical period, the behavioral pattern will not develop properly. In addition to the critical period described above, some animals have a **visual critical period**. If light is not present during this period, visual effectors will not develop properly.

INTRASPECIFIC INTERACTIONS

Intraspecific interactions occur as a means of communication between members of a species.

Behavioral Displays

A display may be defined as an **innate behavior** that has evolved as a signal for **communication** between members of the same species. According to this definition, a song, call, or intentional change in an animal's physical characteristics are considered displays. Categories of displays include:

- **Reproductive displays** are specific behaviors found in all animals including humans. Many animals have evolved a variety of complex actions that function as signals in preparation for mating.
- **Agonistic displays** are such things as a dog's display of appeasement when it wags its tail or the dog's **antagonistic** behavior when it directs its face straight and raises its body.
- Other displays include various **dancing** procedures exhibited by **honeybees**, especially the scout honeybee, to convey information concerning the quality and location of food sources. Displays utilizing auditory, visual, chemical, and tactile elements are often used as a means of communication.

Pecking Order

The relationships among members of the same species living as a contained social group frequently become stable for a period of time. When food, mates, or territory are disputed, a **dominant** member of the species will prevail over a **subordinate** one. The social hierarchy is frequently referred to as the **pecking order**. It minimizes violent intraspecific aggressions by defining stable relationships among members of the group.

Territoriality

Members of most land-dwelling species **defend** a limited area or territory from intrusion by other members of the species. These territories are typically occupied by a male or a male-female pair and are frequently used for mating, nesting, and feeding. Territoriality serves the adaptive function of **distributing** members of the species so that the environmental resources are not depleted in a small region; furthermore, intraspecific competition is reduced. Although there is frequently a minimum size for any species' territory, the territory size varies with the population size and density. The larger the population, the smaller the territories are likely to be.

Response to Chemicals

The **olfactory sense** is immensely important as a means of communication in many animals. Many animals secrete substances called **pheromones** that influence the behavior of other members of the same species. Pheromones can be classified in one of two types:

- **Releaser pheromones** trigger a reversible behavioral change in the recipient. For example, female silkworms secrete a very powerful attracting pheromone, so powerful that a male responds to one ten-millionth of a gram from a distance of two miles or more. **Sex attractant** pheromones are secreted by many animals, including cockroaches, queen honeybees, and gypsy moths. In addition to sex-attracting purposes, releaser pheromones are secreted as **alarm** and **toxic defensive** substances.

- **Primer pheromones** produce long-term behavioral and physiological alterations in recipient animals. For example, pheromones from male **mice** may affect the **estrous cycles** of females. Pheromones have also been shown to limit sexual reproduction in areas of high animal density. Primer pheromones are important in social insects such as ants, bees, and termites where they regulate role determination and reproductive capacities.

REVIEW PROBLEMS

1. When exposed to warm temperatures, a dog will begin to pant. In an experiment, a researcher sings "Like a Virgin" every time a dog is exposed to warm temperatures. Eventually, the dog begins to pant whenever the researcher sings "Like a Virgin." What are the unconditioned stimulus, the unconditioned response, the neutral stimulus, and the conditioned stimulus in this experiment?

2. A baby initially cries whenever a car passes its window. Eventually, the baby no longer responds to cars driving by. This is an example of

   (A) habituation.
   (B) conditioned reflex.
   (C) operant conditioning.
   (D) extinction.

3. Give an example of operant learning with positive reinforcement. Give an example with negative reinforcement.

4. The male fiddler crab will advance against other male fiddler crabs if they move within a certain radius. This is an example of

   (A) agonistic display.
   (B) conditioned reflex.
   (C) reproductive display.
   (D) territoriality.

5. The cocktail party effect is observed when an individual hears and responds to their name amidst many distractions. This automatic response is coordinated by the

   (A) spinal cord.
   (B) efferent neuron.
   (C) olfactory bulb.
   (D) reticular activating system.

SOLUTIONS TO REVIEW PROBLEMS

1. Before the experiment, the dog panted when it was exposed to warm temperatures. The unconditioned stimulus is warm temperature, and the unconditioned response is panting. The neutral stimulus, before the experiment, is the singing of "Like a Virgin" by the researcher. The neutral stimulus becomes the conditioned stimulus when the dog begins to pant in response to it. This experiment uses classical conditioning.

2. **A** Habituation is the gradual suppression of the normal startle responses to a stimuli. Note that extinction refers to the elimination of conditioned responses, not innate startle responses.

3. In operant learning, a behavior is rewarded or reinforced through conditioning. A positive reinforcement is any reward given to promote a desired behavior. A negative reinforcement is anything rewarding a nonaction.

4. **D** Discussed in intraspecific interactions section.

5. **D** Discussed in patterns of animal behavior section.

CHAPTER TWENTY

Ecology

Ecology is the study of the **interactions** between organisms and their environment. The environment encompasses all that is external to the organism and is necessary for its existence. An organism's environment contains two components—the physical (**abiotic**) environment and the living (**biotic**) environment. The physical environment includes climate, temperature, availability of light and water, and the local topology. The biotic environment includes all living things that directly or indirectly influence the life of the organism including the relationships that exist between organisms. The interaction with other species is a major limiting factor in the abundance and distribution of organisms. Furthermore, one individual species can sometimes dramatically influence another species' evolutionary fitness in such a way that both kinds of organisms evolve in a process called coevolution. As one can guess, interaction with the human species is the most powerful biological and evolutionary factor on earth today.

LEVELS OF BIOLOGICAL ORGANIZATION

Organism

The organism is the individual unit of an ecological system, but the organism itself is composed of smaller units. The organism contains many organ systems that are made up of **organs**. Organs are formed from **tissues**, tissues from **cells**, cells from many different **molecules**, molecules from **atoms**, and atoms from subatomic particles.

Population

A population is a group of organisms of the same species **living together** in a given location. Examples of populations include dandelions on a lawn, flies in a barn, minnows of a certain species in a pond, and lions in a grassland area. A **species** is any group of similar organisms that are capable of reproducing. Environmental factors such as nutrients, water, and sunlight limitations aid in maintaining populations at relatively constant levels.

Communities

A community consists of populations of different plants and animal species interacting with each other in a given environment. The term **biotic community** is used to include only the populations and not their physical environment. An **ecosystem** includes the community and the environment. Generally, a community contains populations from all five kingdoms (monerans, protists, plants, fungi, and animals), all depending upon each other for survival. The following are examples of communities:

- A **lawn** contains dandelions, grasses, mushrooms, earthworms, nematodes, and bacteria.
- A **pond** contains dragonflies, algae, minnows, insect larvae, etc.
- A **forest** contains moss, pine trees, bacteria, lichens, ferns, deer, chipmunks, spiders, foxes, etc.
- The **sea** contains fish, whales, plankton, etc.

Ecosystem

An ecosystem or ecological community encompasses the interaction between living **biotic communities** and the **nonliving environment**. In studying the ecosystem, the biologist emphasizes the effects of the biotic community on the environment and the environment on the community. The examples listed above for communities are also examples of ecosystems.

Biosphere

The biosphere includes all portions of the planet that support life—the **atmosphere**, the **lithosphere** (rock and soil surface), and the **hydrosphere** (the oceans). It is a relatively thin zone extending a few feet beneath the earth's surface, several miles down into the deepest sea, and several miles high into the atmosphere.

THE ENVIRONMENT

Physical Environment

Water

Water is the major component of the internal environment of all living things. Water may be readily available, or the organism may possess adaptations for storage and conservation of water. The amount of water that each species needs on a daily basis will vary. Some species such as the camel, can go without consuming water for long periods of time, whereas other species, such as bacteria, expire rapidly when not in the presence of water.

Temperature

Temperature must be maintained at an optimal level. Protoplasm is destroyed at temperatures below 0°C and at high temperatures. Organisms have adaptations necessary for protection against these extremes. The temperature of a geographic location depends upon its latitude and altitude. The same changes in habitat that occur as one approaches the colder polar regions occur as one ascends toward the colder regions of a mountain top.

Sunlight

Sunlight is the ultimate source of energy for all organisms. Green plants must compete for sunlight in forests. They have adapted to capture as much sunlight as possible by growing broad leaves, branching, growing to greater height, or producing vine growths. The **photic zone** in water, the top layer through which light can penetrate, is where all aquatic photosynthetic activity takes place. In the **aphotic zone**, only animal life and other heterotrophic life exist.

Oxygen supply

This poses no problem for **terrestrial** life because the air contains approximately 20 percent oxygen. Aquatic plants and animals use the small amount of oxygen **dissolved** in water. Pollution can significantly lower oxygen content in water and threaten aquatic life.

Substratum (soil or rock)

The substratum determines the nature of plant and animal life in the soil. Soil is affected by a number of factors:

- **Acidity** (pH)—Rhododendrons and pines are more suited for growth in acid soil. Acid rain may make soil pH too low for most plant growth.
- The **texture** of soil and its clay content determine the water holding capacity of the soil. Willows require moist soil. Most plants grow well in **loams** that contain high percentages of each type of soil.
- **Minerals**, including **nitrates** and **phosphates**, affect the type of vegetation that can be supported. Beach sand has been leached of all minerals and is generally unable to support plant life.
- **Humus** quantity is determined by the amount of decaying plant and animal life in the soil.

Biotic Factors in the Environment

Organisms belonging to the same or different species influence each other's development. Living things interact with other living organisms and with their physical environment.

INTERACTIONS WITHIN THE ECOSYSTEM

Complex interactions exist among the constituents of an ecosystem. These interactions involve a cyclic flow of energy and materials.

The Niche

The **niche** defines the functional role of an organism in its ecosystem. The niche is distinct from the **habitat**—the latter is the physical place where an organism lives. The characteristics of the habitat aid in defining the niche, but additional factors must also be considered. The niche describes what the organism eats, where and how it obtains its food, what climatic factors it can tolerate and which are optimal, the nature of its parasites and predators, where and how it reproduces, and so on. The concept of niche embodies every aspect of an organism's existence.

It is implicit in the definition of *niche* that no two species can ever occupy the same niche. Organisms occupying the same niche compete for the same limited resources; food, water, light, oxygen, space, minerals, and reproductive sites. There may be many organisms in this niche, but they are all of the same species and thus have the same requirements. The niche is so specific that a species can be identified by the niche it occupies.

Species occupying similar niches use at least one resource in common. Therefore, they will compete for that resource. This competition can have a number of outcomes:

- One species may be competitively superior to the other and drive the second to **extinction**.
- One species may be competitively superior in some regions, and the other may be superior in other regions under different environmental conditions. This would result in the elimination of one species in some places and the other in other places.
- The two species may rapidly evolve in **divergent** directions under the strong selection pressure resulting from intense competition. Thus, the two species would rapidly evolve greater differences in their niches.

Nutritional Interactions Within the Ecosystem

Autotrophs

Autotrophs are organisms that manufacture their own food. The green plants use the energy of the sun to manufacture food. Chemosynthetic bacteria obtain energy from the oxidation of inorganic sulfur, iron, and nitrogen compounds.

Heterotrophs

Heterotrophs cannot synthesize their own food and must depend upon autotrophs or other heterotrophs in the ecosystem to obtain food and energy.

Herbivores—Herbivores are animals that consume only plants or plant foods. The toughness of **cellulose-containing** plant tissues has led to the development of structures for crushing and grinding that can extract plant fluids. Herbivores have long digestive tracts that provide greater surface area and time for digestion. However, they cannot digest much of the food they consume. **Symbiotic bacteria** capable of digesting cellulose inhabit the digestive tracts of herbivores and allow the breakdown and use of cellulose. Symbiosis is the close interrelationship of two different species.

Herbivores are more adept in **defense** than carnivores because they are often prey. Many herbivores, such as cows and horses, have hoofs instead of toes for faster movement on the grasslands. They have incisors adapted for cutting and molars adapted for grinding their food. Insects or other invertebrates can also be herbivores.

Carnivores—Carnivores are animals that only eat other **animals**. In general, carnivores possess pointed teeth and fang-like canine teeth for tearing flesh. They have shorter digestive tracts because of the easier digestibility of animal food.

Omnivores—Omnivores are animals that eat both plants and animals. Humans are prime examples of omnivores.

Interspecific Interactions

A community is not simply a collection of different species living within the same area. It is an **integrated system** of species that are dependent upon one another for survival. The major types of interspecific interactions are symbiosis, predation, saprophytism, and scavenging.

Symbiosis

Symbionts live together in an intimate, often permanent association, which may or may not be beneficial to both participants. Some symbiotic relationships are **obligatory** (i.e., one or both organisms cannot survive without the other). Symbiotic relationships are classified according to the benefits the symbionts receive. The types of symbiotic relationships include commensalism, mutualism, and parasitism.

Commensalism—Commensalism is when one organism is benefited by the association and the other is not affected. The host neither discourages nor fosters the relationship. Some examples include:

- **Remora and shark**—The remora (sharksucker) attaches itself by a holdfast device to the underside of a shark. Through this association, the remora obtains the food the shark discards, wide geographic dispersal, and protection from enemies. The shark is totally indifferent to the association.

- **Barnacle and whale**—The barnacle is a sessile crustacean that attaches to the whale and obtains wider feeding opportunities through the migrations of the whale.

Mutualism—Mutualism is a symbiotic relationship from which both organisms derive some benefit. Some examples are:

- **Tick bird and rhinoceros**—The bird receives food in the form of ticks on the skin of the rhinoceros. The rhinoceros has its ticks removed and is warned of danger by the rapid departure of the bird.

- **Lichen**—Lichen is a very intimate association between a fungus and an algae. Lichens are found on rocks and tree barks. The green algae produces food for itself and the fungus by **photosynthesis**. The meshes of fungal threads support the algae and conserve rain water. The fungus also provides carbon dioxide and nitrogenous wastes for the algae, all of which are needed for photosynthesis and protein synthesis. Lichens are significant in that they are pioneer organisms in the order of ecological succession on bare rock.

- **Nitrogen-fixing bacteria and legumes**—Nitrogen-fixing bacteria invade the roots of legumes, and infected cells grow to form root nodules. In the nodule, the legume provides nutrients for the bacteria and the bacteria fixes nitrogen (by changing it to a soluble nitrate, a mineral essential for protein synthesis by the plant). These bacteria are a major source of usable nitrogen, which is needed by all plants and animals.

- **Protozoa and termites**—Termites chew and ingest wood but are unable to digest the cellulose. Protozoa in the digestive tract of the termite secrete an enzyme that digests the cellulose. Both organisms share the carbohydrates. Thus, the protozoan is guaranteed protection and a steady food supply while the termite is able to obtain nourishment from the ingested wood.

- **Intestinal bacteria and humans**—Bacteria use some of the food material not fully digested by humans and manufacture vitamin K.

Parasitism—Parasitism is when a parasite benefits at the expense of the host. Parasitism exists when competition for food is most intense. Few autotrophs (green plants) exist as parasites (mistletoe is an exception). Parasitism flourishes among organisms such as bacteria, fungi, and animals. Some parasites cling to the exterior surface of the host (**ectoparasites**) using suckers or clamps. They may bore through the skin and suck out blood and nutrients. Leeches, ticks, and sea lampreys use these techniques. Other parasites (**endoparasites**), live within the host. To gain entry, they must pass through defenses such as skin, digestive juices, antibodies, and white blood cells. Parasites possess special adaptations to overcome these defenses.

Parasitism is advantageous and efficient. The parasite lives with a minimum expenditure of energy. Parasites may even have parasites of their own. Thus, a mammal may have parasitic worms, which, in turn, are parasitized by bacteria, which, in turn, are victims of bacteriophages.

- **Virus and host cell**—All viruses are parasites. They contain nucleic acids surrounded by a protein coat and are nonfunctional outside the host. Upon entry of the viral nucleic acid into the host, the virus takes over the host cell functions and redirects them into replication of itself. The life functions of the bacterial cell slow down or cease.

- **Disease bacteria and animals**—Most bacteria are either chemosynthetic or **saprophytic** (bacteria of decay). Diphtheria is parasitic upon humans, anthrax on sheep, and tuberculosis on cows or on man.

- **Disease fungi and animals**—Most fungi are saprophytic. **Ringworm** is parasitic on man.

- **Worms and animals**—Parasitic relationships exist between the tapeworm and humans. It is interesting to note that successful parasites do not kill their hosts; this would lead to the death of the parasite. The more dangerous the parasite, the less the chance it will survive.

Predation

Predators are free-living organisms that feed on other living organisms. This definition of predation includes both **carnivores** and **herbivores**. The effects of predators on their prey vary. The predator may severely limit the numbers or distribution of the prey, and the prey may become extinct. On the other hand, the predator may only slightly affect the prey because the predator is scarce or often uses another food source. In many cases, the predator aids in controlling the numbers of the prey but not so as to endanger the existence of the prey population. Predator-prey relationships evolve toward a balance in which the predator is a regulatory influence on the prey but not a threat to its survival. Examples of predators include the hawk, lion, humans, and Venus fly trap.

Saprophytism

Saprophytes include those protists and fungi that **decompose** (digest) dead organic matter externally and absorb the nutrients; they constitute a vital link in the cycling of material within the ecosystem. Examples of saprophytes include mold, mushrooms, bacteria of decay, and slime molds.

Scavengers

Scavengers are animals that consume dead animals. They therefore require no adaptations for hunting and killing their prey. Decomposers such as the bacteria of decay may be considered scavengers. Examples of scavengers include the vulture and hyena. The snapping turtle is an organism that may be considered both a scavenger and a predator.

Intraspecific Interactions

Competition is not restricted to **interspecific** interactions (relations between species). Individuals belonging to the same species use the same resources; if a particular resource is limited, then these organisms must compete with one another. Members of the same species compete, but they must also **cooperate**. Intraspecific cooperation may be extensive (formation of societies in animal species) or may be nearly nonexistent. Relationships among individuals within a species are influenced by both **disruptive** and **cohesive** forces. Competition is the chief disruptive force. Cohesive forces include reproduction and protection from predators and destructive weather.

Interactions Between Organisms and Their Environment

Osmoregulation

Animals have developed many adaptations for maintaining their internal osmolarity and conserving water.

- **Saltwater fish** live in a **hyperosmotic** environment, which causes them to lose water and take in salt. They are constantly in danger of dehydration and must compensate by constant drinking and active excretion of salt across their gills.

- **Freshwater fish** live in a **hypoosmotic** environment, which causes intake of excess water and excessive salt loss. These fish correct this condition by seldom drinking, absorbing salts through the gills, and excreting dilute urine.

- **Insects** excrete solid uric acid crystals to conserve water.

- Desert animals possess adaptations for avoiding desiccation (drying up). The **camel** can tolerate a wide range of body temperatures and possesses fat layers in regions that are exposed to solar radiation. The **horned toad** has thick scaly skin, which prevents water loss. Other desert animals burrow in the sand during the day and search for food at night, thereby avoiding the intense heat that causes water loss.

- Plants possess adaptations for conservation of water. Nondesert land plants possess waxy **cuticles** on leaf surfaces and stomata on the lower leaf surfaces only. They shed leaves in winter to avoid water loss. Desert plants have extensive root systems, **fleshy stems** to store water, **spiny leaves** to limit water loss, extra thick cuticles, and few stomata.

Thermoregulation

Cellular respiration only transfers a fraction of the energy derived from the oxidation of carbohydrates into the high-energy bonds of ATP. Roughly **60 percent** of the total energy is given off as heat. The vast majority of animals and plants are cold-blooded or **poikilothermic**, and most of their heat energy escapes to the environment. The body temperature of poikilotherms is very close to that of their surroundings. Because an organism's metabolism is closely tied to its body temperature, the activity of poikilothermic animals is radically affected by environmental temperature changes. As the temperature rises, these organisms become more active. As temperatures fall they become sluggish and lethargic.

Some animals, notably **mammals** and **birds**, are warm-blooded or **homeothermic**. They have evolved physical mechanisms that allow them to make use of the heat produced as a consequence of respiration. Physical adaptations like fat, hair, and feathers retard heat loss. Homeotherms maintain constant body temperatures that are higher than that of the environment. They are less dependent upon environmental temperature than poikilothermic animals and can inhabit a comparatively wider range of environments.

RELATIONSHIPS WITHIN THE ECOSYSTEM

Energy Flow

All living things require energy to carry on their life functions. The complex pathways involved in the transfer of energy through the living components of the ecosystem (biotic community) may be mapped in the form of a **food chain** or **food web**.

Food chain

Energy from the sun enters living systems through the photosynthetic production of glucose by green plants. Within the food chain, energy is transferred from the original sources in green plants through a series of organisms with repeated stages of consumption and finally decomposition. Thus, there are producers, primary consumers, secondary consumers, tertiary consumers and decomposers.

Producers—Producers are the **autotrophic** green plants and **chemosynthetic** bacteria. They use the energy of the sun and simple raw materials (carbon dioxide, water, and minerals) to manufacture carbohydrates, proteins, and lipids. The radiant energy of the sun is captured and stored in the C–H bond. Producers always form the initial step in any food chain. The wheat plant is a typical producer.

Primary consumers—Primary consumers are animals that consume green plants (**herbivores**). Examples include the cow, grasshopper, and elephant.

Secondary consumers—Secondary consumers are animals that consume the primary consumers (**carnivores**). These include frogs, tigers, and dragonflies.

Tertiary consumers—Tertiary consumers are animals that feed on secondary consumers.

Decomposers—Decomposers include **saprophytic** organisms and organisms of decay, which include bacteria and fungi. The producers and consumers concentrate and organize materials of the environment into complex living substances. Living things give off wastes during their lifetime and eventually die. Bacteria and fungi decompose the organic wastes and dead tissues into simpler compounds, such as nitrates and phosphates, which are returned to the environment to be used again by living organisms. These processes are demonstrated in **food webs** and **material cycles** (nitrogen, carbon, and water).

Food web

The food chain is not a simple linear chain but an intricate web. Almost every species is consumed by one or more other species, some of which are on different food chain levels. The result is a series of branches and cross-branches among all the food chains of a community to form a web. The greater the number of pathways in a community food web, the more stable the community. For example, owls eat rabbits. If rabbits died off because of disease, there would be more vegetation available to mice. Mice would thrive and provide substitute food for owls. Meanwhile, the decimated rabbit population would have a better chance of recovering while owls concentrated their predation on mice.

Food pyramids

Without a constant input of **energy** from the sun, an ecosystem would soon run down. As food is transferred from one level of the food chain to the next, a transfer of energy occurs. According to the

second law of thermodynamics, every energy transfer involves a loss of energy. In addition to the energy lost in the transfer, each level of the food chain uses some of the energy it obtains from the food for its own metabolism (i.e., to support life functions) and loses some additional energy in the form of heat. A pyramid of energy is thus a fundamental property of all ecosystems at all levels.

Pyramid of energy

Each member of a food chain uses some of the energy it obtains from its food for its own metabolism (life functions) and loses some additional energy in the form of heat. Because this means a loss of energy at each feeding level, the producer organism at the base of the pyramid contains the greatest amount of energy. Less energy is available for the primary consumer and still less for secondary and tertiary consumers. The smallest amount of available energy is thus at the top of the pyramid.

Pyramid of mass

Because organisms at the upper levels of the food chain derive their food energy from organisms at lower levels, and because energy is lost from one level to the next, each level can support a successively smaller biomass. Three hundred pounds of foliage (producer) may support 125 pounds of insects. This may support 50 pounds of insectivorous hens, who, in turn, will be just the right amount to sustain 25 pounds of hawks.

Pyramid of numbers

Consumer organisms that are higher in the food chain are usually larger and heavier than those further down. Because the lower organisms have a greater total mass, there must be a greater number of lower level organisms. (A large bass eats tiny minnows, but eats many of them.) With the greatest number of organisms at the base (producer level) and the smallest number at the top (final consumer level), we have a pyramid of numbers.

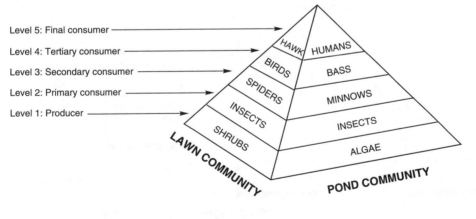

Figure 20.1

Note: Because other factors, such as the generation time and the size of the organisms, must be considered, the pyramids of numbers and biomass do not apply to all levels at all times (unlike the pyramid of energy). In general, as the pyramid is ascended, there is less energy content, less mass, and fewer organisms.

Material Cycles

Material is cycled and recycled between organisms and their environments, passing from inorganic forms to organic forms and then back to the inorganic forms. Many of these cycles are accomplished largely through the action of scavengers (such as hyenas and vultures) and decomposers (saprophytes such as bacteria and fungi).

Nitrogen cycle

Nitrogen is an essential component of amino acids and nucleic acids, which are the building blocks for all living things. Because there is a finite amount of nitrogen on the earth, it is important that it be recovered and reused.

- Elemental nitrogen is chemically inert and cannot be used by most organisms. Lightning and nitrogen-fixing bacteria in the roots of legumes change the nitrogen into the usable, soluble nitrates.

- The nitrates are absorbed by plants and are used to synthesize nucleic acids and plant proteins.

- Animals eat the plants and synthesize specific animal proteins from the plant proteins. Both plants and animals give off wastes and eventually die.

- The nitrogen locked up in the wastes and dead tissues is released by the action of the bacteria of decay, which convert the proteins into ammonia.

- Two fates await the ammonia (NH_3). Some is **nitrified** to nitrites by chemosynthetic bacteria and then to usable nitrates by nitrifying bacteria. The rest is **denitrified**. This means the ammonia (NH_3) is broken down to release free nitrogen, which returns to the beginning of the cycle. Note that four kinds of bacteria are involved in this cycle: **decay**, **nitrifying**, **denitrifying**, and **nitrogen-fixing**. The bacteria have no use for the excretory ammonia, nitrites, nitrates, and nitrogen they produce. These materials are essential, however, for the existence of other living organisms.

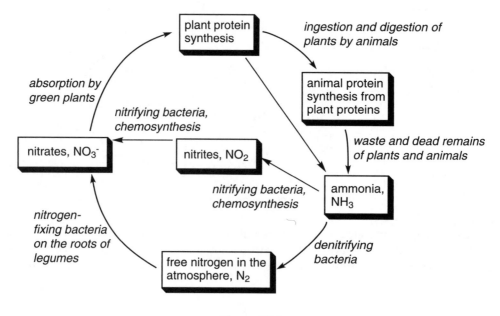

Figure 20.2

Carbon cycle

- **Gaseous CO_2** enters the living world when plants use it to produce glucose via photosynthesis. The carbon atoms in CO_2 are bonded to hydrogen and other carbon atoms. The plant uses the glucose to make starch, proteins, and fat.
- Animals eat plants and use the digested nutrients to form carbohydrates, fats, and proteins characteristic of the species. A part of these organic compounds is used as fuel in respiration in plants and animals.
- The metabolically produced CO_2 is released to the air. The rest of the organic carbon remains locked within an organism until its death (except for wastes given off), at which time decay processes by bacteria return the CO_2 to the air.

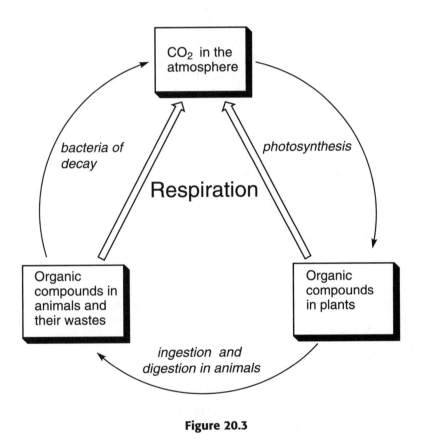

Figure 20.3

Other cycles

Other cycles recycle water, oxygen, and phosphorus. These substances are used by almost all living things and must be returned by the biotic community to the environment so they can be reused.

STABILITY IN THE ECOSYSTEM

Conditions for Stability in an Ecosystem

An ecosystem is self-sustaining and therefore will be stable if there is a relatively stable physical environment (abiotic factors) and a relatively stable biotic community. A stable ecosystem requires a constant **energy source** and a living system incorporating this energy into organic compounds. **Cycling** of materials between the living system and its environment is critical.

The Climax Community

A **climax community** is the stable, living (biotic) part of the ecosystem described above in which populations exist in balance with each other and with the environment. The type of climax community depends upon all the abiotic factors: rainfall, soil conditions, temperature, shade, etc. A climax community persists until a major climatic or geological change disturbs the abiotic factors or a major biotic change (such as disease, mutations, etc.) affects the populations. Once the equilibrium is upset, new climax conditions are produced, and new communities will be established in the ecosystem.

Ecological Succession

Ecological succession is the orderly process by which one biotic community replaces or succeeds another until a climax community is established. Each community stage, or **sere**, in an ecological succession is identified by a **dominant** species—the one that exerts control over the other species that are present. Thus, in a grassland community, grass is the dominant species.

Changes occur because each community that establishes itself changes the **environment**, making it more unfavorable for itself and more favorable for the community that is to succeed it. Successive communities are composed of populations that are able to exist under the new conditions. Finally, a stage arises in which a population alters the environment in such a way that the original conditions giving rise to that population are recreated. Replacement stops, and we have our **climax community**, an ecological steady state. This climax community is permanent in the ecosystem unless the abiotic factors are drastically altered by climatic or geologic upheavals. If this happens, a new series of successions is initiated.

Example 1

Consider a barren rocky area in northeastern United States, barren perhaps as a result of a severe forest fire. Lichen may be the first or **pioneer organism** to resettle this virgin area. Recall that a lichen is an association between an alga and a fungus that can live on a rocky surface. Acids produced by the lichen attack the rocks and help to form bits of soil. Because lichens thrive only on a solid surface, conditions are now worse for the lichen but better for mosses. Airborne spores of mosses land on the soil and germinate. The result is a new sere with the moss as the dominant species in the community. As the remains of the moss build up the soil still more, annual grasses and then perennial grasses with deeper roots become the dominant species. As time marches on, we find shrubs and then trees. The first trees are the sun-loving gray birch and poplar. As more and more trees compete for the sun, these trees are replaced by white pine and, finally, maples and beeches, which grow in deep shade—the climax community.

The growth of maples and beeches produces the same conditions that originally favored their appearance. So this community remains for thousands of years. In the final maple-beech community, you would find foxes, deer, chipmunks, and plant-eating insects. These are animals that would not have been found in the original barren rock terrain. However, one forest fire can kill the entire community. Ecological succession then starts all over again, commencing with the lichen and the bare rock.

It is important to note again that the dominant species of the climax community depends on such physical factors as temperature, nature of the soil, rainfall, etc. Thus the climax community in **New York State** at higher elevations is hemlock-beech-maple, whereas at lower elevations, the climax plant is more often oak-hickory. In cold **Maine**, the climax community is dominated by the pine; in the wet areas of **Wisconsin**, by cypress; in sandy **New Jersey**, by pine; on a cold, windy mountaintop, by scrub oak.

Example 2

Step 1. **Pond:** Plants such as algae and pondweed; animals such asprotozoa, water insects, and small fish

Step 2. **Shallow pond:** Reeds, cattails, and water lilies

Step 3. **Moist land:** Grass, herbs, shrubs, willow trees, frogs, and snakes

Step 4. **Woodland:** Climax tree—perhaps pine or oak

WORLD BIOMES (MAJOR COMMUNITIES)

Terrestrial Biomes

The evolutionary **origin** of plants and animals can be traced to the seas. To survive on land, these organisms had to develop adaptations to face an environment with a 1) relative lack of water, 2) relative lack of food and supporting medium, 3) varying temperature (as compared with the oceans that have a relatively constant temperature), and 4) varying composition of the soil as compared to the definite salt composition in the oceans. The conditions in different terrestrial and climate regions selected for plants and animals possessing suitable adaptations. Each **geographic region** is inhabited by a distinct community called a **biome**.

Land biomes are characterized and named according to the **climax vegetation** of the region. The climax vegetation is the vegetation that becomes dominant and stable after years of evolutionary development. Because plants are important as food producers, they determine the nature of the inhabiting animal population, and thus, the climax vegetation determines the **climax animal population**. Following are some types of terrestrial biomes.

Desert biome

Deserts receive less than ten inches of rain each year; the rain is concentrated within a few heavy cloudbursts. The growing season in the desert is restricted to those days after rainfalls. Generally, small plants and animals inhabit the desert. Most desert plants conserve water actively (cactus, sagebrush, mesquite). Desert animals live in burrows (desert insects and lizards). Few birds and mammals are found in the deserts except those which have developed adaptations for maintaining constant body temperatures. Examples of deserts include the Sahara in Africa and the Gobi in Asia.

Grassland biome

Grasslands are characterized by low rainfall (usually from 10–30 inches per year), although considerably more than the desert biomes receive. Grasslands provide no shelter for **herbivorous mammals** (bison, antelope, cattle, and zebra) from carnivorous predators. Animals that inhabit the grasslands have developed long legs, and many are hoofed. Examples of grasslands include the prairies east of the Rockies, the steppes of the Ukraine, and the pampas of Argentina.

Tropical rain forest biome

Rain forests are "**jungles**" characterized by high temperatures and torrential rains. The climax community includes a dense growth of vegetation that does not shed its leaves. Vegetation such as vines and **epiphytes** (plants growing on other plants) and animals such as monkeys, lizards, snakes, and birds inhabit typical rain forests. Trees grow closely together; sunlight hardly reaches the forest floor. The floor is inhabited by **saprophytes** living off dead organic matter. Tropical rain forests are found in Central Africa, Central America, the Amazon basin, and Southeast Asia.

Temperate deciduous forest biome

Temperate deciduous forests have cold winters, warm summers, and moderate rainfall. Trees such as beech, maple, oaks, and willows shed their leaves during the cold winter months. Animals in temperate deciduous forests include the deer, fox, woodchuck, and squirrel. These biomes are found in the Northeast and Central-Eastern United States and in Central Europe.

Temperate coniferous forest biome

These forests are cold, dry, and inhabited by fir, pine, and spruce trees. Much of the vegetation has evolved adaptations for water conservation such as needle-shaped leaves. These forests are found in the extreme northern part of the United States and in southern Canada.

Taiga biome

Taigas receive less rainfall than the temperate forests, have long, cold winters, and are inhabited by a single coniferous tree—the spruce. The forest floors in the taiga contain moss and lichens. The chief animal inhabitant is the moose; however, the black bear, wolf, and some birds are found there. Taigas exist in the extreme northern parts of Canada and Russia.

Tundra biome

The tundra is a treeless, frozen plain found between the taiga lands and the northern ice sheets. There is only a very short summer and thus a very short growing season during which time the ground becomes wet and marshy. Lichens, moss, polar bears, musk oxen, and arctic hens are found in the tundra.

Polar region

The polar region is a frozen area with no vegetation and terrestrial animals. Animals that do inhabit polar regions generally live near the polar oceans.

Terrestrial Biome and Altitude

The sequence of biome between the equator and the poles is comparable to the sequence of regions on mountains. The nature of those regions is determined by the same decisive factors—temperatures and rainfall. For example, the base of the mountain would resemble the biome of a temperate deciduous area. As one ascends the mountain, one would pass a coniferous-like biome, then taiga-like, tundra-like, and polar-like biomes.

Aquatic Biomes

More than 70 percent of earth's surface is covered by water. Most of the earth's plant and animal life is found in water. As much as 90 percent of the earth's food and oxygen production (**photosynthesis**) takes place in the water. Aquatic biomes are classified according to criteria quite different from the criteria used to classify terrestrial biomes. Plants have little controlling influence in communities of aquatic biomes compared to their role in terrestrial biomes. Aquatic areas are the most stable ecosystems; the conditions affecting temperature, amount of available oxygen and carbon dioxide, and amount of suspended or dissolved materials are stable over very large areas and show little tendency to change. Therefore, aquatic food webs and aquatic communities are balanced. There are two types of major aquatic biomes: **marine** and **freshwater**.

Marine biomes

The oceans connect to form one continuous body of water, which controls the earth's temperature by absorbing solar heat. Water has the distinctive property of being able to absorb or utilize large amounts of heat without undergoing a great temperature change. Marine biomes contain a relatively constant amount of nutrient materials and dissolved salts. Although ocean conditions are more uniform than those on land, distinct zones in the marine biomes exist.

Intertidal zone—This is the region exposed at low tides that undergoes variations in temperature and periods of dryness. Populations in the intertidal zones include algae, sponges, clams, snails, sea urchins, starfish, and crabs.

Littoral zone—This is the region on the continental shelf that contains ocean area with depths up to 600 feet and extends several hundred miles from the shores. Populations in littoral zone regions include algae, crabs, crustacea, and many different species of fish.

Pelagic zone—This is the region typical of the open seas and can be divided into photic and aphotic zones.

- **Photic zone**—The **sunlit layer** of the open sea extending to a depth of 250–600 feet. It contains **plankton**, passively drifting masses of microscopic photosynthetic and heterotrophic organisms, and nekton, active swimmers such as fish, sharks, or whales that feed on plankton and smaller fish. The chief autotroph is the **diatom**, an algae.
- **Aphotic zone**—The region beneath the photic zone that receives **no sunlight**. There is no photosynthesis in the aphotic zone, and only heterotrophs exist here. **Deep-sea organisms** in this zone have adaptations enabling them to survive in very cold water, with high pressures, and in complete darkness. The zone contains **nekton** and **benthos** (the crawling and sessile organisms). Some are scavengers, and some are predators. The habitat of the aphotic zone is fiercely competitive.

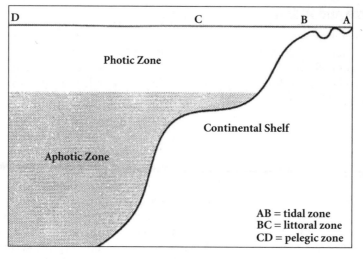

Figure 20.4

Freshwater biomes

Rivers, lakes, ponds, and marshes—the links between the oceans and land—contain freshwater. Rivers are the routes by which ancient marine organisms reached land and evolved terrestrial adaptations. Many forms failed to adapt to land and developed adaptations for freshwater. Others developed special adaptations suitable for both land and freshwater. As in **marine biomes**, factors affecting life in freshwater include **temperature**, **transparency** (illumination because of suspended mud particles), **depth** of water, available **carbon dioxide** and **oxygen**, and most importantly, the **salt concentration**. Freshwater biomes differ from saltwater biomes in three basic ways:

- Freshwater is **hypotonic**, creating a diffusion gradient, which results in the passage of water into the cell. Freshwater organisms have homeostatic mechanisms to maintain water balance by the regular **removal** of the **excess water**. These include the contractile vacuoles of protozoa and excretory systems of fish. Plant cells have rigid cell walls and thus build up cell pressure (cell **turgor**) as water flows in. This pressure counteracts the gradient pressure, stops the influx of water, and establishes a water balance.

- In rivers and streams, strong swift **currents** exist, and thus fish that have developed strong muscles and plants with rootlike **holdfasts** have survived.

- Freshwater biomes, except very large lakes, are affected by variations in climate and weather. Temperature of freshwater bodies varies considerably; they may freeze or dry up, and mud from their floors may be stirred up by storms.

REVIEW PROBLEMS

1. What is the primary difference between a community and an ecosystem?

2. All of the following are examples of communities EXCEPT

   (A) birds, fish, invertebrates, and insects living on a seashore.
   (B) microbes living in a drop of water.
   (C) black bears living in Yosemite.
   (D) fish, mammals, and plankton living in the Pacific Ocean.

3. Describe two differences between the photic and the aphotic zones of marine biomes.

4. What is a niche?

5. Which of the following is NOT an example of a symbiotic relationship?

   (A) Barnacles living on whales
   (B) Bacteria residing in the guts of termites
   (C) Fleas living on a dog
   (D) Mushrooms living on a dead tree trunk

Questions 6–9 refer to the following description of an ecosystem:

A coral reef supports a wide variety of organisms. Coral itself is a colonial cnidarian that produces a calcium carbonate shell. The individual coral polyps contain a photosynthetic organism called zooxanthella. Zooxanthella lives within the gut of the polyp and produces food for the polyp and itself by photosynthesis. The coral polyp can also catch passing photosynthetic plankton with its tentacles. The Stoplight Parrot Fish feeds on green algae that grows on the coral. In doing so, it breaks up the coral and excretes a fine sediment. Barracuda are large predatory fish that may feed on the Parrot Fish.

6. Which of the following is a primary consumer?

   (A) Zooxanthella
   (B) Coral polyps
   (C) Parrot Fish
   (D) A and B
   (E) B and C

7. Which organism is at the top of the food pyramid in the coral reef?

   (A) Zooxanthella
   (B) Coral polyps
   (C) Parrot Fish
   (D) Barracuda

8. Which organisms are involved in a mutualistic relationship?
   (A) Zooxanthella and coral polyps
   (B) Coral polyps and Parrot Fish
   (C) Parrot Fish and barracuda
   (D) Barracuda and plankton

9. How would a sudden increase in the Stoplight Parrot Fish population affect the ecological succession in the coral reef?

10. Draw the carbon cycle. Include the role of bacteria.

SOLUTIONS TO REVIEW PROBLEMS

1. A community includes only the populations of living organisms in an environment, whereas an ecosystem also includes the nonliving, abiotic environment.

2. **C** The black bears living in Yosemite are a population. A community includes all of the species living in a particular area.

3. The photic zone receives light, whereas the aphotic zone does not. This affects the communities living in these regions. The photic zone will support a wide variety of autotrophs and heterotrophs, whereas the aphotic zone can only support heterotrophs.

4. A niche describes an organism's place in its environment. It includes the organism's habitat, food sources, mating procedures, climatic tolerance, parasites and predators, and all other aspects that describe how an organism interacts with its environment.

5. **D** Symbiotic relationships are long-term relationships between two living organisms. Mushrooms and other fungi are saprophytes, living off of dead material and organic waste.

6. **E** A primary consumer feeds on autotrophic producers. The coral polyp feeds on plankton, and the Parrot Fish feeds on algae.

7. **D** Barracudas eat other fish and are therefore secondary consumers and at the top of the food pyramid.

8. **A** Mutualistic relationships are beneficial for both organisms. Zooxanthella produce food for the coral polyp via photosynthesis, and the polyp gives the zooxanthella a safe environment and raw materials.

9. The Parrot Fish eats algae that grows on the coral. In doing so, it destroys the habitat for the algae and reduces its supply of food. If there is an increase in the population of the Parrot Fish, too much coral may be destroyed, and the Parrot Fish may be succeeded by another sere.

10. See Figure 20.3 in this chapter.

CHAPTER TWENTY-ONE

Classification

TAXONOMIC CLASSIFICATION

Taxonomy

Billions of years of evolution have led to the great diversity of living organisms we see today. Scientists have tried to categorize relationships among the vast number of different organisms. The science of classification and the nomenclature used is known as **taxonomy**. Each organism can be placed into a taxonomic group based on its individual genus and species name. A genus is a group of very similar organisms related by a common descent from a relatively recent ancestor, and these organisms share similar physical traits. A species is a unique group within a given genus whose members interbreed. For example, humans belong to the genus name *Homo* and species name *sapiens*; hence, we are *Homo sapiens*. The modern classification system seeks to group organisms on the basic of **evolutionary relationships.** In this system, the bat, whale, horse, and humans are placed in the same class of animals because they have all descended from a common ancestor. Because much of early evolutionary history is not known, there is some disagreement among biologists as to the best classification system to use, particularly with regard to groups of unicellular organisms. Taxonomy takes into account anatomical and structural characteristics, modes of excretion, movement, and digestion, genetic makeup, and biochemical capabilities. Taxonomic organization proceeds from the largest, broadest group to the smaller, more specific subgroups.

Classification and Subdivisions

The modern scheme of taxonomy has **five kingdoms** for all living organisms. Each kingdom is divided into several major **phyla** (in the animal kingdom) or **divisions** (in other kingdoms). A phylum or division has several **subphyla** or **subdivisions** which are further divided into **classes**. Each class includes multiple **orders**. Orders are subdivided into **families**, and each family is made up of many **genera** (singular: genus). The **species** is the final, smallest subdivision. Organisms of the same species can mate with one another to produce fertile offspring.

Kingdom

  Phylum (Division)

    Subphylum (Subdivision)

      Class

        Order

          Family

            Genus

              Species

Figure 21.1

For example, the full classification of humans is: **Kingdom**: Animal, **Phylum**: Chordata, **Subphylum**: Vertebrata, **Class**: Mammalia, **Order**: Primates, **Family**: Hominidae, **Genus**: *Homo*, **Species**: *sapiens*.

Assignment of Scientific Names

All organisms are assigned a scientific name consisting of the **Genus** and **species** name of that organism. Thus, humans are *Homo sapiens,* and the common house cat is *Felis domestica*. This follows a scheme originated by the biologist Carolus Linnaeus.

CLASSIFICATION INTO KINGDOMS (A MODERN APPROACH)

Biologists originally divided all living things into two categories: plants and animals. This division ignored a number of different organisms. One type of modern classification system recognizes five different kingdoms: Monera, Protista, Plantae, Fungi, and Animalia. Another classification system uses three kingdoms: Monera, Plantae (including Fungi), and Animalia (including Protista).

Viruses

Viruses are generally not considered to be living organisms. They cannot function outside of a host cell and are dependent upon the host's reproductive machinery to replicate. Therefore, they have not been placed in any of the five kingdoms.

Kingdom Monera

Monerans are **prokaryotes**. They lack a nucleus or any membrane-bound organelles. All monerans are single-celled organisms that reproduce asexually.

Protista

The Protist kingdom contains primitive **eukaryotic** organisms with both plantlike and animal-like characteristics. These organisms are either single cells, or colonies of similar cells with no differentiation of specialized tissues. Each protist cell possesses the capability to carry out all of the life processes. The Protist kingdom contains all simple eukaryotes that cannot be classified as plants or animals. For example, the protist **Euglena** demonstrates the motility of animals and the photosynthetic capability of plants.

Fungi

Fungi may be considered nonphotosynthetic plants (i.e., they resemble plants in that they are **multicellular**, **differentiated**, and **nonmotile**). Fungi are either **saprophytic** (e.g., bread mold) or **parasitic** (e.g., athlete's foot fungus). Their modes of reproduction are varied and unique. In addition, their cell walls are composed of chitin, not cellulose (as in plants).

Plantae

The plant kingdom includes multicellular organisms that exhibit **differentiation** of tissues and are **nonmotile** and **photosynthetic**. Many plants exhibit an alternation of generations and a distinct embryonic phase.

Animalia

The animal kingdom contains the **multicellular**, generally **motile**, **heterotrophic** organisms that have **differentiated** tissues (and organs in higher forms).

VIRUSES

Viruses do not carry out physiological or biochemical processes outside of a host. They may be considered **nonliving**, although they are highly advanced parasites. Viruses are capable of taking over their host's cellular machinery and directing the replication of the viral genome and protein cost. Viruses have **lytic** and **lysogenic** life cycles. They contain either DNA or RNA and some essential enzymes surrounded by a protein coat. Viruses that exclusively infect bacteria are called **bacteriophages**.

The classic example of a virus is HIV. The pathogenic mechanisms of the HIV infection are both multifactorial and multiphasic. The hallmark of AIDS is a profound immunodeficiency resulting from the progressive quantitative and qualitative deficiency of "helper T" or "inducer T" cells, which are a subset of the T lymphocytes. These T cells are defined phenotypically by the CD4 molecules on the surface of the cells. The CD4 molecules are the primary cellular receptor of HIV. A number of mechanisms, concerning the cytopathicity and immune dysfunction, have been proposed. However, it is still not known which mechanism or combination of mechanisms is primarily responsible for the progressive depletion and functional impairment of the helper T cells. As the number of CD4 cells decrease to less than a "certain level," the patient is at an increasingly high risk for developing any number of opportunistic infections. These opportunistic infections are the primary reasons for mortality secondary to AIDS.

KINGDOM MONERA

Monerans, also called **bacteria**, are **prokaryotic** cells. They may exist as single cells or as aggregates of cells that stick together after division. All of these prokaryotic cells have an outer cell wall, inner plasma membrane, and a noncompartmentalized cytoplasm that contains ribosomes. Members of this kingdom lack organelles that are enclosed by a membrane. Bacteria can be classified as being heterotrophs because they consume organic nutrients or autotrophs because they can make their own nutrients. There are three primary phyla of monera:

1. **Archaeobacteria** (such as halophiles)—These organisms are known as methane produces and can withstand salty, hot, and acidic environments.

2. **Cyanophytes** (such as blue green algae)—These organisms use chlorophyll.

3. **Schizophyta** (such as various types of bacteria, actinomycetes, eubacteria [gram-negative, gram-positive bacteria], rickettsiae, mycoplasma, and spirochetes)—These organisms are the most commonly found monera with respect to medical problems. The majority of pharmaceutical agents are developed to treat infectious diseases arising from this phylum.

Cyanobacteria

Cyanobacteria, also called blue-green algae, live primarily in freshwater but also exist in marine environments. They possess a cell wall and **photosynthetic pigments** but have no flagella, true nucleus, chloroplasts, or mitochondria. They can withstand extreme temperatures and are believed to be directly descended from the first organisms that developed photosynthetic capabilities.

Other Bacteria

Bacteria are single-celled **prokaryotes** with a single double-stranded circular loop of DNA that is not enclosed by a nuclear membrane. Almost all forms have **cell walls**. They play active roles in **biogeochemical cycles**: the recycling of various chemicals such as carbon, nitrogen, phosphorous, and sulfur. Bacteria may be classified by their **morphological** appearances: **cocci** (round), **bacilli** (rods), and **spirilla** (spiral). Some forms are **duplexes** (diplococci), **clusters** (staphylococci), and **chains** (streptococci). Bacteria are ubiquitous, and many possess a wide variety of complex biochemical pathways.

Note: Much of the information that follows concerning eukaryotic classification is presented to improve your background in the features of living things. The general trends should be understood, but the specific details need not be memorized, with the exception of the classification of higher vertebrates.

KINGDOM PROTISTA

Most protists are unicellular, but there exist some colonial forms as well as some simple multicellular organisms that are neither plants nor animals. Protists are **eukaryotes** and possess a membrane-bound nucleus and organelles. The kingdom Protista includes two major categories—**protozoa** and **algae**. The kingdom is divided into many phyla that fall primarily into these two categories.

Protozoa

Traditionally, protozoans are considered those single-celled organisms that are **heterotrophic**, like little animals. This category of protists includes a number of phyla. The **rhizopods**, including amoebas, move with cellular extensions called pseudopods. The **ciliophors** have cilia that are used for feeding and locomotion.

Algae

Algae are primarily **photosynthetic** organisms. They include the **phytoplankton**, which are important sources of food for many marine organisms. The **euglena** may be considered an algal protist because it photosynthesizes. The euglena can also act as a heterotroph and move about with its flagellum. The blue, green, and red algae can be multicellular and are sometimes placed in the animal kingdom.

Protists Resembling Fungi

The slime molds are often placed in Kingdom Fungi. However, they appear to be more directly related to the protists. They are arranged in a **coenocytic** (many nuclei) mass of **protoplasm**. The slime mold undergoes a unique life cycle containing animal-like and plantlike stages. These stages include fruiting bodies and unicellular flagellated spores. Slime molds reproduce asexually by sporulation.

KINGDOM FUNGI

Fungi are **eukaryotes** and primarily multicellular. All fungi are **heterotrophs**. This differentiates them from members of the plant kingdom. They may be **saprophytic**, decomposing dead organic material, or **parasitic**. In either case, fungi **absorb** their food from their environment. Fungi reproduce by asexual **sporulation** or by intricate sexual processes. Some varieties of eumycophyta utilize extracellular digestion. Notable types are mushrooms, yeast, and lichens. The fungi in this kingdom are the causes of "classical" fungal infections in humans.

THE PLANT KINGDOM

All plants are multicellular, nonmotile, photosynthetic autotrophs.

Differentiation of Tissues

Plants have developed complex, differentiated tissues to adapt to a terrestrial life. **Photosynthetic tissue** layers contain chloroplasts for the manufacture of carbohydrates. **Supportive tissues** provide mechanical support, facilitating the typical upright radial construction of plants. **Absorptive tissues** like specialized **rhizoids** or complex roots project into soil for absorption of water and minerals. **Conducting** or **vascular tissues** include specialized "tubes" that transport water, minerals, and nutrients to all parts of the plant. **Waxy cuticles** on exposed surfaces minimize loss of water while permitting the transmittance of light. Cells are in direct contact with the external environment by means of **air spaces** and **stomata**; therefore, elaborate respiratory and excretory systems are unnecessary.

Reproduction

Specialized sex organs in the gametophyte include the **archegonium** that produces eggs. The sporophyte contains a **sporangium** that manufactures spores. Plants undergo **alternation of generations** with a sexual gametophyte (haploid) stage followed by an asexual sporophyte (diploid) stage.

Division Bryophyta

Bryophytes are simple plants with few specialized organs and tissues. They lack the water-conducting woody material (xylem), which functions support in as **tracheophytes**, and retain flagellated sperm cells, which must swim to the eggs. Bryophytes have never become successful terrestrial plants and must live in moist places.

Bryophytes undergo alternation of generations. The **gametophyte** is the dominant generation; it is the "main plant," larger and nutritionally independent. The **sporophyte** is small, short-lived, and attached to the gametophyte, and it grows from the **archegonium**. It resembles a heterotrophic parasite in that it obtains organic and inorganic material from the independent autotrophic gametophyte. There are two types of bryophytes: mosses and liverworts.

Mosses

Mosses are primitive bryophytes in which the sporophyte and gametophyte generations grow together. The gametophyte has a filamentous protonema (young moss plant) from which grows a vertical "stem" with radial leaves and a short sporophyte consisting of a foot, stalk, and a capsule filled with spores. The sporophyte grows out of the archegonium at the tip of the gametophyte.

Liverworts

Liverworts are flat, horizontal, leaflike plants with differentiated dorsal and ventral surfaces. The lower surface contains rhizoids, the middle provides for the storage of food, and the upper surface is photosynthetic.

Division Tracheophyta

Vascular plants (tracheophytes) are complex plants with a great degree of cell differentiation. They contain vascular tissues: **xylem** (water conducting) and **phloem** (food conducting). Tracheophytes have radial symmetry about a main vertical axis and are anchored by deep roots instead of rhizoids. Their extensive woody or nonwoody support system allows them to grow to great heights. They have developed excellent provisions for water conservation (waxy surfaces) and gas exchange (stomata). Cellular water storage creates turgid cells.

In contrast to bryophytes, in vascular plants, the sporophyte generation is dominant. The gametophyte is short-lived and independent in primitive tracheophytes (fern), small and parasitic in more advanced tracheophytes (seed plants).

There are four divisions of vascular plants, three of which are almost extinct. Those that remain are evidence of prior evolutionary linkage to the bryophytes.

Division psilophyta

Psilophytes are the most primitive of the tracheophytes and contain rhizoids instead of roots and one vascular bundle (microphyll) in the leaves (e.g., psilotum).

Division lycophyta

Lycophytes belong to an ancient subdivision, have roots, are nonwoody, and contain microphyll leaves (e.g., club mosses).

Division sphenophyta

Sphenophytes possess roots, microphyll leaves, and hollow-jointed stems. Whorls of leaves occur on each joint (e.g., equisetum, or horsetail).

Division pterophyta

Pterophytes are the largest division and include the familiar fern. They evolved from early psilopsids. Pteropsida contain large leaves (megaphylls), which possess many vascular bundles. Ferns grow lengthwise, not in diameter, and contain xylem as **tracheids**, not vessels. They do not produce seeds, and their short-lived gametophyte generation possesses heart-shaped leaves. Sperm are flagellated and thus require water or moisture to facilitate fertilization. The fern's leaves are part of the sporophyte generation. They grow from an underground stem called the rhizome. Sporangium on the underside of the leaves produce monoploid spores, which germinate to form gametophytes.

Division Coniferophyta

Conifers are the largest grouping of **gymnosperms**, naked-seeded plants. They include cycads, pines, spruce, and firs. Conifers have cones, spiral clusters of modified leaves. There are two different types of cones: large female cones whose sporangia produce **megaspores** and small male cones whose sporangia produce **microspores**.

The gametophyte stage of gymnosperms is short-lived and microscopic. The male microspore produces pollen that can be carried by the wind; thus, the requirement of a water environment for flagellated sperm is eliminated, and the gymnosperms are truly terrestrial. Sperm nuclei fertilize the egg with the aid of a pollen tube, and the embryo develops within the exposed seed.

The presence of a specialized cambium tissue allows for secondary growth—secondary xylem (wood) and secondary phloem. Gymnosperms can grow in diameter as well as in length and are woody, not herbaceous (green with soft stems) plants. Most gymnosperms are evergreens (nondeciduous).

Division Anthophyta

This division includes the flowering plants known as **angiosperms**. They have covered seeds and are the most abundant of all plants.

Angiosperms have flowers, not cones, as their principal **reproductive structure**. The **anther** of the male **stamen** produces microspores (pollen grains) while the **ovary** of the female **pistil** produces megaspores. Successful pollination results in the germination of pollen tubes, which aid in fertilization of female eggs in the gametophyte. The embryo develops into a seed within the ovary. The ovary eventually ripens into fruit—the means by which the seeds are dispersed. Xylem-conducting cells are in the form of vessels as well as tracheids, allowing for better conduction of water.

Subclasses of the angiosperms

- **Dicotyledons** (dicots)—Have "net-veined" leaves and vascular bundles about a ring within the central cylinder. Dicotyledons contain two cotyledons (seed leaves) within the seed. Many have cambium and can be woody. They have flower parts in multiples of four or five. Some examples of dicotyledons are the maple and apple trees, potatoes, carrots, goldenrods, and buttercups.

- **Monocotyledons** (monocots)—Contain leaves with parallel veins, scattered vascular bundles, and seeds with single cotyledons (seed leaves). Most monocots do not possess cambium and therefore are nonwoody (herbaceous). They contain flower parts in multiples of three. Some examples are grasses such as wheat, corn, rye, and rice. Other monocots include sugar cane, pineapple, irises, bananas, orchids, and palms (woody monocots).

THE ANIMAL KINGDOM

The animal kingdom encompasses a wide variety of vertebrates and invertebrates. Most people think of animals as being those with a "backbone" or vertebrates; however, more than 95 percent of all animal species are invertebrates, or those without a backbone.

General Characteristics of All Animals (Metazoa)

Differentiation of tissues, organs, and organ systems

Simple multicellular animals such as sponges, coelenterates, and flatworms have minimal differentiation. Most of their cells are in direct contact with the outside environment. In these organisms, few systems (such as the digestive systems and the reproductive systems) are required to support the life processes. In more advanced animals, specialized tissues and systems facilitate digestion, locomotion, circulation, message conduction (nervous system), and support.

Alimentation

All animals, except some parasites like the tapeworm, ingest bulk foods (holotrophic), digest them, and then eliminate the remains.

Locomotion

All animals employ some form of locomotion to acquire nutrients. Some are **sessile** (stationary) and create currents to trap food. Locomotion is also important for protection, mate selection, and reproduction.

Bilateral symmetry

Most animals have right and left sides that are mirror images. The head is directed **anteriorly**. However, some animals, such as the echinoderms and cnidarians, are radially symmetrical.

Nervous system

Animals possess a system enabling them to receive stimuli and control their actions. They have sense organs, specialized conductors, and higher brain centers for coordination and learning.

Chemical coordinating system

Animals secrete chemicals (hormones) that operate in conjunction with the nervous system to maintain a steady state or homeostasis.

Porifera (Sponges)

The sponges have two layers of cells, and they have pores. They are sessile and have a low degree of cellular specialization. These animals have saclike bodies that are asymmetrical, and no cephalization occurs. Interestingly, there are no evolutionary descendants for this invertebrate.

Cnidarians

Cnidarians, also called coelenterates, contain a digestive sac that is sealed at one end (gastrovascular cavity). Two layers of cells are present—the **ectoderm** and the **endoderm**. Cnidarians have many specialized features including tentacles, stinging cells, and net nerves (e.g., hydra, jellyfish, sea anemone, coral).

Platyhelminthes (Flatworms)

Flatworms are ribbonlike and **bilaterally symmetrical** and possess three layers of cells including a solid mesoderm. They do not have circulatory systems, and their nervous system consists of eyes, an anterior brain ganglion, and a pair of longitudinal nerve cords. The life cycles of these animals are often very complex and frequently include two or more hosts.

Nematoda (Roundworms)

Roundworms possess long digestive tubes and an anus. A solid mesoderm is present. Nematodes lack circulatory systems. They possess nerve cords and an anterior nerve ring (e.g., hookworm, trichina, free-living soil nematodes). These invertebrates are commonly found as parasites on plants and animals.

Annelida (Segmented Worms)

Segmented worms possess a **coelom** (a true body cavity) contained in the mesoderm. Annelids have well-defined systems including nervous, circulatory, and excretory systems (e.g., earthworms, leeches). The annelida possess bilateral symmetry and possess a hydroskeleton. These animals help to aerate the soils of the earth.

Mollusca

Mollusks are soft-bodied and possess mantles that often secrete calcareous (**calcium carbonate**) exoskeletons. They breathe by gills and contain chambered hearts, blood sinuses, and a pair of ventral nerve cords (e.g., clams, snails, and squid).

Arthropoda

Arthropods have jointed appendages, chitinous exoskeletons, and open circulatory systems (sinuses). The three most important classes of arthropods are insects, arachnids, and crustaceans. This is the most diverse phylum on earth.

- **Insects**—Possess three pair of legs, spiracles, and tracheal tubes designed for breathing outside of an aquatic environment.
- **Arachnids**—Have four pairs of legs and "book lungs" (e.g., scorpion, spider).
- **Crustaceans**—Have a segmented body with a variable number of appendages and possess gills (e.g., lobster, crayfish, shrimp).

Echinoderms

Echinoderms (e.g., starfish, sea urchin) are spiny and **radially** symmetrical. They contain a water-vascular system and possess the capacity for regeneration of parts. Evolutionary evidence suggests a link between echinoderms and chordates.

Chordates

Chordates are characterized by a stiff dorsal rod called the **notochord** present at some stage of embryologic development. They have paired gill slits and a tail extending beyond the anus at some point during development. The **lancelets** and **tunicates** (like **amphioxus**) are chordates but not vertebrates.

Vertebrates are the most advanced subphylum of the chordates. Vertebrates include **amphibians, reptiles, birds, fish,** and **mammals**. In addition to the chordate characteristics described above, vertebrates also possess bones called vertebrae that form the **backbone**. Bony vertebrae replace the notochord of the embryo and protect the nerve cord; a bony case (i.e., the skull) protects the brain. Vertebrates can be divided into the following classes.

Fish

All fish possess a two-chambered heart and gills and use external fertilization for reproduction.

- **Jawless fish** are eel-like, retain the notochord throughout life, have a cartilaginous internal skeleton, and have no jaws and a sucking mouth. Jawless fish include the class agnatha. Examples include the lamprey and hagfish.
- **Cartilaginous fish** possess jaws and teeth. A reduced notochord exists as segments between cartilaginous vertebrae (e.g., shark).
- **Bony fish** are the most prevalent type of fish. They have scales and lack a notochord in the adult form. During development, cartilage is replaced by a bony skeleton (e.g., sturgeon, trout, and tuna).

Amphibia

The larval stage, known as the **tadpole**, is found in water and possesses gills and a tail and has no legs. The adult amphibian lives on land, has **lungs**, two pairs of legs, no tail, a three-chambered heart, no scales. It utilizes external fertilization. Eggs are laid in water with a jellylike secretion (e.g., frog, salamander, toad, and newt).

Reptiles

Reptiles are **terrestrial** animals. They breathe air by means of **lungs**, lay leathery **eggs**, and use **internal fertilization**. Reptiles are cold-blooded (**poikilothermic**) and have scales and a three-chambered heart (e.g., turtle, lizard, snake, and crocodile).

Birds

Birds possess a four-chambered heart. They are **warm-blooded** (homeothermic), and their eggs are surrounded by shells (e.g., hen and eagle).

Mammals

Mammals are warm-blooded animals that feed their offspring with milk produced in mammary glands.

- **Monetremes** lay leathery eggs, have horny bills, and milk (mammary) glands with numerous openings but no nipples. Examples include the duckbill platypus and spiny anteater.
- **Marsupials** are pouched mammals. The embryo begins development in the uterus and completes development while attached to nipples in the abdominal pouch (e.g., kangaroo and opossum).
- **Placental mammals** have embryos that develop fully in the uterus. The placenta attaches the embryo to the uterine wall and provides for the exchange of food, oxygen, and waste material. Examples include the bat, whale, mouse, and humans.

REVIEW PROBLEMS

1. Which of the following correctly lists the hierarchy of the taxonomic system from largest grouping to most specific grouping?

    (A) Kingdom, Phylum, Subphylum, Genus, Class, Order, Family, Species

    (B) Kingdom, Phylum, Subphylum, Class, Order, Family, Genus, Species

    (C) Kingdom, Phylum, Subphylum, Order, Class, Family, Genus, Species

    (D) Kingdom, Phylum, Subphylum, Class, Order, Genus, Family, Species

2. Discuss two ways in which conifers differ from angiosperms.

3. All of the following are arthropods EXCEPT

    (A) clams.

    (B) lobsters.

    (C) crabs.

    (D) butterflies.

4. Which of the following phyla have radial symmetry?

    I. Echinodermata

    II. Arthropoda

    III. Cnidaria

    IV. Chordata

    (A) I and II

    (B) II and III

    (C) I and III

    (D) II and IV

5. Why are blue-green algae considered monerans and more correctly called cyanobacteria?

6. Discuss the differences between fungi and plants.

7. Which of the following pairs of species and phyla is correct?

    (A) wheat–coniferophyta

    (B) moss–bryophyta

    (C) hookworm–annelida

    (D) gibbon–mammalia

SOLUTIONS TO REVIEW PROBLEMS

1. **B** Discussed in taxonomic classification section.

2. Conifers have naked seeds, whereas angiosperm seeds are encased in a shell that blocks loss of water. Angiosperms have flowers as their primary sexual organs, whereas conifers have cones that produce spores.

3. **A** Clams are mollusks.

4. **C** Both cnidarians (jellyfish) and echinoderms (starfish) exhibit radial symmetry.

5. Cyanobacteria have no nucleus, chloroplasts, or mitochondria. They have a cell wall. These are characteristics of prokaryotic bacteria and not of eukaryotic cells like true algae. The Kingdom Monera includes all prokaryotes.

6. Both plants and fungi are nonmotile, multicellular organisms with differentiated tissues. However, there are some significant differences. All plants are autotrophic, whereas all fungi are heterotrophic. Fungi acquire their nutrients through the breakdown of organic material and the absorption of the breakdown products. The cell walls of fungi are composed of chitin, whereas those of plants are composed of cellulose.

7. **B** Moss belongs to the division Bryophyta. (A) is incorrect because wheat are flowering plants and belong to the Anthophyta division. Hookworms are round worms (Nematoda). Gibbons are mammals but belong to the phylum Chordata; Mammalia is a class.

CHAPTER TWENTY-TWO

Evolution

The change in the genetic makeup of a population with time is termed *evolution*. Evolution is explained by the constant propagation of new variations in the genes of a species, some of which impart an adaptive advantage. In summary, all living things (past and present) are descendents from some common ancestor. Each of these organisms arose as a direct result of some genetic alteration in the species that lived before them, and this process is called evolution. It is important to note that most evolutionary changes occur slowly over a long period of time.

EVIDENCE OF EVOLUTION

Fossil Record

Fossils are the most direct evidence of evolutionary change. They represent the remains of an extinct ancestor. Fossils are generally found in sedimentary rocks.

Types of fossils

Many types of fossils can provide information. Paleontologists can find **actual remains**, including teeth, bones, etc., rock, tar pits, ice, and amber (the fossil resin of trees). **Petrification** is the process in which minerals replace the cells of an organism. **Imprints** are impressions left by an organism (e.g., footprints). **Molds** form in hollow spaces of rocks, as the organisms within decay. **Casts** are formed by minerals deposited in molds.

Significant fossil remains found

The **trilobite** is a primitive crustacean (relative of the lobster), which was a dominant form of the early **Paleozoic** era. **Dinosaurs** were ancient animals similar to both reptiles and birds. Various forms lived on land, in the air and in water. They were a dominant form of the **Mesozoic** era. **Eohippus**, the dawn horse, was a primitive horse the size of a fox with four toes and short teeth with pointed cusps for feeding on soft leaves. Fossil evidence indicates a gradual change to the modern horse which has one toe (hoof) and two vestigial toes as side splints, flat teeth with ridges for grinding grain and tough prairie grass, and long legs for running. The **woolly mammoth** was a hairy elephant found in the Siberian ice. **Saber-tooth tigers** have been preserved in asphalt tar pits. Insects have been discovered preserved in **amber** (fossilized resin that oozed from trees). **Archaepteryx**, the missing link between reptiles (has teeth and scales) and birds (also has feathers), has been found in fossil evidence.

Comparative Anatomy

Homologous structures

Homologous structures have the same basic anatomical features and **evolutionary origins**. They demonstrate similar evolutionary patterns with late divergence of form due to differences in exposure to evolutionary forces. Examples of homologous structures include the wings of a bat, the flipper of a whale, the forelegs of horses, and the arms of man.

Analogous structures

Analogous structures have **similar functions** but may have different evolutionary origins and entirely different patterns of development. The wings of a fly (membranous) and the wings of a bird (bony and covered with feathers) are analogous structures. Analogous organs demonstrate a superficial resemblance that cannot be used as a basis for classification.

Comparative Embryology

The **stages of development** of the embryo resemble the stages in an organism's evolutionary history. The human embryo passes through the stages that demonstrate common ancestry. The **two-layer gastrula** is similar to the structure of the hydra, a cnidarian. The three-layer gastrula is similar in structure to the flatworm. Gill slits in the embryo indicate a common ancestry with fish.

The similarity of stages suggests a common ancestry and development history, rather than an identical early development to that of the hydra, flatworm, and fish. The earlier the stage at which the development begins to diverge, the more dissimilar the adult organisms will be. Thus, it is difficult to differentiate between the embryo of a human and that of a gorilla until relatively late in the development of each embryo.

Embryological development suggests other evidence of evolution. The avian embryo has teeth, suggesting a reptile stage. The larvae of some mollusks resemble annelids. Human embryos possess a tail.

Comparative Biochemistry (Physiology)

Most organisms demonstrate the same basic needs and **metabolic processes**. They require the same nutrients and contain similar cellular organelles and energy storage forms (ATP). For example, **respiratory processes** are very similar in most organisms. The similarity of the enzymes involved in these processes suggests that all organisms must contain some DNA sequences in common. The closer the organisms in the evolutionary scheme, the greater the similarity of their chemical constituents (enzymes, hormones, antibodies, blood) and **genetic information**. Thus, we can conclude that all organisms are descended from a common, primitive ancestral form. The chemical similarity of the blood of different organisms very closely parallels the evolutionary pattern. A chimpanzee's blood shows close similarity to that of a human but is quite different from that of a rabbit or fish. Thus, the more time that has elapsed since the **divergence** of two species, the more different their biochemical characteristics.

Vestigial Structures

Vestigial structures appear to be useless but apparently had some ancestral function. There are many examples of vestigial structures in humans, other animals, and plants:

- In humans, the **appendix** is small and useless. In herbivores, it assists in the digestion of cellulose.
- In humans, the **tail** is reduced to a few useless bones (coccyx) at the base of the spine.
- **Splints** on legs of horses are the vestigial remains of the two side toes of eohippus.
- The python has "legs" that are reduced to useless bones embedded in the sides of the adult. The whale has similar hind-limb bones.

Geographic Barriers

Species multiplication is generally accompanied by **migration** to lessen **intraspecific competition**. Separation of a widely distributed population by emerging geographic barriers increases the likelihood of genetic adaptations on either side of the barrier. Each population may evolve specific adaptations to the environment in which it lives, in addition to the accumulation of neutral (random, nonadaptive) changes. These adaptations will remain unique to the population in which they evolve—provided that interbreeding is prevented by the barrier. In time, genetic differences will reach the point where interbreeding becomes impossible between the populations and **reproductive isolation** would be maintained even if the barrier were removed. Following are two examples:

1. **Marsupials**—A line of pouched mammals paralleling the development of placental mammals developed on the **Australian** side of a large water barrier. The geographic barrier protected the more primitive pouched mammals from competition with modern placental mammals. This barrier resulted in the development of uniquely Australian plants and animals; e.g. the kangaroo, duckbill platypus, pouched wolves, and eucalyptus tree.
2. **Darwin's finches**—Over a comparatively short period of time, a single species of finch underwent adaptive radiation to form **13 different species** of finches. Slight variations in the beak, for example, favored ground or tree feeding. Such adaptations minimized the competition among the birds, enabling each emerging species to become firmly entrenched in its environmental **niche**.

THEORIES OF EVOLUTION

Lamarckian Evolution

This discredited theory held that new organs or changes in existing ones arose because of the needs of the organism. The amount of change was thought to be based on the **use or disuse** of the organ. The theory of use and disuse was based upon a fallacious understanding of genetics. Any useful characteristic acquired in one generation was thought to be transmitted to the next. An example was that of the early giraffes that supposedly stretched their necks to reach for leaves on higher branches of trees. The offspring were believed to inherit the valuable trait of longer necks as a result of this excessive use.

Modern genetics has disproved theories of acquired characteristics. **Only changes in the DNA of the sex cells can be inherited.** Changes acquired during an individual's life are changes in the characteristics and organization of somatic cells. Weissman showed that these changes are not inherited in an experiment in which he cut off the tails of mice for 20 generations (somatic change) only to find that the 21st generation was born with tails.

Darwin's Theory of Natural Selection

In Charles Darwin's theory, pressures in the environment select for the organism most fit to survive and reproduce. Darwin essentially concluded that a member of a particular species that is equipped with beneficial traits, allowing it to cope effectively with the immediate environment, will produce more offspring with the same traits then individuals with less favorable genetic traits. Darwin subsequently chose the words *natural selection* to describe his theory because nature selects the best set of parents for the next generation. Darwin outlined a number of basic agents leading to evolutionary change.

Overpopulation

More offspring are produced than can survive. Thus, there is insufficient food, air, light, and space to support the entire population.

Variations

Offspring naturally show differences (variations) in their characteristics compared to their parents'. Darwin did not know the source of these differences. Hugo De Vries later suggested mutations as the cause of variations. Some mutations are beneficial, although most are harmful.

Competition (struggle for survival)

The developing population must compete for the necessities of life. Many young must die, and the number of adults in the population generally remains constant from generation to generation.

Natural selection

Some organisms in a species have variations that give them an advantage over other members of the species. In the struggle for existence, these organisms may have adaptations that are advantageous for survival. For example, a giraffe with a variation of a longer neck would be able to get more food from higher branches of a tree and would be more fit for survival. This principle is encapsulated in the phrase "survival of the fittest."

Inheritance of the variations

The individuals that survive (those with the favorable variations) live to adulthood, reproduce their own kind, and thus **transmit** these favorable variations or adaptations to their offspring. These favored genes gradually dominate the gene pool.

Evolution of new species

Over many generations of natural selection, the favorable changes (adaptations) are perpetuated in the species. The accumulation of these favorable changes eventually results in such significant changes of the gene pool that we can say a new species has evolved. These physical changes in the gene pool were perpetuated or selected for by environmental conditions. For example:

- The rapid evolution of **DDT-resistant** insects illustrates the theory of natural selection. A change in the environment such as the introduction of DDT, constitutes a favorable change for the DDT-resistant mutant flies. These mutants existed before the environmental change. Now, conditions select for survival of DDT-resistant mutants.

FORCES OF EVOLUTION

Population Genetics

A **population** includes all members of a particular species inhabiting a given location. The **gene pool** of a population is the sum total of all the alleles for any given trait in the population. **Gene frequency** is the decimal fraction representing the presence of an allele for all members of a population that have this particular gene locus. The letter p is used for the frequency of the **dominant allele** of a particular gene locus. The letter q represents the frequency of the **recessive allele**. For a given gene locus, p + q = 1.

The Hardy-Weinberg Principle

Evolution can be viewed as a result of changing gene frequencies within a population. Gene frequency is the relative frequency of a particular allele. When the gene frequencies of a population are not changing, the gene pool is stable, and the population is not evolving. However, this is true only in ideal situations in which the following conditions are met:

- The population is very large.
- No mutations affect the gene pool.
- Mating between individuals in the population is random.
- There is no net migration of individuals into or out of the population.
- The genes in the population are all equally successful at reproducing.

Under these idealized conditions, a certain equilibrium will exist among all of the genes in a gene pool, which is described by the **Hardy-Weinberg equation**.

For a gene locus with only two alleles, T and t, p = the frequency of allele T and q = the frequency of allele t. By definition, for a given gene locus, $p + q = 1$, since the combined frequencies of the alleles must total 100 percent. Thus $(p + q)^2 = (1)^2$ and

$$p^2 + 2pq + q^2 = 1$$

where p^2 = frequency of TT (dominant homozygotes)

$2pq$ = frequency of Tt (heterozygotes)

q^2 = frequency of tt (recessive homozygotes)

The Hardy-Weinberg equation may be used to determine gene frequencies in a large population in the absence of microevolutionary change (defined by the five conditions given above). For example, individuals from a nonevolving population can be randomly crossed to demonstrate that the gene frequencies remain constant from generation to generation. Assume that in the original gene pool, the gene frequency of the dominant gene for tallness, T, is .80 and the gene frequency of the recessive gene for shortness, t, is .20. Thus, p = .80 and q = .20. In a cross between two heterozygotes, the resulting F_1 genotype frequencies are: 64% TT, 16% + 16% = 32% Tt, and 4% tt (see the Punnett square below).

	$p = .80\ (T)$	$q = .20\ (t)$
$p = .80\ (T)$	$(p^2 = .64)$ $TT = 64\%$	$(pq = .16)$ $Tt = 16\%$
$q = .20\ (t)$	$(pq = .16)$ $Tt = 16\%$	$(q^2 = .04)$ $tt = 4\%$

The gene frequencies of the F1 generation can be calculated as follows:

64% *TT* = 64% *T* allele + 0% *t* allele

32% *Tt* = 16% *T* allele + 16% *t* allele

4% *tt* = 0% *T* allele + 4% *t* allele

Gene frequencies = 80% *T* allele + 20% *t* allele

Thus, $p = .80$ and $q = .20$. These frequencies are the same as those in the parent generation, demonstrating Hardy-Weinberg equilibrium in a nonevolving population.

Microevolution

No population can be represented indefinitely by the Hardy-Weinberg equilibrium because such idealized conditions do not exist in nature. Real populations have **unstable** gene pools and **migrating** populations. The agents of microevolutionary change—natural selection, mutation, assortive mating, genetic drift, and gene flow—are all deviations from the five conditions of a Hardy-Weinberg population.

Natural Selection

Genotypes with favorable variations are selected through natural selection, and the frequency of favorable genes increases within the gene pool. Genotypes with low adaptive values tend to disappear.

Mutation

Gene mutations change allele frequencies in a population, shifting gene equilibria. These gene mutations can either be favorable or detrimental for the offspring.

Assortive Mating

If mates are not randomly chosen but rather selected according to criteria such as phenotype and proximity, the relative genotype ratios will be affected and will depart from the predictions of the Hardy-Weinberg equilibrium. On the average, the allele frequencies in the gene pool remain unchanged.

Genetic drift

Genetic drift refers to changes in the composition of the gene pool due to chance. Genetic drift tends to be more pronounced in small populations, where it is sometimes called the **founder effect**.

Gene flow

Migration of individuals between populations will result in a loss or gain of genes, thus changing the composition of a population's gene pool.

Speciation

Speciation is the evolution of new species, which are groups of individuals who can interbreed freely with each other but not with members of other species. Different selection pressures act upon the gene pools of each group, causing them to evolve independently. Changes in the environment change the survival value of certain traits, and the gene frequencies for these traits change accordingly. Eventually the populations will become sufficiently different from each other as to become **reproductively isolated**. They are then considered to be distinct species.

Demes

A deme is a **small local population**. For example, all the beavers along a specific portion of a river form a deme. There may be many demes belonging to a specific species. Members of a deme resemble one another more closely than they resemble the members of other demes. They are closely related genetically since mating between members of the same deme occurs more frequently. They are influenced by similar environmental factors and thus are subject to the same selection processes.

Development of new species

If the gene pools within a species become sufficiently different so that two individuals cannot mate and produce fertile offspring, two different species have developed. Gene flow is impossible between two different species. Genetic **variation**, changes in the **environment**, **migration** to new environments, **adaptation** to new environments, **natural selection**, and **isolation** are all factors that lead to speciation.

Adaptive radiation

Adaptive radiation is the emergence of a number of lineages from a **single ancestral species**. A single species may **diverge** into a number of distinct species; the differences between them are those adaptive to a distinct lifestyle, or niche. A classic example is Darwin's finches of the Galapagos island chain. Over a comparatively short period of time, a single species of finch underwent adaptive radiation, resulting in 13 separate species of finches, some of them on the same island. Such adaptations minimized competition among the birds, enabling each emerging species to become firmly established in its own environmental niche.

Evolutionary history

Dissimilar species have been found to have evolved from a common ancestor. Biologists seek to understand evolutionary relationships among the species alive today. This evolutionary history is termed **phylogeny**. Evolutionary history may be visualized as a branching tree, where the common ancestor is found at the trunk and the modern species at the tips of the branches. It is interesting to note that groups within the branches develop in similar ways when exposed to similar environments. This is known as **convergent evolution**. For example, fish and dolphins have come to resemble one another physically, although they belong to different classes of vertebrates. They evolved certain similar features in adapting to the conditions of aquatic life.

Descendants of an ancestral **pouched mammal** include the pouched wolf, anteater, mouse, and mole. They have developed **parallel** to the placental wolf, anteater, mouse, and mole. These pouched mammals and their placental counterparts faced similar, though geographically separate environments; thus, they developed similar adaptations.

The concepts of **adaptive radiation** and **phylogeny** form the basis for the methods employed in developing a system for the classification of living things.

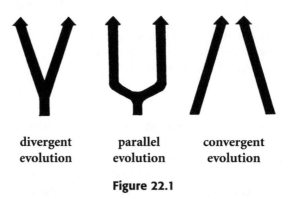

divergent   parallel   convergent
evolution   evolution   evolution

Figure 22.1

Isolation

Genetic isolation often results from the geographic isolation of a population. When groups are isolated from each other, there is no gene flow between them. Any difference arising from mutations or new combinations of genes will be maintained in the isolated population. Over time, these genetic differences may become significant enough to make mating impossible. In this way, a new species is formed.

ORIGIN AND EARLY EVOLUTION OF LIFE

The Heterotroph Hypothesis

The first forms of life lacked the ability to synthesize their own nutrients; they required preformed molecules. These "organisms" were **heterotrophs**, which depended upon outside sources for food. The primitive seas contained **simple inorganic** and **organic** compounds such as salts, methane, ammonia, hydrogen, and water. **Energy** was present in the form of **heat, electricity, solar radiation**, including **X rays** and **ultraviolet light, cosmic rays**, and **radioactivity**.

The presence of these building blocks and energy may have led to the synthesis of simple organic molecules such as sugars, amino acids, purines, and pyrimidines. These molecules dissolved in the "**primordial soup**," and after many years, the simple monomeric molecules combined to form a supply of macromolecules.

Evidence of organic synthesis

In 1953, **Stanley L. Miller** set out to demonstrate that the application of ultraviolet radiation, heat, or a combination of these to a mixture of methane, hydrogen, ammonia, and water could result in the formation of complex organic compounds. Miller set up an apparatus in which the four gases were continuously circulated past electrical discharges from tungsten electrodes.

After circulation of the gases for one week, Miller analyzed the liquid in the apparatus and found that an amazing variety of organic compounds, including **urea, hydrogen cyanide, acetic acid,** and **lactic acid** had been synthesized.

Formation of primitive cells

Colloidal protein molecules tend to clump together to form **coacervate droplets** (a cluster of colloidal molecules surrounded by a shell of water). These droplets tend to absorb and incorporate substances from the surrounding environment. In addition, the droplets tend to possess a definite internal structure. It is highly likely that such droplets developed on the early earth. Although these coacervate droplets were not living, they did possess some properties normally associated with living organisms.

Most of these systems were **unstable**; however, a few systems may have arisen that were **stable** enough to survive. A small percentage of the droplets possessing favorable characteristics eventually developed into the first primitive cells. These first primitive cells probably possessed **nucleic acid polymers** and became capable of reproduction.

Development of Autotrophs

The primitive heterotrophs slowly evolved complex **biochemical pathways**, which enabled them to use a wider variety of nutrients. They evolved **anaerobic respiratory processes** to convert nutrients into energy. However, these organisms required nutrients at a faster rate than they were being synthesized. Life would have ceased to exist if **autotrophic nutrition** had not developed. The pioneer autotrophs developed primitive **photosynthetic** pathways, capturing solar energy and using it to synthesize carbohydrates from carbon dioxide and water.

Development of Aerobic Respiration

The primitive autotrophs fixed **carbon dioxide** during the synthesis of carbohydrates and released molecular oxygen as a waste product. The addition of molecular oxygen to the atmosphere converted the atmosphere from a **reducing** to an **oxidizing** one. Some molecular oxygen was converted to ozone, which functions in the atmosphere to block high-energy radiation. In this way, living organisms **destroyed** the conditions that made their development possible. Once molecular oxygen became a major component of the earth's atmosphere, both heterotrophs and autotrophs evolved the biochemical pathways of aerobic respiration. Now equilibrium exists between oxygen-producing and oxygen-consuming organisms.

General Categories of Living Organisms

All living organisms can be divided into four basic categories. The **autotrophic anaerobes** include chemosynthetic bacteria. The **autotrophic aerobes** include the green plants and photoplankton. The **heterotrophic anaerobes** include yeasts. The **heterotrophic aerobes** include amoebas, earthworms, and humans.

REVIEW PROBLEMS

1. Can the muscular strength that a weight lifter gains be inherited by the athlete's children?

2. Which organism has a greater evolutionary fitness: one that lives 70 years and has 5 fertile offspring, or one that lives 40 years and has 10 fertile offspring?

3. Homologous structures are
   (A) similar in function but not in origin.
   (B) similar in origin but not in function.
   (C) completely dissimilar.
   (D) found only in mammals.

4. Will chance variation have a greater effect in a large or a small population? What is this effect called?

5. As the climate got colder during the Ice Age, a particular species of mammal evolved a thicker layer of fur. This is an example of what kind of selection?

6. At what point are two populations descended from the same ancestral stock considered separate species?

7. In a nonevolving population, there are two alleles, R and r, which code for the same trait. The frequency of R is 30 percent. What are the frequencies of all the possible genotypes?

8. As the ocean became saltier, whales and fish independently evolved mechanisms to maintain the concentration of salt in their bodies. This can be explained by
   (A) homologous evolution.
   (B) analogous evolution.
   (C) convergent evolution.
   (D) divergent evolution.
   (E) parallel evolution.

9. In a particular Hardy-Weinberg population, there are only two eye colors: brown and blue. Thirty-six percent of the population has blue eyes, the recessive trait. What percentage of the population is heterozygous for brown eyes?

10. In a certain population, 64 percent of individuals are homozygous for curly hair (CC). The gene for curly hair is dominant to the gene for straight hair, c. Use the Hardy-Weinberg equation to determine what percentage of the population has curly hair.

11. Which of the following was NOT a belief of Darwin's?

    (A) Evolution of species occurs gradually and evenly over time.
    (B) There is a struggle for survival among organisms.
    (C) Genetic mutation and recombination are the driving forces of evolution.
    (D) Those individuals with fitter variants will survive and reproduce.

12. The proposed "primordial soup" was composed of organic precursor molecules formed by interactions between all of the following gases EXCEPT

    (A) oxygen.
    (B) helium.
    (C) nitrogen.
    (D) carbon.
    (E) hydrogen.

SOLUTIONS TO REVIEW PROBLEMS

1. No. The only characteristics that are inherited are those genetically coded for, not those acquired through the use or disuse of body parts. Therefore, the musculature of the weight lifter an acquired characteristic, cannot be inherited by that athlete's children.

2. The organism that lives 40 years and has 10 fertile offspring has the greater evolutionary fitness because it makes a greater genetic contribution to the next generation. It has twice as many direct descendants as the organism that lives 70 years and has 5 fertile offspring.

3. **B** Homologous structures are similar in origin but not similar in function. Analagous structures are similar in function but not in origin. Homologous structures are not limited to mammals; e.g., the forelimbs of crocodiles and birds are homologous structures.

4. Chance variation will have a greater effect in a small population because any one variant individual is a greater percentage of the whole population. This effect is called genetic drift.

5. This is an example of directional selection; in directional selection, the phenotypic norm of a particular species shifts toward an extreme to adapt to a selective pressure, such as an increasingly colder environment. Only those individuals with a thick layer of fur were able to survive during the Ice Age, thus shifting the phenotypic norm.

6. Two populations are considered separate species when they can no longer interbreed and produce viable, fertile offspring.

7. The frequency of R = 30%. Thus, $p = .30$. The frequency of recessive gene r = 100% − 30% = 70%. Thus, q = 0.70. Frequency of genotypes = $p^2 + 2pq + q^2 = 1$, where $p^2 =$ RR, $2pq =$ Rr, and $q^2 =$ rr.

p^2	=	$(.3)^2$	=	.09	=	9% RR
$2pq$	=	2(.3)(.7)	=	.42	=	42% Rr
q^2	=	$(.7)2$	=	.49	=	49% rr

8. **C** Whales and fish have similar body structures (streamlined body with fins and tail), although they belong to different classes of vertebrates. When organisms that differ phylogenetically develop in similar ways when exposed to similar environments, the process is known as convergent evolution.

9. The percentage of the population with blue eyes (genotype = bb) = 36% = $q^2 = .36$; therefore, q = .6. Because p + q = 1, p = .4. The frequency of heterozygous brown eyes is $2pq = 2(.4)(.6) = .48$. So 48% of the population is heterozygous for brown eyes.

10. *P* represents the frequency of the dominant allele (C), and *q* represents the frequency of the recessive allele (c). The CC frequency is 64%, which means that $p2 = .64$, or $p = .8$. Because $p + q = 1, q = 1 - .8 = .2$.

The problem asks for the percentage of the population with curly hair; this includes both homozygotes and heterozygotes (CC and Cc). The genotype frequencies can be found using the equation $p2 + 2pq + q2$.

CC	=	$p2$	=	(.8)2	=	.64	=	64% homozygous curly
Cc	=	$2pq$	=	2(.8)(.2)	=	.32	=	32% heterozygous curly
cc	=	$q2$	=	(.2)2	=	.04	=	4% straight hair

Therefore, the percentage of the population with curly hair is 64% + 32% = 96%.

11. C Darwin believed the driving force behind evolution was the fitness of the organism for its particular environment.

12. B He, as a noble gas, is inert and does not form molecules with other atoms.

CHAPTER TWENTY-THREE

Reading Skills

Preparing for Reading Comprehension is an interesting task. There aren't any lengthy calculations, and you don't need to memorize complex science concepts. Instead, you need to practice with the exercises we give you and read on your own time. Do the exercises under testlike conditions, and carefully read through all of the question explanations. Familiarity with the questions will increase your score because you'll know what to expect on Test Day.

In addition to completing the exercises, you should read material with subject matter similar to that of exam passages. Most of the passages in the Reading Comprehesion portion of the exam contain medical topics and natural science subjects. Read through some recent editions of journals, such as the *Journal of the American Pharmaceutical Association*, and magazines, such as *National Geographic, Science*, and *Scientific American,* to increase your familiarity with this type of material.

Even if you love reading, you might not be an expert on Reading Comprehension. To do well on Reading Comprehension, you need to read critically and understand why the author presents certain information.

Can you tell the difference between fact and opinion?

Of course you know the difference. But under the pressure of an examination, some test takers lose sight of the difference, and their critical reading skills become blunted. You'll want to recognize the difference instantly on Test Day.

- FACT is an unbiased observation or something that is irrefutable.
- OPINION interjects the author's feelings on, or evaluation of, a subject.

Recognizing Key Words

Key words provide structure to text. They also serve as clues for shifts in ideas, examples, or contrasting viewpoints. Understanding the function of key words can greatly improve your ability to understand a Reading Comprehension passage. Review the following types of key words. Can you think of any more?

Continuation key words announce that more of the same is about to come up. Some of the most common words and phrases include:

also	*futhermore*	*in addition*	*as well as*
moreover	*plus*	*at the same time*	*equally*

Also (there's a signal for you), the colon sort of does the same job: it usually tells you that what follows expands upon, or continues, what came before.

Illustration key words signal that an example is about to arrive. *For example* and *for instance* are the most obvious. But think about these:

In the words of Hannah Arendt	*According* to these experts
As Maya Angelou *says*	*For* historians
To Proust	Toynbee *claims* that

In each case, what's about to follow is an example of that person's thinking.

Contrast key words, of course, signal an opposition or shift. There are lots of these words:

but	*however*	*although*	*not*
nevertheless	*despite*	*alternatively*	*unless*
though	*by contrast*	*yet*	*still*
otherwise	*while*	*notwithstanding*	

Contrast key words are among the most significant in Verbal Reasoning because so many passages are based on contrast or opposition. Almost certainly, something important is happening when a contrast keyword shows up.

Sequence key words are the author telling you "Hey, there's some sort of order at work here." Some examples are:

second (and third, fourth, etc.)	*next*	*finally*
on the one hand	*recently*	

Conclusion key words signal that the author is about to sum up or announce the thesis. The most common one is *therefore*, to which we can add:

thus	*consequently*	*hence*	*in conclusion*
it can be seen that	*so*	*we can conclude that*	

Because these key words have to do with the author's logic, it's no wonder that they are especially crucial for Verbal Reasoning.

Evidence key words tell you that the author is about to provide support for a point. Here are the "big four" evidence key words:

because	*for*	*since*	*the reason is that*

Emphasis key words, when all is said and done, may be the most welcome. If we're supposed to read for the author's point of view—and we are—what better way than to stumble across words and phrases whose sole purpose is to announce "I, the author, find this important"? Note these well:

above all	*most of all*	*primarily*	*in large measure*
essentially	*especially*	*particularly*	*indeed*

PRACTICE EXERCISES

Passage 1

Directions: Each of the following sets of questions is preceded by descriptive material. After reading the material, select the best answer to each question.

One of the basic principles of ecology is that population size is to some extent a function of available food resources. Recent field experiments demonstrate that the interrelationship may be far more complex than hitherto imagined. Specifically, the browsing of certain rodents appears to trigger biochemical reactions in the plants they feed on that help regulate the size of the rodent populations. Two such examples of phytochemical regulation (regulation involving plant chemistry) have been reported so far.

Patricia Berger and her colleagues at the University of Utah have demonstrated the instrumentality of 6-methoxybenzoxazolinone (6-MBOA) in triggering reproductive behavior in the montane vole (*Microtus montanus*), a small rodent resembling the field mouse. 6-MBOA forms in young mountain grasses in response to browsing by predators such as voles. The experimenters fed rolled oats coated with 6-MBOA to nonbreeding winter populations of *Microtus*. After three weeks, the sample populations revealed a high incidence of pregnancy among the females and pronounced swelling of the testicles among the males. Control populations receiving no 6-MBOA revealed no such signs. Since the timing of reproductive effort is crucial to the short-lived vole in an environment in which the onset of vegetative growth can vary by as much as two months, the phytochemical triggering of copulatory behavior in *Microtus* represents a significant biological adaptation.

A distinct example is reported by John Bryant of the University of Alaska. In this case, plants seem to have adopted a form of phytochemical self-defense against the depredations of the snowshoe hare (*Lepus americanus*) of Canada and Alaska. Every 10 years or so, for reasons that are not entirely understood, the *Lepus* population swells dramatically. The result is intense overbrowsing of early and midsuccessional deciduous trees and shrubs. Bryant has shown that, as if in response, four common boreal forest trees favored by *Lepus* produce adventitious shoots high in terpene and phenolic resins, which effectively discourage hare browsing. He treated mature nonresinous willow twigs with resinous extracts from the adventitious shoots of other plants and placed treated and untreated bundles at hare feeding stations, weighing them at the end of each day. Bryant found that bundles containing only half the resin concentration of natural twigs were left untouched. The avoidance of these unpalatable resins, he concludes, may play a significant role in the subsequent decline in the *Lepus* population to its normal level.

These results suggest obvious areas for further research. For example, observational data should be reviewed to see whether the periodic population explosions among the prolific lemming (like the vole and the snowshoe hare, a small rodent in a marginal northern environment) occur during years in which there is an early onset of vegetative growth; if so, a triggering mechanism similar to that found in the vole may be involved.

1. The author of the passage primarily wants to

   (A) review some findings suggesting biochemical regulation of predator populations by their food sources.

   (B) outline the role of 6-MBOA in regulating the population of browsing animals.

   (C) summarize available data on the relationship between food resources and population size.

   (D) argue that earlier researchers have misunderstood the relationship between food supply and population size.

2. The passage describes the effect of 6-MBOA on voles as a "significant biological adaptation" because it

   (A) limits reproductive behavior in times of food scarcity.

   (B) leads the vole population to seek available food resources.

   (C) tends to ensure the survival of the species in a situation of fluctuating food supply.

   (D) maximizes the survival prospects of individual voles.

3. It can be inferred that the study of lemmings proposed by the author would probably

   (A) fully explain the interrelationship between food supply and reproductive behavior in northern rodent populations.

   (B) disprove the conclusions of Berger and her colleagues.

   (C) be irrelevant to the findings of Berger and her colleagues.

   (D) provide evidence indicating whether the conclusions of Berger and her colleagues can be generalized.

4. The statement, "The interrelationship may be far more complex than hitherto imagined," suggests that scientists previously believed that

   (A) the amount of food available is the only food factor that affects population size.

   (B) reproductive behavior is independent of environmental factors.

   (C) food resources biochemically affect reproduction and the lifespan of some species.

   (D) population size is not influenced by available food resources.

5. The experiments described in the passage involved all of the following EXCEPT

   (A) measuring alterations in reproductive organs after a specific compound was ingested.

   (B) testing whether breeding behavior could be induced in normally nonbreeding animals by a change in diet.

   (C) measuring animals' consumption of treated and untreated foods.

   (D) measuring changes in the birth rate of test animals as opposed to control animals.

6. Bryant's interpretation of the results of his experiment depends on which of the following assumptions?

   (A) The response of *Lepus* to resinous substances in nature may be different from its response under experimental conditions.

   (B) The decennial rise in the *Lepus* population is triggered by an unknown phytochemical response.

   (C) Many *Lepus* will starve to death rather than eat resinous shoots or change their diet.

   (D) *Lepus* learns to search for alternative food sources once resinous shoots are encountered.

7. The experiments performed by Berger and Bryant BOTH study

    I. the effect of diet on reproduction in rodents.

    II. a relationship between food source and population size.

    III. phytochemical phenomena in northern environments.

    (A) II only

    (B) III only

    (C) I and II only

    (D) II and III only

8. The author provides specific information to answer which of the following questions?

    (A) Why does 6-MBOA form in response to browsing?

    (B) Why is the timing of the voles' reproductive effort important?

    (C) Are phytochemical reactions found only in northern environments?

    (D) How does 6-MBOA trigger reproductive activity in the montane vole?

Passage 2

The foxglove (*Digitalis purpurea*) of the Scrophylariaceae family is a plant found in wooded areas throughout central Europe, primarily in Hungary and the Harz mountains. The botanical name *Digitalis purpurea* comes from two Latin words, *digitus* and *purpura*. *Digitus* refers to the finger-shaped corolla of the plant. *Purpurea* refers to the purple color of the flowering part of the plant. The products derived from the foxglove have been used for hundreds of years because of their remarkable effects on the heart.

Currently the *Digitalis purpurea* is commercially grown and harvested to obtain its useful by-products. The yearly crop is harvested during the months of September and October. The commercial products with therapeutic benefits are obtained only from the first year's leaves of each plant because each season after the first yields a product with decreased potency. A portion of the first season's crop is unharvested to allow for the development of a flowering stalk to grow in the second season. Inside the stalk are seeds, which will be cultivated into new plants each year.

At the end of each harvest, the leaves are dried and subsequently processed into therapeutic products, named cardiac glycosides. The structure of these cardiac glycosides contains a steroid nucleus with sugar moieties attached. The sugar portions of the plant products are responsible for the term *glycoside* being used. There are over 30 different glycosides processed from the first-year leaves; however, only 3 are used therapeutically: digitoxin, gitoxin, and gitaloxin. The potency and relative concentrations of each of the three glycosides may vary with each harvest depending on the environmental conditions in which the plants were grown.

The foxglove has been used for centuries to treat many different ailments. The first recorded use was by the Anglo-Saxons, who named the plant *foxes glofa*. Physicians of that time used a mixture of the plant leaves and honey to purge the body of illness. The claim of the mixture was that it aided in removing harmful obstructions from the liver and spleen. These obstructions were believed to be the cause of many illnesses and their associated sequelae. For example, the modern-day flu presents with aches and gastrointestinal problems. The first recorded use of the foxglove for its effect on the heart was in 1775 by an English physician. He used digitoxin as a "cardiotonic" because of its stimulating effect on the heart. Digitoxin also has mild diuretic effects. This tonic was used to treat cases of dropsy, commonly referred to as congestive heart failure.

Digitoxin is the glycoside obtained from the foxglove currently used in the treatment of congestive heart failure and various arrhythmias. However, in treating these conditions, toxicity may occur; therefore, when using the foxglove products, the individual should be under medical supervision to ensure optimal outcomes. When used properly, this natural medication may alleviate many ailments of the heart.

9. The author mentions in paragraph 3 that the potency and relative concentrations of the three glycosides may vary in order to

   (A) keep the amount of sunlight and water constant from season to season.
   (B) discredit the therapeutic benefits of the plant.
   (C) imply that testing the plant after each harvest is necessary to ensure that the amount of glycoside given to each person will be constant.
   (D) promote giving large doses of the plant products to each person to ensure that enough drug is given.

10. Based on the passage, it can be inferred that

    (A) the foxglove may be used to treat many minor modern-day ailments.
    (B) the amount of digitoxin obtained from each leaf will be in the same proportions after each harvest.
    (C) use of the foxglove may produce more harm than good if it is not used carefully.
    (D) only one glycoside obtained from the foxglove has therapeutic properties.

11. Based on the passage which of the following is TRUE?

    (A) The seeds of the first-season plants are used to grow second-season plants.
    (B) The older the plant gets, the more potent the products derived from it.
    (C) The plant's products are generally harvested in the fall season.
    (D) The plant's products, which have medical value, are obtained from the stalk.

12. The name "foxglove" was probably derived from

    (A) Latin.
    (B) English.
    (C) Anglo-Saxon.
    (D) Italian.

13. Congestive heart failure is a condition where the heart is unable to pump blood properly; therefore, digitoxin must act by

    (A) increasing the amount of blood in the body.
    (B) stimulating the heart to pump blood more effectively.
    (C) removing obstructions in the liver and spleen.
    (D) promoting the condition of dropsy.

14. Which of the following is most structurally related to digitoxin?

    (A) Fats
    (B) Carbohydrates
    (C) Proteins
    (D) Triglycerides

15. Based on the passage, when does the foxglove normally produce flowers?

    (A) Never
    (B) Winter
    (C) First season
    (D) Second season

16. Which of the following is not mentioned in the passage as a use of the foxglove?

    (A) Proarrhythmic
    (B) Treatment of congestive heart failure
    (C) Removing obstructions from the spleen
    (D) Aid in treating gastrointestinal problems

17. The central thrust of the passage is that

    (A) the foxglove products are naturally harvested medications and will have a therapeutic effect on the user.
    (B) harvesting the foxglove is so difficult that it is hardly ever used even though it has many beneficial therapeutic effects.
    (C) naturally derived medications can still be used today and may be superior to synthetic medications.
    (D) only one of the foxglove products (digitoxin) is therapeutically beneficial.

Passage 3

It is notorious that breakthroughs in science often come in tandem: the same, or almost the same, theoretical advance is made simultaneously by two or more investigators. Watson and Crick "raced" Linus Pauling to verify the helical structure of DNA; Darwin and Alfred Wallace announced the essentials of evolutionary theory simultaneously in 1858. Why should this occur? Why—to take another example—should Newton and Leibniz have worked out the differential calculus independently and in isolation from one another, when they were not even working on the same sorts of problems?

Newton's work on the calculus stemmed from his interest in the physical problem of the measurement of continuously changing quantities. Take, for example, the problem of determining the velocity of a freely falling body at a given instant. The body is constantly accelerating due to gravity. An approximate velocity at any time may be found by measuring the distance travelled over a very brief time interval such as a hundredth of a second; if one reduces the time interval measured until it approaches zero, the approximate velocity over the interval approaches the actual velocity at any instant as a limit. Newton's genius was to grasp how to calculate such a change over an infinitesimal time period through a mathematical operation known as differentiation.

For various reasons, Newton delayed publishing a clear account of his calculus for nearly 40 years. In the meantime, Leibniz approached the calculus from a completely different standpoint, that of the formal geometric problem of determining the tangent to a curve (and later, for the integral calculus, the area under a curve). This geometric problem was mathematically equivalent to Newton's consideration of bodies in motion, however, since the changing position of such a body over time can be plotted graphically as a curve in which the tangent to the curve at any point represents the velocity of the body at a given instant. Thus, Leibniz's formal geometric approach duplicated Newton's results.

This phenomenon of simultaneous discovery is surprising only to a public that views such breakthroughs as solitary acts of genius. In reality, Newton and Leibniz's ground had been thoroughly prepared in advance. In the century before Newton's birth, Europe had seen an explosion of scientific inquiry. Copernicus, Kepler, and others had formulated the laws of planetary motion and celestial mechanics. More specifically, when he began his mathematical work, Newton was already familiar with Descartes's coordinate geometry, the mathematics of infinitesimal intervals recently developed by John Wallis, and the method of finding tangents through differentiation worked out by Isaac Barrow. Thus, both the scientific problems and the conceptual tools that stimulated and facilitated Newton's astonishingly rapid development of the differential calculus were already the common property of science. Given Newton's delay in publishing his work, an independent discovery of the calculus by some other genius became not only possible but likely.

18. The primary purpose of this passage is to

    (A) present mathematical discoveries.

    (B) clarify a recurring phenomenon in scientific history.

    (C) solve a long-standing puzzle in intellectual history.

    (D) describe a period of rapid scientific change.

19. It can be inferred from the passage that

    I. Newton based his calculus in part on the work of Descartes.

    II. Leibniz worked out the differential calculus without knowing of Newton's work.

    III. Leibniz approached the differential calculus from a standpoint similar to Newton's.

    (A) I only

    (B) II only

    (C) I and II only

    (D) II and III only

20. According to the author, Newton devised the differential calculus in an attempt to understand

    (A) why falling bodies accelerate.

    (B) how to measure continuously varying quantities.

    (C) how to measure the area under a curve.

    (D) the relationship between average and actual speed.

21. It can be inferred that the author regards the development of the calculus as

    (A) an outgrowth of previous intellectual developments.

    (B) a unique act of genius.

    (C) an achievement whose significance has been overestimated.

    (D) an unusual case of near-simultaneous discovery.

22. The passage implies that Newton and Leibniz arrived at similar results because

    (A) they used similar approaches.

    (B) they knew of each other's work.

    (C) no one had previously considered the problem of continuous motion.

    (D) the problems they considered were mathematically equivalent.

23. The author suggests that cases of simultaneous discovery

    (A) cannot really be called breakthroughs, since the important work has been done by others.

    (B) are extremely rare in science.

    (C) are made by individuals unaware of the historical influences on their thought.

    (D) seem remarkable to a public influenced by an inaccurate notion of genius.

24. In the final paragraph, the author draws connections between the work of Leibniz and Newton and the work of Copernicus and Kepler primarily to

    (A) provide support for the "great man" view of scientific history.

    (B) argue that the work of most scientific geniuses reveals unusually coincidental patterns of discovery.

    (C) expose the myth of independent scientific discovery.

    (D) describe the evolutionary nature of scientific achievement.

EXPLANATIONS TO PRACTICE EXERCISES

Passage 1

1. **A** The answer to a Main Idea question has to be broad enough to cover the entire passage without being too broad. Choice C, for example, is wrong because, although the author does summarize some data on the relationship between food sources and population size, it would be impossible for the passage to cover all available data on the subject. B, on the other hand, is not broad enough; 6-MBOA is discussed in only one of the paragraphs. D is off base because the author never argues against the conclusions of earlier researchers. She just says that things are more complex than was previously thought and leaves it at that. Choice A summarizes the passage nicely and is the correct answer.

2. **C** This Inference question contains a line reference which leads you to the end of paragraph 2. The biological adaptation to which the sentence is referring is the "phytochemical triggering of copulatory behavior" in voles—that is, the chemical MBOA in young mountain grasses causes voles to reproduce at just the right time, when there is a lot of grass for voles to feed on. This is important because the amount of available grass varies considerably. 6-MBOA, then, ensures the survival of voles in a situation of fluctuating food supply (choice C). 6-MBOA doesn't limit reproduction; it encourages reproduction, so A is wrong. Use your common sense to eliminate choice B: seeking available food resources comes pretty naturally to animals. D is wrong because a biological adaptation maximizes the survival of the entire species, not just individual voles.

3. **D** The author recommends research on the reproductive behavior of lemmings because lemmings are similar in kind and in habitat to voles. Knowing whether lemmings have a reproductive trigger mechanism similar to that of voles would allow us to determine whether Berger's findings about voles are true of other species as well. This idea is captured by choice D. Choices B and C contradict this notion entirely. Choice A goes way too far: there is no way one study of lemmings could tell us all there is to know about the interrelationship between food supply and reproductive behavior in northern rodent populations.

4. **A** Ecologists have long thought, according to the first sentence of the paragraph, that population size is a function of available food (this, by the way, rules out choice D). They just didn't realize that the interrelationship of food and population size was so complex. In other words, they thought that the amount of available food was the only food factor that affected population (choice A); they didn't know about food that biochemically encouraged or discouraged reproduction (which eliminates choice C). We don't know what scientists formerly thought about the link between environmental factors and reproductive behavior, so B is not an option.

5. **D** In this All/Except question, you have to identify the choice that is not an element of either experiment. Choice A is mentioned in the middle of paragraph 2 as part of the mountain vole experiment. Choice B was part of that experiment as well, as indicated at the beginning of paragraph 2. Measuring consumption of treated and untreated foods (choice C) was the method used in the experiment on hares. Choice D is the one choice that was not an element of either experiment discussed in the passage. The passage does discuss the use of a control group in the 6-MBOA experiment, but this experiment was not measuring changes in the birth rate of the animals, so D is the correct answer.

6. **C** This question asks for the assumption upon which Bryant's interpretation rests. Bryant concluded from his experiment that avoidance of unpalatable resins in the natural food source of Lepus may play a role in the decline in the Lepus population. He is assuming that hares will not eat anything at all, and thus starve to death, if they find resin on their food. The gist of this is captured in choice C. Certainly choice A is not an underlying assumption. Bryant's experiment would be worthless if the hares' behavior in the experiment didn't give us an idea of how they behaved in nature. Choice B is out because Bryant's experiment does not investigate the reasons for the decennial rise in hare population. Choice D makes no sense because if the hares learned to look for new sources of food once they couldn't eat the resinous shoots, their population wouldn't decrease.

7. **D** This Roman Numeral question is a bit reminiscent of Question 5 in that you are once again considering what was or was not part of both studies. Statement I is not true because the effect of diet on reproduction is part of Berger's study only. Both studies investigate the relationship between food source and population size, so Statement II is true. Statement III is clearly true as well, so choice D is the answer you want.

8. **B** This is a very general question about the passage, so let's look at the answer choices to see if some of them can be ruled out. Choices A and D are wrong because we never find out why 6-MBOA forms in response to browsing or exactly how it triggers reproductive activity in the vole. Nor do we know whether phytochemical reactions can be found anywhere besides northern environments, which eliminates choice C. That leaves us with choice B, and sure enough, the importance of the timing of the voles' reproductive effort is explained in the last sentence of paragraph 2.

Passage 2

9. **C** The purpose of the author's making a special note of the fact that the potency and relative concentrations of the glycosides may vary was to ensure that the reader understands that a standard extraction and distribution of the drug should not occur. The foxglove products may be very toxic if overdosed. If someone were to administer a set weight of foxglove products, the receiver would most likely receive different amounts of medication. Careful testing of each harvest needs to occur to maximize therapeutic benefit and minimize toxicity (choice C is correct, and choices A and B are incorrect). In a controlled environment, choice A could occur; however, the plants are grown in the wild, and humans cannot control nature.

10. **C** The foxglove has been used for centuries to treat various aliments; however, it is currently used to treat congestive heart failure and arrhythmias (choice A is incorrect). In supervised doses, the medication may be beneficial; however, in large doses, it can cause detrimental effects to the user (choice C is correct). Three glycosides are beneficial and may vary from harvest to harvest depending on the environmental factors (choices B and D are incorrect).

11. **C** The foxglove products are primarily harvested in the fall months of September and October (choice C is correct). In harvesting the plants, the seeds of the second season are used in the next season to produce new plants (choice A is incorrect). The reason why new plants need to be planted each year is because with each successive season the leaves produce less potent products (choices B and D are incorrect).

12. **C** The Anglo-Saxons named the plant *foxes glofa*, which is similar to the current name foxglove (choice C is correct). The Latin words *digitus* and *purpurea* are the word origins of the botanical name (choice A is incorrect based on the question). The English and Italian languages had no part in naming the plant (choices B and D are incorrect).

13. **B**   When treating a medical condition, the goal is usually to reverse the pathologic state. For example in congestive heart failure, the heart is unable to effectively pump blood throughout the body; therefore, treatment with digitalis would be used to stimulate the heart to pump blood more efficiently (choice B is correct). Digitoxin does not increase the amount of blood in the body or remove obstructions from the liver (choices A and C are incorrect). If dropsy was promoted, then the congestive heart failure would be worsened (choice D is incorrect).

14. **B**   Digitoxin is a glycoside that is derived from plants. It has a steroid component, which has sugar moieties attached to it. Sugars are most structurally related to carbohydrates (choice B is correct).

15. **D**   The foxglove is harvested in the months of September and October. The first season yields the most potent products from the leaves. It is not until the second season that a flowering stalk is seen (choice D is correct).

16. **A**   Some of the older uses for the foxglove include aiding in the removal of obstructions from the spleen and liver and to treat gastrointestinal disorders (choices C and D are incorrect). It is important to note that the previously mentioned uses were never proven effective and should not be used to treat these conditions now. The foxglove products are currently used in the treatment of congestive heart failure (choice B is incorrect). Any drug that is a proarrhythmic will promote arrhythmias, and the foxglove products are NOT used to promote these conditions (choice A is correct).

17. **A**   The main idea of the paragraph is that the foxglove is a plant that is commercially harvested to produce a product that has been used for therapeutic purposes for many years (choice A is correct). Choice B is incorrect because it suggests that the purpose of the passage is to argue that the cost of harvesting the product greatly outweighs the benefit. Choice C is incorrect because it references synthetic products, which are not mentioned in the passage. Choice D is incorrect because the passage specifically states in paragraph 3 that the foxglove provides three products that provide therapeutic benefit; only digitoxin is described in detail.

Passage 3

18. **B**   The opening paragraph raises the Newton-Leibniz discoveries in the context of two other examples (DNA, evolution) of simultaneous discovery, something the author says happens "often." After going through the specifics in paragraphs 2–3, the author returns to the broader point in the last paragraph, stressing the dependence of great scientific breakthroughs on earlier step-by-step work. So the purpose of the whole passage is to clarify the phenomenon of simultaneous discovery (choice B). Choices A and D omit the broader context; the author is interested in the calculus (choice A) and the scientific advances of Newton's time (choice D) only insofar as they illustrate the broader points about how great discoveries are made. The author never implies that the "puzzle" of Newton and Leibniz's simultaneous discovery is "long-standing" or that he/she is going to "solve" it (choice C).

19. **C**   The last paragraph states that Newton was familiar with Descartes's work, and implies that this was one of the "conceptual tools" he brought to his work on the calculus (I). Paragraph 1 states that Leibniz worked "independently and in isolation" from Newton (II). Both this paragraph and paragraph 3 make it clear that Leibniz's approach was "completely different" from Newton's, contrary to III.

20. **B** This choice is stated explicitly in the first sentence of paragraph 2. Choice A is wrong because the acceleration of falling bodies is mentioned by the author as an example of the problem of continuous motion; it is not clear that this was the specific problem Newton was working on or that Newton didn't understand "why" falling bodies accelerate. Choice C is mentioned as one of Leibniz's concerns (paragraph 3); Choice D is not mentioned at all. Paragraph 2 mentions approximate—not average—velocity; it's not implied that Newton was trying to understand the relationship between this and the actual velocity.

21. **A** The main question raised by the passage is: why do simultaneous discoveries occur? The answer, given in the last paragraph, is: because the groundwork is prepared in advance. This point is made specifically in relation to Newton and Leibniz in the second sentence of paragraph 4. This idea is paraphrased in choice A. The fact that Newton and Leibniz discovered the calculus independently rules out choice B. The author doesn't question the significance of the achievement (choice C)—only the misconceived idea of "solitary acts of genius." The first sentence of the passage says that such cases are not unusual (choice D).

22. **D** Paragraph 3 states that although Leibniz's approach was "completely different" from Newton's (ruling out choice A), the geometric problem he considered was "mathematically equivalent" to Newton's and "thus ... duplicated Newton's results." Choice D sums this up. Leibniz and Newton worked independently, ruling out choice B. Choice C is not stated and wouldn't explain their similar results anyway.

23. **D** This choice paraphrases the first sentence of the last paragraph. Choice A goes too far—the author does stress the preliminary work done by others but doesn't suggest that the discovery of the calculus (or similar discoveries) was not a breakthrough. Choice B, as we've seen before, is contradicted in the first paragraph. Choice C is not implied—we don't know what influences Leibniz, Newton, Darwin, et al. may have been aware of.

24. **D** Copernicus and Kepler are mentioned in the fourth sentence of the last paragraph in the context of the series of scientific and mathematical advances that "prepared the ground" for Newton and Leibniz. So the point is that science builds on earlier work—it is evolutionary (choice D) even when making great advances. Of the wrong choices, choice C is probably trickiest; one's first impulse is to say "Yes, this is what the author is doing, but 'expose the myth' goes too far." On reflection, you should realize that the author doesn't think independent discovery is a myth at all. Newton and Leibniz are examples of independent discovery. Neither one, of course, was wholly "independent" of previous developments, but their discoveries were made on their own. The "great man" view in choice A probably refers to the misconception that breakthroughs are "solitary acts of genius" (first sentence of paragraph 4); this is not the author's view. Choice B is a big overstatement; the passage says that simultaneous discoveries occur often, not all the time.

CHAPTER TWENTY-FOUR

Arithmetic

NUMBER OPERATIONS

Important terms and concepts to be familiar with for the test:

- **Real number**—All numbers on the number line. All numbers that appear on this test are real.
- **Integers**—All numbers with no fractional or decimal parts, including negative whole numbers and zero; multiples of 1. See the number line below.
- **Operations**—A process that is performed on one or more numbers. The four basic arithmetic operations are addition, subtraction, multiplication, and division.
- **Sum**—The result of addition
- **Difference**—The result of subtraction
- **Product**—The result of multiplication
- **Reciprocal**—The result of switching the numerator and denominator of a fraction. The reciprocal of $\frac{3}{5}$ is $\frac{5}{3}$. The reciprocal of 2 is $\frac{1}{2}$ because 2 can be considered to be the fraction $\frac{2}{1}$.

Numbers and the Number Line

A number line is a straight line, extending infinitely in either direction, on which real numbers are represented as points. Decimals and fractions can also be depicted on a number line, as can numbers such as $\sqrt{2}$.

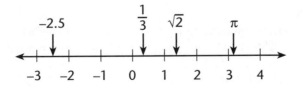

The values of numbers get larger as you move to the right along the number line. Numbers to the right of zero are **positive**; numbers to the left of zero are **negative**. **Zero** is neither positive nor negative. Any positive number is larger than any negative number. For example, –300 is less than 4.

Laws of Operations

Commutative laws of addition and multiplication

$$a + b = b + a$$
$$a \times b = b \times a$$

Addition and multiplication are both **commutative**; switching the order of any two numbers being added or multiplied together does not affect the result. For example, $5 + 8 = 8 + 5$; both sums equal 13. Similarly $2 \times 6 = 6 \times 2$; both products equal 12.

Subtraction and division are *not* commutative; switching the order of the numbers changes the result. For instance, $3 - 2 \neq 2 - 3$; the left side yields a result of 1, whereas the right side yields a result of -1.

Similarly, $6 \div 2 \neq 2 \div 6$; the left side gives us 3, whereas the right side gives us $\frac{1}{3}$.

Associative laws of addition and multiplication

$$(a + b) + c = a + (b + c)$$
$$(a \times b) \times c = a \times (b \times c)$$

Addition and multiplication are both **associative**.

Example:
$$(3 + 5) + 8 = 3 + (5 + 8)$$
$$8 + 8 = 3 + 13$$
$$16 = 16$$

Example:
$$(4 \times 5) \times 6 = 4 \times (5 \times 6)$$
$$20 \times 6 = 4 \times 30$$
$$120 = 120$$

Because addition and multiplication are both commutative and associative, numbers can be added or multiplied in any order. Subtraction and division are *not* associative.

Example: $7 - (10 - 4) = 7 - 6 = 1$, whereas $(7 - 10) - 4 = -3 - 4 = -7$.
So $7 - (10 - 4) \neq (7 - 10) - 4$.

Example: $24 \div (12 \div 3) = 24 \div 4 = 6$, whereas $(24 \div 12) \div 3 = 2 \div 3 = \frac{2}{3}$.
So $24 \div (12 \div 3) \neq (24 \div 12) \div 3$.

Distributive law

The distributive law of multiplication allows you to "distribute" a factor over a group of numbers that is being added or subtracted by multiplying that factor by each number in the group.

In general, $a(b + c) = ab + ac$

Example:

$$4(3 + 7) = ?$$
$$= (4 \times 3) + (4 \times 7)$$
$$4 \times 10 = 12 + 28$$
$$40 = 40$$

Division can be distributed in a similar way, because dividing by a number is equivalent to multiplying by that number's reciprocal.

Example:

$$\frac{3 + 5}{2} = \frac{1}{2}(3 + 5) = \frac{1}{2}(3) + \frac{1}{2}(5)$$
$$= \frac{1}{2}(8) \qquad = \frac{3}{2} + \frac{5}{2}$$
$$= \frac{8}{2} \qquad = \frac{8}{2}$$

Don't get carried away, though. When the sum or difference is in the denominator—that is, when you're dividing by a sum or difference—no distribution is possible.

$\frac{9}{4 + 5}$ is NOT equal to $\frac{9}{4} + \frac{9}{5}$; $\frac{9}{4 + 5} = \frac{9}{9} = 1$. But $\frac{9}{4}$ and $\frac{9}{5}$ are both greater than 1, so their sum certainly can't equal 1.

Operations with signed numbers

Numbers can be treated as though they had two parts: a positive or negative sign and a number part. For example, the sign of the number −3 is negative, and the number part is 3. Numbers without any sign are understood to be positive.

To add two numbers that have the same sign, add the number parts and keep the sign.

Example: What is the sum of −6 and −3?

To find (−6) + (−3), add 6 and 3, and then attach the negative sign from the original numbers to the sum: (−6) + (−3) = −9

To add two numbers that have different signs, find the difference between the number parts and keep the sign of the number whose number part is larger.

Example: What is the sum of −7 and +4?

To find (−7) + (+4), subtract 4 from 7 to get 3. 7 > 4; that is, the number part of −7 is greater than the number part of +4, so the final sum will be negative. (−7) + (+4) = −3

Subtraction is the opposite of addition. You can rephrase any subtraction problem as an addition problem by changing the operation sign from a minus to a plus and switching the sign on the second number. For instance, 8 − 5 = 8 + (−5). There's no real advantage to rephrasing if you are subtracting a smaller positive number from a larger positive number. But the concept comes in very handy when you are subtracting a negative number from any other number, a positive number from a negative number, or a larger positive number from a smaller positive number.

To subtract a negative number, rephrase as an addition problem and follow the rules for addition of signed numbers.

For instance, $9 - (-10) = 9 + 10 = 19$.

Here's another example: $(-5) - (-2) = (-5) + 2$. The difference between 5 and 2 is 3, and the number with the larger number part is -5, so the answer is -3.

To subtract a positive number from a negative number or from a smaller positive number, change the sign of the number that you are subtracting from positive to negative and follow the rules for addition of signed numbers.

For example, $(-4) - 1 = (-4) + (-1) = -5$.

Example: Subtract 8 from 2.

$2 - 8 = 2 + (-8)$. The difference between the number parts is 6, and the -8 has the larger number part, so the answer is -6.

Multiplication and division of signed numbers. Multiplying or dividing two numbers with the same sign gives a positive result.

$$(-4) \times (-7) = +28$$
$$(-50) \div (-5) = +10$$

Multiplying or dividing two numbers with different signs gives a negative result.

$$(-2) \times (+3) = -6$$
$$8 \div (-4) = -2$$

Properties of Zero, 1, and −1

Properties of zero
Adding zero to or subtracting zero from a number does not change the number.

$$x + 0 = x$$
$$0 + x = x$$
$$x - 0 = x$$

Example:

$$5 + 0 = 5$$
$$0 + (-3) = -3$$
$$4 - 0 = 4$$

Notice, however, that subtracting a number from zero switches the number's sign. It's easy to see why if you rephrase the problem as an addition problem.

Example: Subtract 5 from 0.

$0 - 5 = -5$. That's because $0 - 5 = 0 + (-5)$, and according to the properties of zero, $0 + (-5) = -5$.

The product of zero and any number is zero.

$$0 \times z = 0$$
$$z \times 0 = 0$$

Example:

$$0 \times 12 = 0$$

Division by zero is undefined. For practical purposes, that translates as "it can't be done." Because fractions are essentially division (that is, $\frac{1}{4}$ means $1 \div 4$), any fraction with zero in the denominator is also undefined.

Properties of 1 and –1

Multiplying or dividing a number by 1 does not change the number.

$$a \times 1 = a$$
$$1 \times a = a$$
$$a \div 1 = a$$

Example:

$$4 \times 1 = 4$$
$$1 \times (-5) = -5$$
$$(-7) \div 1 = -7$$

Multiplying or dividing a nonzero number by –1 changes the sign of the number.

$$a \times (-1) = -a$$
$$(-1) \times a = -a$$
$$a \div (-1) = -a$$

Example:

$$6 \times (-1) = -6$$
$$(-3) \times (-1) = 3$$
$$(-8) \div (-1) = 8$$

Order of Operations

Whenever you have a string of operations, be careful to perform them in the proper order. Otherwise, you will probably get the wrong answer.

PEMDAS

The acronym PEMDAS stands for the correct order of operations:

Parentheses

Exponents

Multiplication
Division $\Big\}$ in order from left to right

Addition
Subtraction $\Big\}$ in order from left to right

If you have trouble remembering PEMDAS, you can think of the mnemonic phrase: Please Excuse My Dear Aunt Sally.

Example:

$$66 \times (3 - 2) \div 11$$

If you were to perform all the operations sequentially from left to right, without regard to the rules for the order of operations, you would arrive at the answer $\frac{196}{11}$. To do this correctly, do the operation inside the parentheses first: $3 - 2 = 1$. Now we have

$$66 \times 1 \div 11 = 66 \div 11 = 6$$

Example:

$$30 - 5 \times 4 + (7 - 3)^2 \div 8$$

First perform any operations within parentheses. (If the expression has parentheses within parentheses, work from the innermost out.)

$$30 - 5 \times 4 + 4^2 \div 8$$

Next, do the exponent.

$$30 - 5 \times 4 + 16 \div 8$$

Then, do all multiplication and division in order from left to right.

$$30 - 20 + 2$$

Last, do all addition and subtraction in order from left to right.

$$10 + 2$$

The answer is 12.

FRACTIONS

Fast Fractions Overview

$$\frac{7}{8} \quad \begin{array}{l} \to \text{Numerator} \\ \to \text{Denominator} \end{array}$$

Multiplying fractions: Multiply numerators by each other and denominators by each other.

$$\frac{3}{4} \times \frac{9}{7} = \frac{3 \times 9}{4 \times 7} = \frac{27}{28}$$

Dividing fractions: Flip the numerator and denominator of the fraction you're dividing by, then multiply.

$$\frac{1}{5} \div \frac{4}{11} = \frac{1}{5} \times \frac{11}{4} = \frac{1 \times 11}{5 \times 4} = \frac{11}{20}$$

Adding fractions: You can add fractions only when they have the same denominator. When you add, add only the numerators, NOT the denominators.

$$\frac{2}{3} + \frac{5}{3} = \frac{2 + 5}{3} = \frac{7}{3}$$

If you don't have a common denominator, you have to find one. The fastest way to get a common denominator is to multiply each fraction by a fraction whose numerator and denominator are the same as the denominator of the other fraction. (You can do this because any fraction with the same numerator and denominator is equal to 1, and multiplying any number by 1 doesn't change the value of the number.)

$$\frac{1}{3} + \frac{2}{5} = \left(\frac{1}{3} \times \frac{5}{5}\right) + \left(\frac{2}{5} \times \frac{3}{3}\right) = \frac{5}{15} + \frac{6}{15} = \frac{11}{15}$$

Subtracting fractions: This works the same way as adding fractions, except you subtract the numerators instead of adding them.

$$\frac{6}{7} - \frac{1}{2} = \left(\frac{6}{7}\right)\left(\frac{2}{2}\right) - \left(\frac{1}{2}\right)\left(\frac{7}{7}\right) = \frac{12}{14} - \frac{7}{14} = \frac{5}{14}$$

Remember, parentheses can be used to indicate multiplication instead of the "×" sign.

Reducing fractions: Whenever there is a common factor in the numerator and denominator, you can reduce the fraction by removing the factor from both parts of the fraction. You can do this because dividing the numerator and denominator by the same number doesn't change the value of the fraction as a whole. This will often make working with the fraction much easier because you'll be using smaller numbers.

$$\frac{4}{12} = \frac{1 \times 4}{3 \times 4} = \frac{1}{3} \times 1 = \frac{1}{3}$$

Obviously, you don't have to write out all this math. We're just doing it to show you exactly what's going on. On the test, you should do easy fractions like these in one step like in the next example.

You can reduce $\frac{42}{28}$ by canceling like this: $\dfrac{\overset{6}{\cancel{42}}}{\underset{4}{\cancel{28}}} = \dfrac{\overset{3}{\cancel{6}}}{\underset{2}{\cancel{4}}} = \dfrac{3}{2}$

Let's look more closely at how we reduced $\frac{42}{28}$. Because both 42 and 28 are divisible by 7, we can divide both the numerator (42) and the denominator (28) by 7. Thus, $\frac{42}{28}$ was reduced to $\frac{6}{4}$. Because both 6 and 4 are divisible by 2, we can divide both the numerator (6) and the denominator (4) by 2. Thus, $\frac{6}{4}$ was reduced to $\frac{3}{2}$.

Canceling: Whenever you have to multiply two or more fractions, you should cancel common factors before you multiply. This is a lot like reducing and has the same advantages, $\frac{1}{7} \times \frac{7}{3}$ can be cancelled like this:

$$\frac{1}{\cancel{7}^{1}} \times \frac{\cancel{7}^{1}}{3} = \frac{1}{1} \times \frac{1}{3} = \frac{1}{3}$$

$\frac{4}{5} \times \frac{15}{12}$ can be cancelled like this:

$$\frac{\cancel{4}^{1}}{\cancel{5}_{1}} \times \frac{\cancel{15}^{3}}{\cancel{12}_{3}} = \frac{1}{1} \times \frac{3}{3} = 1$$

Notice that we divided both the 5 in the denominator of the first fraction and the 15 in the numerator of the second fraction by 5. We also divided the 4 in the numerator of the first fraction and the 12 in the denominator of the second fraction by 4.

Comparing Fractions

One way to compare fractions is to re-express them with a **common denominator.** $\frac{3}{4} = \frac{21}{28}$ and $\frac{5}{7} = \frac{20}{28}$. $\frac{21}{28}$ is greater than $\frac{20}{28}$, so $\frac{3}{4}$ is greater than $\frac{5}{7}$. Another way to compare fractions is to convert them both to decimals. $\frac{3}{4}$ converts to 0.75, and $\frac{5}{7}$ converts to approximately 0.714.

Mixed Numbers and Fractions

A mixed number consists of an integer and a fraction. For example, $3\frac{1}{4}$, $12\frac{2}{5}$, and $5\frac{7}{8}$ are all mixed numbers.

To convert an improper fraction (a fraction whose numerator is greater than its denominator) to a mixed number, divide the numerator by the denominator. The number of "whole" times that the denominator goes into the numerator will be the integer portion of the mixed number; the remainder will be the numerator of the fractional portion.

Example: Convert $\frac{23}{4}$ to a mixed number.

Dividing 23 by 4 gives you 5 with a remainder of 3, so $\frac{23}{4} = 5\frac{3}{4}$.

To change a mixed number to a fraction, keep the denominator of the fraction. To figure out the numerator, multiply the integer portion of the mixed number by the number in the denominator. Then add this result to the numerator of the mixed number.

Example: Convert $2\frac{3}{7}$ to a fraction.

$$2\frac{3}{7} = \frac{(2 \times 7) + 3}{7} = \frac{17}{7}$$

Example: Convert $5\frac{8}{9}$ to a fraction.

$$5\frac{8}{9} = \frac{(5 \times 9) + 8}{9} = \frac{53}{9}$$

Adding and Subtracting Mixed Numbers

Adding or subtracting mixed numbers whose fractional parts have the same denominator will probably be on the test.

Example: $3\frac{12}{17} + 4\frac{10}{17} = ?$

First, add the integer parts: $3 + 4 = 7$.

Next, add the fractional parts: $\frac{12}{17} + \frac{10}{17} = \frac{22}{17}$.

Now, $\frac{22}{17} = 1\frac{5}{17}$.

Therefore, $3\frac{12}{17} + 4\frac{10}{17} = 7 + 1\frac{5}{17} = 8\frac{5}{17}$.

Example: $4\frac{5}{8} - 2\frac{7}{8} = ?$

The wrinkle here is that the fractional part of the first number is smaller than the fractional part of the second number (i.e., $\frac{5}{8}$ is smaller then $\frac{7}{8}$). What we need to do, therefore, is to borrow from the integer part of the first number to make the fractional part of the first number bigger. We'll borrow 1 from the integer part and add it to the fractional part (remembering that 1 can be rewritten as $\frac{8}{8}$).

So $4\frac{5}{8} = 3 + \frac{8}{8} + \frac{5}{8} = 3\frac{13}{8}$. So the problem of finding $4\frac{5}{8} - 2\frac{7}{8}$ has been replaced with the problem of finding $3\frac{13}{8} - 2\frac{7}{8}$, which is easier because the fractional part of the first number is greater than the fractional part of the second number.

Notice that all we've done is replace $4\frac{5}{8}$ with $3\frac{13}{8}$, which is equal to $4\frac{5}{8}$. To find $3\frac{13}{8} - 2\frac{7}{8}$, first subtract the integer parts: $3 - 2 = 1$. Next subtract the fractional parts: $\frac{13}{8} - \frac{7}{8} = \frac{6}{8} = \frac{3}{4}$. So $4\frac{5}{8} - 2\frac{7}{8} = 1\frac{3}{4}$.

Example: $5\frac{1}{4} - 1\frac{3}{4} = ?$

$$5\frac{1}{4} - 1\frac{3}{4} = 5 + \frac{1}{4} - 1\frac{3}{4} = \left(4 + \frac{4}{4}\right) + \frac{1}{4} - 1\frac{3}{4} = 4\frac{5}{4} - 1\frac{3}{4} = 3\frac{2}{4} = 3\frac{1}{2}$$

When you gain experience with this, you'll be able to skip some of the steps and do this type of problem more quickly.

Example: $8\frac{3}{25} - 4\frac{12}{25} = ?$

$$8\frac{3}{25} - 4\frac{12}{25} = 7 + \frac{25}{25} + \frac{3}{25} - 4\frac{12}{25} = 7\frac{28}{25} - 4\frac{12}{25} = 3\frac{16}{25}$$

RATIOS

Setting up a ratio

To find a ratio, put the number associated with the word *of* on top and the quantity associated with the word *to* on the bottom and reduce. The ratio of 20 oranges to 12 apples is $\frac{20}{12}$, which reduces to $\frac{5}{3}$.

Part-to-part ratios and part-to-whole ratios

If the parts add up to the whole, a part-to-part ratio can be turned into two part-to-whole ratios by putting each number in the original ratio over the sum of the numbers. If the ratio of males to females is 1 to 2, then the males-to-people ratio is $\frac{1}{1+2} = \frac{1}{3}$ and the females-to-people ratio is $\frac{2}{1+2} = \frac{2}{3}$. In other words, $\frac{2}{3}$ of all the people are female.

Solving a proportion

To solve a proportion, **cross-multiply**:

$$\frac{x}{5} = \frac{3}{4}$$

$$4x = 5 \times 3$$

$$x = \frac{15}{4} = 3.75$$

An important point about ratios

Notice that if you are given a ratio, you can't determine how many there are of each item represented by a number of the ratio. For example, if you are told that the ratio of the number of pencils to the number of pens in a drawer is 5 to 4, you don't know that there are 5 pencils and 4 pens in the drawer. All you know is that for every 5 pencils, there are 4 pens. There might be 50 pencils and 40 pens, or there might be 10 pencils and 8 pens in the drawer.

Example: The ratio of dogs to cats in an apartment building is 3 to 2. If there are a total of 50 animals in the apartment building and all of the animals in the building are dogs or cats, how many dogs are in the apartment building?

The fraction of animals that are dogs is $\frac{3}{3+2}$, or $\frac{3}{5}$. So the number of dogs in the building is $\frac{3}{5} \times 50$, or 30.

DECIMALS

There are two different ways to express numbers that are not integers: as fractions and as decimals. Fractions we've already discussed; now it's time to talk about decimals.

When a number is expressed in decimal form, it has two parts: the whole number part and the decimal fraction part. The two parts are separated by the decimal point (.). The whole number part is to the left of the decimal point; the decimal fraction part is the decimal point and the numbers to the right of the decimal point. For example, in 4.56, the whole number is 4, and the decimal fraction is 0.56.

You are certainly familiar with decimals from dealing with money: $12.45 is an example of a decimal. The part to the left of the decimal point is the whole number part: 12 in this case. The decimal fraction part is 0.45 in this case.

Let's see how decimals work by looking at dollars and cents. What fraction of a dollar is 1 cent? That's 0.01 dollars. Well there are 100 cents in a dollar, so 1 cent must represent $\frac{1}{100}$ of a dollar. So we know that the fraction $\frac{1}{100}$ is equivalent to the decimal 0.01.

Now, what fraction of a dollar is 10 cents, or 0.10 dollars? That's equal to a dime, and there are 10 dimes in a dollar, so 10 cents must be $\frac{1}{10}$ of a dollar. So we also know that $\frac{1}{10}$ is equivalent to the decimal 0.10.

Now notice this: the fraction $\frac{1}{10}$ is ten times as much as the fraction $\frac{1}{100}$. Similarly, the decimal 0.10 is ten times as much as the decimal 0.01. This should reassure you that we aren't changing the values of the fractions, only the way they're expressed.

Let's backtrack. You can tell the value of a digit in a number by its place value. For instance, in the number 27,465, the number 6 has a value of 60, because it's in the tens place. Each place is worth 10 times as much as the place to its right:

$$
\begin{aligned}
27,465 &= 2 \times 10,000 \\
&= + 7 \times 1,000 \\
&= + 4 \times 100 \\
&= + 6 \times 10 \\
&= + 5 \times 1
\end{aligned}
$$

Decimals work the same way. You know the value of each digit in a decimal by its place relative to the decimal point. The first place to the right of the decimal point is worth $\frac{1}{10}$ (thus we call it the tenths place). The second place is worth $\frac{1}{100}$ (thus we call it the hundredths place). The third place is worth $\frac{1}{1,000}$ (thus we call it the thousandths place). The fourth place is worth $\frac{1}{10,000}$ (thus we call it the ten-thousandths place), and so on.

As before, each place is worth 10 times as much as the place to its right. That's why 0.10 means $\frac{1}{10}$, and 0.01 means $\frac{1}{100}$. By the way, the decimal point is small and has a habit of getting lost (is that a decimal or a bug?); for this reason, it's best to put the 0 before the decimal. That doesn't change the value; 0.01 is the same as .01. Also, zeros to the right of a decimal don't change the value: 0.10 is the same as 0.1; they're both $\frac{1}{10}$. Similarly, 7.59 and 7.59000 have the same value; they're both $7\frac{59}{100}$.

Changing Fractions to Decimals

It's easy to change a fraction into a decimal—all you do is divide the denominator of the fraction into the numerator.

Example: Change $\frac{415}{3,220}$ into a decimal.

First write the fraction as long division.

$$3,220\overline{)415}$$

3,220 is much bigger than 415. So what we do is add a zero to the 415 to make the division work out. The only way we can do this without changing the value of 415 is if we add a decimal point after the 5. Then we're just changing 415 to 415.00—and those zeros don't change the value of anything. We divide normally, but we put a decimal point in the quotient (the answer) directly above the decimal point in 415.

```
         .12
3,220)415.000
      4150
      3220
       9300
       6440
      28600
```

How far we should go depends on how much accuracy we need, but at this point, we can tell that the answer is going to be close to 0.13.

Changing Decimals to Fractions

How do you express 0.5 as a fraction? Well, 0.1 represents $\frac{1}{10}$, and 0.5 is five times as much as 0.1, so 0.5 must represent 5 times $\frac{1}{10}$ or $\frac{5}{10}$. Of course, we can reduce $\frac{5}{10}$ to $\frac{1}{2}$.

How do you express 0.55 as a fraction? Well—let's think of it in terms of dollars and cents. $0.01 is one cent, and that's $\frac{1}{100}$ of a dollar. $0.55 is 55 cents, and that's 55 times as much, so $0.55 must be $\frac{55}{100}$ of a dollar. We can reduce this by dividing the top and bottom by 5, giving us $\frac{11}{20}$. That's the fractional equivalent of 0.55.

Hopefully by this point you recognize a pattern:

$$0.1 = 1 \times \frac{1}{10} \text{ or } \frac{1}{10}$$

$$0.11 = 11 \times \frac{1}{100} \text{ or } \frac{11}{100}$$

$$0.111 = 111 \times \frac{1}{1,000} \text{ or } \frac{111}{1,000}$$

$$0.1111 = 1,111 \times \frac{1}{10,000} \text{ or } \frac{1,111}{10,000}$$

and so on.

What we did on the previous page to change these decimals that are between 0 and 1 to fractions was to put the digits to the right of the decimal point in the numerator. To figure out the denominator, we put a 1 in the denominator and followed it with as many zeros as there were digits to the right of the decimal point.

Example: Change 0.564 to a fraction.

There are three digits to the right of the decimal point, so the denominator of our fraction will be 1,000 (a 1 followed by three zeros). The numerator of the fraction is 564.

$$0.564 = \frac{564}{1,000}$$

But notice that $\frac{564}{1,000}$ can be reduced. Because both 564 and 1,000 are divisible by 4, we can divide both the numerator and the denominator by 4; therefore, $\frac{564}{1,000} = \frac{564 \div 4}{1,000 \div 4} = \frac{141}{250}$.

Addition and Subtraction of Decimals

You add and subtract decimals the same way you add and subtract whole numbers. Just make sure the decimal points are lined up and add. In the answer, put the decimal point directly below the other decimal points.

$$
\begin{aligned}
0.456 + 1.234 = \quad &0.456 \\
+\ &1.234 \\
\hline
1.690 = \ &1.69
\end{aligned}
$$

If one of the terms you are adding or subtracting is longer than another (has more digits to the right of the decimal point), it helps to add zeros to the shorter number.

$$
\begin{aligned}
6.97 - 3.567 = \quad &6.970 \\
-\ &3.567 \\
\hline
&3.403
\end{aligned}
$$

Multiplication of Decimals

As with addition and subtraction, you multiply decimals as if they were whole numbers and worry about the decimal points later. You don't need to add zeros to make the numbers the same length when you multiply, however.

$$
\begin{array}{r}
4.5 \times 3.2 = 4.5 \\
\times\, 3.2 \\
\hline
90 \\
1\,3\,5 \\
\hline
1,440
\end{array}
$$

To place the decimal point in the answer, count the number of digits to the right of the decimal point in each number. Here we have 1 decimal place in 4.5, and 1 in 3.2, for a total of $1 + 1$ or 2 places. Put the decimal point 2 places from the right in the answer: 14.40.

It's a good idea when you get the answer to see whether it makes sense and to check that you put the decimal point in the right place. Here the answer should be a little bigger than 4×3 or 12. So 14.40 should be about right. If you placed the decimal point incorrectly and ended up with 144, you would know that was wrong.

Division of Decimals

It's easiest to discuss division of decimals if we express the division in fractional form.

Example: $\quad 4.15 \div 32.2 = \dfrac{4.15}{32.2}$

Make both the numerator and the denominator of the fraction whole numbers; to do this, multiply both top and bottom by a sufficient power of 10. In our example, we need to multiply by 100; this will make the denominator 3,220 and the numerator 415. We're left with

$$
\frac{4.15}{32.2} = \frac{415}{3,220}
$$

Now divide 3,220 into 415. You should get approximately 0.129.

Rounding Decimals to the Nearest Place

To round a decimal to the nearest place, look at the digit immediately to the right of that place. If that digit is 5, 6, 7, 8, or 9, then round up the place you are rounding to. If the digit immediately to the right of the place you are rounding to is 0, 1, 2, 3, or 4, then don't change the digit at the place you are rounding to. In either case, in the rounded-off number, there will be no digits to the right of the place you are rounding off to.

Example: Round 0.12763 to the nearest thousandth.

The digit in the thousandths place is 7. The digit immediately to the right of the 7 is a 6. Because 6 is among the digits that are 5 or more, we round up the thousandths digits from 7 to 8. So 0.12763 rounded to the nearest thousandth is 0.128.

Example: Round 0.5827 to the nearest hundredth.

The digit in the hundredths place is 8. Immediately to the right of the 8 is a 2. Because 2 is among the digits 0 through 4, we keep the digit in the hundredths place the same. So 0.5827 rounded to the nearest hundredth is 0.58.

Example: Round $\frac{5}{37}$ to the nearest hundredth.

$$
\begin{array}{r}
0.135 \\
37\overline{)5.000} \\
50 \\
\underline{37} \\
130 \\
\underline{111} \\
190 \\
\underline{185} \\
5
\end{array}
$$

Because the digit in the thousandths place is a 5, the hundredths digit is rounded up from 3 to 4. So $\frac{5}{37}$ rounded to the nearest hundredth is 0.14.

Scientific Notation

Scientific notation is a convention for expressing numbers that simplifies computation and standardizes results. To write a nonzero number in scientific notation, write the number in the form $a \times 10^n$, where n is an integer and $1 \leq a < 10$ or $-10 < a \leq -1$.

Example: $123 = 1.23 \times 10^2$

1.23 is the **coefficient** and 2 is the **exponent**.

Example: $0.042 = 4.2 \times 10^{-2}$

One can easily obtain products and quotients of numbers expressed in scientific notation. When multiplying, one simply multiplies the coefficients and adds the exponents to find the new coefficient and exponent of the answer. Some additional conversion may be necessary so that the new coefficient a is such that $1 \leq a_1 < 10$ or $-10 < a_1 \leq -1$, as in the third example on the next page.

Example: $(1.1 \times 10^6)(5.0 \times 10^{17}) = ?$

Multiply the coefficients 1.1 and 5.0 and add the exponents 6 and 17.

The answer is 5.5×10^{23}.

The quotient of two numbers expressed in scientific notation is obtained by dividing the coefficient in the numerator by the coefficient in the denominator and subtracting the exponent in the denominator from the exponent in the numerator.

Example: $\dfrac{6.2 \times 10^5}{2.0 \times 10^{-7}}$

Divide 6.2 by 2.0 and subtract −7 from 5 (note that $5 - (-7) = 5 + 7 = 12$).

The answer is 3.1×10^{12}.

When a number expressed in scientific notation is raised to an exponent, the coefficient is raised to that exponent, and the original exponent is multiplied by that exponent.

Example: $(6.0 \times 10^4)^2$

Square the 6.0 and multiply the exponent by 2.

$$(6.0)^2 \times 10^{4 \times 2} = 36.0 \times 10^8 = 3.6 \times 10^9$$

Note that when we move the decimal point one place to the left, we must increase the power of ten by one, from 8 to 9.

When adding or subtracting numbers expressed in scientific notation, they must have the **same** exponent; when they do not, the appropriate conversion must be made first.

Example: $3.7 \times 10^4 + 1.5 \times 10^3 = ?$

First, convert 1.5×10^3 to 0.15×10^4 so both numbers have the same exponent. Then, $3.7 \times 10^4 + 0.15 \times 10^4 = 3.85 \times 10^4$, which can be rounded to 3.9×10^4.

PERCENTS

Percents are a special kind of ratio. Any percent can be expressed as a fraction with a denominator of 100 (*cent* means "one hundred," so *percent* means "per one hundred"). Because of this, it is very easy to convert percents into decimals as well as fractions. When you see the symbol %, think of its being the factor $\frac{1}{100}$. Thus, $70\% = 70\left(\frac{1}{100}\right)$.

To convert a percent to a fraction or decimal, just divide the percent by 100%. Because $100\% = 1$, we are dividing the percent by 1, so we are not changing the value of the percent. (To convert to decimals, the shortcut is simply to drop the percent symbol and move the decimal point two places to the left.)

Percent to fraction: $\qquad 78\% = \dfrac{78\%}{100\%} = \dfrac{78}{100}$

Note that in going from $\frac{78\%}{100\%}$ to $\frac{78}{100}$, the percent symbol was cancelled, which is the factor $\frac{1}{100}$, from the numerator and denominator.

Percent to decimal: $\qquad 78\% = 0.78$

$$\frac{78}{100} = 0.78$$

To convert any fraction or decimal to a percent, just multiply by 100%. For decimals, just move the decimal point two places to the right and add a percent sign. For fractions, remember to reduce if you can before you multiply.

Decimal to percent: $\qquad 0.29 = 0.29 \times 100\% = 29\%$

$$0.3 = 0.30 \times 100\% = 30\%$$

$$1.45 = 1.45 \times 100\% = 145\%$$

Fraction to percent: $\dfrac{3}{5} = \dfrac{3}{5} \times 100\% = \dfrac{3(100)}{5}\% = 3(20)\% = 60\%$

Know these common conversions. They come up frequently on the test, and you can avoid errors and save time by memorizing them instead of having to calculate them on the test.

In general, a digit with a bar over it means that the digit repeats indefinitely. In the table below, $0.3\overline{3}$ means that the 3 with the bar over it repeats indefinitely. Thus, $0.3\overline{3} = 0.3333\ldots$

Fraction	Decimal	Percent
$\dfrac{1}{1}$	1.0	100%
$\dfrac{3}{4}$	0.75	75%
$\dfrac{2}{3}$	$0.\overline{66}$	$66\dfrac{2}{3}\%$
$\dfrac{1}{2}$	0.5	50%
$\dfrac{1}{3}$	$0.3\overline{3}$	$33\dfrac{1}{3}\%$
$\dfrac{1}{4}$	0.25	25%
$\dfrac{1}{5}$	0.2	20%
$\dfrac{1}{8}$	0.125	$12\dfrac{1}{2}\%$
$\dfrac{1}{10}$	0.1	10%
$\dfrac{1}{20}$	0.05	5%

The percent formula

The percent formula is commonly expressed in two different ways that are mathematically identical. Memorize and use whichever version of the formula you prefer. Notice how easy it is to get from one formula to the other—just multiply or divide both sides of the equation by the Whole.

$$\textbf{Percent} = \frac{\textbf{Part}}{\textbf{Whole}}$$

or

$$\textbf{Percent} \times \textbf{Whole} = \textbf{Part}$$

If the Part is 3 and the Whole is 4, then the Percent $= \dfrac{3}{4} = 0.75 = 75\%$.

If the Percent is 20% and the Whole is 8, then the Part $= 20\%(8) = (0.2)(8) = 1.6$.

If the Percent is 60% and the Part is 12, then $60\% \times (\text{Whole}) = 12$. So:

$$\text{Whole} = \frac{12}{60\%} = \frac{12}{\left(\dfrac{6}{10}\right)} = 12\left(\frac{10}{6}\right) = 20$$

Translating

Translating percent word problems into math is relatively easy. Whenever you see the phrase "what percent *of* . . . *is* . . .?," whatever follows the word *of* is the Whole and whatever follows the verb (often *is* or *are*) is the Part.

Example: 25% of 48 is 12.

$$\frac{\text{(part) } 12}{\text{(whole) } 48} = 25\%$$

Example: What percent of the songbirds are Cardinals?

You don't really have to know what the question is talking about to know that the Whole is the number of songbirds and the Part is the number of Cardinals.

Percent increase/decrease

Once you understand percents, percent increase and decrease are not as difficult as they may seem.

$$\% \text{ increase} = \frac{\textbf{Amount of increase}}{\textbf{Original whole}} \times 100\%$$

$$\% \text{ decrease} = \frac{\textbf{Amount of decrease}}{\textbf{Original whole}} \times 100\%$$

New Whole = Original whole ± Amount of change

Look at the first equation above. To find a percent increase, divide the amount of increase by the original whole. Then multiply this fraction by 100%.

Example: If a number increases from 50 to 70, what is the percent increase?

The amount of increase is 70 − 50, or 20. The original whole is 50. So the percent increase is $\frac{20}{50} \times 100\% = \frac{2}{5} \times 100\%$. What you learned reducing fractions can help here.

$$\frac{2}{5} \times 100\% = 2 \times 20\% = 40\%$$

If the new price of an item is 130% of its previous price, then it has increased in price by 30%. If an item goes on sale at 60% of its previous price, then it has decreased in price by 40%.

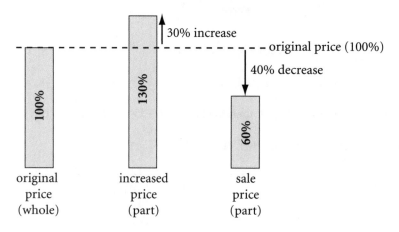

The percent increase or decrease is just the difference in percent from the whole (which is always equal to 100%).

When you come across the following phrases, use the percent increase/decrease formula:

percent increase	percent decrease
percent higher than	percent lower than
percent greater than	percent less than
percent gain	percent loss
percent more than	percent less than

If X is 10% greater than Y, then X is 110% of Y.

If X is 70% less than Y, then X is 30% of Y.

Example: If the value of a certain piece of property now is 350% of its original value when Kim purchased it, by what percent has the value of the property increased since Kim purchased it?

The percent increase is the difference from 100%. So there was a $350\% - 100\% = 250\%$ increase.

AVERAGES

Formula for computing averages

To find the average of a set of numbers, add them up and divide by the number of terms (the number of numbers).

$$\text{Average} = \frac{\text{Sum of the terms}}{\text{Number of terms}}$$

To find the average of the five numbers 12, 15, 23, 40, and 40, first add them: $12 + 15 + 23 + 40 + 40 = 130$. Then divide the sum by 5: $130 \div 5 = 26$.

Using the average to find the sum

$$\text{Sum} = (\text{Average}) \times (\text{Number of terms})$$

If the average of 10 numbers is 50, then they add up to 10×50, or 500.

Finding the missing number

To find a missing number when you're given the average, **use the sum**. If the average of four numbers is 7, then the sum of those four numbers is 4×7, or 28. Suppose that three of the numbers are 3, 5, and 8. These three numbers add up to 16 of that 28, which leaves $28 - 16 = 12$ for the fourth number.

REVIEW PROBLEMS

1. The average of 3, 15, 18, and 8 is

   (A) 5   (B) 9   (C) 11   (D) 18   (E) 21

2. Which of the following fractions is largest?

   (A) $\dfrac{2}{5}$ (B) $\dfrac{1}{2}$ (C) $\dfrac{2}{7}$ (D) $\dfrac{2}{10}$ (E) $\dfrac{4}{16}$

3. $\dfrac{2}{7} + \dfrac{1}{4} =$

   (A) $\dfrac{13}{11}$ (B) $\dfrac{15}{28}$ (C) $\dfrac{2}{28}$ (D) $\dfrac{7}{8}$ (E) $\dfrac{2}{11}$

4. $6\dfrac{1}{7} - 3\dfrac{4}{7} =$

   (A) $2\dfrac{4}{7}$ (B) $3\dfrac{3}{7}$ (C) $2\dfrac{3}{7}$ (D) $3\dfrac{4}{7}$ (E) $3\dfrac{1}{7}$

5. Which of the following numbers is smallest?

   (A) 0.1
   (B) 0.01
   (C) 0.0407
   (D) 0.03995
   (E) 1.00001

6. What is the value of $5\dfrac{1}{4} \div 7$?

   (A) $\dfrac{5}{7}$ (B) 3   (C) $\dfrac{3}{4}$ (D) $3\dfrac{4}{7}$ (E) $3\dfrac{3}{7}$

7. $16 + 0.267 + 36.78 =$

   (A) 52.047
   (B) 8.26
   (C) 5.347
   (D) 54.47
   (E) 53.047

8. What is the cost of a blouse that is priced at $50.00 with a tax of 7%?

   (A) $35.00
   (B) $50.35
   (C) $85.00
   (D) $53.50
   (E) $535.00

9. If a pencil costs $0.26, what is the cost of 96 pencils?

   (A) $12.
   (B) $24.
   (C) $2.49
   (D) $249.60
   (E) $24.96

10. What is the value of 2,886 ÷ 37?

   (A) 780   (B) 708   (C) 7,008   (D) 78   (E) 7,800

SOLUTIONS TO REVIEW PROBLEMS

1. **C**

$$\text{Average} = \frac{\text{Sum of the terms}}{\text{Number of terms}}$$

Here, the average is $\dfrac{3 + 15 + 18 + 8}{4} = \dfrac{44}{4} = 11$.

2. **B** Begin by comparing choice (A), $\dfrac{2}{5}$, and choice (B), $\dfrac{1}{2}$. $\dfrac{2}{5}$ has a numerator that is less than half of its denominator, so choice (A) is less than $\dfrac{1}{2}$. Choice (A) can be eliminated. Each of choices (C), (D), and (E) also has a numerator that is less than half of its denominator, so these three choices are also less than $\dfrac{1}{2}$ and can therefore also be eliminated. This means that choice (B), $\dfrac{1}{2}$, is the largest.

3. **B** $\dfrac{2}{7} + \dfrac{1}{4} = \dfrac{2}{7} \times \dfrac{4}{4} + \dfrac{1}{4} \times \dfrac{7}{7} = \dfrac{8}{28} + \dfrac{7}{28} = \dfrac{8 + 7}{28} = \dfrac{15}{28}$

4. **A** $6\dfrac{1}{7} - 3\dfrac{4}{7} = 5 + 1 + \dfrac{1}{7} - 3\dfrac{4}{7} = 5 + \dfrac{7}{7} + \dfrac{1}{7} - 3\dfrac{4}{7} = 5\dfrac{8}{7} - 3\dfrac{4}{7} = 2\dfrac{4}{7}$

5. **B** Notice that choice (E), 1.00001, is greater than 1 while all of the other choices are less than 1, so choice (E) can be eliminated right away. Choice (A) has a tenths digit of 1, while choices (B), (C), and (D) each have a tenths digit of 0. So choice (A) can be eliminated. Looking at the hundredths digits of choices (B), (C), and (D), we see that 0.01 has a hundredths digit of 1, 0.0407 has a hundredths digit of 4, and 0.03995 has a hundredths digit of 3. Since choice (B), 0.01, has the smallest hundredths digit, it must be the smallest of choices (B), (C), and (D), and since we've already eliminated choices (A) and (E), choice (B), 0.01, is the smallest of all the choices.

6. **C** When you divide one fraction by another, you invert the second fraction and multiply.

Think of the integer 7 as the fraction $\dfrac{7}{1}$, so that you can invert it to get the fraction $\dfrac{1}{7}$.

Rewrite $5\dfrac{1}{4}$ as an improper fraction. $5\dfrac{1}{4} = \dfrac{5 \times 4 + 1}{4} = \dfrac{21}{4}$.

Then $5\dfrac{1}{4} \div 7 = \dfrac{21}{4} \div \dfrac{7}{1} = \dfrac{21}{4} \times \dfrac{1}{7} = \dfrac{21 \times 1}{4 \times 7} = \dfrac{21}{28} = \dfrac{3}{4}$.

7. **E** Write the numbers in a column, making sure to align the decimal points. Write 16 as 16.000 and write 36.78 as 36.780.

$$
\begin{array}{r}
16.000 \\
0.267 \\
\underline{36.780} \\
53.047
\end{array}
$$

8. **D** Add 7% of 50 to 50. 7% of 50 is $\dfrac{7}{100} \times 50 = \dfrac{7}{2} \times 1 = \dfrac{7}{2} = 3\dfrac{1}{2} = 3.5$. So the cost of the blouse is $50 + 3.50$, or \$53.50.

9. **E** Multiply the cost of one pencil by the number of pencils. The cost of all the pencils is $\$0.26 \times 96 = \$24.96$.

10. **D**

$$
\begin{array}{r}
78 \\
37\overline{)2{,}886} \\
259 \\
\hline
296 \\
296 \\
\hline
0
\end{array}
$$

CHAPTER TWENTY-FIVE

Algebra

EXPONENTS—KEY OPERATIONS

You can't be adept at algebra unless you're completely at ease with exponents. Here's what you need to know:

Multiplying powers with the same base: To multiply powers with the same base, keep the base and add the exponents:

$$x^3 \times x^4 = x^{3+4} = x^7$$

Dividing powers with the same base: To divide powers with the same base, keep the base and subtract the exponents:

$$y^{13} \div y^8 = y^{13-8} = y^5$$

Raising a power to an exponent: To raise a power to an exponent, keep the base and multiply the exponents:

$$(x^3)^4 = x^{3 \times 4} = x^{12}$$

Multiplying powers with the same exponent: To multiply powers with the same exponent, multiply the bases and keep the exponent:

$$(3^x)(4^x) = 12^x$$

Dividing powers with the same exponent: To divide powers with the same exponent, divide the bases and keep the exponent:

$$\frac{6^x}{2^x} = 3^x$$

Example: For all $xyz \neq 0$, $\dfrac{6x^2y^{12}z^6}{(2x^2yz)^3} =$

There's nothing tricky about this question if you know how to work with exponents. The first step is to eliminate the parentheses. Everything inside gets cubed:

$$\frac{6x^2y^{12}z^6}{(2x^2yz)^3} = \frac{6x^2y^{12}z^6}{8x^6y^3z^3}$$

The next step is to look for factors common to the numerator and denominator. The 6 on top and the 8 on bottom reduce to 3 over 4. The x^2 on top cancels with the x^6 on bottom, leaving x^4 on the bottom. You're actually subtracting the exponents: $2 - 6 = -4$, since x^{-4} is the same as $\dfrac{1}{x^4}$. The y^{12} on top cancels with the y^3 on bottom, leaving y^9 on top. And the z^6 on top cancels with the z^3 on bottom, leaving z^3 on top:

$$\frac{6x^2y^{12}z^6}{8x^6y^3z^3} = \frac{3y^9z^3}{4x^4}$$

ADDING, SUBTRACTING, AND MULTIPLYING POLYNOMIALS

Algebra is the basic language of mathematics, and you will want to be fluent in that language. You might not get a whole lot of questions that ask explicitly about such basic algebra procedures as combining like terms, multiplying binomials, or factoring algebraic expressions, but you will do all of those things in the course of working out the answers to more advanced questions. So it's essential that you be at ease with the mechanics of algebraic manipulations.

Combining like terms: To combine like terms, keep the variable part unchanged while adding or subtracting the coefficients:

$$2a + 3a = (2 + 3)a = 5a$$

Adding or subtracting polynomials: To add or subtract polynomials, combine like terms:

$$(3x^2 + 5x - 7) - (x^2 + 12) =$$
$$(3x^2 - x^2) + 5x + (-7 - 12) =$$
$$2x^2 + 5x - 19$$

Multiplying monomials: To multiply monomials, multiply the coefficients and the variables separately:

$$2x \times 3x = (2 \times 3)(x \times x) = 6x^2$$

Multiplying binomials: To multiply binomials, use FOIL. To multiply $(x + 3)$ by $(x + 4)$, first multiply the First terms: $x \times x = x^2$. Next the Outer terms: $x \times 4 = 4x$. Then the Inner terms: $3 \times x = 3x$. And finally the Last terms: $3 \times 4 = 12$. Then add and combine like terms:

$$x^2 + 4x + 3x + 12 = x^2 + 7x + 12$$

Multiplying polynomials: To multiply polynomials with more than two terms, make sure you multiply each term in the first polynomial by each term in the second. (FOIL works only when you want to multiply two binomials.)

$$(x^2 + 3x + 4)(x + 5) = x^2(x + 5) + 3x(x + 5) + 4(x + 5)$$
$$= x^3 + 5x^2 + 3x^2 + 15x + 4x + 20$$
$$= x^3 + 8x^2 + 19x + 20$$

After multiplying two polynomials together, the number of terms in your expression before simplifying should equal the number of terms in one polynomial multiplied by the number of terms in the second. In the example above, you should have $3 \times 2 = 6$ terms in the product before you simplify like terms.

DIVIDING POLYNOMIALS

To divide polynomials, you can use long division. For example, to divide $2x^3 + 13x^2 + 11x - 16$ by $x + 5$:

$$x + 5 \overline{)2x^3 + 13x^2 + 11x - 16}$$

The first term of the quotient is $2x^2$, because that's what will give you a $2x^3$ as a first term when you multiply it by $x + 5$:

$$
\begin{array}{r}
2x^2 \\
x + 5 \overline{)2x^3 + 13x^2 + 11x - 16} \\
2x^3 + 10x^2
\end{array}
$$

Subtract and continue in the same way as when dividing numbers:

$$
\begin{array}{r}
2x^2 + 3x - 4 \\
x + 5 \overline{)2x^3 + 13x^2 + 11x - 16} \\
2x^3 + 10x^2 \\
\hline
3x^2 + 11x \\
3x^2 + 15x \\
\hline
-4x - 16 \\
-4x - 20 \\
\hline
4
\end{array}
$$

The result is $2x^2 + 3x - 4$ with a remainder of 4.

Example: When $2x^3 + 3x^2 - 4x + k$ is divided by $x + 2$, the remainder is 3. What is the value of k?

To answer this question, start by cranking out the long division:

$$
\begin{array}{r}
2x^2 - x - 2 \\
x + 2 \overline{)2x^3 + 3x^2 - 4x + k} \\
2x^3 + 4x^2 \\
\hline
-x^2 - 4x \\
-x^2 - 2x \\
\hline
-2x + k \\
-2x - 4 \\
\hline
\end{array}
$$

The question says that the remainder is 3, so whatever k is, when you subtract -4 from it, you get 3:

$$k - (-4) = 3$$
$$k + 4 = 3$$
$$k = -1$$

FACTORING

Performing operations on polynomials is largely a matter of cranking it out. Once you know the rules, adding, subtracting, multiplying, and even dividing is automatic. Factoring algebraic expressions is a different matter. To factor successfully, you have to do more thinking and less cranking. You have to try to figure out what expressions multiplied will give you the polynomial you're looking at. Sometimes that means having a good eye for the test makers' favorite factorables:

- Factor common to all terms
- Difference of squares
- Square of a binomial

Factor common to all terms: A factor common to all the terms of a polynomial can be factored out. This is essentially the distributive property in reverse. For example, all three terms in the polynomial $3x^3 + 12x^2 - 6x$ contain a factor of $3x$. Pulling out the common factor yields $3x(x^2 + 4x - 2)$.

Difference of squares: You will want to be especially keen at spotting polynomials in the form of the difference of squares. Whenever you have two identifiable squares with a minus sign between them, you can factor the expression like this:

$$a^2 - b^2 = (a + b)(a - b)$$

$4x^2 - 9$, for example, factors to $(2x + 3)(2x - 3)$.

Squares of binomials: Learn to recognize polynomials that are squares of binomials:

$$a^2 + 2ab + b^2 = (a + b)^2$$
$$a^2 - 2ab + b^2 = (a - b)^2$$

A polynomial such as those seen above can be expressed as a product of two or more polynomials of lower positive degree. Each of these polynomials is referred to as a factor or the given polynomial. To factor a given polynomial over a designated factor set, you express it as a product of polynomials belonging to the factor set. Unless stated in the question otherwise, one can assume only integral coefficients for the factors of a polynomial with integral coefficients.

For example, $4x^2 + 12x + 9$ factors to $(2x + 3)^2$, and $a^2 - 10a + 25$ factors to $(a - 5)^2$.

Sometimes you'll want to factor a polynomial that's not in any of these classic factorable forms. When that happens, factoring becomes a kind of logic exercise with some trial and error thrown in. To factor a quadratic expression, think about what binomials you could use FOIL on to get that quadratic expression. For example, to factor $x^2 - 5x + 6$, think about what **First** terms will produce x^2, what **Last** terms will produce $+6$, and what **Outer** and **Inner** terms will produce $-5x$. Some common sense—and a little trial and error—will lead you to $(x - 2)(x - 3)$.

Example: For all $x \neq \pm 3$, $\dfrac{3x^2 - 11x + 6}{9 - x^2} =$

(A) $\dfrac{2x - 3}{x + 3}$ (B) $\dfrac{2 - 3x}{x + 3}$ (C) $\dfrac{2x - 3}{x - 3}$ (D) $\dfrac{3x - 2}{x + 3}$ (E) $\dfrac{3x - 2}{x - 3}$

To reduce a fraction, you eliminate factors common to the top and bottom. So the first step in reducing an algebraic fraction is to *factor the numerator and denominator.* Here the denominator is easy since it's the difference of squares: $9 - x^2 = (3 - x)(3 + x)$. The numerator takes some thought and some trial and error. For the first term to be $3x^2$, the first terms of the factors must be $3x$ and x. For the last term to be $+6$, the last terms must be either $+2$ and $+3$, or -2 and -3, or $+1$ and $+6$, or -1 and -6. After a few tries, you should come up with: $3x^2 - 11x + 6 = (3x - 2)(x - 3)$. Now the fraction looks like this:

$$\frac{3x^2 - 11x + 6}{9 - x^2} = \frac{(3x - 2)(x - 3)}{(3 - x)(3 + x)}$$

In this form there are no precisely common factors, but there is a factor in the numerator that's the opposite (negative) of a factor in the denominator: $x - 3$ and $3 - x$ are opposites. Factor -1 out of the numerator and get:

$$\frac{(3x - 2)(x - 3)}{(3 - x)(3 + x)} = \frac{(-1)(3x - 2)(3 - x)}{(3 - x)(3 + x)}$$

Now $(3 - x)$ can be eliminated from both the top and the bottom:

$$\frac{(-1)(3x - 2)(3 - x)}{(3 - x)(3 + x)} = \frac{-(3x - 2)}{3 + x} = \frac{-3x + 2}{3 + x}$$

That's the same as choice (B):

$$\frac{-3x + 2}{3 + x} = \frac{2 - 3x}{x + 3}$$

Alternative method: Here's another way to answer this question. *Pick a number for x and see what happens.* One of the answer choices will give you the same value as the original fraction, no matter what you plug in for x. Pick a number that's easy to work with—like 0.

When you plug $x = 0$ into the original expression, any term with an x drops out, and you end up with $\dfrac{6}{9}$, or $\dfrac{2}{3}$. Now plug $x = 0$ into each answer choice to see which ones equal $\dfrac{2}{3}$. Eliminate any answer choices that do not equal $\dfrac{2}{3}$ when $x = 0$.

When you get to (B), it works, but you can't stop there. It might just be a coincidence. When you pick numbers, *look at every answer choice.* Choice (E) also works for $x = 0$. At least you know one of those is the correct answer, and you can decide between them by picking another value for x.

This is not a sophisticated approach, but who cares? You don't get points for elegance. You get points for right answers.

Example: Factor the following polynomial: $8xy + 18y^2$.

One can easily see that $2y$ is the monomial of greatest coefficent and degree that is a factor of each term in the polynomial. Therefore, by the distributive law, we can factor

$$8xy + 18y^2 = 2y\,(4x + 9y)$$

In this example, $2y$ is referred to as the greatest monomial factor of the given polynomial because it is the monomial with the greatest numerical coefficient and the greatest degree that is a factor of each term of the polynomial. The other factor, $4x + 9y$, cannot be reduced to a product of factors of lower positive degree and therefore is irreducible. Moreover, the greatest monomial factor is 1. A polynomial is said to be completely factored when it is expressed as a product of a constant and one or more irreducible polynomials, each of which has 1 as its greatest monomial factor.

THE GOLDEN RULE OF EQUATIONS

You probably remember the basic procedure for solving algebraic equations: *do the same thing to both sides*. You can do almost anything you want to one side of an equation as long as you preserve the equality by doing the same thing to the other side. Your aim in whatever you do to both sides is to get the variable (or expression) you're solving for all by itself on one side.

Example: If $\sqrt[3]{8x + 6} = -3$, what is the value of x?

To solve this equation for x means to do whatever you have to to both sides of the equation to get x all by itself on one side. Layer by layer you want to peel away all those extra symbols and numbers around the x. First you want to get rid of that cube-root symbol. The way to undo a cube root is to cube both sides:

$$\sqrt[3]{8x + 6} = -3$$
$$(\sqrt[3]{8x + 6}\,)^3 = (-3)^3$$
$$8x + 6 = -27$$

The rest is easy. Subtract 6 from both sides and divide both sides by 8:

$$8x + 6 = -27$$
$$8x = -27 - 6$$
$$8x = -33$$
$$x = -\frac{33}{8} = -4.125$$

The test makers have a couple of favorite equation types that you should be prepared to solve. Solving linear equations is usually pretty straightforward. Generally it's obvious what to do to isolate the unknown. But when the unknown is in a denominator or an exponent, how to proceed might not be so obvious.

UNKNOWN IN A DENOMINATOR

The basic procedure for solving an equation is the same even when the unknown is in a denominator: do the same thing to both sides. In this case, you multiply to undo division.

If you wanted to solve $1 + \dfrac{1}{x} = 2 - \dfrac{1}{x}$, you would multiply both sides by x :

$$1 + \frac{1}{x} = 2 - \frac{1}{x}$$

$$x\left(1 + \frac{1}{x}\right) = x\left(2 - \frac{1}{x}\right)$$

$$x + 1 = 2x - 1$$

Now you have an equation with no denominators, which is easy to solve:

$$x + 1 = 2x - 1$$

$$x - 2x = -1 - 1$$

$$-x = -2$$

$$x = 2$$

Another good way to solve an equation with the unknown in the denominator is to *cross multiply*. That's the best way to do the following example.

Example: If $\dfrac{5}{x+3} = \dfrac{1}{x} + \dfrac{1}{2x}$, what is the value of x?

Before you can cross multiply, you need to re-express the right side of the equation as a single fraction. That means giving the two fractions a common denominator and adding them. The common denominator is $2x$:

$$\frac{5}{x+3} = \frac{1}{x} + \frac{1}{2x}$$

$$\frac{5}{x+3} = \frac{2}{2x} + \frac{1}{2x}$$

$$\frac{5}{x+3} = \frac{3}{2x}$$

Now you can cross multiply:

$$\frac{5}{x+3} = \frac{3}{2x}$$

$$(5)(2x) = (x+3)(3)$$

$$10x = 3x + 9$$

$$10x - 3x = 9$$

$$7x = 9$$

$$x = \frac{9}{7}$$

UNKNOWN IN AN EXPONENT

The procedure for solving an equation when the unknown is in an exponent is a little different. What you want to do in this situation is to re-express one or both sides of the equation so that the two sides have the same base.

Example: If $8^x = 16^{x-1}$, then $x =$

(A) $\dfrac{1}{8}$ 　　　　 (B) $\dfrac{1}{2}$ 　　　　 (C) 2 　　　　 (D) 4 　　　　 (E) 8

In this case, the base on the left is 8 and the base on the right is 16. They're both powers of 2, so you can reexpress both sides as powers of 2:

$$(2^3)^x = (2^4)^{x-1}$$
$$2^{3x} = 2^{4(x-1)} = 2^{4x-4}$$

Thus, $2^{3x} = 2^{4x-4}$. Now that both sides have the same base, you can simply set the exponent expressions equal and solve for x:

$$3x = 4x - 4$$
$$3x - 4x = -4$$
$$-x = -4$$
$$x = 4$$

Alternative method: Here's another way to answer this question. Nobody says you have to figure out the answer to the question and then look for your solution among the answer choices. If you don't see how to do it the front way, try working backwards. Try plugging the answer choices back into the problem until you find the one that works. Here, if you start with (C) and $x = 2$, you get $8^x = 8^2 = 64$ on the left side of the equation and $16^{x-1} = 16^1 = 16$ on the right side. It's not clear whether (C) was too small or too large, so you should probably try (D) next—it's easier to work with than (B), which is a fraction. If $x = 4$, then $8^x = 8^4 = 4{,}096$ on the left, and $16^{x-1} = 16^3 = 4{,}096$. No need to do any more. (D) works, so it's the answer.

Don't depend on backsolving too much. Lots of math questions can't be backsolved at all. And most that *can* be backsolved are almost certainly more *quickly* solved by a more direct approach.

QUADRATIC EQUATIONS

To solve a quadratic equation, put it in the $ax^2 + bx + c = 0$ form, factor the left side (if you can), and set each factor equal to 0 separately to get the two solutions. To solve $x^2 + 12 = 7x$, first rewrite it as $x^2 - 7x + 12 = 0$. Then factor the left side:

$$x^2 - 7x + 12 = 0$$
$$(x - 3)(x - 4) = 0$$
$$x - 3 = 0 \text{ or } x - 4 = 0$$
$$x = 3 \text{ or } x = 4$$

Sometimes the left side may not be obviously factorable. You can always use the *quadratic formula*. Just plug in the coefficients a, b, and c from $ax^2 + bx + c = 0$ into the formula:

$$x = \frac{-b \pm \sqrt{b^2 - 4ac}}{2a}$$

To solve $x^2 + 4x + 2 = 0$, plug $a = 1$, $b = 4$, and $c = 2$ into the formula:

$$x = \frac{-4 \pm \sqrt{4^2 - 4 \cdot 1 \cdot 2}}{2 \cdot 1}$$

$$= \frac{-4 \pm \sqrt{8}}{2} = \frac{-4 \pm 2\sqrt{2}}{2} = -2 \pm \sqrt{2}$$

For all real numbers b and c, and all nonzero real numbers a, the quadratic equation $ax^2 + bx + c = 0$ has:

- Two different real roots if $b^2 - 4ac > 0$
- One double real root if $b^2 - 4ac = 0$
- Two imaginary complex conjugate roots if $b^2 - 4ac < 0$

"IN TERMS OF"

So far in this chapter, solving an equation has meant finding a numerical value for the unknown. When there's more than one variable, it's generally impossible to get numerical solutions. Instead, what you do is solve for the unknown *in terms of* the other variables.

To solve an equation for one variable in terms of another means to isolate the one variable on one side of the equation, leaving an expression containing the other variable on the other side of the equation.

For example, to solve the equation $3x - 10y = -5x + 6y$ for x in terms of y, isolate x:

$$3x - 10y = -5x + 6y$$
$$3x + 5x = 6y + 10y$$
$$8x = 16y$$
$$x = 2y$$

Example: If $a = \dfrac{b + x}{c + x}$, what is the value of x in terms of a, b, and c ?

You want to get x on one side by itself. First thing to do is eliminate the denominator by multiplying both sides by $c + x$:

$$a = \frac{b + x}{c + x}$$
$$a(c + x) = \left(\frac{b + x}{c + x}\right)(c + x)$$
$$ac + ax = b + x$$

Next move all terms with x to one side and all terms without to the other:

$$ac + ax = b + x$$
$$ax - x = b - ac$$

Now factor x out of the left side and divide both sides by the other factor to isolate x:

$$ax - x = b - ac$$
$$x(a - 1) = b - ac$$
$$x = \frac{b - ac}{a - 1}$$

SIMULTANEOUS EQUATIONS

You can get numerical solutions for more than one unknown if you are given more than one equation. Simultaneous Equations questions take a little thought to answer. Solving simultaneous equations almost always involves combining equations, but you have to figure out what's the best way to combine the equations.

You can solve for two variables only if you have two distinct equations. Two forms of the same equation will not be adequate. Combine the equations in such a way that one of the variables cancels out. For example, to solve the two equations $4x + 3y = 8$ and $x + y = 3$, multiply both sides of the second equation by -3 to get $-3x - 3y = -9$. Now add the two equations; the $3y$ and the $-3y$ cancel out, leaving $x = -1$. Plug that back into either one of the original equations and you'll find that $y = 4$.

Example: If $2x - 9y = 11$ and $x + 12y = -8$, what is the value of $x + y$?

If you just plow ahead without thinking, you might try to answer this question by solving for one variable at a time. That would work, but it would take a lot more time than this question needs. As usual, the key to this Simultaneous Equations question is to combine the equations, but combining the equations doesn't necessarily mean losing a variable. Look what happens here if you just add the equations as presented:

$$2x - 9y = 11$$
$$+[x + 12y = -8]$$
$$3x + 3y = 3$$

Suddenly you're almost there! Just divide both sides by 3 and you get $x + y = 1$.

ABSOLUTE VALUE AND INEQUALITIES

To solve an equation that includes absolute value signs, think about the two different cases. For example, to solve the equation $|x - 12| = 3$, think of it as two equations:

$$x - 12 = 3 \text{ or } x - 12 = -3$$
$$x = 15 \text{ or } 9$$

To solve an inequality, do whatever is necessary to both sides to isolate the variable. Just remember that when you multiply or divide both sides by a negative number, you must reverse the sign. To solve $-5x + 7 < -3$, subtract 7 from both sides to get $-5x < -10$. Now divide both sides by -5, remembering to reverse the sign: $x > 2$.

Example: What is the solution set of $|2x - 3| < 7$?

    (A) $\{x: -5 < x < 2\}$
    (B) $\{x: -5 < x < 5\}$
    (C) $\{x: -2 < x < 5\}$
    (D) $\{x: x < -5 \text{ or } x > 2\}$
    (E) $\{x: x < -2 \text{ or } x > 5\}$

What does it mean if $|2x - 3| < 7$? It means that if the expression between the absolute value bars is positive, it's less than +7, or if the expression between the bars is negative, it's greater than −7. If the expression between the absolute value bars is 0, its absolute value is less than 7. In other words, $2x - 3$ is between −7 and +7:

$$-7 < 2x - 3 < 7$$
$$-4 < 2x < 10$$
$$-2 < x < 5$$

In fact, there's a general rule that applies here: to solve an inequality in the form $|\text{whatever}| < p$, where $p > 0$, just put that "whatever" inside the range $-p$ to p:

$$|\text{whatever}| < p \text{ means: } -p < \text{whatever} < p$$

For example, $|x - 5| < 14$ becomes $-14 < x - 5 < 14$.

And here's another general rule: to solve an inequality in the form $|\text{whatever}| > p$, where $p > 0$, just put that "whatever" outside the range $-p$ to p:

$$|\text{whatever}| > p \text{ means: whatever} < -p \text{ OR whatever} > p$$

For example, $\left|\dfrac{3x + 9}{2}\right| > 7$ becomes $\dfrac{3x + 9}{2} < -7 \text{ OR } \dfrac{3x + 9}{2} > 7$.

LOGARITHMS

The properties of logarithms are dependent upon the laws of exponents; therefore, a review of exponents is necessary before the introduction of logarithms.

In the equation:

$$b^c = x$$

b is the base

c is the exponent

x is b raised to the exponent c, where b is positive and not equal to 1.

In the equation above, the exponent c may be an integer, a fraction, or an irrational number. The value of c may be positive, negative, or 0.

In the equation $b^c = x$, the exponent c is the exponent that b must be raised to obtain the number x. This relationship is described by the statement "The logarithm of x to the base b," which means, if $b^c = x$, then the logarithm to the base b of x is c. In other words:

The logarithm to the base b of a positive number x is equal to the exponent to which b must be raised to obtain x.

$$\text{Log}_b(x) = c \rightarrow b^c = x$$

Examples:

$$\log_4(16) = 2, \text{ since } 4^2 = 16$$
$$\log_{10}(10{,}000) = 4, \text{ since } 10^4 = 10{,}000$$
$$\log_{25}(5) = \frac{1}{2}, \text{ since } 25^{\frac{1}{2}} = 5$$

If one of the three numbers in the equation $\log_b x = c$ is unknown, then the unknown number can be calculated using the properties of logarithms and exponents. This can be done because $\log_b(x) = c$ means that $b^c = x$.

Example: If $\log_5(x) = 3$, then $x = ?$

The expression $\log_5(x) = 3$ means that $5^3 = x$; therefore, $x = 125$.

Example: If $\log_b(36) = 2$, then $b = ?$

The expression $\log_b(36) = 2$ means that $b^2 = 36$; therefore, $b = 6$.

Example: If $\log_{10}(100) = c$, then $c = ?$

The expression $\log_{10}(100) = c$ means that $10^c = 100$; therefore, $c = 2$.

Properties of Logs

The logarithm of the product of two numbers equals the sum of the individual logarithms:

$$\log_b(st) = \log_b(s) + \log_b(t)$$

The logarithm of a quotient of two numbers is the logarithm of the numerator minus the logarithm of the denominator:

$$\log_b\left(\frac{s}{t}\right) = \log_b(s) - \log_b(t)$$

The logarithm of a power with a positive base is equal to the exponent of the power multiplied by the logarithm of the base of that power:

$$\log_b(s^p) = p \cdot \log_b(s)$$

Log Base 10

Most commonly, logs are expressed in "base 10," which means that multiples of the log operate on a 10-digit scale. This also means that an increase of one logarithmic unit (in base 10) corresponds to a multiplication of 10 of the actual total.

$$\log_{10}(100) = 2, \text{ since } 10^2 = 100$$
$$\log_{10}(1,000) = 3, \text{ since } 10^3 = 1,000$$

In base 10, logarithms are often expressed as decimal numbers. In these cases, the base of 10 is understood. The integer is called the **characteristic** and the decimal fraction is called the **mantissa**. Shifting the decimal point to the right or left in a number increases or decreases the characteristic of the logarithm of that number by a factor of 1, as seen below:

Example: log 42.6 = 1.62941

log 426 = 2.62941

log 4.26 = 0.62941

REVIEW PROBLEMS

1. If $x = 3 - y^2$ and $y = -2$, what is the value of x?

   (A) -2 (B) -1 (C) 1 (D) 2 (E) 25

2. For all x, $2^x + 2^x + 2^x + 2^x =$

   (A) 2^{x+2} (B) 2^{x+4} (C) 2^{3x} (D) 2^{4x} (E) 2^{5x}

3. For all $x \neq \pm \dfrac{1}{2}$, $\dfrac{6x^2 - x - 2}{4x^2 - 1} =$

   (A) $\dfrac{2 - 3x}{2x + 1}$

   (B) $\dfrac{3x + 2}{2x + 1}$

   (C) $\dfrac{3x + 2}{2x - 1}$

   (D) $\dfrac{3x - 2}{2x + 1}$

   (E) $\dfrac{3x - 2}{2x - 1}$

4. When $3x^3 - 7x + 7$ is divided by $x + 2$, the remainder is:

   (A) -5 (B) -3 (C) 1 (D) 3 (E) 5

5. If $\sqrt[4]{\dfrac{x + 1}{2}} = \dfrac{1}{2}$, then $x =$

   (A) -0.969 (B) -0.875 (C) 0 (D) 0.875 (E) 0.969

6. If $\dfrac{19}{5x + 17} = \dfrac{19}{31}$, then $x =$

   (A) 0.4 (B) 1.4 (C) 2.8 (D) 3.4 (E) 3.8

7. If $(3^{x^2})(9^x)(3) = 27$ and $x > 0$, what is the value of x?

   (A) 0.268 (B) 0.414 (C) 0.732 (D) 1.414 (E) 1.464

8. If $y \neq 4a$, and $x = \dfrac{y + a^2}{y - 4a}$, what is the value of y in terms of a and x?

   (A) $\dfrac{4a - 4a^2 x}{x + 1}$

   (B) $\dfrac{a^2 - 4ax}{x + 1}$

   (C) $\dfrac{a^2 + 4ax}{x + 1}$

   (D) $\dfrac{a^2 + 4ax}{x - 1}$

   (E) $\dfrac{a^2 - 4ax}{x - 1}$

9. If $4x + ky = 15$ and $x - ky = -25$, which of the following could be the values of x and y?

   (A) $x = -3$ and $y = -5$
   (B) $x = -2$ and $y = 3$
   (C) $x = 0$ and $y = -2$
   (D) $x = 2$ and $y = 3$
   (E) $x = 3$ and $y = 5$

10. How many integers are in the solution set of $\left| 4x + 3 \right| < 8$?

   (A) None
   (B) Two
   (C) Three
   (D) Four
   (E) Infinitely many

SOLUTIONS TO REVIEW PROBLEMS

1. **B** Substitute -2 for y into the equation $x = 3 - y^2$:

$$x = 3 - y^2 = 3 - (-2)^2 = 3 - 4 = -1$$

2. **A** The sum of 4 identical quantities is 4 times one of those quantities, so the sum of the four terms 2^x is 4 times 2^x:

$$2^x + 2^x + 2^x + 2^x = 4(2^x) = 2^2(2^x) = 2^{x+2}$$

3. **E** Factor the top and the bottom and cancel the factors they have in common:

$$\frac{6x^2 - x - 2}{4x^2 - 1} = \frac{(2x+1)(3x-2)}{(2x+1)(2x-1)}$$
$$= \frac{3x-2}{2x-1}$$

4. **B** Use long division. Watch out: The expression that goes under the division sign needs a place-holding $0x^2$ term:

$$
\begin{array}{r}
3x^2 - 6x + 5 \\
x + 2 \overline{)3x^3 + 0x^2 - 7x + 7} \\
\underline{3x^3 + 6x^2} \\
-6x^2 - 7x \\
\underline{-6x^2 - 12x} \\
5x + 7 \\
\underline{5x + 10} \\
-3
\end{array}
$$

The remainder is -3.

5. **B** To undo the fourth-root symbol, raise both sides to the exponent 4:

$$\sqrt[4]{\frac{x+1}{2}} = \frac{1}{2}$$
$$\left(\sqrt[4]{\frac{x+1}{2}}\right)^4 = \left(\frac{1}{2}\right)^4$$
$$\frac{x+1}{2} = \frac{1}{16}$$

Now cross multiply:

$$\frac{x+1}{2} = \frac{1}{16}$$

$$(x+1)(16) = (2)(1)$$

$$16x + 16 = 2$$

$$16x = -14$$

$$x = -\frac{14}{16} = -\frac{7}{8} = -0.875$$

6. **C** This might look at first glance like a candidate for cross multiplication, but that would just make things more complicated. Notice that the fractions on both sides have the same numerator, 19. If the two fractions are equal and they have the same numerator, then they must have the same denominator, so just write an equation that says that one denominator is equal to the other denominator:

$$\frac{19}{5x + 17} = \frac{19}{31}$$

$$5x + 17 = 31$$

$$5x = 31 - 17$$

$$5x = 14$$

$$x = \frac{14}{5} = 2.8$$

7. **C** Watch what happens when you express everything as powers with a base of 3:

$$(3^{x^2})(9x)(3) = 27$$

$$(3^{x^2})(3^{2x})3^1 = 3^3$$

The left side of the equation is the product of powers with the same base, so just add the exponents:

$$3^{x^2}(3^{2x})3^1 = 3^3$$

$$3^{x^2 + 2x + 1} = 3^3$$

Now the two sides of the equation are powers with the same base, so you can just set the exponents equal:

$$3^{x^2 + 2x + 1} = 3^3$$

$$x^2 + 2x + 1 = 3$$

$$(x + 1)^2 = 3$$

$$x + 1 = \pm\sqrt{3}$$

The positive value is $-1 + \sqrt{3}$, which is approximately 0.732.

8. **D** First multiply both sides by $y - 4a$ to clear the denominator:

$$x = \frac{y + a^2}{y - 4a}$$

$$x(y - 4a) = y + a^2$$

$$xy - 4ax = y + a^2$$

Now move all terms with y to the left and all terms without y to the right:

$$xy - 4ax = y + a^2$$

$$xy - y = a^2 + 4ax$$

Now factor the left side and divide to isolate y :

$$xy - y = a^2 + 4ax$$
$$y(x - 1) = a^2 + 4ax$$
$$y = \frac{a^2 + 4ax}{x - 1}$$

9. **B** With only two equations, you won't be able to get numerical solutions for three unknowns. But apparently you can get far enough to rule out four of the five answer choices. How? Look for a way to combine the equations that leads somewhere useful. Notice that the first equation contains $+ky$ and the second equation contains $-ky$, so if you add the equations as they are, you'll lose those terms:

$$
\begin{aligned}
4x + ky &= 15 \\
\underline{x - ky} &= \underline{-25} \\
5x &= -10 \\
x &= -2
\end{aligned}
$$

There's not enough information to get numerical solutions for k or y, but you do know that $x = -2$, so the correct answer is the only choice that has an x-value of -2.

10. **D** If the absolute value of something is less than 8, then that something is between -8 and 8:

$$\left| 4x + 3 \right| < 8$$
$$-8 < 4x + 3 < 8$$
$$-11 < 4x < 5$$
$$-\frac{11}{4} < x < \frac{5}{4}$$
$$-2\frac{3}{4} < x < 1\frac{1}{4}$$

There are four integers in that range: $-2, -1, 0,$ and 1.

CHAPTER TWENTY-SIX

Probability and Statistics

WHAT IS PROBABILITY?

Probability is the branch of mathematics concerned with calculating the likelihood that an event will or will not occur. This likelihood is assigned a numeric value between 0 and 1 inclusive, where 0 means there's *no* chance and 1 means the event will *definitely* happen.

Probability can be expressed as a percent (e.g., there's a 50% chance of getting heads in a fair coin toss), as a fraction (e.g., the probability of getting heads is $\frac{1}{2}$...) or as a decimal (e.g., there's a 0.5 chance of getting heads). What does this value mean? It's simply a statement of what's *likely* to happen and not a guarantee of what will actually happen. It's certainly possible, for example, to flip a coin 10 times and get 10 tails.

WHAT'S BEHIND PROBABILITY?

Now, how did we arrive at the conclusion that there's a 50% chance of getting heads? What we did was figure out how many different outcomes there were for the coin toss (2—heads or tails) and then figure out how many of those outcomes would give a result of heads (just 1). So 1 out of the 2 possible outcomes (or 50% of them) would result in heads. That's the basic formula for probability:

$$\text{probability} = \frac{\text{desired outcomes}}{\text{possible outcomes}}$$

We can see now that probability is a fraction, with desired outcomes on the top and possible outcomes on the bottom. In other words, probability is just a way of predicting the likelihood of a specific outcome by figuring out what fraction of all possible outcomes have the characteristic you're looking for. So in every probability question, your first goal is to find the total possible outcomes and desired outcomes. Keep in mind as well that "desired" here means only that these are the outcomes that have the characteristic we're interested in, not that we necessarily want these outcomes to happen.

Example:

A bag contains 10 identical balls numbered 1 through 10 inclusive. If a ball is drawn from the bag at random, what is the probability (as a percentage) that it bears a number less than 4?

Let's see… if there are 10 numbers in the bag, and we're picking only one ball, then there are 10 possible outcomes. So we now have the bottom of our probability fraction. What we still need to do is to figure out the number of desired outcomes. We're interested in numbers less than 4, and the only ones that have this characteristic are 1, 2, and 3, so 3 out of the 10 balls would give us a number less than 4. That's $\frac{3}{10}$ or 30%. So to find a probability for a single event:

1) Figure out how many outcomes are possible overall.

2) Figure out how many of the possible outcomes have the characteristic you're looking for.

3) Plug these numbers into the probability formula.

So as you can see, every probability problem starts with two basic things:

1. Total possible outcomes
2. Desired outcomes

Because they're so important, let's practice finding them.

DESIRED AND POSSIBLE OUTCOMES

Example:

A regular six-sided die is thrown. What is the probability that it lands with an even number facing up?

Desired outcomes = 3

Total possible outcomes = 6

How do we know this?

A regular six-sided die has six numbers (1, 2, 3, 4, 5, and 6) on its faces. That gives us a total of six possible outcomes. We're interested only in the even numbers, of which there are three (2, 4, and 6). So the number of desired outcomes is three. This gives us a probability of $\frac{3}{6}$, or $\frac{1}{2}$.

Example:

A woman has exactly 5 tickets for a certain raffle for which exactly 1,000 tickets exist. If the raffle has only one prize, what is the probability that the woman will win?

Desired outcomes = 5

Total possible outcomes = 1,000

There are 1,000 tickets available for the raffle, which means that there are 1,000 chances to win the prize. So the total number of possible outcomes is 1,000. The woman in the question, though, has only 5 of those possible chances. So the desired outcome here is 5. That gives us a probability of $\frac{5}{1,000}$, or $\frac{1}{200}$.

Example:

A certain pet store has exactly 13 mice in a single tank. Five of the mice are white, and 8 of the mice are brown. If the store clerk reaches into the mice's tank to select a mouse at random, what is the probability that the mouse is white?

Desired outcomes = 5

Total possible outcomes = 13

If there are 13 mice total, then the total possible outcomes is 13. Only 5 of the mice are white, so the number of desired outcomes is 5. This gives us a probability of $\frac{5}{13}$.

Now that we've seen how to find the probability of a single event, let's look at what happens when we're interested in more than one event.

MULTIPLE-EVENT PROBABILITY

The probability for a single event is just $\frac{\text{desired outcomes}}{\text{possible outcomes}}$. But what if we're interested in the probability that *two* different events both happen? Or in the probability that one of the events happens and the other does not? In those cases, it's not enough just to figure out the probabilities of the individual events—we have to combine the probabilities somehow.

Let's start off with the situation where we want to know the probability that *either* one *or* the other of two events happens, but not both.

One or the Other

Some probability questions might test your ability to figure out the probability of what are known technically as **mutually exclusive events**. You don't need to know this term for your exam, but you do need to know the concept it represents.

Mutually exclusive events are those where the occurrence of one event eliminates the possibility of the other event (in other words, where the two events "exclude" each other).

For example, what is the probability that a certain machine randomly fills a box with all pennies *or* with all dimes? If the box contains all pennies, then it can't contain all dimes. If it contains all dimes, it can't contain all pennies. So these two events are mutually exclusive, in that the occurrence of one means the other can't happen at the same time.

Let's continue with the box example. If we wanted to figure out the probability that a box contains either all pennies or all dimes, the first thing we'd need is the probabilities of the two events separately.

Let's say that the probability that the machine fills the box with all pennies is $\frac{1}{2}$ and the probability that the machine fills the box with all dimes is $\frac{1}{3}$. To calculate the probability that one or the other of these two events occurs, we need to add their respective probabilties:

$$\frac{1}{2} + \frac{1}{3} = \frac{3}{6} + \frac{2}{6} = \frac{5}{6}$$

So the probability that the box contains all pennies *or* all dimes is $\frac{5}{6}$.

Remember, to calculate the probability that either event A *or* event B occurs (but not both), find the probabilities of A and B separately and then *add* them together.

Why do we need to add in such cases?

Let's take the pennies/dimes example again. If the probability that the machine fills the box with all pennies is $\frac{1}{2}$, then $\frac{1}{2}$ of all boxes filled by the machine should (in theory) contain all pennies. And if the probability that the machine fills the box with all dimes is $\frac{1}{3}$, this means that $\frac{1}{3}$ of all boxes filled by the machine should (in theory) contain all dimes. So if $\frac{1}{2}$ of all the boxes should contain all pennies and $\frac{1}{3}$ of all the boxes should contain all dimes, then these two events (all pennies or all dimes) should account for $\frac{1}{2} + \frac{1}{3}$ or $\frac{5}{6}$ of all the boxes. So $\frac{5}{6}$ of all the boxes should contain either all pennies **or** all dimes, which is the same as saying that the probability that any given box contains all pennies **or** all dimes is $\frac{5}{6}$.

Example:
A bag contains 20 identical plastic tiles. Eleven of the tiles are marked with the numbers 1 through 11 inclusive. The remaining 9 tiles are marked with the letters A through I inclusive. If a single tile is drawn at random from the bag, what is the probability that it bears either an even number or a vowel?

To find the probability of getting either an even number *or* a vowel, we need to find the probability of each of these occurrences separately and then add them together. Let's start off with the even numbers. There are 20 tiles in the bag, so we know that the number of total possible outcomes is 20. The even numbers in the bag are 2, 4, 6, 8, and 10. So there are five desired outcomes. So the probability of withdrawing an even number is $\frac{5}{20}$ (we're not going to reduce the fraction yet, you'll see why). Now for the vowels, the number of possible outcomes is still 20. There are three vowels in the bag (A, E, and I). So there are three desired outcomes and the probability of withdrawing a vowel is $\frac{3}{20}$, and the probability of withdrawing an even number *or* a vowel is $\frac{3}{20} + \frac{5}{20}$ (this is why we didn't want to reduce before), which sums to $\frac{8}{20}$, or $\frac{2}{5}$.

Now let's see what happens when we need to find the probability that two events *both* happen…

Independent Events

Some probability questions might ask you to find the probability that event A *and* event B both occur. Technically, these are known as **independent events**, because the occurrence of one is independent of the other. This means that the occurrence of one event does *not* eliminate the possibility of the other event is occurring. For example, imagine that the probability is $\frac{1}{2}$ that it will rain in Chicago tomorrow and that the probability is $\frac{1}{4}$ that it will be sunny in Boston. If it rains in Chicago, it may still be sunny in Boston, and vice versa. So these two events are independent because the occurrence of one doesn't prevent the other from happening as well. Now we already know how to find the probability of Event A *or* Event B, but what about the probability of Event A *and* Event B?

To find the probability that event A and event B both happen, we need to find the individual probabilties of these events and then multiply them. So if the probability of rain in Chicago is $\frac{1}{2}$ and the probability of sun in Boston is $\frac{1}{4}$, then the probability of rain in Chicago *and* sun in Boston is $\frac{1}{2} \times \frac{1}{4}$ or $\frac{1}{8}$. Why do we need to multiply in such cases?

Example:

Let's imagine that the probability of finding a pearl in any given oyster is $\frac{1}{3}$ and that the probability of any given pearl's being black is $\frac{2}{5}$. This means that $\frac{1}{3}$ of all oysters should (in theory) contain a pearl and that $\frac{2}{5}$ of all pearls should (in theory) be black. So what's the probability that if we crack open a randomly chosen oyster, we'll find a black pearl? Well, in $\frac{1}{3}$ of the cases when we crack open an oyster, we'll find a pearl. And in $\frac{2}{5}$ of the cases when we find a pearl, that pearl will be black. So in how many cases will we find a black pearl? Well, it should happen in $\frac{2}{5}$ of $\frac{1}{3}$ of the times that we open an oyster, which is $\frac{2}{5} \times \frac{1}{3}$ or $\frac{2}{15}$ of all the times that we open an oyster. So the probability of finding a pearl *and* having the pearl be black is $\frac{2}{15}$.

Example:

A bag contains 10 identically shaped plastic tiles. Six of the tiles are red, 3 are blue, and 1 is black. If two tiles are drawn at random from the bag, without replacement, what is the probability that the first tile drawn is red and the second tile drawn is black?

First we need to find the individual probabilities of drawing a red tile and then drawing the black tile.

For the first tile drawn, there are 10 tiles in the bag and 6 of them are red, so the probability of drawing a red tile first is $\frac{6}{10}$ or $\frac{3}{5}$. For the second tile, there are only 9 tiles left in the bag and 1 of them is black, so the probability of getting a black tile on the second draw is $\frac{1}{9}$. Now we need to find the probability of getting a red tile on the first draw *and* a black tile on the second draw. To do so, we multiply the individual probabilities: $\frac{3}{5} \times \frac{1}{9} = \frac{3}{45} = \frac{1}{15}$.

SUMMARY COMPARISON: AND/OR

We've seen two different ways to calculate probabilities for situations involving more than one event. It's essential that you understand which method to use in any given probability question. To recap:

- To find the probability of event A *or* event B, find the probability of A and the probability of B and then *add* these two probabilities. (The same rule applies if you're trying to figure out A *or* B *or* C, etc.)

- To find the probability of event A *and* event B, find the probability of A and the probability of B and then *multiply* these two probabilities. (The same rule applies if you're trying to figure out A *and* B *and* C, etc.)

REVIEW PROBLEMS

1. A certain school has 50 students assigned randomly to five distinct classes, and each student is assigned to only one class. If the numbers of students in the classes are consecutive, what is the probability that a given student is in one of the two largest classes?

   (A) 48%   (B) 46%   (C) 42%   (D) 38%   (E) 34%

2. A certain machine produces toy cars in an infinitely repeating cycle of blue, red, green, yellow, and black. If six consecutively produced cars are selected at random, what is the probability that two of the cars selected are red?

   (A) $\frac{1}{6}$ (B) $\frac{1}{5}$ (C) $\frac{1}{3}$ (D) $\frac{2}{5}$ (E) $\frac{1}{2}$

3. A certain circular stopwatch has exactly 60 second marks and a single hand. If the hand of the watch is randomly set to one of the marks and allowed to count exactly 10 seconds, what is the probability that the hand will stop less than 10 marks from the 53-second mark?

   (A) $\frac{1}{6}$ (B) $\frac{19}{60}$ (C) $\frac{1}{3}$ (D) $\frac{29}{60}$ (E) $\frac{1}{2}$

4. A certain board game is played by rolling a pair of fair six-sided dice and then moving one's piece forward the number of spaces indicated by the sum showing on the dice. A player is "frozen" if her opponent's piece comes to rest in the space already occupied by her piece. If player A is about to roll and is currently six spaces behind player B, what is the probability that player B will be frozen after player A rolls?

   (A) $\frac{1}{12}$ (B) $\frac{5}{36}$ (C) $\frac{1}{6}$ (D) $\frac{1}{3}$ (E) $\frac{17}{36}$

5. A machine is made up of two components, A and B. Each component either works or fails. The failure or nonfailure of one component is independent of the failure or nonfailure of the other component. The machine works if at least one of the components works. If the probability that each component works is $\frac{2}{3}$, what is the probability that the machine works?

   (A) $\frac{1}{9}$ (B) $\frac{4}{9}$ (C) $\frac{1}{2}$ (D) $\frac{2}{3}$ (E) $\frac{8}{9}$

SOLUTIONS TO THE REVIEW PROBLEMS

1. **B**   The correct answer is 46%. To find the probability, we need possible outcomes and desired outcomes. The possible outcomes here are just the total number of students we have to choose from. The desired outcomes will be the number of students in the two largest classes. How can we find that, though? The key to this problem is the fact that the numbers of students in the classes are consecutive. Whenever you see *consecutive* in a math problem, it's there for a specific reason. It tells you that each number in the series is separated from the next by a fixed amount. Consecutive integers are separated by 1, consecutive even integers by 2, etc. So here we know that if we add up all the classes, we'll get 50 students. We also know that the numbers of students in the classes are separated by 1. So let's call the smallest class x. The next largest class would be $x + 1$, then $x + 2$, $x + 3$, and $x + 4$. If we added these up, we'd get $5x + 10 = 50$. Now we can solve for x: subtract 10 from both sides to get $5x = 40$; divide both sides by 5 to get $x = 8$. So the smallest class has 8 students, and the two largest classes then will have $8 + 3$ and $8 + 4$ students respectively, which gives us a total of 23 students in the two largest classes. So that's $\frac{23}{50} \times \frac{2}{2} = \frac{46}{100} = 46\%$.

2. **B**   The correct answer is $\frac{1}{5}$. We need to find possible and desired outcomes. What are the possible outcomes here? Well, we're going to be randomly selecting six consecutively produced cars, and we want to know what the probability is that two of those cars will be red. How many different groups of six consecutive cars are there? Well, we've got five colors, so any one of them could be the first in the string of six that we choose. That gives us five different strings of six. So five is the number of possible outcomes here. What about desired outcomes? We need to know how many of those five strings have two red cars. What does getting two red cars depend on? It depends on the color of the first car of the string of six. For example, if blue is the first car of the string, then you'd get blue, red, green, yellow, black, and then blue again. So, the only way to get two red cars is if the first car of the string is red, because then we'd have red, green, yellow, black, blue, and then red again as the sixth car. So one out of the five strings will contain two red cars, so that's a probability of $\frac{1}{5}$.

3. **B**   The correct answer is $\frac{19}{60}$. The setup in this question may seem a little weird, but if we think about the situation for a few seconds, the question begins to make sense. There's a watch with a single hand and 60 second marks. Say we randomly spin the hand so it points to one of those marks and then we let the watch count 10 seconds. What are the chances that the hand will end up pointing to a mark that's less than 10 marks from the 53-second mark? What would it depend on? It would depend on the mark the hand began counting from. Well, how many marks are less than 10 marks from 53 seconds? This is a good question for scrap paper. If we jot down 53 and then count 9 in either direction (remember, we need less than 10, so we don't want to count 10), we start with 44 seconds and count all the way past 53 and the 1-minute mark to 2 seconds. This gives us 19 marks that are less than 10 marks from 53 seconds. So to end up less than 10 marks from 53 seconds, we need to end up on one of those 19 marks. Now each one of those 19 marks corresponds to another mark that's exactly 10 seconds earlier than it, which would be marks 34–52. If the hand begins counting

from any of the 19 marks between 34 and 52, it will end up on a mark between 44 and 02. So there are 19 marks that have the characteristic we're looking for. That's 19 out of 60, or $\frac{19}{60}$.

4. B The correct answer is $\frac{5}{36}$. This is a weird setup, but let's think about the situation for a second. In this game, a player is "frozen" whenever another player lands on the spot where the first player already has her piece. Then the question asks for the probability that player B will be frozen by player A, who's six spaces behind. What does it depend on? It depends on whether player A gets a roll of exactly 6 on the dice. So what's the probability of getting 6 on the dice? First, let's figure out the total possible outcomes for the roll. Since there are six numbers on each die, the total number of possible rolls will be 6×6, or 36. So there are 36 possible rolls. How many of them would allow player A to move exactly six spots? Well, any roll that adds up to 6. So we could have $\frac{1}{5}$, $\frac{2}{4}$, and $\frac{3}{3}$. But remember that since there are two dice, there are two ways to get $\frac{1}{5}$ and $\frac{2}{4}$ because either die could get the 1 or the 5, etc. So there's $\frac{1}{5}, \frac{5}{1}, \frac{2}{4}, \frac{4}{2}$, and $\frac{3}{3}$. That's five rolls that add up to exactly 6. So 5 out of the 36 possible rolls would allow player A to "freeze" player B, which gives us a probability of $\frac{5}{36}$.

5. E The fastest way to do this is to find the probability that neither component works, and subtract that from 1. Since the probability of a component working is $\frac{2}{3}$, the probability of a component not working is $1 - \frac{2}{3} = \frac{1}{3}$. Therefore, the probability that neither component works is $\frac{1}{3} \times \frac{1}{3} = \frac{1}{9}$, and the probability that the machine works is $1 - \frac{1}{9} = \frac{8}{9}$.

CHAPTER TWENTY-SEVEN

Precalculus and Calculus

In this chapter, we will begin by covering some important concepts in precalculus. Following, we will lead into a discussion of calculus derivatives and integrals, focusing on key concepts for success on the PCAT. While these topics frighten many test takers, remember that the PCAT is testing your math skills for a career in pharmacy. You don't have to be a calculus whiz to do well—you just have to know the following basic concepts.

FUNCTIONS

A function is simply an equation that states that one variable depends on another. For example, when the variable y is dependent on the value of x, we say "y is a function of x." Based on this, we refer to y as the dependent variable and x as the independent variable.

We may rewrite the equation $y = 3x + 5$ as $f(x) = 3x+5$. Further, we may be asked to define the function for the domain, where the set of values in domain A is equal to {2,4,6,8}. The domain of a function is the set of values of x for which that function is valid.

Example: $$\text{i.e. } f(x) = 3x + 5$$
$$A = \{2,4,6,8\}$$

The ordered pairs for this domain are: (2,11), (5,17), (6,23), and (8,29).

All we had to do was plug in each value of the domain for the value of x and determine the value of y.

You can also combine two functions. For example, if you have $f(x) = 3x + 5$ and $g(x) = 9x$, then you can define your domain as $g(x)$. In other words, you plug in $g(x)$ for the value of x in the function $f(x)$. If you did this, you would notate it as $f(g(x))$. Mathematically, you plug in $9x$ for the value of x in f(x). Hence, f(g(x)) would equal 3(9x) + 5.

GRAPHS

When you graph a function, you may be graphing a polynomial. Hence, the function may be first order, second order, third order, etc. A first-order function is one in which the exponent of x is 1, a second-order function is one in which the exponent of x is 2, and likewise, the exponent of a third-order function is 3. Generally on the PCAT, you will not need to go above third order. A second-order function is often referred to as the squared function.

Example:

$$\text{First order: } f(x) = x$$
$$\text{Second order: } f(x) = x^2$$
$$\text{Third order: } f(x) = x^3$$

You should be able to recognize the graph for each of these functions.

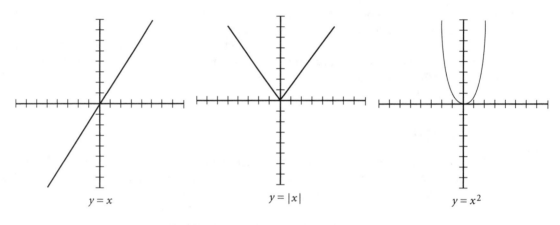

$y = x$	$y = |x|$	$y = x^2$
Figure 27.1	**Figure 27.2**	**Figure 27.3**

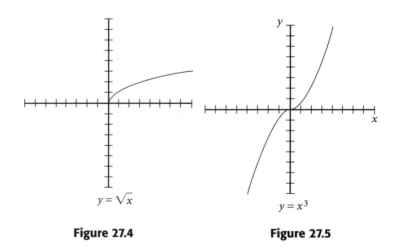

$y = \sqrt{x}$	$y = x^3$
Figure 27.4	**Figure 27.5**

Calculus problems on the PCAT generally will deal with squared, square root, and cubic functions.

LINES

It is important to understand lines, equations of lines, and the slope of a line.

Lines are graphed on a coordinate plane based on an equation. The general form of the equation is $y = mx + b$, where m is the slope of the line and b is the y-intercept.

The slope of the line, m, can be calculated and is equal to:

$$\Delta y \backslash \Delta x = y_2 - y_1 \backslash x_2 - x_1 = \textbf{Change in } y\textbf{-coordinate}\backslash\textbf{Change in } x\textbf{-coordinate}$$

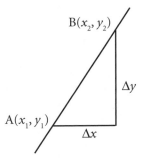

Figure 27.6

The slope of a horizontal line will always be zero. The slope of a vertical line is undefined because there is no change in the x-value.

Parallel Lines: Lines are said to be **parallel** to each other when they have the same slope.

Perpendicular Lines: Lines are **perpendicular** to each other when their slopes are negative inverses of each other. For example, if line 1 has a slope of 2, then the line that is perpendicular to line 1 will have a slope of $-\frac{1}{2}$.

FIRST DERIVATIVE

We will now look at how to calculate first and second derivatives through differentiation, as well as how to interpret them as slopes and rates of change.

For the purposes of the PCAT, you must be able to calculate the derivative of a function. The functions on the PCAT will be relatively simple. Do not worry about learning the derivatives of the trigonometric functions or logarithmic functions. However, it is important to understand the different possible notations for functions so you are not surprised on Test Day.

One standard form is $f(x)$, which is called "f of x."

If $f(x) = x^n$, then $f'(x) = nx^{n-1}$.

For any $f(x)$, the derivative of this function is $f'(x)$, which is often called "f prime of x." Specifically, this is called the first derivative of $f(x)$.

$f'(x)$ is the first derivative of $f(x)$.

We will see later that there is also a second derivative. For a function consisting of x raised to the power of n, the first derivative is given by nx^{n-1}. Try to see a visual operation of pulling the exponent, n, down and putting it in front of the x. Afterwards, subtract 1 from the original exponent to find the new exponent.

The other notation is the dx notation. For a function $y = x^n$, the derivative is written dy over dx. Similarly the derivative of $f(x)$ can be written as $df(x)$ over dx. Don't be confused by the different notations; they all mean exactly the same thing—the first derivative of a function.

Example:

$$f'(x) = \frac{df(x)}{dx} = nx^{n-1}.$$

$$\text{For } y = x^n, \frac{dy}{dx} = nx^{n-1}.$$

The derivative of a constant is 0. One way to look at this is that a constant term is actually a number times x to the zero power. When you take the derivative of something to the zero power, you pull down the exponent and multiply. Since the exponent is zero in this case, the derivative is zero.

$$\text{For } f(x) = c, f'(x) = 0.$$

DERIVATIVES AT A POINT

In many problems, you will need to evaluate the derivative at a point. Often this is written "f prime of b," where b is some value like 3 or 6 or 2π. All this means is that you plug the value b into the formula for $f'(x)$.

Example:

$$\text{For } f(x), f'(b) = f'(x) \text{ when } x = b.$$
$$\text{For } f(x) = 4x^3, \text{ what is } f'(5)?$$

To find the derivative at a point, the first step is to find the expression for $f'(x)$. Pull down the exponent, 3, and put it before the expression. Then subtract 1 from the exponent. This gives $f'(x) = 12x^2$.

$$f'(x) = 4(3)x^{3-1} = 12x^2$$

To find $f'(5)$, plug $x = 5$ into the expression for $f'(x)$. This gives 300.

$$f'(5) = 12(5)^2 = 12(25) = 300$$

DERIVATIVES OF A POLYNOMIAL

For a polynomial, which is a function consisting of several terms of varying powers of x, find the derivative by treating each term separately.

Example:

$$\text{For } y = 2x^2 + 4x^{-1} + 2, \text{ what is } dy/dx?$$

$$dy/dx = 2(2)x^{2-1} + 4(-1)x^{-1-1} + 0$$

$$dy/dx = 4x - 4x^{-2}$$

This problem has different notation than the last problem. Remember, a function can be written as $f(x)$ or as y. dy/dx is the derivative of the function. Find the derivative of each term separately, using the same method as before. Do not be confused by the negative exponent in the second term. Just remember the formula: pull down the exponent, multiply, and then subtract one from the exponent. The constant term, 2, has a derivative of 0.

GRAPHICAL INTERPRETATION OF DERIVATIVES

Let's move on to the interpretation of the derivative. First, consider the graphical meaning of the derivative.

For $f(x)$, $f'(b)$ is the slope of $f(x)$ at $x = b$.

The derivative at a point is equal to the slope of a function at that point. $f'(b)$ is the slope of $f(x)$ at $x = b$.

Consider this graph of a parabola, which is U-shaped. There are three distinct sections to this graph. On the left side, the graph is sloping down to the right. This means the derivative of the function is negative. At the bottom of the U, the function is horizontal, which is indicated by the dotted line. When the slope is horizontal like this, the derivative is zero. To the right of this point, the graph starts sloping up to the right. Here the derivative is positive.

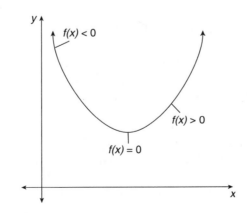

Since the derivative is the same as the slope, the sign of the derivative tells you the sign of the slope of the graph at any given point. A positive derivative means a positive slope, a negative derivative means a negative slope, and when the derivative is zero, the slope is zero, and the graph is horizontal, or flat.

The slope of a function is the rate of change of that function. For ordinary graphs of y versus x, we define the slope as the change in y over the change in x, often called "rise over run" in algebra classes. The slope tells you how y changes because of changes in x. This is referred to as the change in y with respect to x. Since the derivative is the same as the slope, another way to look at derivatives is in terms of rates. The derivative of $f(x)$ is the rate of change of $f(x)$ with respect to x.

$\dfrac{dy}{dx} > 0$: positive slope

$\dfrac{dy}{dx} < 0$: negative slope

$\dfrac{dy}{dx} = 0$: zero slope (horizontal)

Thus, a positive derivative indicates a positive slope, which means $f(x)$ is increasing. A negative derivative indicates a negative slope, which means $f(x)$ is decreasing. Zero slope means the function is horizontal, which means it is neither increasing nor decreasing. The function is constant.

$\dfrac{dy}{dx} > 0$: positive slope, function is *increasing*

$\dfrac{dy}{dx} < 0$: negative slope, function is *decreasing*

$\dfrac{dy}{dx} = 0$: zero slope (horizontal), function is constant

SECOND DERIVATIVE

$f''(x)$, "f double prime of x," is the second derivative of $f(x)$.

Example:

$$f''(x) = \frac{d^2 f(x)}{dx^2} = \frac{df'(x)}{dx}$$

$f''(x)$ is the derivative of $f'(x)$

The notation for second derivatives can be quite confusing at first glance. Remember that the second derivative of $f(x)$ is the derivative of the first derivative. The number of primes indicates the *order* of the derivative. There are also such things as third derivatives and higher. They are notated by the number of primes.

Let's say that you start with a cubic function: $f(x) = x^3$. The first derivative will be a parabolic function $f'(x) = x^2$, and the second derivative will be a linear graph $f''(x) = 2x$. The third derivative will be a horizontal line $f'''(x) = 2$. At this point, if you wished, you could take a fourth derivative, but since the derivative is simply the slope of the previous equation, the fourth derivative would be zero because the slope of a horizontal line is zero.

The graphical interpretation of second derivates is shown. $f''(x)$ indicates the concavity of the function.

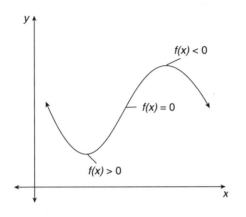

There are three distinct sections to this graph. On the left half, the function is said to be concave-up. Concave-up means U-shaped. In this section of the graph, the slope is increasing everywhere. Think about it for a second. On the far left side, the slope is negative, because the function is decreasing. At the bottom of the U, the slope is zero, and to the right of this point the slope is positive. The second derivative is the change in $f'(x)$, which is the slope, and since the slope is increasing everywhere, $f''(x)$ is positive. Thus, a positive $f''(x)$ means concave-up.

Similarly, the right half the graph shows a decreasing slope, so $f''(x)$ is negative. The point in the middle of the graph is where $f''(x) = 0$, which is where the slope is neither increasing nor decreasing. Here, the slope is constant.

$f''(x) > 0$: concave up (U-shaped); slope is *increasing*

$f''(x) < 0$: concave down; slope is *decreasing*

$f''(x) = 0$: constant slope

GRAPHICAL INTERPRETATIONS OF SECOND DERIVATIVES

Now that we know the graphical interpretations of first and second derivatives, we can use them in a very useful way, finding the extreme values of a function.

In the graph shown, point A is a **local minimum** and point B is a **local maximum**. Point A is the not lowest point on the graph, which is why it is only a local minimum instead of an absolute, or global, minimum. Similarly, point B is not the highest point on the graph. These points are both called local extreme values, or local extrema.

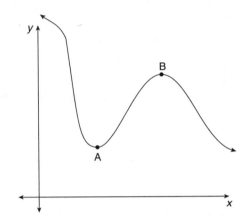

The first tool in finding local extreme values is realizing that any extreme value will have a slope of zero. This is because the graph always flattens out at the top of a peak or the bottom of a valley. Thus, for points A and B, $f'(x) = 0$.

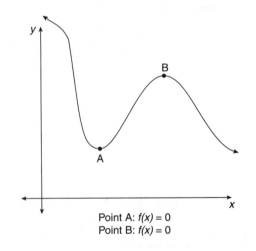

Point A: $f(x) = 0$
Point B: $f(x) = 0$

At point A, the function is concave-up, or U-shaped, so $f''(x) > 0$. At point B, the function is concave down, so $f''(x) < 0$. Thus, local maxima have $f''(x) < 0$, and local minima have $f''(x) > 0$.

LOCAL MINIMA AND MAXIMA

There is a clear step-by-step process to finding local minima and maxima.

First, find the first derivative of the function and locate the points where $f'(x)$ is zero. This is often called the first derivative test.

Next, find the second derivative of the function and determine the sign of $f''(x)$ at the points from step 1.

Example:

Which point is a local maximum of $f(x) = -3x^2 + 12x$?

First, find points where $f'(x)$ is zero. $f'(x)$, the derivative of the function $f(x)$, is $-6x + 12$.

Set $f'(x) = 0$ and solve for x.

$-6x + 12 = 0$

$x = 2$

Next, find $f''(x)$ and check the sign.

$f''(x) = -6(1) + 0 = -6$.

$f''(x) = -6$, which means that $f''(x)$ is negative everywhere. Since $f''(x) < 0$, the point is a local maximum.

Since $f''(x)$ is always negative, this means that the point we are talking about is the absolute maximum of the function. Plug $x = 2$ into the function to find the value of y at this point.

$f(2) = -3(2)^2 + 12(2) = -12 + 24 = 12$

$f(2) = 12$

Thus, the point of the maximum value of the function is (2,12).

INDEFINITE INTEGRALS

It is important to know the relationship between derivatives and integrals and to be able to go backwards and forwards between the two. An integral simply reverses the derivative. For example, if you take the derivative of a parabolic function at $x = 1$, you will get the equation for the line tangent to the parabola at $x = 1$. Then if you integrate the equation for the slope of that line, you will get the equation for the parabola. Hence, you can think of the integral as the antiderivative.

The process of finding an integral is called integration. The first type of integral we will discuss is the indefinite integral.

The integral of $f(x)$, with a lowercase f, is denoted by $F(x)$, with an uppercase F. This notation is only necessary when writing out formulas and is often ignored when working problems. There is a special symbol for the integration operation. It is the somewhat S-shaped symbol. To integrate a function, you always also need to have dx. The reason for this is fairly complicated and relies on understanding the technical meaning of an integral. For the time being, do not worry about the presence of the dx term. Sometimes it is omitted for simplicity. For the purposes of the PCAT, this will not be of importance.

Since integration and differentiation are inverse operations, instead of lowering the power of the exponent, in integration you raise the power of the exponent. Also, instead of multiplying by the old exponent, you divide by the new exponent.

One exception to this is when the exponent is –1. This does not follow the regular rule for integration. You cannot simply find the integral of x^{-1}. After a lengthy derivation, it can be shown that the integral of x^{-1} is the natural log of x, but you do not need to know this for Test Day.

Example:

What is $\int 8x^{-2}dx$?

Raise the power of the exponent from –2 to –1, then divide by –1. The integral is $-8x^{-1}$. It is important to very careful with signs when doing integrals of functions with negative powers.

$$\int 8x^{-2}dx = \frac{8x^{-2+1}}{(-2+1)} = \frac{8x^{-1}}{(-1)} = -8x^{-1}$$

Just as with derivatives, to find the integral of a polynomial, which is a function that has several x terms with different powers, simply find the integral of each term separately.

$$F(x) = \int (f(x) + g(x)), \, dx = \int (f(x)dx + \int g(x)dx$$

INDEFINITE INTEGRALS OF POLYNOMIALS

Example:

What is $\int (x^2 - 2x + 5)dx$?

To find the integral of the function, find the integral of each term separately by applying the integration rule. Remember to raise the exponent and then divide by the new exponent. This causes the fraction 1/3 and causes the 2 in front of x to cancel out. Remember that the constant term can be treated as 5 times x to the zero power. This means that the integral of 5 is $5x$.

$$\int (x^2 - 2x + 5)dx$$

$$\frac{1}{3}x^3 - x^2 + 5x$$

$$\int (x^2 - 2x + 5)dx = \int x^2\,dx + \int -2xdx + \int 5dx$$

$$\frac{x^{2+1}}{3} - 2\frac{x^{1+1}}{2} + 5\frac{x^{0+1}}{1} = \frac{1}{3}x^3 - x^2 + 5x$$

DEFINITE INTEGRALS

The next topic is definite integrals. As we saw, the indefinite integral of a function is another function, just like the derivative of a function is another function. We also saw that we could evaluate the derivative at a certain point. For integration, we do not evaluate at a certain point; we evaluate over a range defined by two points, a and b. The endpoints a and b are written at the bottom and top of the integral sign, as shown. To do this, find the indefinite integral as before. Then evaluate it at $x = a$ and $x = b$. Finally, subtract the value for $x = a$ from the value for $x = b$.

For $f'(x) = x^n$, $F(x) = \int_a^b x^n\,dx = \dfrac{x^{n+1}}{n+1}\Big|_a^b \; \dfrac{b^{n+1}}{n+1} = \dfrac{a^{n+1}}{n+1}$

When we do this, we are finding the definite integral of the function, evaluated from a to b.

$$\int_a^b x^n\,dx = \text{is the integral of } x^n, \text{ evaluated form } x = a \text{ to } x = b.$$

Example:

$\int_{-2}^{1} (4x^3 + 4x)\,dx = ?$

The first step is to find the indefinite integral of the function. The indefinite integral is $x^4 + 2x^2$. Next, evaluate the function at $x = -2$ and $x = 1$. Subtract the value at $x = -2$ from the value at $x = 1$. Be very careful with the signs here. The final answer is -21.

$\int_{-2}^{1} (4x^3 + 4x)\,dx = \dfrac{4x^4}{4} + 4\dfrac{x^2}{2}\Big|_{-2}^{1} = x^4 + 2x^2\Big|_{-2}^{1}$

$= [(1)^4 + 2(1)^2] - [(-2)^4 + 2(-2)^2] = [1 + 2] - [16 + 8]$

$= 3 - 24 = -21$

GRAPHICAL INTERPRETATION

Next, we consider the graphical meaning of integrals. The definite integral of a function from a to b is the area under the curve of that function from a to b.

Example:

$\int_a^b f(x)\,dx$

The graph of $y = 2x$ is shown. The shaded area is the area under the curve from $x = 3$ to $x = 7$. Rather than calculate the integral of this function, it would be easier to simply find the areas of the rectangular portion and the triangular portion and add them. However, when the function has a curve, rather than a straight line, it is necessary to integrate to find the area.

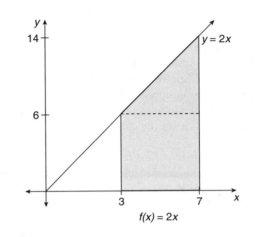

$f(x) = 2x$

What is the area of the shaded portion of the graph shown below?

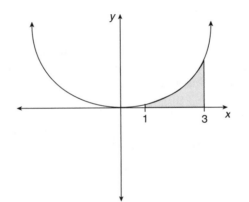

The shaded section is the area under the curve of the function $y = x^2$. To find the area, find the definite integral of $y = x^2$, evaluated from $x = 1$ to $x = 3$.

$$\text{Area} = \int_a^b f(x)dx = \int_1^3 x^2 dx$$

Follow the procedure for finding the definite integral. First find the indefinite integral of x^2, which is $\frac{1}{3} \times 3$. Next evaluate at $x = 1$ and $x = 3$. Subtract the value at $x = 1$ from the value at $x = 3$. The area is $8\frac{2}{3}$.

$$\int_1^3 x^2 dx = \frac{1}{3} x^3 \Big|_1^3 = \left[\frac{1}{3}(3)^3\right] - \left[\frac{1}{3}(1)^3\right] = \frac{1}{3}(27) - \frac{1}{3}(1) = 9 - \frac{1}{3} = 8\frac{2}{3}$$

It is helpful to understand how integration and differentiation are inverse operations, because test questions can be structured to make use of this fact.

Now we will look more closely at the relationship between derivatives and integrals.

Example:

Consider the function $f(x) = 3x^2$.

The derivative of $f(x)$ is $f'(x) = 3(2)x = 6x$.

Now integrate $f'(x)$.

$$\int f'(x)d(x) = \int 6x dx = \frac{6x^2}{2} = 3x^2$$

The integral of $f'(x) = 3x^2$. The integral of the derivative of a function is the original function.

However, in the workshop so far, we have overlooked an aspect of integration, the constant C.

THE CONSTANT OF INTEGRATION

Consider this function, $g(x) = 3x^2 + 5$.

$g(x) = 3x^2 + 5$

$g'(x) = 3(2)x + 0 = 6x$

$g'(x) = 6x$, which is the same as $f(x)$.

Now integrate $g'(x)$. In this case, the integral of $g'(x)$ does not equal $g(x)$! The constant term, 5, is missing.

$$\int g'(x)d(x) = \int 6x dx = \frac{6x^2}{2} = 3x^2 + C$$

This example shows a technicality in finding integrals. Anytime you calculate an integral, there is an unknown constant term left over, which is usually called C. This is for the reason we just showed. When you integrate the derivative of a function, you have to account for the fact that the original function may have had a constant term that disappeared when the differentiation was applied.

REVIEW PROBLEMS

1.

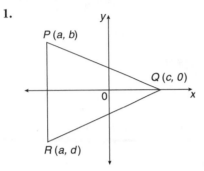

In the rectangular coordinate system above, the area of $\triangle PQR$ is

(A) $\dfrac{ac}{2}$ (B) $\dfrac{(c-a)(b-d)}{2}$ (C) $\dfrac{(c+a)(b+d)}{2}$ (D) $\dfrac{c(b-d)}{2}$ (E) $\dfrac{c(b+d)}{2}$

2. Line A is perpendicular to the line with the equation $y = -\dfrac{1}{5}x$, and the point $(3, -10)$ is on line A. Which of the following is the equation of line A?

(A) $y = -\dfrac{1}{5}x - \dfrac{47}{5}$

(B) $y = -\dfrac{1}{5}x - \dfrac{53}{5}$

(C) $y = 5x$

(D) $y = 5x - 5$

(E) $y = 5x - 25$

3. What is $f'(x)$ for $f(x) = 5x^4 + 3x^2 - 5$?

(A) $15x^3 + 3x$ (B) $5x^3 + 3x$ (C) $20x^3 + 6x$ (D) $20x^3 + 6x - 5$

4. What is the slope of $y = 3x^3$ when $y = 24$?

(A) 2 (B) 6 (C) 24 (D) 36

5. At $x = 0$, the function $f(x) = 4x^3 - 15x^2$ is

(A) concave up.

(B) concave down.

(C) increasing.

(D) decreasing.

6. The slope of $f(x) = x^3 + 2x + 2$ is _____ at $x = 3$.

    (A) increasing (B) decreasing (C) constant (D) zero

7. $\int 4x^{-5}dx = ?$
    (A) $-5x^{-4} + C$
    (B) $-\left(\dfrac{4}{5}\right)x^{-4} + C$
    (C) $-x^{-4} + C$
    (D) $-24x^{-6} + C$

8. What is the area of the shaded section of the graph of $f(x) = -x^2 + 10$, shown below?

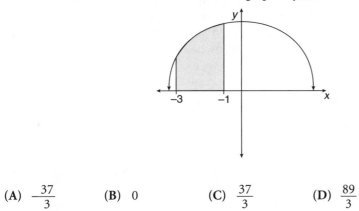

    (A) $-\dfrac{37}{3}$ (B) 0   (C) $\dfrac{37}{3}$ (D) $\dfrac{89}{3}$

9. Which of the following is equivalent to $\int (x^{-4} + x^4)dx$?
    (A) $\dfrac{x^5}{5} - \dfrac{x^{-3}}{3}$?
    (B) 0
    (C) $-4x^{-5} + 4x^3$
    (D) $\dfrac{x^5}{4} - \dfrac{x^{-3}}{4}$

SOLUTIONS TO THE REVIEW PROBLEMS

1. **B** To find the area of a triangle, we need to find the length of its base and the length of its height. For triangle *PQR*, we can use segment *PR* to represent its base and the portion of the *x*-axis that cuts through the triangle (ending in vertex *Q*) as its height.

    First let's find the length of base *PR*. Above the *x*-axis, *PR* ends in coordinate (a, b). In this case *b* is positive, so the distance from the *x*-axis to point (a, b) is of length (B). Below the *x*-axis, *PR* ends in coordinate (a, d). In this case *d* is a negative number, so we must subtract *d* from *b* to find the length of *PR*. If we were to add a negative number to *b*, *b* would become smaller. In this instance, we need to add the magnitude, or size, of *d* but not the sign of (D) Therefore, the length of *PR* is *b*–*d*.

    Now for the height. Vertex Q has coordinates $(c, 0)$, so the distance from the *y*-axis to this vertex is represented by (C) This does not account for the entire height, however—we also must consider the length of the height to the left of the *y*-axis. This length runs from the *y*-axis to a point on side PR. This point, being on both the *x*-axis and PR, must have coordinates $(a, 0)$. Once again, *a* is negative, so we must subtract it from *c* to get the length of the height: $c - (A)$.

    Substituting the base and height into the formula for an area of a triangle, we find:
    $$\frac{1}{2}\,bh = \frac{1}{2}\,(b - d)(c - a) = \frac{(c - a)(b - d)}{2}$$

2. **E** If a line has a nonzero slope of *m*, any line perpendicular to the line has a slope which is the negative reciprocal of *m*—that is, any line perpendicular to this line has a slope of $-\dfrac{1}{m}$.

    Since the slope of the line with the equation $y = -\dfrac{1}{5}x = \dfrac{-1}{5}$, the slope of any line perpendicular to this line has a slope of $\dfrac{-1}{\left(\dfrac{1}{5}\right)} = -(-5) = 5$. Therefore, line *A*, which is perpendicular to the line with the equation $y = -\dfrac{1}{5}x$, has a slope of 5. So line *A* has an equation of the form $y = 5x + b$.

    We also know that line *A* passes through the point $(3, -10)$. If we substitute $x = 3$ and $y = -10$ into $y = 5x + b$ and then solve for *b*, we can find the correct equation for line *A*:

    $y = 5x + b$

    $\rightarrow -10 = 5(3) + b$

    $\rightarrow -10 = 15 + b$

    $\rightarrow -25 = b$

    The equation of line *A* is $y = 5x - 25$.

3. **C** To find the derivative of a polynomial, find the derivative of each term separately. Remember the formula $\frac{df(x)}{dx} = nx^{n-1}$. So $f'(x) = 5(4)x^3 + 3(2)x + 0 = 20x^3 + 6x$. The derivative of a constant term is always zero. Choice (C) is correct.

4 **D** This is a two-part problem. First, you need to find an expression for the derivative of the function. $f'(x) = 3(3)x^2 = 9x^2$. Secondly, you need to find the value of x that gives $y = 24$. Plug into the original function and solve.

$24 = 3x^3$

$8 = x^3$

$2 = x$

Thus, $x = 2$ gives $y = 24$. Plug $x = 2$ into the expression for the derivative: $f'(2) = 9(2)^2 = 9(4) = 36$. Choice (D) is correct.

5. **B** The first derivative tells you whether the function is increasing, decreasing, or constant. The second derivative tells you the concavity of the function.

Find the first derivative: $f'(x) = (4)(3)x^2 - 2(15)x = 12x^2 - 30x$.

$f'(0) = 12(0) - 30(0) = 0$.

The first derivative is zero, so the function is constant at $x = 0$, meaning it is neither increasing nor decreasing. So we have to look at the second derivative.

$f''(x) = (2)(12)x - 30 = 24x - 30$

$f''(0) = 24(0) - 30 = -30$

When the second derivative is negative, this means the function is concave down. Choice (B) is correct.

6. **A** The first derivative, $f'(x)$, is the slope of the function. The second derivative, $f''(x)$, is the rate of change of the slope, $f'(x)$. Find $f''(x)$ at $x = 3$:

$f'(x) = 3x^2 + 2 + 0 = 3x^2 + 2$

$f''(x) = 3(2)x + 0 = 6x$

$f''(3) = 6(3) = 18$

$f''(x) > 0$ at $x = 3$, which means $f'(x)$ is increasing. Since $f'(x)$ is the slope, the slope is increasing at $x = 3$. Choice (A) is correct.

7. **C** Remember the formula for finding integrals: if $f(x) = xn$, $F(x) = \int 4x^{-5}dx = \int x^n dx + C$. So $\frac{x^{n+1}}{n+1} = 4\left(\frac{1}{-4}\right)x^{-4} + C = -x^{-4} + C$. Choice (C) is correct.

8. **C** The shaded section of the graph is the area under the curve. Thus, you are being asked to find the definite integral of $f(x) = -x^2 + 10$, evaluated from $x = -3$ to $x = -1$.

$$\int_{-3}^{-1}(-x^2 + 10)dx =$$

$$\frac{x^3}{3} + 10x \Big|_{-3}^{-1} = \left[-\frac{(-1)^3}{3} + 10(-1)\right] - \left[-\frac{(-3)^3}{3} + 10(-3)\right] = \left[-\frac{-1}{3} - 10\right] - \left[-\frac{-27}{3} - 30\right]$$

$$= \left[\frac{1}{3} - 10\right]$$

If you are short on time, narrow down the answer choices by realizing that since the shaded section is above the *x*-axis, the area must be positive. This eliminates choices (A) and (B). Choice (C) is correct.

9. **A** $\int(x^{-4} + x^4)dx = \frac{x^{-3}}{-3} + \frac{x^5}{5} = \frac{x^5}{5} - \frac{x^{-3}}{-3}$

The correct answer is choice (A).

CHAPTER TWENTY-EIGHT

Atomic Structure

Chemistry is the study of the nature and behavior of matter. The **atom** is the basic building block of matter, representing the smallest unit of a chemical element. An atom in turn is composed of subatomic particles called **protons**, **neutrons**, and **electrons**. The protons and neutrons in an atom form the **nucleus**, the core of the atom. The electrons exist outside the nucleus in characteristic regions of space called **orbitals**. All atoms of an **element** show similar chemical properties and cannot be further broken down by chemical means.

SUBATOMIC PARTICLES

In the early 1800s, an English scientist by the name of John Dalton formulated a specific theory of invisible building blocks of matter that are now called atoms. Dalton's atomic theory marks the beginning of the modern era of chemistry. Below is a summary of the key points of his hypotheses:

- All **elements** are composed of very small particles called atoms. All atoms of a given element are identical in size, mass, and chemical properties. The atoms of one element are different from atoms of all other elements.
- All **compounds** are composed of atoms of more than one element. For any given compound, the ratio of the numbers of atoms of any two of the elements present is either an integer or a simple fraction.
- A given **chemical reaction** involves only the separation, combination, or rearrangement of atoms; it does NOT result in the creation or destruction of atoms.

Protons

Protons carry a single positive charge and have a mass of approximately one **atomic mass unit**, or amu (see below). The **atomic number** (Z) of an element is equal to the number of protons found in an atom of that element. All atoms of a given element have the same atomic number. These positively charged particles carry the same "quantity of charge" as an electron; however, they have a weight that is approximately 1,840 times heavier than that of an electron. The mass of the nucleus of an atom comprises almost the entire weight of an atom; however, it occupies only $1/10^{13}$ of the volume of the atom. Putting this in perspective, if the entire atom was the size of a football stadium that seats 80,000 to 100,000 people, the volume of the actual nucleus would be that of a small marble.

Neutrons

Neutrons carry no charge and have a mass only slightly larger than that of protons. Different isotopes of one element have different numbers of neutrons but the same number of protons. The **mass number** of an atom is equal to the total number of protons and neutrons. The convention $^A_Z X$ is used to show both the atomic number and mass number of an X atom, where Z is the atomic number and A is the mass number.

Electrons

Electrons carry a charge equal in magnitude but opposite in sign to that of protons. An electron has a very small mass, approximately 1/1,837th the mass of a proton or neutron, which is negligible for most purposes. The electrons farthest from the nucleus are known as **valence electrons**. The farther the valence electrons are from the nucleus, the weaker the attractive force of the positively charged nucleus and the more likely the valence electrons are to be influenced by other atoms. Generally, the valence electrons and their activity determine the reactivity of an atom. In a neutral atom, the number of electrons is equal to the number of protons. A positive or negative charge on an atom is due to a loss or gain of electrons; the result is called an **ion**.

Some basic features of the three subatomic particles are shown in the table below.

Subatomic Particle	Symbol	Relative Mass	Charge	Location
Proton	$^1_1 H$	1	+1	Nucleus
Neutron	$^1_0 n$	1	0	Nucleus
Electron	e–	0	–1	Electron orbitals

Example: Determine the number of protons, neutrons, and electrons in a Nickel-58 atom and in a Nickel-60 2+ cation.

Solution: ^{58}Ni has an atomic number of 28 and a mass number of 58. Therefore, ^{58}Ni will have 28 protons, 28 electrons, and 58 – 28, or 30, neutrons.

In the $^{60}Ni^{2+}$ species, the number of protons is the same as in the neutral ^{58}Ni atom. However, $^{60}Ni^{2+}$ has a positive charge because it has lost 2 electrons, so Ni^{2+} will have 26 electrons. Also the mass number is two units higher than for the ^{58}Ni atom, and this difference in mass must be due to 2 extra neutrons, thus it has a total of 32 neutrons.

ATOMIC WEIGHTS AND ISOTOPES

Atomic Weights

The atomic mass of an atom is the relative mass of that atom compared to the mass of a **carbon-12 atom**, which is used as a standard with an assigned mass of 12.000. Atomic masses are expressed in terms of atomic mass units (amu), with one amu being defined as exactly one-twelfth the mass of the carbon-12 atom, approximately 1.66×10^{-24} grams (g). A more common convention used to define the mass of an atom is **atomic weight**. The atomic weight is the weight in grams of one mole (mol) of a given element and is expressed in terms of g/mol. A **mole** is a unit used to count particles and is represented by **Avogadro's number**, 6.022×10^{23} particles. For example, the atomic weight of carbon is 12.0 g/mol, which means that 6.022×10^{23} carbon atoms weigh 12.0 g (see Chapter 31, Compounds and Stoichiometry).

All atoms can be identified by the number of protons and neutrons that they contain. The **atomic number (Z)** is the number of protons in the nucleus of each atom of a given element. In a neutral atom, the number of protons and neutrons are equal. Therefore, the atomic number indicates the number of electrons in an atom. The **mass number (A)** equals the total number of neutrons and protons present in the nucleus of an atom of an element.

The mass number = number of protons + number of neutrons
= atomic number + number of neutrons

Isotopes

For a given element, multiple species of atoms with the same number of protons (same atomic number) but different numbers of neutrons (different mass numbers) exist; these are called **isotopes** of the element. Isotopes are referred to either by the convention described above or, more commonly, by the name of the element followed by the mass number. For example, carbon-12 ($^{12}_{6}C$) is a carbon atom with 6 protons and 6 neutrons, while carbon-14 ($^{14}_{6}C$) is a carbon atom with 6 protons and 8 neutrons. Since isotopes have the same number of protons and electrons, they generally exhibit the same chemical properties.

In nature, almost all elements exist as a collection of two or more isotopes, and these isotopes are usually present in the same proportions in any sample of a naturally occurring element. The presence of these isotopes accounts for the fact that the accepted atomic weight for most elements is not a whole number. The masses listed in the periodic table are weighted averages that account for the relative abundance of various isotopes.

Example: Element Q consists of three different isotopes, A, B, and C. Isotope A has an atomic mass of 40 amu and accounts for 60% of naturally occurring Q. The atomic mass of isotope B is 44 amu and accounts for 25% of Q. Finally, isotope C has an atomic mass of 41amu and a natural abundance of 15%. What is the atomic weight of element Q?

Solution: 0.60(40 amu) + 0.25(44 amu) + 0.15(41 amu) = 24.00 amu + 11.00 amu + 6.15 amu
= 41.15 amu

The atomic weight of element Q is 41.15 g/mol.

BOHR'S MODEL OF THE HYDROGEN ATOM

In 1911, Ernest Rutherford provided experimental evidence that an atom has a dense, positively charged nucleus that accounts for only a small portion of the volume of the atom. In 1900, Max Planck developed the first **quantum theory**, proposing that energy emitted as electromagnetic radiation from matter comes in discrete bundles called **quanta**. The energy value of a quantum is given by the equation E = hf, where h is a proportionality constant known as **Planck's constant**, equal to 6.626×10^{-34} J·s, and f (sometimes designated ν) is the **frequency** of the radiation.

The Bohr Model

In 1913, Niels Bohr used the work of Rutherford and Planck to develop his model of the electronic structure of the hydrogen atom. Starting from Rutherford's findings, Bohr assumed that the hydrogen atom consisted of a central proton around which an electron travelled in a circular orbit, and that the centripetal force acting on the electron as it revolved around the nucleus was the electrical force between the positively charged proton and the negatively charged electron.

Bohr's model used the quantum theory of Planck in conjunction with concepts from classical physics. In classical mechanics, an object, such as an electron, revolving in a circle may assume an infinite number of values for its radius and velocity. Therefore, the **angular momentum** (L = mvr) and **kinetic energy** ($KE = mv^2/2$) can take on any value. However, by incorporating Planck's quantum theory into his model, Bohr placed conditions on the value of the angular momentum. Like Planck's energy, the angular momentum of an electron is quantized according to the following equation:

angular momentum = nh/2π

where h is Planck's constant and n is a quantum number that can be any positive integer. Since h, 2, and π are constants, the angular momentum changes only in discrete amounts with respect to the quantum number, n.

Bohr then equated the allowed values of the angular momentum to the energy of the electron. He obtained the following equation:

$$E = -R_H/n^2$$

where R_H is an experimentally determined constant (known as the **Rydberg constant**) equal to 2.18×10^{-18} J/electron. Therefore, like angular momentum, the energy of the electron changes in discrete amounts with respect to the quantum number.

A value of zero energy was assigned to the state in which the proton and electron were separated completely, meaning that there was no attractive force between them. Therefore, the electron in any of its quantized states in the atom would have a negative energy as a result of the attractive forces between the electron and proton. This explains the negative sign in the above equation for energy.

Applications of the Bohr Model

In his model of the structure of hydrogen, Bohr postulated that an electron can exist only in certain fixed-energy states. In terms of quantum theory, the energy of an electron is **quantized**. Using this model, certain generalizations concerning the characteristics of electrons can be made. The energy of the electron is related to its **orbital radius**: the smaller the radius, the lower the energy state of the electron. The smallest orbit (radius) an electron can have corresponds to $n = 1$, which is the ground state of the hydrogen electron. At the **ground state** level, the electron is in its lowest energy state. The Bohr model is also used to explain the atomic emission spectrum and atomic absorption spectrum of hydrogen, and it is helpful in interpretation of the spectra of other atoms.

Atomic emission spectra

At room temperature, the majority of atoms in a sample are in the ground state. However, electrons can be excited to higher energy levels, by heat or other energy, to yield the excited state of the atom. Because the lifetime of the excited state is brief, the electrons will return rapidly to the ground state, emitting energy in the form of photons. The electromagnetic energy of these photons may be determined using the following equation:

$$E = hc/\lambda$$

where h is Planck's constant, c is the velocity of light (3.00×10^8 m/s), and λ is the wavelength of the radiation.

The different electrons in an atom will be excited to different energy levels. When these electrons return to their ground states, each will emit a photon with a wavelength characteristic of the specific transition it undergoes. The quantized energies of light emitted under these conditions do not produce a continuous spectrum (as expected from classical physics). Rather, the spectrum is composed of light at specific frequencies and is thus known as a **line spectrum**, where each line on the emission spectrum corresponds to a specific electronic transition. Because each element can have its electrons excited to different distinct energy levels, each one possesses a unique **atomic emission spectrum**, which can be used as a fingerprint for the element. One particular application of atomic emissions spectroscopy is in the analysis of stars; while a physical sample can not be taken, the light from a star can be resolved into its component wavelengths, which are then matched to the known line spectra of the elements.

The Bohr model of the hydrogen atom explained the atomic emission spectrum of hydrogen, which is the simplest emission spectrum among all the elements. The group of hydrogen emission lines corresponding to transitions from upper levels $n > 2$ to $n = 2$ is known as the **Balmer series** (four wavelengths in the visible region), while the group corresponding to transitions between upper levels $n > 1$ to $n = 1$ is known as the **Lyman series** (higher energy transitions in the UV region). Below is a summary of the various series in atomic emission spectrum where n_f and n_i are the final and initial states, respectively.

Series	n_f	n_i	Spectrum region
Lyman	1	2, 3, 4….	Ultraviolet
Balmer	2	3, 4, 5….	Visible and ultraviolet
Paschen	3	4, 5, 6….	Infrared
Brackett	4	5, 6, 7….	Infrared

When the energy of each frequency of light observed in the emission spectrum of hydrogen was calculated according to Planck's quantum theory, the values obtained closely matched those expected from energy level transitions in the Bohr model. That is, the energy associated with a change in the quantum number from an initial value n_i to a final value n_f is equal to the energy of Planck's emitted photon. Thus:

$$E = hc/\lambda = -R_H[1/(n_i)^2 - 1/(n_f)^2]$$

and the energy of the emitted photon corresponds to the precise difference in energy between the higher-energy initial state and the lower-energy final state.

Atomic absorption sectra

When an electron is excited to a higher energy level, it must absorb energy. The energy absorbed as an electron jumps from an orbital of low energy to one of higher energy is characteristic of that transition. This means that the excitation of electrons in a particular element results in energy absorptions at specific wavelengths. Thus, in addition to an emission spectrum, every element possesses a characteristic **absorption spectrum**. Not surprisingly, the wavelengths of absorption correspond directly to the wavelengths of emission since the energy difference between levels remains unchanged. Absorption spectra can thus be used in the identification of elements present in a gas phase sample.

QUANTUM MECHANICAL MODEL OF ATOMS

While the concepts put forth by Bohr offered a reasonable explanation for the structure of the hydrogen atom and ions containing only one electron (such as He^{1+} and Li^{2+}), they did not explain the structures of atoms containing more than one electron. This is because Bohr's model does not take into consideration the repulsion between multiple electrons surrounding one nucleus. Modern quantum mechanics has led to a more rigorous and generalized study of the electronic structure of atoms. The most important difference between the Bohr model and modern quantum mechanical models is that Bohr's assumption that electrons follow a circular orbit at a fixed distance from the nucleus is no longer considered valid. Rather, electrons are described as being in a state of rapid motion within regions of space around the nucleus, called **orbitals**. An orbital is a representation of the **probability** of finding an electron within a given region. In the current quantum mechanical description of electrons, pinpointing the exact location of an electron at any given point in time is impossible. This idea is best described by the **Heisenberg uncertainty principle**, which states that it is impossible to determine, with perfect accuracy, the momentum (defined as mass times velocity) and the position of an electron simultaneously. This means that if the momentum of the electron is being measured accurately, its position will change, and vice versa.

Quantum Numbers

Modern atomic theory states that any electron in an atom can be completely described by four **quantum numbers**: n, ℓ, m_ℓ, and m_s. Furthermore, according to the **Pauli exclusion principle**, no two electrons in a given atom can possess the same set of four quantum numbers. The position and energy of an electron described by its quantum numbers is known as its **energy state**. The value of n limits the values of ℓ, which in turn limit the values of m_ℓ. The values of the quantum numbers qualitatively give information about the orbitals: n about the size, ℓ about the shape, and m_ℓ about the orientation of the orbital. All four quantum numbers are discussed below.

Principal quantum number

The first quantum number is commonly known as the **principal quantum number** and is denoted by the letter n. This is the quantum number used in Bohr's model that can theoretically take on any positive integer value. The larger the integer value of n, the higher the energy level and radius of the electron's orbit. The maximum number of electrons in energy level n (electron shell n) is $2n^2$. The difference in energy between adjacent shells decreases as the distance from the nucleus increases, since it is related to the expression $1/n_2^2 - 1/n_1^2$. For example, the energy difference between the third and fourth shells ($n = 3$ to $n = 4$) is less than that between the second and third shells ($n = 2$ to $n = 3$).

Azimuthal quantum number

The second quantum number is called the **azimuthal (angular momentum) quantum number** and is designated by the letter ℓ. This number tells us the "shape" of the orbitals. The second quantum number refers to the **subshells** or **sublevels** that occur within each principal energy level. For any given n, the value of ℓ can be any integer in the range of 0 to $n - 1$. The four subshells corresponding to $\ell = 0, 1, 2$, and 3 are known as the s, p, d, and f subshells, respectively. The maximum number of electrons that can exist within a subshell is given by the equation $4\ell + 2$. The greater the value of ℓ, the greater the energy of the subshell. However, the energies of subshells from different principal energy levels may overlap. For example, the 4s subshell will have a lower energy than the 3d subshell because its average distance from the nucleus is smaller.

Magnetic quantum number

The third quantum number is the **magnetic quantum number** and is designated m_ℓ. This number describes the orientation of the orbital in space. An orbital is a specific region within a subshell that may contain no more than two electrons. The magnetic quantum number specifies the particular orbital within a subshell where an electron is highly likely to be found at a given point in time. The possible values of m_ℓ are all integers from ℓ to $-\ell$, including 0. Therefore, the s subshell, where there is one possible value of m_ℓ (0), will contain one orbital; likewise, the p subshell will contain three orbitals, the d subshell will contain five orbitals, and the f subshell will contain seven orbitals. The shape and energy of each orbital are dependent upon the subshell in which the orbital is found. For example, a p subshell has three possible m_ℓ values (−1, 0, +1). The three dumbbell-shaped orbitals are oriented in space around the nucleus along the x, y, and z axes and are often referred to as p_x, p_y, and p_z.

Spin quantum number

The fourth quantum number is also called the **spin quantum number** and is denoted by m_s. The spin of a particle is its intrinsic angular momentum and is a characteristic of a particle, like its charge. In classical mechanics, an object spinning about its axis has an angular momentum; however, this does not apply to the electron. Classical analogies often are inapplicable in the quantum world.

In any case, the two spin orientations are designated $+\dfrac{1}{2}$ and $-\dfrac{1}{2}$.

Whenever two electrons are in the same orbital, they must have opposite spins. Electrons in different orbitals with the same m_s values are said to have **parallel** spins.

The quantum numbers for the orbitals in the second principal energy level, with their maximum number of electrons noted in parentheses, are shown in the following table. Electrons with opposite spins in the same orbital are often referred to as **paired**.

n	2(8)				
ℓ	0(2)			1(6)	
m_ℓ	0(2)	+1(2)		0(2)	−1(2)
m_s	$+\dfrac{1}{2}, -\dfrac{1}{2}$	$+\dfrac{1}{2}, -\dfrac{1}{2}$		$+\dfrac{1}{2}, -\dfrac{1}{2}$	$+\dfrac{1}{2}, -\dfrac{1}{2}$

Electron Configuration and Orbital Filling

For a given atom or ion, the pattern by which subshells are filled and the number of electrons within each principal level and subshell are designated by an **electron configuration**. In electron configuration notation, the first number denotes the principal energy level, the letter designates the subshell, and the superscript gives the number of electrons in that subshell. For example, $2p^4$ indicates that there are four electrons in the second (p) subshell of the second principal energy level.

When writing the electron configuration of an atom, it is necessary to remember the order in which subshells are filled. Subshells are filled from lowest to highest energy, and each subshell will fill completely before electrons begin to enter the next one. The $(n + \ell)$ **rule** is used to rank subshells by increasing energy. This rule states that the lower the values of the first and second quantum numbers, the lower the energy of the subshell. If two subshells possess the same $(n + \ell)$ value, the subshell with the lower n value has a lower energy and will fill first. The order in which the subshells fill is shown in the following chart.

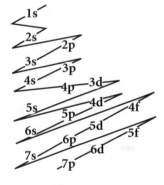

Figure 28.1

Example: Which will fill first, the $3d$ subshell or the $4s$ subshell?

Solution: For $3d$, $n = 3$ and $\ell = 2$, so $(n + \ell) = 5$. For $4s$, $n = 4$ and $\ell = 0$, so $(n + \ell) = 4$. Therefore, the $4s$ subshell has lower energy and will fill first. This can also be determined from the chart by examination.

To determine which subshells are filled, you must know the number of electrons in the atom. In the case of uncharged atoms, the number of electrons equals the atomic number. If the atom is charged, the number of electrons is equal to the atomic number plus the extra electrons if the atom is negative, or the atomic number minus the electrons if the atom is positive.

In subshells that contain more than one orbital, such as the $2p$ subshell with its 3 orbitals, the orbitals will fill according to **Hund's rule**. Hund's rule states that within a given subshell, orbitals are filled such that there are a maximum number of half-filled orbitals with parallel spins. Electrons "prefer" empty orbitals to half-filled ones, because a pairing energy must be overcome for two electrons carrying repulsive negative charges to exist in the same orbital.

Example: What are the written electron configurations for nitrogen (N) and iron (Fe) according to Hund's rule?

Solution: Nitrogen has an atomic number of 7, thus its electron configuration is $1s^2 \, 2s^2 \, 2p^3$. According to Hund's rule, the two s orbitals will fill completely, while the three p orbitals will each contain one electron, all with parallel spins.

$$\underset{1s^2}{\underline{\uparrow\downarrow}} \qquad \underset{2s^2}{\underline{\uparrow\downarrow}} \qquad \underset{2p^3}{\underline{\uparrow}\;\underline{\uparrow}\;\underline{\uparrow}}$$

Iron has an atomic number of 26, and its 4s subshell fills before the 3d. Using Hund's rule, the electron configuration will be:

$$\underset{1s^2}{\underline{\uparrow\downarrow}} \qquad \underset{2s^2}{\underline{\uparrow\downarrow}} \quad \underset{2p^6}{\underline{\uparrow\downarrow}\,\underline{\uparrow\downarrow}\,\underline{\uparrow\downarrow}} \quad \underset{3s^2}{\underline{\uparrow\downarrow}} \quad \underset{3p^6}{\underline{\uparrow\downarrow}\,\underline{\uparrow\downarrow}\,\underline{\uparrow\downarrow}} \quad \underset{3d^6}{\underline{\uparrow\downarrow}\,\underline{\uparrow}\,\underline{\uparrow}\,\underline{\uparrow}\,\underline{\uparrow}} \quad \underset{4s^2}{\underline{\uparrow\downarrow}}$$

Iron's electron configuration is written as $1s^2 \, 2s^2 \, 2p^6 \, 3s^2 \, 3p^6 \, 3d^6 \, 4s^2$. Subshells may be listed either in the order in which they fill (e.g., $4s$ before $3d$) or with subshells of the same principal quantum number grouped together, as shown here. Both methods are correct.

The presence of paired or unpaired electrons affects the chemical and magnetic properties of an atom or molecule. If the material has unpaired electrons, a magnetic field will align the spins of these electrons and weakly attract the atom. These materials are said to be **paramagnetic**. Materials that have no unpaired electrons and are slightly repelled by a magnetic field are said to be **diamagnetic**.

Valence Electrons

The valence electrons of an atom are those electrons that are in its outer energy shell or that are available for chemical bonding. For elements in Groups IA and IIA, only the outermost s electrons are valence electrons. For elements in Groups IIIA through VIIIA, the outermost s and p electrons in the highest-energy shell are valence electrons. For transition elements, the valence electrons are those in the outermost s subshell and in the d subshell of the next-to-outermost energy shell. For the inner transition elements, the valence electrons are those in the s subshell of the outermost energy shell, the d subshell of the next-to-outermost energy shell, and the f subshell of the energy shell two levels below the outermost shell.

IIIA–VIIA elements beyond Period II might, under some circumstances, accept electrons into their empty d subshell, which gives them more than eight valence electrons.

Example: Which are the valence electrons of elemental iron, elemental selenium, and the sulfur atom in a sulfate ion?

Solution: Iron has 8 valence electrons: 2 in its $4s$ subshell and 6 in its $3d$ subshell.

Selenium has 6 valence electrons: 2 in its $4s$ subshell and 4 in its $4p$ subshell. Selenium's $3d$ electrons are not part of its valence shell.

Sulfur in a sulfate ion has 12 valence electrons: its original 6 plus 6 more from the oxygens to which it is bonded. Sulfur's $3s$ and $3p$ subshells can only contain 8 of these 12 electrons; the other 4 electrons have entered the sulfur atom's $3d$ subshell, which in elemental sulfur is empty.

REVIEW PROBLEMS

1. The Mg^{2+} ion has how many electrons?

    (A) 12

    (B) 10

    (C) 14

    (D) 24

2. It can be shown using mass spectrometry that the ratio of naturally occurring chlorine-35 to its isotope chlorine-37 is 3:1. Assuming that no other isotopes existed, what would be the atomic weight of chlorine?

3. A student represents electrons within the same orbital as having parallel spins. This goes against which of the following principles?

    (A) Bohr's model of the hydrogen atom

    (B) Pauli exclusion principle

    (C) Heisenberg's uncertainty principle

    (D) Planck's quantum theory

4. What are the four quantum numbers? Discuss how they are related and to what each one refers.

5. The maximum number of electrons in a shell with the principal quantum number equal to 4 is

    (A) 2

    (B) 10

    (C) 16

    (D) 32

6. In Bohr's model of the hydrogen atom, the energy of an electron is directly dependent on

    (A) the spin quantum number (m_s).

    (B) Planck's constant.

    (C) the principal quantum number (n).

    (D) the angular momentum quantum number (ℓ).

7. Which of the following describes the excitation exhibited when an electron jumps from its ground state to a higher energy level?

    (A) Balmer series

    (B) Atomic absorption spectrum

    (C) Lyman series

    (D) Atomic emission spectrum

8. The Pauli exclusion principle states that

   (A) no two electrons can have the same four quantum numbers.
   (B) it is impossible to determine simultaneously the momentum and the position of an electron.
   (C) energy is emitted from matter as quantized units.
   (D) an electron will enter an empty orbital in a subshell before entering half-filled orbitals.
   (E) electrons travel around the nucleus with orbits of known radii.

9. Atoms with the same atomic number but with different atomic weights are known as

   (A) elements.
   (B) isomers.
   (C) ions.
   (D) isotopes.

10. If the principal quantum number of a shell is equal to 2, what types of orbitals will be present?

    (A) s
    (B) s and p
    (C) s, p, and d
    (D) s, p, d, and f

11. What is the amount of energy emitted when a hydrogen electron relaxes from $n = 3$ to $n = 2$? ($R_H = 2.18 \times 10^{-18}$ J)

12. What wavelength (in nm) corresponds to the energy calculated in Question 11? ($c = 3 \times 10^8$ m/s)

13. What is the total number of electrons that could be held in a sublevel with angular momentum number equal to 2?

    (A) 2
    (B) 6
    (C) 8
    (D) 10

14. An element with an atomic number of 26 has how many electrons in the $3d$ orbital?

    (A) 0
    (B) 2
    (C) 6
    (D) 8
    (E) 10

15. An energy of −328 kJ/mol corresponds to the energy of an electron in which principal energy level? (R_H = 1,312 kJ/mol)

    (A) 1
    (B) 2
    (C) 3
    (D) 4
    (E) 5

16. In going from $1s^2 \, 2s^2 \, 2p^6 \, 3s^2 \, 3p^6 \, 4s^1$ to $1s^2 \, 2s^2 \, 2p^6 \, 3s^2 \, 3p^5 \, 4s^2$, an electron would

    (A) absorb energy.
    (B) emit energy.
    (C) relax to the ground state.
    (D) bind to another atom.
    (E) undergo no change in energy.

17. The values of the spin quantum number are directly related to

    (A) the principal quantum number.
    (B) the angular momentum quantum number.
    (C) the magnetic quantum number.
    (D) none of the above.

18. Which of the following orbitals has the lowest energy?

    (A) $2p$
    (B) $3s$
    (C) $3d$
    (D) $4s$
    (E) $3p$

19. Which of the following correctly represents the excited state of scandium?

    (A) $1s^2 \, 2s^2 \, 2p^6 \, 3s^2 \, 3p^6 \, 3d^1 \, 4s^2$
    (B) $1s^2 \, 2s^3 \, 2p^5 \, 3s^2 \, 3p^6 \, 3d^1 \, 4s^2$
    (C) $1s^2 \, 2s^2 \, 2p^6 \, 3s^2 \, 3p^6 \, 3d^2 \, 4s^1$
    (D) $1s^2 \, 2s^2 \, 2p^6 \, 3s^2 \, 3p^6 \, 3d^2 \, 4s^2$
    (E) $1s^2 \, 2s^2 \, 2p^6 \, 3s^2 \, 3p^8 \, 3d^1 \, 4s^0$

20. The photon frequency of red light is $4.51 \times 10^{14} \, s^{-1}$. What is the energy of the photon? Is this enough energy to cause a hydrogen electron to be excited from $n = 1$ to $n = 3$?

SOLUTIONS TO REVIEW PROBLEMS

1. **B** Magnesium has an atomic number of 12, meaning that it has 12 protons and 12 electrons. However, the Mg^{2+} ion has a positive charge because it has lost 2 electrons. Therefore, the Mg^{2+} ion has 10 electrons.

2. **35.5**

    Mass spectrometry shows that three out of every four chlorine atoms are Cl-35 and one is Cl-37. Thus, 75% of all chlorine atoms are Cl-35 and 25% are Cl-37. Using this information and the atomic weights of the isotopes (Cl-35 = 35 g/mol, Cl-37 = 37 g/mol), the atomic weight of chlorine can be determined as follows:

    (0.75)(35 g/mol) + (0.25)(37 g/mol)

    = (26.25 + 9.25) g/mol

    = 35.5 g/mol

3. **B** Discussed in the section on quantum numbers.

4. Discussed in the section on quantum numbers.

5. **D** The number of electrons within a principal energy level is given by the equation $2n^2$. Therefore, a shell with the principal quantum number equal to 4 will hold a maximum of 32 electrons.

6. **C** In the Bohr model for hydrogen, the energy of the electron is given by the equation $E = -R_H/n^2$, where R_H is a theoretically determined constant. Therefore, the energy of the electron is dependent only on n, the principal quantum number.

7. **B** For electrons to jump from ground state to higher energy levels, they must absorb energy. Therefore, the movements from ground state to excited state are characterized by an atomic absorption spectrum.

8. **A** Discussed in the section on quantum numbers.

9. **D** Atomic weight equals the number of protons (atomic number) plus the number of neutrons. If two atoms have the same atomic number but different atomic weights, then the number of neutrons must be different. This is the definition of an isotope.

10. **B** When the principal quantum number is equal to 2, then the angular momentum quantum number will have values of $\ell = 0$ and 1. When $\ell = 0$, the subshell is an s subshell, and when $\ell = 1$, the subshell is a p subshell. Therefore, the second principal energy level contains an s subshell and a p subshell.

11. **3.03×10^{-19} J**

To calculate the energy emitted when a hydrogen electron relaxes from $n = 3$ to $n = 2$, the equation $E = -R_H[1/(n_i)^2 - 1/(n_f)^2]$ is used, where $R_H = 2.18 \times 10^{-18}$ J and n_i and n_f are equal to 3 and 2, respectively. The calculation is done as follows:

$$E = -2.18 \times 10^{-18} \text{ J} \left(\frac{1}{3}^2 - \frac{1}{2}^2\right)$$

$$E = -2.18 \times 10^{-18} \text{ J} \left(\frac{1}{9} - \frac{1}{4}\right)$$

$$E = -2.18 \times 10^{-18} \text{ J} \left(\frac{4}{36} - \frac{9}{36}\right)$$

$$E = -2.18 \times 10^{-18} \text{ J} \left(-\frac{5}{36}\right)$$

$$E = 3.03 \times 10^{-19} \text{ J}$$

The value of the energy is positive because energy is released when an electron falls from an excited state back to the ground state.

12. **656 nm**

The wavelength in nm of a photon that carries 3.03×10^{-19} J of energy found in Question 11 can be determined as follows:

$E = \dfrac{hc}{\lambda}$, thus by rearrangement, $\lambda = \dfrac{hc}{e}$

$$\lambda = \frac{(6.6262 \times 10^{-34})\,(36 \times 10^8 \text{m/s})}{3.03 \times 10^{-19}\text{J}}$$

$$= 656 \text{ nm}$$

13. **D** The angular momentum number 2 corresponds to the sublevel or subshell d, and the d sublevel is capable of holding a maximum of $4(2) + 2$ electrons or 10 electrons.

14. **C** An element with an atomic number of 26 will have 6 electrons in its $3d$ subshell. This can be determined by writing the electron configuration for the element: $1s^2\ 2s^2\ 2p^6\ 3s^2\ 3p^6\ 3d^6\ 4s^2$. The number of electrons must equal 26; recall that the $4s$ subshell must be filled before the $3d$ because it has the lower energy. Thus, $3d$ will carry 6 electrons.

15. **B** To determine which of the principal energy levels has an energy of -328 kJ/mol, the equation $E = -R_H/n^2$ is used ($R_H = 1{,}312$ kJ/mol). Solving for n:

-328 kJ/mol $= -1{,}312$ kJ/mol $/ n^2$

$$n^2 = 4$$

$$n = 2$$

Therefore, the second principal energy level has an energy of -328 kJ/mol.

16. **A** The difference between the first and second electron configurations is that in the second configuration one electron has moved from the $3p$ subshell to the $4s$ subshell. Although the $3p$ and $4s$ subshells have the same $(n + \ell)$ value, the $3p$ subshell fills first because it is slightly lower in energy. For an electron to move from the $3p$ subshell to the $4s$ subshell, it must absorb energy.

17. **D** The spin quantum number is the intrinsic angular momentum of an electron in an orbital. The spin number can be either $+\dfrac{1}{2}$ or $-\dfrac{1}{2}$. These numbers are arbitrary and are not dependent on the other three quantum numbers.

18. **A** To determine which subshell has the lowest energy, the $(n + \ell)$ rule must be used. The values of the first and second quantum numbers are added together, and the subshell with the lowest $(n + \ell)$ value has the lowest energy. The sums of the five choices are $(2 + 1) = 3, (3 + 0) = 3, (3 + 2) = 5, (4 + 0) = 4, (3 + 1) = 4$. (A) and (B) have the same $(n + \ell)$ value, so the subshell with the lower principal quantum number has the lower energy. This is the $2p$ subshell.

19. **C** Scandium has 21 electrons. When it is in its excited state, one or more of the electrons will be present in a subshell with a higher energy than the one in which it is usually located. The number of electrons and ordering of subshells will not vary from the ground state electron configuration of scandium. (C) has one of the $4s$ electrons present in the $3d$ orbital. This represents an excited state because energy is required to cause an electron to jump from $4s$ to $3d$.

20. **$2.988 \times 10{-}19$ J; No**

To determine the energy of a photon with a frequency (ν) of $4.51 \times 10^{14}\ s^{-1}$, the following calculations are performed:

$E = h\nu$

$E = 6.626 \times 10^{-34}\ J \cdot s \times 4.51 \times 10^{14}\ s^{-1}$

$E = 2.988 \times 10^{-19}\ J$

The energy from red light will not be sufficient to excite a hydrogen electron from $n = 1$ to $n = 3$. This is because the energy necessary to perform that excitation is:

$E = -(2.179 \times 10^{-18}\ J)(1/(1)^2 - 1/(3)^2)$

$E = -(2.179 \times 10^{-18}\ J)(8/9)$

$E = -1.937 \times 10^{-18}\ J$

which is greater than the energy of red light.

CHAPTER TWENTY-NINE

The Periodic Table

In 1869, the Russian chemist Dmitri Mendeleev published the first version of his periodic table, in which he showed that ordering the elements according to atomic weight produced a pattern where similar properties periodically recurred. This table was later revised, using the work of the physicist Henry Moseley, to organize the elements on the basis of increasing atomic number. Using this revised table, the properties of certain elements that had not yet been discovered were predicted: a number of these predictions were later borne out by experimentation. The substance of this work is summarized in the **periodic law**, which states that the chemical properties of the elements are dependent, in a systematic way, upon their atomic numbers.

In the periodic table used today, the elements are arranged in **periods** (rows) and **groups** (columns). There are seven periods, representing the principal quantum numbers $n = 1$ to $n = 7$, and each period is filled sequentially. Groups represent elements that have the same electronic configuration in their **valence**, or outermost shell, and share similar chemical properties. The electrons in the outermost shell are called **valence electrons**. They are involved in chemical bonding and determine the chemical reactivity and properties of the element. The Roman numeral above each group represents the number of valence electrons. There are two sets of groups, designated A and B. The A elements are the **representative elements**, which have either s or p sublevels as their outermost orbitals. These representative elements are those in Groups 1A through 7A, all of which have incompletely filled s or p subshells of the highest principal number. Note: With the exception of the noble gases (Group 8), elements all have a completely filled p subshell. The B elements are the **nonrepresentative elements**, including the **transition elements**, which have partly filled d sublevels, and the **lanthanide** and **actinide** series, which have partly filled f sublevels. The electron configuration for the valence electrons is given by the Roman numeral and letter designations. For example, an element in Group VA will have a valence electron configuration of s^2p^3 ($2 + 3 = 5$ valence electrons).

PERIODIC PROPERTIES OF THE ELEMENTS

The properties of the elements exhibit certain trends, which can be explained in terms of the position of the element in the periodic table or in terms of the electron configuration of the element. All elements seek to gain or lose valence electrons so as to achieve the stable octet formation possessed by the **inert** or **noble gases** of Group VIII. Two other important trends exist within the periodic table. First, as one goes from left to right across a period, electrons are added one at a time; the electrons of the outermost shell experience an increasing amount of nuclear attraction, becoming closer and more tightly bound to the nucleus. Second, as one goes down a given column, the outermost electrons become less tightly bound to the nucleus. This is because the number of filled principal energy levels (which shield the outermost electrons from attraction by the nucleus) increases downward within each group. These trends help explain elemental properties such as atomic radius, ionization potential, electron affinity, and electronegativity.

Atomic Radii

The atomic radius of an element is equal to one-half the distance between the centers of two atoms of that element that are just touching each other. For example, the atomic radius of a metal is one-half the distance between the two nuclei in two adjacent atoms. In general, the atomic radius decreases across a period from left to right and increases down a given group; the atoms with the largest atomic radii will be located at the bottom of groups, and in Group I.

As one moves from left to right across a period, electrons are added one at a time to the outer energy shell. Electrons within a shell cannot shield one another from the attractive pull of protons. Therefore, since the number of protons is also increasing, producing a greater positive charge attracting the valence electrons, the effective nuclear charge increases steadily across a period. This causes the atomic radius to decrease.

As one moves down a group of the periodic table, the number of electrons and filled electron shells will increase, but the number of valence electrons will remain the same. Thus, the outermost electrons in a given group will feel the same amount of effective nuclear charge, but electrons will be found farther from the nucleus as the number of filled energy shells increases. Thus, the atomic radii will increase.

The **ionic radium** is the radius of a cation or an anion. The ionic radius will affect the physical and chemical properties of an ionic compound. For example, the three-dimensional infrastructure of a given ionic compound will depend largely upon the relative sizes of the cations and anions. If a neutral atom, for example, is converted into an ion, one would expect the radius to increase secondary to the repulsion of the additional electrons that will increase the size of the electron cloud.

Ionization Energy

The ionization energy (IE), or **ionization potential**, is the energy required to remove an electron completely from a gaseous atom or ion. Removing an electron from an atom always requires an input of energy (is endothermic; see Chapter 33, Thermochemistry). The closer and more tightly bound an electron is to the nucleus, the more difficult it will be to remove and the higher the ionization energy will be. The **first ionization energy** is the energy required to remove one valence electron from the parent atom, the **second ionization energy** is the energy needed to remove a second valence electron from the univalent ion to form the divalent ion, and so on. Successive ionization energies grow increasingly large; i.e., the second ionization energy is always greater than the first ionization energy.

For example:

$$Mg\,(g) \longrightarrow Mg^+(g) + e^- \quad \text{First Ionization Energy} = 7.646\,\text{eV}$$

$$Mg^+\,(g) \longrightarrow Mg^{2+}(g) + e^- \quad \text{Second Ionization Energy} = 15.035\,\text{eV}$$

Ionization energy increases from left to right across a period as the atomic radius decreases. Moving down a group, the ionization energy decreases as the atomic radius increases. Group I elements have low ionization energies because the loss of an electron results in the formation of a stable octet.

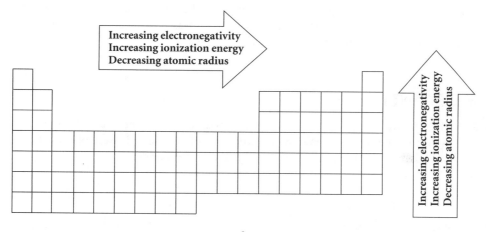

Figure 29.1

Electron Affinity

Electron affinity is the energy change that occurs when an electron is added to a gaseous atom, and it represents the ease with which the atom can accept an electron. The stronger the attractive pull of the nucleus for electrons (**effective nuclear charge, or Z_{eff}**), the greater the electron affinity will be. In discussing electron affinities, two sign conventions are used. The more common one states that a positive electron affinity value represents energy release when an electron is added to an atom; the other states that a negative electron affinity represents a release of energy. In this discussion, the first convention will be used.

Electron affinity can be best represented by the following equation, where X is an atom of a given element in the gaseous state (g):

$$X_{(g)} + e^- \longrightarrow X^-_{(g)}$$

Generalizations can be made about the electron affinities of particular groups in the periodic table. For example, the Group IIA elements, or **alkaline earths**, have low electron affinity values. These elements are relatively stable because their s subshell is filled. Group VIIA elements, or **halogens**, have high electron affinities because the addition of an electron to the atom results in a completely filled shell, which represents a stable electron configuration. Achieving the stable octet involves a release of energy, and the strong attraction of the nucleus for the electron leads to a high energy change. The Group VIII elements, or **noble gases**, have electron affinities on the order of zero because they already possess a stable octet and cannot readily accept an electron. Elements of other groups generally have low values of electron affinity.

Electronegativity

Electronegativity is a measure of the attraction an atom has for electrons in a chemical bond. The greater the electronegativity of an atom, the greater its attraction for bonding electrons. Electronegativity values are not determined directly. The most common electronegativity scale is the **Pauling electronegativity scale** where the values range from 0.7 for the most electropositive elements, like cesium, to 4.0 for the most electronegative element, fluorine. Electronegativities are related to ionization energies: Elements with low ionization energies will have low electronegativities because their nuclei do not attract electrons strongly, while elements with high ionization energies will have high electronegativities because of the strong pull the nucleus has on electrons. Therefore, electronegativity increases from left to right across periods. In any group, the electronegativity decreases as the atomic number increases, as a result of the increased distance between the valence electrons and the nucleus (i.e., greater atomic radius).

TYPES OF ELEMENTS

The elements of the periodic table may be classified into three categories: **metals**, located on the left side and in the middle of the periodic table; **nonmetals**, located on the right side of the table; and **metalloids** (**semimetals**), found along a diagonal line between the other two.

Metals

Metals are shiny solids (except for mercury) at room temperature and generally have high melting points and densities. Metals have the characteristic ability to be deformed without breaking. The ability of a metal to be hammered into shapes is called **malleability**, and the ability to be drawn into wires is called **ductility**. Many of the characteristic properties of metals, such as large atomic radius, low ionization energy, and low electronegativity, are due to the fact that the few electrons in the valence shell of a metal atom can easily be removed. Because the valence electrons can move freely, metals are good conductors of heat and electricity. Group IA and IIA represent the most reactive metals and will be discussed below. The transition elements, also discussed later, are metals that have partially filled *d* orbitals.

Nonmetals

Nonmetals are generally brittle in the solid state and show little or no metallic luster. They have high ionization energies and electronegativities and are usually poor conductors of heat and electricity. Most nonmetals share the ability to gain electrons easily, but otherwise they display a wide range of chemical behaviors and reactivities. The nonmetals are located on the upper right side of the periodic table; they are separated from the metals by a line cutting diagonally through the region of the periodic table containing elements with partially filled *p* orbitals.

Metalloids

The metalloids or semimetals are found along the line between the metals and nonmetals in the periodic table, and their properties vary considerably. Their densities, boiling points, and melting points fluctuate widely. The electronegativities and ionization energies of metalloids lie between those of metals and nonmetals; therefore, these elements possess characteristics of both those classes. For example, silicon has a metallic luster, yet it is brittle and is not an efficient conductor. The reactivity of metalloids is dependent upon the element with which they are reacting. For example, boron (B) behaves as a nonmetal when reacting with sodium (Na) and as a metal when reacting with fluorine (F). The elements classified as metalloids are boron, silicon, germanium, arsenic, antimony, and tellurium.

THE CHEMISTRY OF GROUPS

Hydrogen

There is no suitable place for hydrogen in the periodic table. Hydrogen does resemble alkali metals because it has a single s valence electron and forms the H^+ ion, which is hydrated in solution. However, it can also form the hydride ion (H^-), which is far too reactive to exist in water. In this respect, hydrogen resembles the halogens.

Alkali metals

The alkali metals are the elements of **Group IA**. They possess most of the physical properties common to metals, yet their densities are lower than those of other metals. The alkali metals have only one loosely bound electron in their outermost shell, giving them the largest atomic radii of all the elements in their respective periods. Their metallic properties and high reactivity are determined by the fact that they have low ionization energies; they easily lose their valence electron to form univalent cations. Alkali metals have low electronegativities and react very readily with nonmetals, especially halogens.

Alkaline Earths

The alkaline earths are the elements of **Group IIA** and also possess many characteristically metallic properties. Like the alkali metals, these properties are dependent upon the ease with which they lose electrons. The alkaline earths have two electrons in their outer shell and thus have smaller atomic radii than the alkali metals. However, the two valence electrons are not held very tightly by the nucleus, so they can be removed to form divalent cations. Alkaline earths have low electronegativities and positive electron affinities.

Halogens

The halogens, **Group VIIA**, are highly reactive nonmetals with seven valence electrons (one short of the favored octet configuration). Halogens are highly variable in their physical properties. For instance, the halogens range from gaseous (F_2 and Cl_2) to liquid (Br_2) to solid (I_2) at room temperature. Their chemical properties are more uniform: the electronegativities of halogens are very high, and they are particularly reactive towards alkali metals and alkaline earths, which "want" to donate electrons to the halogens to form stable ionic crystals. Fluorine (F) has the highest electronegativity of all the elements.

Noble Gases

The noble gases, also called the **inert gases**, are found in **Group VIII** (also called Group O). They are fairly nonreactive because they have a complete valence shell, which is an energetically favored arrangement. This gives them little or no tendency to gain or lose electrons, high ionization energies, and no real electronegativities. They possess low boiling points and are gases at room temperature.

Transition Elements

The transition elements, **groups IB to VIIIB**, are all considered metals; hence, they are also called the **transition metals**. These elements are very hard and have high melting points and boiling points. As one moves across a period, the five d orbitals become progressively more filled. The d electrons are held only loosely by the nucleus and are relatively mobile, contributing to the malleability and high electrical conductivity of these elements. Chemically, transition elements have low ionization energies and may exist in a variety of positively charged forms or **oxidation states**. This is because transition elements are capable of losing various numbers of electrons from the s and d orbitals of their valence shell. Theoretically, the transition metals in Group VIIIB could have eight different oxidation states, from +1 to +8; however, they typically do not exhibit so many. For instance, copper (Cu), in group IB, can exist in either the +1 or the +2 oxidation state, and manganese (Mn), in Group VIIB, occurs in the +2, +3, +4, +6, or +7 state. Because of this ability to attain positive oxidation states, transition metals form many different ionic and partially ionic compounds. The dissolved ions can form **complex ions** either with molecules of water (**hydration complexes**) or with nonmetals, forming highly colored solutions and compounds (e.g., $CuSO_4.5H_2O$, or chalcanthhite), and this complexation may enhance the relatively low solubility of certain compounds (e.g., AgCl is insoluble in water but quite soluble in aqueous ammonia due to the formation of the complex ion $[Ag(NH_3)_2]^+$). The formation of complexes causes the d orbitals to be split into two energy sublevels. This enables many of the complexes to absorb certain frequencies of light—those containing the precise amount of energy required to raise electrons from the lower to the higher d sublevel. The frequencies not absorbed—known as the **subtraction frequencies**—give the complexes their characteristic colors.

REVIEW PROBLEMS

1. Elements in a given period have the same

   (A) atomic weight.
   (B) maximum azimuthal quantum number.
   (C) maximum principal quantum number.
   (D) valence electron structure.
   (E) atomic number.

2. Arrange the following species in terms of increasing atomic (or ionic) radius: Sr, P, Mg, Mg^{2+}.

3. The Ca^{2+} species is electronically similar to the elements in

   (A) Group IIA.
   (B) Group IA.
   (C) Group IVB.
   (D) Group O.

4. What is the electron configuration for the outermost electrons of elements found in Group IVB?

   (A) $s^2 p^6 d^4$
   (B) $s^2 d^2$
   (C) $s^2 d^4$
   (D) $s^2 p^4$
   (E) $s^2 p^2$

5. Which of the following elements has the lowest electronegativity?

   (A) Cesium
   (B) Strontium
   (C) Calcium
   (D) Barium
   (E) Potassium

6. Arrange the following calcium species in terms of increasing size: Ca, Ca^+, Ca^{2+}, Ca^{3+}, Ca^-, Ca^{2-}.

7. The order of the elements in the periodic table is based on

   (A) the number of neutrons.
   (B) the radius of the atom.
   (C) the atomic number.
   (D) the atomic weight.
   (E) the number of oxidation states.

8. The elements within each column of the periodic table
   (A) have similar valence electron configurations.
   (B) have similar atomic radii.
   (C) have the same principal quantum number.
   (D) will react to form stable elements.
   (E) have no similar chemical properties.

9. Discuss the properties of nonmetals and give four examples of nonmetallic elements.

10. Arrange the following elements in terms of increasing first ionization energy: Ga, Ba, Ru, F, N.

11. Explain why the Group O elements are so unreactive.

12. Arrange the following elements in terms of decreasing electronegativity: Ca, Cl, Fr, P, Zn.

13. Which group contains an element with an electron configuration of $1s^2\ 2s^2\ 2p^6\ 3s^2\ 3p^6\ 4s^2\ 3d^{10}\ 4p^6\ 4d^5\ 5s^2$?
    (A) VA
    (B) VIIA
    (C) VB
    (D) VIIB
    (E) VIIIB

14. Discuss the trends in the atomic radii of different elements. How does the atomic number affect the atomic radius of an element?

15. Which element has the greatest electronegativity?
    (A) Chlorine
    (B) Oxygen
    (C) Sulfur
    (D) Phosphorus
    (E) Fluorine

16. The change in energy that occurs when an electron is added to an atom is known as the
    (A) electronegativity.
    (B) metallic character.
    (C) electron affinity.
    (D) ionization energy.
    (E) oxidation state.

17. Discuss the properties of metalloids and give three examples of elements exhibiting metalloid behavior.

18. Which of the following elements is most electronegative?

    (A) S
    (B) Cl
    (C) Na
    (D) Mg
    (E) P

19. Transition metal compounds generally exhibit bright colors because

    (A) the electrons in the partially filled *d* orbitals are easily promoted to excited states.
    (B) the metals become complexed in water.
    (C) the metals conduct electricity, producing colored light.
    (D) the electrons in the *d* orbitals emit energy as they relax.
    (E) their valence electrons cause them to bind to other metals.

20. Discuss the properties of metals and give four examples of metallic elements.

21. Identify the following elements as metal, nonmetal, or semimetal:

    (A) Fr
    (B) Pd
    (C) I
    (D) B
    (E) Sc
    (F) Si
    (G) S

SOLUTIONS TO REVIEW PROBLEMS

1. **C** Discussed in the introduction to this chapter.

2. **Mg 2+ < P < Mg < Sr**

   The trends in atomic radii are as follows. Going from left to right across a period, the atomic radii decrease because the atomic number increases. The increasing number of protons in the nucleus will have a stronger attraction for the outermost electrons, causing them to be held closer and more tightly to the nucleus. Going down a group, the atomic radius will increase because more filled principal energy levels separate the nucleus and the outermost electrons, shielding the attractive force between them. P has a small radius because it lies far to the right and high in a group. The magnesium species will have smaller radii than the strontium species because they are higher in Group II. Finally, positive ions have smaller atomic radii than the corresponding neutral molecules, because the loss of electrons leads to a decrease in electron-electron repulsion within the atom, which in turn allows the electrons to move in closer to the nucleus. Therefore, Mg^{2+} will be smaller than Mg. Mg^{2+} has a smaller radius than P because Mg^{2+} has no electrons in orbitals of the third principal energy level.

3. **D** The Ca^{2+} ion is electronically similar to atoms in Group O because its outermost valence shell is a complete octet. It is isoelectronic to argon.

4. **B** The electron configuration of the different groups can be written as long as a few basic rules are applied. First, the Roman numeral represents the number of electrons that will lie outside of the noble gas core configuration. Second, the letters A and B tell whether the atom is a representative or a nonrepresentative element. Representative elements will successively fill the *s* and *p* orbitals, while the nonrepresentative elements will successively fill the *s*, *d*, and maybe *f* orbitals. Thus, elements in Group IVB are nonrepresentative elements and will have four electrons outside their respective rare gas cores. The correct standard electron configuration for Group IVB elements is thus s^2d^2.

   Using *G* to represent any noble gas, the full electron configuration of a nonspecified group IVB element can be abbreviated as $[G](n-1)d^2ns^2$.

5. **A** The least electronegative elements are located at the bottom left of the periodic table. Cesium has the lowest ionization energy, so it is the least electronegative. Note that Francium (Fr) would be lower still but is is not a stable, naturally occurring element.

6. $Ca^{3+}, Ca^{2+}, Ca^{+}, Ca, Ca^{-}, Ca^{2-}$

   Positive ions will have smaller radii than the corresponding neutral atoms, and the greater the positive charge, the smaller the ionic radius. Negative ions will have larger radii than the corresponding neutral atoms, and the greater the negative charge, the larger the ionic radius (see answer to Question 2, above).

7. **C** Discussed in the introduction to this chapter.

8. **A** Discussed in the introduction to this chapter.

9.   Nonmetals are brittle, lusterless elements possessing high ionization energies and high electronegativities. They tend to gain electrons to form negative ions. They are poor conductors of heat and electricity. The nonmetals are located on the upper right side of the periodic table.

10.   **Ba < Ru < Ga < N < F**

Two common trends should be remembered when ordering atoms according to their ionization energies. First, the ionization energy increases toward the right across a period, because the elements are less willing to give up an electron as the attractive pull (Z_{eff}) of the nucleus increases. Second, the ionization energy decreases down a group, because the distance separating the valence electrons from the nucleus increases. Therefore, to order the elements according to their first ionization energy, it is necessary to go from the bottom left of the periodic table, where the lowest values are, across to the top right of the periodic table, where the highest values are.

11.   Group O elements are also known as the noble, rare, or inert gases. They are very unreactive because their outermost shell contains the complete, stable octet formation. There is no reason for these elements to attempt to gain or lose electrons to other atoms because they are electronically stable on their own.

12.   **Cl > P > Zn > Ca > Fr**

The two trends to remember with electronegativity are that it increases across a period and decreases down a group. Therefore, chlorine, which is farthest to the top and right, will have the highest value. Francium lies farthest to the left and bottom, so it will have the lowest electronegativity.

13. **D**   This element has seven electrons in its outermost shell so its Roman numeral designation is VII; because the *d* orbital is being filled, it is a nonrepresentative, or B, element. Thus, it is found in Group VIIB.

14.   There are two major trends concerning the atomic radii of elements. The first of these is that the atomic radius decreases across a period. This can be explained by the fact that the atomic number (i.e., the number of protons within the nucleus) increases. Thus, the electrostatic force between the valence electrons and the nucleus increases, and the outermost electrons will be pulled closer to the nucleus, making the atom smaller. The second trend concerning atomic radii is that the atomic radius increases down a group. This can be explained by the fact that with every subsequent element down a group, a filled principal energy level has been added. This increases the distance between the nucleus and the valence electrons, as orbital size increases with increasing principal quantum number.

15. **E**   The most electronegative elements are located at the top right of the periodic table.

16. **C**   Discussed in the section on periodic properties.

17.   Metalloids are elements that possess characteristics of both metals and nonmetals. Their electronic characteristics, such as ionization energies and electronegativities, lie between those of the metals and nonmetals. When undergoing reactions, the metalloids may act as either metals or nonmetals depending upon the species with which they are reacting. The elements classified as metalloids are boron, silicon, germanium, arsenic, antimony, and tellurium.

18.   **B**   Chlorine has the greatest electronegativity because, out of all the choices, it lies farthest to the right and top of the periodic table. Chlorine has a great attraction for electrons in a chemical bond because it needs only one more electron to complete a stable octet formation. Therefore, it has a high electronegativity.

19.   **A**   The closely spaced split *d* orbitals allow for relatively low energy transitions; these transitions often occur in the visible region of the electromagnetic spectrum, as do other electronic transitions from the transition metal *d* subshell to other nearby, empty subshells.

20.   Metals are shiny, lustrous solids that have high melting points and densities. The ease with which metals lose electrons contributes to their high thermal and electrical conductivities, their malleability and ductility, and the ease with which they form compounds with reactive nonmetals. All of the elements on the left side of the periodic table (except H) and all of the transition elements are metals.

21.   **A**   Fr: metal

    B   Pd: metal

    C   I: nonmetal

    D   B: semimetal

    E   Sc: metal

    F   Si: semimetal

    G   S: nonmetal

CHAPTER THIRTY

Bonding and Chemical Reactions

The atoms of many elements can combine to form **molecules**. The atoms in most molecules are held together by strong attractive forces called **chemical bonds**. These bonds are formed via the interaction of the valence electrons of the combining atoms. The chemical and physical properties of the resulting molecules are often very different than those of their constituent elements. In addition to the very strong forces within a molecule, there are weaker **intermolecular forces** between molecules. These intermolecular forces, although weaker than the intramolecular chemical bonds, are of considerable importance in understanding the physical properties of many substances.

BONDING

Many molecules contain atoms bonded according to the **octet rule**, which states that an atom tends to bond with other atoms until it has eight electrons in its outermost shell, thereby forming a stable electron configuration similar to that of the Group VIII (noble gas) elements. **Exceptions** to this rule are as follows: **hydrogen**, which can have only two valence electrons (the configuration of He), **lithium** and **beryllium**, which bond to attain two and four valence electrons, respectively; **boron** which bonds to attain six; and elements beyond the second row, such as phosphorus and sulfur, which can expand their octets to include more than eight electrons by incorporating *d* orbitals.

When classifying chemical bonds, it is helpful to introduce two distinct types: ionic bonds and covalent bonds. In **ionic bonding**, an electron(s) from an atom with a smaller ionization energy is transferred to an atom with a greater electron affinity, and the resulting ions are held together by electrostatic forces. In **covalent bonding**, an electron pair is shared between two atoms. In many cases, the bond is partially covalent and partially ionic; we call such bonds **polar covalent bonds**.

IONIC BONDS

When two atoms with large differences in electronegativity react, there is a complete transfer of electrons from the less electronegative atom to the more electronegative atom. The atom that loses electrons becomes a positively charged ion, or **cation**, and the atom that gains electrons becomes a negatively charged ion, or **anion**. For this transfer to occur, the difference in electronegativity must be greater than 1.7. In general, the elements of Groups I and II (low electronegativities) bond ionically to elements of Group VII (high electronegativities). Elements of Groups I and II give up their electrons to achieve a noble gas configuration, while Group VII elements gain an electron to achieve the noble gas configuration. For example, $Na + Cl \longrightarrow Na+ Cl-$ (sodium chloride). The electrostatic force of attraction between the charged ions is called an **ionic** or **electrovalent bond**.

Ionic compounds have characteristic physical properties. They have high melting and boiling points due to the strong electrostatic forces between the ions. They can conduct electricity in the liquid and aqueous states, though not in the solid state. Ionic solids form crystal lattices consisting of infinite arrays of positive and negative ions in which the attractive forces between ions of opposite charge are maximized, while the repulsive forces between ions of like charge are minimized.

COVALENT BONDS

When two or more atoms with similar electronegativities interact, the energy required to form ions is greater than the energy that would be released upon the formation of an ionic bond (i.e., the process is not energetically favorable). However, since a complete transfer of electrons cannot occur, such atoms achieve a noble gas electron configuration by **sharing** electrons in a covalent bond. The binding force between the two atoms results from the attraction that each electron of the shared pair has for the two positive nuclei.

Covalent compounds contain discrete molecular units with weak intermolecular forces. Consequently, they are low-melting solids and do not conduct electricity in the liquid or aqueous states.

Properties of Covalent Bonds

Atoms can share more than one pair of electrons. Two atoms sharing one, two, or three electron pairs are said to be joined by a **single**, **double**, or **triple covalent bond**, respectively. The number of shared electron pairs between two atoms is called the **bond order**; hence a single bond has a bond order of one, a double bond has a bond order of two, and a triple bond has a bond order of three.

A covalent bond can be characterized by two features: bond length and bond energy.

Bond length

Bond length is the average distance between the two nuclei of the atoms involved in the bond. As the number of shared electron pairs increases, the two atoms are pulled closer together, leading to a decrease in bond length. Thus, for a given pair of atoms, a triple bond is shorter than a double bond, which is shorter than a single bond.

Bond energy

Bond energy is the energy required to separate two bonded atoms. For a given pair of atoms, the strength of a bond (and therefore the bond energy) increases as the number of shared electron pairs increases. (Bond energy is further discussed in Chapter 33, Thermochemistry.)

Covalent Bond Notation

The shared valence electrons of a covalent bond are called the **bonding electrons**. The valence electrons not involved in the covalent bond are called **nonbonding electrons**. The unshared electron pairs can also be called **lone electron pairs**. A convenient notation, called a **Lewis structure**, is used to represent the bonding and nonbonding electrons in a molecule, facilitating chemical "bookkeeping." The number of valence electrons attributed to a particular atom in the Lewis structure of a molecule is not necessarily the same as the number would be in the isolated atom, and the difference accounts for what is referred to as the **formal charge** of that atom. Often, more than one Lewis structure can be drawn for a molecule; this phenomenon is called **resonance**. Lewis structures, formal charge, and resonance are discussed in detail below.

Lewis structures

When different atoms interact to form a bond, only their outermost regions come in contact. Hence, only the valence electrons are involved. One of the easiest ways to follow the valence electrons in a chemical reaction is with **Lewis dot symbols**. A Lewis dot symbol contains the symbol of an element and one "dot" for each valence electron in an atom. For example, sodium (Na) is a Group 1A element and has one valence electron. The first ionization can be written in the following manner:

$$\cdot Na \lozenge Na^+ + e^-$$

Magnesium, for example, belongs to Group 2A and has two valence electrons (:Mg) and so on. Note: Because the transitional metals lanthanides and actinides all have incompletely filled inner shells, Lewis dot symbols are not written for these elements.

·Li	Lithium	$\ddot{N}$	Nitrogen
·Be·	Beryllium	·Ö:	Oxygen
·B·	Boron	·F̈:	Fluorine
·Ċ·	Carbon	:N̈e:	Neon

Just as a Lewis symbol is used to represent the distribution of valence electrons in an atom, it can also be used to represent the distribution of valence electrons in a molecule. For example, the Lewis symbol of an F ion is :F̈:⁻ ; the Lewis structure of an F_2 molecule is :F̈—F̈: .

Certain steps must be followed in assigning a Lewis structure to a molecule. These steps are outlined below, using HCN as an example.

Write the skeletal structure of the compound (i.e., the arrangement of atoms). In general, the least electronegative atom is the central atom. Hydrogen (always) and the halogens F, Cl, Br, and I (usually) occupy the end position.

In HCN, H must occupy an end position. Of the remaining two atoms, C is the least electronegative and therefore occupies the central position. The skeletal structure is as follows:

$$H—C—N$$

Count all the valence electrons of the atoms. The number of valence electrons of the molecule is the sum of the valence electrons of all atoms present:

> H has 1 valence electron;
>
> C has 4 valence electrons;
>
> N has 5 valence electrons; therefore,
>
> HCN has a total of 10 valence electrons.

Draw single bonds between the central atom and the atoms surrounding it. Place an electron pair in each bond (bonding electron pair).

$$H:C:N$$

Each bond has 2 electrons, so $10 - 4 = 6$ valence electrons remain.

Complete the octets (8 valence electrons) of all atoms bonded to the central atom, using the remaining valence electrons still to be assigned. (Recall that H is an exception to the octet rule since it can have only 2 valence electrons.) In this example H already has 2 valence electrons in its bond with C.

Place any extra electrons on the central atom. If the central atom has less than an octet, try to write double or triple bonds between the central and surrounding atoms using the nonbonding, unshared lone electron pairs.

$$H:C:\ddot{\underset{\cdot\cdot}{N}}:$$

The HCN structure above does not satisfy the octet rule for C because C possesses only 4 valence electrons. Therefore, 2 lone electron pairs from the N atom must be moved to form two more bonds with C, creating a triple bond between C and N. Finally, bonds are drawn as lines rather than pairs of dots.

$$H–C{\equiv}N:$$

Now, the octet rule is satisfied for all three atoms because C and N have 8 valence electrons and H has 2 valence electrons.

Formal charges

The number of electrons officially assigned to an atom in a Lewis structure does not always equal the number of valence electrons of the free atom. The difference between these two numbers is the **formal charge** of the atom. Formal charge can be calculated using the following formula:

$$\text{Formal charge} = V - \frac{1}{2} N_{bonding} - N_{nonbonding}$$

where V is the number of valence electrons in the free atom, $N_{bonding}$ is the number of bonding electrons, and $N_{nonbonding}$ is the number of nonbonding electrons.

The formal charge of an ion or molecule is equal to the sum of the formal charges of the individual atoms comprising the ion or molecule.

Example: Calculate the formal charge on the central N atom of $[NH_4]^+$.

Solution: The Lewis structure of $[NH_4]^+$ is

$$\begin{bmatrix} & H & \\ & | & \\ H - & N & - H \\ & | & \\ & H & \end{bmatrix}^+$$

Nitrogen is in group VA; thus, it has 5 valence electrons. In $[NH_4]^+$, N has 4 bonds (i.e., 8 bonding electrons and no nonbonding electrons).

So $V = 5$; $N_{bonding} = 8$; $N_{nonbonding} = 0$

Formal charge $= 5 - \dfrac{1}{2}(8) - 0 = +1$

Thus, the formal charge on the N atom in $[NH_4]^+$ is +1.

Resonance

For some molecules, two or more nonidentical Lewis structures can be drawn; these are called **resonance structures**. A resonance structure is one of two or more Lewis structures for a single molecule that is unable to be described fully with only one Lewis structure. Furthermore, the term *resonance* actually means using two or more Lewis structures to represent a given molecule. The molecule doesn't actually exist as either one of the resonance structures but is rather a composite, or hybrid, of the two. For example, SO_2 has three resonance structures, two of which are minor: $O = S—O$ and $O—S = O$. The actual molecule is a hybrid of these three structures (spectral data indicate that the two S—O bonds are identically equivalent). This phenomenon is known as resonance, and the actual structure of the molecule is called the **resonance hybrid**. Resonance structures are expressed with a double-headed arrow between them:

$$\ddot{O} = \ddot{S} = \ddot{O} \longleftrightarrow \ddot{O} = \ddot{S} - \ddot{O}: \longleftrightarrow :\ddot{O} - \ddot{S} = \ddot{O}$$

represents the resonance structures of SO_2.

The last two resonance structures of sulfur dioxide shown above have equivalent energy or stability. Often, nonequivalent resonance structures may be written for a molecule. In these cases, the more stable the structure, the more that structure contributes to the character of the resonance hybrid. Conversely, the less stable the resonance structure, the less that structure contributes to the resonance hybrid. The structure on the left of the diagram is the most stable. Formal charges are often useful for qualitatively assessing the stability of a particular resonance structure, and the following guidelines are used.

- A Lewis structure with small or no formal charges is preferred over a Lewis structure with large formal charges.
- A Lewis structure in which negative formal charges are placed on more electronegative atoms is more stable than one in which the formal charges are placed on less electronegative atoms.

Example: Write the resonance structures for [NCO]⁻.

Solution: C is the least electronegative of the three given atoms, N, C, and O. Therefore the C atom occupies the central position in the skeletal structure of [NCO]⁻.

N C O

N has 5 valence electrons;

C has 4 valence electrons;

O has 6 valence electrons; and the species itself has one negative charge.

Total valence electrons = 5 + 4 + 6 + 1 = 16

Draw single bonds between the central C atom and the surrounding atoms, N and O. Place a pair of electrons in each bond.

N:C:O

Complete the octets of N and O with the remaining 16 − 4 = 12 electrons.

:N̈:C:Ö:

The C octet is incomplete. There are three ways in which double and triple bonds can be formed to complete the C octet. Two lone pairs from the O atom can be used to form a triple bond between the C and O atoms:

:N̈—C≡O:

Or one lone electron pair can be taken from both the O and the N atoms to form two double bonds, one between N and C and the other between O and C:

:N̈=C=Ö:

Or two lone electron pairs can be taken from the N atom to form a triple bond between the C and N atoms:

:N≡C—Ö:

These three are all resonance structures of [NCO]⁻.

Assign formal charges to each atom of each resonance structure.

The most stable structure is:

:N≡C—Ö:

since the negative formal charge is on the most electronegative atom, O.

Exceptions to the octet rule

Atoms found in or beyond the third period can have more than eight valence electrons, since some of the valence electrons may occupy *d* orbitals. These atoms can be assigned more than four bonds in Lewis structures. When drawing the Lewis structure of the sulfate ion, for example, giving the sulfur 12 valence electrons permits three of the five atoms to be assigned a formal charge of zero. The sulfate ion can be drawn in six resonance forms, each with the two double bonds attached to a different combination of oxygen atoms.

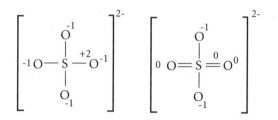

Figure 30.1

Types of Covalent Bonding

The nature of a covalent bond depends on the relative electronegativities of the atoms sharing the electron pairs. Covalent bonds are considered to be polar or nonpolar depending on the difference in electronegativities between the atoms.

Polar covalent bond

Polar covalent bonding occurs between atoms with small differences in electronegativity, generally in the range of 0.4 to 1.7 Pauling units. The bonding electron pair is not shared equally but is pulled more towards the element with the higher electronegativity. As a result, the more electronegative atom acquires a partial negative charge, d–, and the less electronegative atom acquires a partial positive charge, d+, giving the molecule a partially ionic character. For instance, the covalent bond in HCl is polar because the two atoms have a small difference in electronegativity (approx. 0.9). Chlorine, the more electronegative atom, attains a partial negative charge, and hydrogen attains a partial positive charge. This difference in charge between the atoms is indicated by an arrow crossed (like a plus sign) at the positive end pointing to the negative end, as shown below.

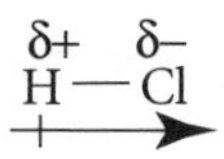

$$\overset{\delta+}{H} - \overset{\delta-}{Cl}$$

Figure 30.2

A molecule that has such a separation of positive and negative charges is called a **polar molecule**. The **dipole moment** itself is a vector quantity μ, defined as the product of the charge magnitude (q) and the distance between the two partial charges (r):

$$\mu = qr$$

The dipole moment is denoted by an arrow pointing from the positive to the negative charge and is measured in **Debye units** (coulomb-meters).

Nonpolar covalent bond

Nonpolar covalent bonding occurs between atoms that have the same electronegativities. The bonding electron pair is shared equally, with no separation of charge across the bond. Not surprisingly, nonpolar covalent bonds occur in diatomic molecules such as H_2, Cl_2, O_2, and N_2.

Coordinate covalent bond

In a coordinate covalent bond, the shared electron pair comes from the lone pair of one of the atoms in the molecule. Once such a bond forms, it is indistinguishable from any other covalent bond. Distinguishing such a bond is useful only in keeping track of the valence electrons and formal charges. Coordinate bonds are typically found in Lewis acid-base compounds (see Chapter 37, Acids and Bases). A **Lewis acid** is a compound that can accept an electron pair to form a covalent bond; a **Lewis base** is a compound that can donate an electron pair to form a covalent bond. For example, in the reaction between borontrifluoride (BF_3) and ammonia (NH_3):

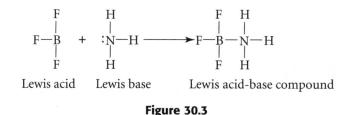

Lewis acid   Lewis base   Lewis acid-base compound

Figure 30.3

NH_3 donates a pair of electrons to form a coordinate covalent bond; thus, it acts as a Lewis base. BF3 accepts this pair of electrons to form the coordinate covalent bond; thus, it acts as a Lewis acid.

Geometry and Polarity of Covalent Molecules

The valence shell electron-pair repulsion theory

The valence shell electron-pair repulsion (VSEPR) theory uses Lewis structures to predict the molecular geometry of covalently bonded molecules. It states that the three-dimensional arrangement of atoms surrounding a central atom is determined by the repulsions between the bonding and the nonbonding electron pairs in the valence shell of the central atom. These electron pairs arrange themselves as far apart as possible, thereby minimizing repulsion.

The following steps are used to predict the geometrical structure of a molecule using the VSEPR theory:

1. Draw the Lewis structure of the molecule.
2. Count the total number of bonding and nonbonding electron pairs in the valence shell of the central atom.
3. Arrange the electron pairs around the central atom so that they are as far apart from each other as possible. For example, the compound AX2 has the Lewis structure, X : A : X. A has two bonding electron pairs in its valence shell. To make these electron pairs as far apart as possible, their geometric structure should be linear:

$$X - A - X$$

Valence electron arrangements are summarized in the following table.

regions of electron density	example	geometric arrangement of electron pairs around the central atom	shape	angle between electron pairs
2	$BeCl_2$	X—A—X	linear	$180°$
3	BH_3		trigonal planar	$120°$
4	CH_4		tetrahedral	$109.5°$
5	PCl_5		trigonal bipyramidal	$90°, 120°, 180°$
6	SF_6		octahedral	$90°, 180°$

Example: Predict the geometry of NH_3.

Solution: The Lewis structure of NH_3 is:

$$H-\underset{..}{N}-H$$
with an H above N

The central atom, N, has three bonding electron pairs and one nonbonding electron pair, for a total of four electron pairs.

The four electron pairs will be farthest apart when they occupy the corners of a tetrahedron. Since one of the four electron pairs is a lone pair, the observed geometry is trigonal bipyramidal.

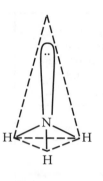

Figure 30.4

In describing the shape of a molecule, only the arrangement of atoms (not electrons) is considered. Even though the electron pairs are arranged tetrahedrally, the shape of NH_3 is pyramidal. It is not trigonal planar because the lone pair repels the three bonding electron pairs, causing them to move as far away as possible.

Example: Predict the geometry of CO_2.

Solution: The Lewis structure of CO_2 is $:O::C::O:$.

The double bond behaves just like a single bond for purposes of predicting molecular shape. This compound has two groups of electrons around the carbon. According to the VSEPR theory, the two sets of electrons will orient themselves 180° apart, on opposite sides of the carbon atom, minimizing electron repulsion. Therefore, the molecular structure of CO_2 is linear: $:O=C=O:$

Polarity of molecules

A molecule with a net dipole moment is called polar, as previously mentioned, because it has positive and negative poles. The polarity of a molecule depends on the polarity of the constituent bonds and on the shape of the molecule. A molecule with nonpolar bonds is always nonpolar; a molecule with polar bonds may be polar or nonpolar depending on the orientation of the bond dipoles.

A molecule of two atoms bound by a polar bond must have a net dipole moment and therefore be polar. The two equal and opposite partial charges are localized at the ends of the molecule on the two atoms. A molecule consisting of more than two atoms bound with polar bonds may be either polar or nonpolar, since the overall dipole moment of a molecule is the vector sum of the individual bond dipole moments. If the molecule has a particular shape such that the bond dipole moments cancel each other (i.e., if the vector sum is zero), then the result is a nonpolar molecule. For instance, CCl_4 has four polar C-Cl bonds. According to the VSEPR theory, the shape of CCl_4 is tetrahedral. The four bond dipoles point to the vertices of the tetrahedron and cancel each other, resulting in a nonpolar molecule.

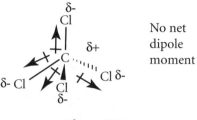

No net
dipole
moment

Figure 30.5

However, if the orientation of the bond dipoles are such that they do not cancel out, the molecules will have a net dipole moment and therefore be polar. For instance, H_2O has two polar O–H bonds. According to the VSEPR model, its shape is angular. The two dipoles add together to give a net dipole moment to the molecule, making the H_2O molecule polar.

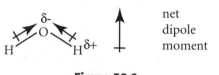

net
dipole
moment

Figure 30.6

Atomic and Molecular Orbitals

A description of the quantum numbers has already been given in Chapter 28. The azimuthal quantum number ℓ describes the orbitals of each n shell. The shapes of these orbitals represent the probability of finding an electron at any given instant. When $\ell = 0$, the orbital is an *s* orbital, and *s* orbitals are spherically symmetric. The 1*s* orbital (n =1, $\ell = 0$) is plotted below.

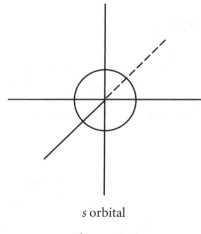

s orbital

Figure 30.7

When $\ell = 1$, there are three possible orbitals (since the magnetic quantum number, m_ℓ, may equal –1, 0, or 1). These are called *p* orbitals and have a dumbbell shape. The three *p* orbitals, designated p_x, p_y, and p_z, are oriented at right angles to each other; the p_x orbital is plotted below.

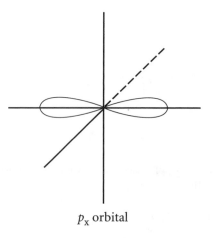

p_x orbital

Figure 30.8

Plus and minus signs, determined from the mathematics of the wave function, are assigned to each lobe of the *p* orbitals. The shapes of the five d orbitals ($\ell = 2$, m$\ell = -2, -1, 0, 1, 2$) and the seven *f* orbitals ($\ell = 3$, m$\ell = -3, -2, -1, 0, 1, 2, 3$) are more complex and need not be memorized. When two atoms bond to form a molecule, the atomic orbitals interact to form a molecular orbital that describes the probability of finding the bonding electrons. Molecular orbitals are obtained by adding the wave functions of the atomic orbitals. Qualitatively, this is described by the overlap of two atomic orbitals. If the signs of the two atomic orbitals are the same, a **bonding orbital** is formed. If the signs are different, an **antibonding orbital** is formed. In addition, two different types of overlap are possible. When orbitals overlap head-to-head, the resulting bond is called a **sigma (s) bond**. When the orbitals are parallel, a **pi (p) bond** is formed.

THE INTERMOLECULAR FORCES

The attractive forces that exist between molecules are collectively known as intermolecular forces. These include **dipole-ion interactions**, **dipole-dipole interactions**, **hydrogen bonding**, and **dispersion forces**. In order of decreasing strength, these are as follows:

dipole-ion > hydrogen bonding > dipole-dipole > dispersion (London) forces

Dipole-Dipole Interactions

Polar molecules tend to orient themselves such that the positive region of one molecule is close to the negative region of another molecule. This arrangement is energetically favorable because an attractive dipole force is formed between the two molecules.

Dipole-dipole interactions are present in the solid and liquid phases but become negligible in the gas phase because the molecules are generally much farther apart. Polar species tend to have higher boiling points than nonpolar species of comparable molecular weight.

Hydrogen Bonding

Hydrogen bonding is a specific, unusually strong form of dipole-dipole interaction, which may be either intra- or intermolecular. When hydrogen is bound to a highly electronegative atom such as fluorine, oxygen, or nitrogen, the hydrogen atom carries little of the electron density of the covalent bond. This positively charged hydrogen atom interacts with the partial negative charge located on the electronegative atoms of nearby molecules. Substances that display hydrogen bonding tend to have unusually high boiling points compared with compounds of similar molecular formula that do not hydrogen bond. The difference derives from the energy required to break the hydrogen bonds. Hydrogen bonding is particularly important in the behavior of water, alcohols, amines, and carboxylic acids (see Chapter 40, Organic Chemistry, for further discussion).

Dispersion Forces

The bonding electrons in covalent bonds may appear to be shared equally between two atoms, but at any particular point in time, they will be located randomly throughout the orbital. This permits unequal sharing of electrons, causing rapid polarization and counterpolarization of the electron cloud and formation of short-lived dipoles. These dipoles interact with the electron clouds of neighboring molecules, inducing the formation of more dipoles. The attractive interactions of these short-lived dipoles are called dispersion or **London forces**.

Dispersion forces are generally weaker than other intermolecular forces. They do not extend over long distances and are therefore most important when molecules are close together. The strength of these interactions within a given substance depends directly on how easily the electrons in the molecules can move (i.e., be polarized). Large molecules in which the electrons are far from the nucleus are relatively easy to polarize and therefore possess greater dispersion forces. If not for dispersion forces, the noble gases would not liquefy at any temperature since no other intermolecular forces exist between the noble gas atoms. The low temperature at which the noble gases liquefy is to some extent indicative of the magnitude of dispersion forces between the atoms.

Carbon-Carbon Bonding

Carbon-carbon bonds can be categorized based on length and energy level, as well as hybridization. In Chapter 40 we will review the hybridization of carbon-carbon bonds. The table below compares the bond length and energy levels of the different carbon-carbon bonds.

	Bond Length	**Bond Energy**
C–C	longest	lowest
C=C	middle	middle
C≡C	shortest	highest

REVIEW PROBLEMS

1. Is Cl– an anion or a cation?

2. Consider the following reaction:

$$H_2\ (g) + F_2\ (g) \longrightarrow 2\ HF\ (g)$$

Is the HF bond more or less polar than an H—H bond?

3. Arrange the following compounds in terms of increasing polarity:

$$HCN,\ NaCl,\ Cl_2$$

4. (A) Which has a greater C–C bond distance, C_2H_4 or C_2H_2?
   (B) Which has a greater C–C bond energy?

5. Which of the following compounds would you expect to be weakly drawn into a magnetic field?

$$H_2,\ NaCl,\ NO,\ NO_2,\ BF_3,\ PCl_5,\ SO_2$$

6. Which represents the proper Lewis structure of
   (A) $CHCl_3$?

   1.

   $$H:\overset{..}{\underset{..}{C}}l:$$

   2. $H=\overset{..}{C}-\overset{..}{\underset{..}{C}}l-\overset{..}{\underset{..}{C}}l-\overset{..}{\underset{..}{C}}l:$

   3.

   4.

(**B**) N$_2$?

1. N≡N

2. N̈=N̈

3. :N̈=N̈:

4. Ṅ≡Ṅ

(**C**) [ClO$_4$]$^-$?

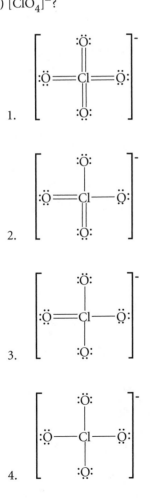

7. Which is not a resonance form of

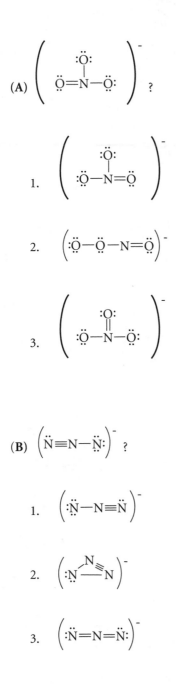

(A) $\left(\begin{array}{c} :\ddot{O}: \\ | \\ \ddot{O}=N-\ddot{O}: \end{array} \right)^{-}$?

1. $\left(\begin{array}{c} :\ddot{O}: \\ | \\ :\ddot{O}-N=\ddot{O} \end{array} \right)^{-}$

2. $\left(:\ddot{O}-\ddot{O}-N=\ddot{O} \right)^{-}$

3. $\left(\begin{array}{c} :O: \\ \| \\ :\ddot{O}-N-\ddot{O}: \end{array} \right)^{-}$

(B) $\left(\ddot{N}\equiv N-\ddot{N}: \right)^{-}$?

1. $\left(:\ddot{N}-N\equiv\ddot{N} \right)^{-}$

2. $\left(:\ddot{N}\overset{N\!\!\equiv}{\diagup\!\!\diagdown}N \right)^{-}$

3. $\left(:\ddot{N}=N=\ddot{N}: \right)^{-}$

8. Label formal charges and predict which is the most likely resonance structure for N_2O.

   (A) $:N≡N=\ddot{O}:$

   (B) $:\ddot{N}=O=\ddot{N}:$

   (C) $:\ddot{N}=N=\ddot{O}:$

   (D) $:N≡N-\ddot{\underset{..}{O}}:$

9. Draw Lewis structures of the most likely ions of the elements from Na to Ca.

10. Draw Lewis structures for each of the following:
    (A) Nitrate ion ($[NO_3]^-$)
    (B) Phosphoric acid (H_3PO_4)
    (C) Aluminum chloride ($AlCl_3$)
    (D) Sodium phosphate (Na_3PO_4)

11. A hydride is a compound containing hydride ion, H^-. Predict two elements whose hydrides would contain incomplete octets.

12. Which of the following sets of molecules contains only nonpolar species?
    (A) BH_3, NH_3, AlH_3
    (B) NO_2, CO_2, ClO_2
    (C) HCl, HNO_2, $HClO_3$
    (D) BH_3, H_2S, BCl_3
    (E) BeH_2, BH_3, CH_4

13. Arrange the following compounds in order of increasing boiling point: C_2H_6, CH_3OH, LiF, HCl.

SOLUTIONS TO REVIEW PROBLEMS

1. Cl– is an anion. Negative ions are called anions, and positive ions are called cations.

2. The HF bond is more polar than an H – H bond. *Polar* denotes unequal sharing of electrons; H—H must have equal sharing because the two atoms are the same. H and F are different atoms, with different electronegativities, and so the electrons are unequally shared.

3. $Cl_2 < HCN < NaCl$

    Cl_2 is the least polar because it contains two identical atoms that must share electrons equally. HCN is a linear molecule with a triple bond between C and N; it has a dipole moment pointing from the relatively electropositive H atom toward the rather electronegative N atom. Still, we should expect HCN to be less polar than NaCl; the bond between Na and Cl, a metal and a nonmetal whose electronegativities differ greatly, is completely ionic.

4. A C_2H_4 has greater bond distance because it is a double bond and is therefore held less closely than C_2H_2, which is a triple bond.

    B C_2H_2 has a greater bond energy because it is a triple bond and more energy is needed to break it.

5. NO and NO_2 would be weakly drawn into a magnetic field because they are paramagnetic. All paramagnetic molecules are weakly drawn into a magnetic field, and any compound with an odd number of valence electrons is paramagnetic. Thus:

    NO: N has 5 valence electrons, O has 6; 6 + 5 = 11, so NO is paramagnetic.

    NO_2: 5 + (2)(6) = 17, so NO_2 is paramagnetic.

    BF_3: B has 3 valence electrons, F has 7; 3 + 3(7) = 24, so BF_3 is not paramagnetic.

6. A 4

    Choice 4 is correct. Choice 2 has an impossible configuration; H can never be double-bonded to anything since the maximum number of electrons it may possess is 2. Choice 3 is also impossible since having four bonds around H would imply 8 electrons.

    B 2

    Choices 1 and 3 must be wrong because, although they satisfy the octet rule, they have the wrong total number of electrons; choice 1 has 8 valence electrons, whereas choice 3 has 12. Given two N atoms, there can be (2)(5) = 10 valence electrons, as in correct choice 2. (Choice 1 is also wrong because quadruple bonding is impossible due to orbital geometries.) Choice 4 is doubly wrong because, in addition to only having 8 total electrons, the octet rule is not satisfied as each nucleus has 7, not 8, valence electrons.

    C 4

    Choice 4 is the preferred structure because four of the five atoms have a formal charge of zero. Since Cl is in the third period, its number of valence electrons can exceed 8.

7. **A** 2

    In resonance forms, only the electrons change place; atoms are not rearranged. Choices 1 and 3 are both resonance structures. Choice 2 requires rearrangement of the atoms.

    B 2

    By the same reasoning as above.

8. **D** There is no formal charge on the structure of choice A; therefore, this structure should be the more likely resonance structure. However, the expanded octet on N makes the structure impossible. Choice C is incorrect because the negative formal charge is on N, which is not the most electronegative atom. Choice B is incorrect because O, which is the most electronegative atom, has a formal charge of +2. Choice D is most likely because the negative formal charge is on O, the more electronegative element.

9. Na^+ Mg^{2+} Al^{3+} Si^{4+} $:\ddot{P}:^{3-}$ $:\ddot{S}:^{2-}$ $:\ddot{Cl}:^-$ (**Ar has none**)
      K^+ Ca^{2+}

     Note that a correct ionic Lewis structure must always show the charge on the ion.

10. **A** $[NO_3]^-$

	has	needs
charge:	1 electron	
N:	5 electrons	8 electrons
3 O:	18 electrons	24 electrons
	24 electrons	32 electrons

    $(32 - 24)$ electrons = 8 electrons = 4 bonds

    Place N at the center:

    (N and O both have a formal charge.)

They cannot be reduced because the N octet cannot be expanded. However, since resonance will be present, a better version might be:

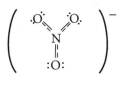

B H_3PO_4

	has	needs
3 H	3 electrons	3(2) = 6 electrons
P	5 electrons	8 electrons (at least)
4 O	24 electrons	32 electrons
	32 electrons	46 electrons

(46 − 32) electrons = 14 electrons = 7 bonds (at least).

Place the P at the center, the 4 oxygens around it, and hydrogens on 3 of the oxygens with single bonds between them; this will use all 7 bonds.

Now check the formal charges:

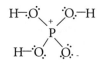

The P has a formal charge of +1 and the O has a formal charge of −1. These can be eliminated by moving a pair of electrons around from the O into a second bond:

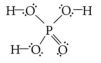

C   Both aluminum chloride and sodium phosphate are ionic.

$AlCl_3$

$$\left(:\ddot{C}l:\right)^-$$

$$Al^{+3} \qquad \left(:\ddot{C}l:\right)^-$$

$$\left(:\ddot{C}l:\right)^-$$

D Na_3PO_4

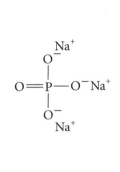

11.   Be and B, because they can join to only two or three hydrogens, respectively, since they have fewer than 4 valence electrons. The elements Mg and Al may also do this, as could Na, Ca, and the other active metals of groups I and II.

12. **E**

   A. NH_3 is polar (positive end at base of pyramid, negative end at N).

   B. NO_2 and ClO_2 are both angular molecules; therefore, it is polar.

   C. All three are polar.

   D. H_2S is angular due to the two lone pairs on S; therefore, it is polar.

13. C_2H_6, HCl, CH_3OH, LiF
       C_2H_6: van der Waals (dispersion)
       HCl: dipole-dipole
       CH_3OH: H-bonding
       LiF: ionic

CHAPTER THIRTY-ONE

Compounds and Stoichiometry

A **compound** is a pure substance that is composed of two or more elements in a fixed proportion. Compounds can be broken down chemically to produce their constituent elements or other compounds. All elements, except for some of the noble gases, can react with other elements or compounds to form new compounds. These new compounds can react further to form yet different compounds.

MOLECULES AND MOLES

A molecule is a combination of two or more atoms held together by covalent bonds. It is the smallest unit of a compound displaying the properties of that compound. Molecules may contain two atoms of the same element, as in N_2 and O_2, or may be comprised of two or more different atoms, as in CO_2 and $SOCl_2$. Molecules are usually discussed in terms of **molecular weights** and **moles**.

Ionic compounds do not form true molecules. In the solid state, they can be considered to be a nearly infinite, three-dimensional array of the charged particles of which the compound is composed. Because no actual molecule exists, molecular weight becomes meaningless, and the term **formula weight** is used in its place.

Molecular Weight

Like atoms, molecules can be characterized by their weight. The molecular weight is the sum of the atomic weights (in amu) of the atoms in the molecule. Similarly, the formula weight of an ionic compound is found by adding up the atomic weights according to the empirical formula of the substance.

Example: What is the molecular weight of $SOCl_2$?

Solution: To find the molecular weight of $SOCl_2$, add together the atomic weights of each of the atoms.

$$1S \ = \ 1 \times 32 \text{ amu} \ = \ 32 \text{ amu}$$
$$1O \ = \ 1 \times 16 \text{ amu} \ = \ 16 \text{ amu}$$
$$2Cl \ = \ 2 \times 35.5 \text{ amu} \ = \ \underline{71 \text{ amu}}$$
$$\text{molecular weight} \ = \ 119 \text{ amu}$$

Mole

A mole is defined as the amount of a substance that contains the same number of particles that is found in a 12.000 g sample of carbon-12. This quantity, **Avogadro's number,** is equal to 6.022×10^{23}. One mole of a compound has a mass in grams equal to the molecular weight of that compound in amu and contains 6.022×10^{23} molecules of the compound. For example, 62 g of H_2CO_3 represents one mole of carbonic acid and contains 6.022×10^{23} H_2CO_3 molecules. The mass of 1 mole of a compound is called its **molar weight** or **molar mass** and is usually expressed as g/mol. Therefore, the molar mass of H_2CO_3 is 62 g/mol.

The following formula is used to determine the number of moles present:

$$\text{Mol} = \frac{\textbf{Weight of Sample(g)}}{\textbf{Molar Weight (g/mol)}}$$

Example: How many moles are in 9.52 g of $MgCl_2$?

Solution: First find the molar mass of $MgCl_2$.

1(24.31 g/mol) + 2(35.45 g/mol) = 95.21 g/mol

Now solve for the number of moles.

$$\frac{9.52}{95.21 \text{ g/mol}} = 0.10 \text{ mol of } MgCl_2$$

Equivalent Weight

For some substances, it is useful to define a measure of reactive capacity. This expresses the fact that some molecules are more potent than others in performing certain reactions. An example of this is the ability of different acids to donate protons (H^+ ions) in solution (see Chapter 37, Acids and Bases). For instance, 1 mole of HCl can donate 1 mol of hydrogen ions, while 1 mol of H_2SO_4 can donate 2 moles of hydrogen ions. This difference is expressed using the term **equivalent:** 1 mole of HCl contains 1 equivalent of hydrogen ions while 1 mol of H_2SO_4 contains 2 equivalents of hydrogen ions. To determine the number of equivalents a compound contains, a new measure of weight, called **gram-equivalent weight (GEW),** was developed.

$$\text{equivalents} = \frac{\textbf{weight of compound}}{\textbf{gram equivalent weight}}$$

and

$$\text{gram equivalent weight} = \frac{\textbf{molar mass}}{\textbf{\textit{n}}}$$

where n is usually either the number of **hydrogens** used per molecule of acid in a reaction or the number of **hydroxyl groups** used per molecule of base in a reaction. This value is strictly dependent on reaction conditions. By using equivalents, it is possible to say that one equivalent of acid will neutralize one equivalent of base, a statement that may not necessarily be true when dealing with moles.

REPRESENTATION OF COMPOUNDS

Law of Constant Composition

The law of constant composition states that any sample of a given compound will contain the same elements in the identical mass ratio. For instance, every sample of H_2O will contain two atoms of hydrogen for every atom of oxygen or, in other words, one gram of hydrogen for every eight grams of oxygen.

Empirical and Molecular Formulas

There are two ways to express a formula for a compound. The **empirical formula** gives the simplest whole number ratio of the elements in the compound. The **molecular formula** gives the exact number of atoms of each element in the compound and is usually a multiple of the empirical formula. For example, the empirical formula for benzene is CH, whereas the molecular formula is C_6H_6. For some compounds, the empirical and molecular formulas are the same, as in the case of H_2O. An ionic compound, such as NaCl or $CaCO_3$, will have only an empirical formula.

Percent Composition

The percent composition by mass of an element is the weight percent of the element in a specific compound. To determine the percent composition of an element X in a compound, the following formula is used:

$$\text{\% Composition} = \frac{\text{Mass of X in Formula}}{\text{Formula Weight of Compound}} \times 100\%$$

The percent composition of an element may be determined using either the empirical or molecular formula. If the percent compositions are known, the empirical formula can be derived. It is possible to determine the molecular formula if both the percent compositions and molecular weight of the compound are known.

Example: What is the percent composition of chromium in $K_2Cr_2O_7$?

Solution: The formula weight of $K_2Cr_2O_7$ is:
2(39 g/mol) + 2(52 g/mol) + 7(16 g/mol) = 294 g/mol

$$\text{\% composition of Cr} = \frac{2(52 \text{ g/mol})}{294 \text{ g/mol}} \times 100\%$$

$$= 0.354 \times 100\%$$

$$= 35.4\%$$

Example: What are the empirical and molecular formulas of a compound that contains 40.9% carbon, 4.58% hydrogen, and 54.52% oxygen and has a molecular weight of 264 g/mol?

Method One: First, determine the number of moles of each element in the compound by assuming a 100-gram sample; this converts the percentage of each element present directly into grams of that element. Then convert grams to moles:

$$\text{\# mol of C} = \frac{40.9 \text{ g}}{12 \text{ g/mol}} = 3.41 \text{ mol}$$

$$\text{\# mol of H} = \frac{4.58 \text{ g}}{1 \text{ g/mol}} = 4.58 \text{ mol}$$

$$\text{\# mol of O} = \frac{54.52 \text{ g}}{16 \text{ g/mol}} = 3.41 \text{ mol}$$

Next, find the simplest whole number ratio of the elements by dividing the number of moles by the smallest number obtained in the previous step:

$$\text{C:} \frac{3.41}{3.41} = 1.00 \qquad \text{H:} \frac{4.58}{3.41} = 1.33 \qquad \text{O:} \frac{3.41}{3.41} = 1.00$$

Finally, the empirical formula is obtained by converting the numbers obtained into whole numbers (multiplying them by an integer value).

$$C_1H_{1.33}O_1 \times 3 = C_3H_4O_3$$

$C_3H_4O_3$ is the empirical formula. To determine the molecular formula, divide the molecular weight by the weight represented by the empirical formula. The resultant value is the number of empirical formula units in the molecular formula.

The empirical formula weight of $C_3H_4O_3$ is:

$3(12 \text{ g/mol}) + 4(1 \text{ g/mol}) + 3(16 \text{ g/mol}) = 88 \text{ g/mol}$

$$\frac{264 \text{ g/mol}}{88 \text{ g/mol}} = 3$$

$C_3H_4O_3 \times 3 = C_9H_{12}O_9$ is the molecular formula.

Method Two: When the molecular weight is given, it is generally easier to find the molecular formula first. This is accomplished by multiplying the molecular weight by the given percentages to find the grams of each element present in one mole of compound, then dividing by the respective atomic weights to find the mole ratio of the elements:

$$\text{\# mol of C} = \frac{(.409)(264) \text{ g}}{12 \text{ g/mol}} = 9 \text{ mol}$$

$$\text{\# mol of H} = \frac{(.0458)(264) \text{ g}}{1 \text{ g/mol}} = 12 \text{ mol}$$

$$\text{\# mol of O} = \frac{(.5452)(264) \text{ g}}{16 \text{ g/mol}} = 9 \text{ mol}$$

Thus, the molecular formula, $C_9H_{12}O_9$, is the direct result.

The empirical formula can now be found by reducing the subscript ratio to the simplest integral values.

TYPES OF CHEMICAL REACTIONS

There are many ways in which elements and compounds can react to form other species; memorizing every reaction would be impossible as well as unnecessary. However, nearly every inorganic reaction can be classified into at least one of four general categories.

Combination Reactions

Combination reactions are reactions in which two or more **reactants** form one **product**. The formation of sulfur dioxide by burning sulfur in air is an example of a combination reaction.

$$S\ (s) + O2\ (g) \rightarrow SO_2\ (g)$$

Combination reactions can also occur when two compounds react to form a new compound. For example, in the equation below, ammonia in the gaseous state is reacted with hydrogen chloride in the gaseous state to form ammonium chloride.

$$NH_3(g) + HCl(g) \rightarrow NH_4Cl(s)$$

Decomposition Reactions

A decomposition reaction is defined as one in which a compound breaks down into two or more substances, usually as a result of heating or electrolysis. When most compounds are heated, for example, most of these compounds will decompose to form molecular oxygen. **Electrolysis** is a process that causes the decomposition of a compound by passing an electric current through the reactant. An example of a decomposition reaction is the breakdown of mercury (II) oxide (the sign Δ represents the addition of heat).

$$2\ HgO\ (s) \overset{\Delta}{\rightarrow} 2\ Hg\ (\ell) + O_2\ (g)$$

Single Deplacement Reactions

Single displacement reactions occur when an atom (or ion) of one compound is replaced by an atom of another element. For example, zinc metal will displace copper ions in a copper sulfate solution to form zinc sulfate.

$$Zn\ (s) + CuSO_4\ (aq) \rightarrow Cu\ (s) + ZnSO_4\ (aq)$$

Single displacement reactions are often further classified as **redox** reactions. (These will be discussed in more detail in Chapter 38, Redox Reactions and Electrochemistry.)

Double Deplacement Reactions

In double displacement reactions, also called **metathesis reactions**, elements from two different compounds displace each other to form two new compounds. This type of reaction occurs when one of the products is removed from the solution as a precipitate or gas, or when two of the original species combine to form a weak electrolyte that remains undissociated in solution. For example, when solutions of calcium chloride and silver nitrate are combined, insoluble silver chloride forms in a solution of calcium nitrate.

$$CaCl_2\ (aq) + 2\ AgNO_3\ (aq) \rightarrow Ca(NO_3)_2\ (aq) + 2\ AgCl\ (s)$$

Net Ionic Equations

Because reactions such as displacements often involve ions in solution, they can be written in ionic form. In the example where zinc is reacted with copper sulfate, the **ionic equation** would be:

$$Zn\ (s) + Cu^{2+}\ (aq) + SO_4^{2-}\ (aq) \rightarrow Cu\ (s) + Zn^{2+}\ (aq) + SO_4^{2-}\ (aq)$$

When displacement reactions occur, there are usually **spectator ions** that do not take part in the overall reaction but simply remain in solution throughout. The spectator ion in the equation above is sulfate, which does not undergo any transformation during the reaction. A **net ionic reaction** can be written showing only the species that actually participate in the reaction:

$$Zn\ (s) + Cu^{2+}\ (aq) \rightarrow Cu\ (s) + Zn^{2+}\ (aq)$$

Net ionic equations are important for demonstrating the actual reaction that occurs during a displacement reaction.

Neutralization Reactions

Neutralization reactions are a specific type of double displacement that occurs when an acid reacts with a base to produce a solution of a salt and water. For example, hydrochloric acid and sodium hydroxide will react to form sodium chloride and water.

$$HCl\ (aq) + NaOH\ (aq) \rightarrow NaCl\ (aq) + H_2O\ (l)$$

(This type of reaction will be discussed further in Chapter 37, Acids and Bases.)

BALANCING EQUATIONS

Chemical equations express how much and what type of reactants must be used to obtain a given quantity of product. From the **law of conservation of mass**, the mass of the reactants in a reaction must be equal to the mass of the products. More specifically, chemical equations must be balanced so that there are the same number of atoms of each element in the products as there are in the reactants. **Stoichiometric coefficients** are used to indicate the number of moles of a given species involved in the reaction. For example, the reaction for the formation of water is:

$$2\ H_2\ (g) + O_2\ (g) \rightarrow 2\ H_2O\ (g)$$

The coefficients indicate that two moles of H_2 gas must be reacted with one mole of O_2 gas to produce two moles of water. In general, stoichiometric coefficients are given as whole numbers.

Example: Balance the following reaction:
$$C_4H_{10}\ (l) + O_2\ (g) \rightarrow CO_2\ (g) + H_2O\ (l)$$

Solution: First, balance the carbons in reactants and products.
$$C_4H_{10} + O_2 \rightarrow 4\ CO_2 + H_2O$$

Second, balance the hydrogens in reactants and products.

$$C_4H_{10} + O_2 \rightarrow 4\ CO_2 + 5\ H_2O$$

Third, balance the oxygens in the reactants and products.

$$2\ C_4H_{10} + 13\ O_2 \rightarrow 8\ CO_2 + 10\ H_2O$$

Finally, check that all of the elements, and the total charges, are balanced correctly. If there is a difference in total charge between the reactants and products, then the charge will also have to be balanced. Instructions for balancing charge are found in Chapter 38.

Applications of Stoichiometry

Once an equation has been balanced, the ratio of moles of reactant to moles of products is known, and that information can be used to solve many types of stoichiometry problems. It is important to use proper units when solving such problems. If and when you are faced with doing the calculations, the units should cancel out, so that the units obtained in the answer represent those asked for in the problem.

Example: How many grams of calcium chloride are needed to prepare 72 g of silver chloride according to the following equation?

$$CaCl_2\ (aq) + 2AgNO_3\ (aq) \rightarrow Ca(NO_3)_2\ (aq) + 2AgCl\ (s)$$

Solution: Noting first that the equation is balanced, one mole of $CaCl_2$ yields two moles of AgCl when it is reacted with two moles of $AgNO_3$. The molar mass of $CaCl_2$ is 110 g, and the molar mass of AgCl is 144 g.

$$72\ AgCl \times \frac{1\ mol\ AgCl}{144\ g\ AgCl} \times \frac{1\ mol\ CaCl_2}{2\ mol\ AgCl} \times \frac{110\ g\ CaCl_2}{1\ mol\ CaCl_2} = 27.5\ g\ of\ CaCl_2$$

Thus, 27.5 g of $CaCl_2$ are needed to produce 72 g of AgCl.

Limiting reactant

When reactants are mixed, they are seldom added in the exact stoichiometric proportions as shown in the balanced equation. Therefore, in most reactions, one of the reactants will be consumed first. This reactant is known as the limiting reactant because it limits the amount of product that can be formed in the reaction. The reactant that remains after all of the limiting reactant is used up is called the **excess reactant**.

Example: If 28 g of Fe react with 24 g of S to produce FeS, what would be the limiting reactant? How many grams of excess reactant would be present in the vessel at the end of the reaction? The balanced equation is: $Fe + S \xrightarrow{\Delta} FeS$.

Solution: First, the number of moles for each reactant must be determined.

$$28 \text{ g Fe} \times \frac{1 \text{ mol Fe}}{56 \text{ g}} = 0.5 \text{ mol Fe}$$

$$24 \text{ g S} \times \frac{1 \text{ mol S}}{32 \text{ g}} = 0.75 \text{ mol S}$$

Since one mole of Fe is needed to react with one mole of S, and there are 0.5 moles Fe for every 0.75 moles S, the limiting reagent is Fe. Thus, 0.5 moles of Fe will react with 0.5 moles of S, leaving an excess of 0.25 moles of S in the vessel. The mass of the excess reactant will be:

$$\text{mass of S} = 0.25 \text{ mol S} \frac{32 \text{ g}}{1 \text{ mol S}}$$
$$= 8 \text{ g of S}$$

Yields

The yield of a reaction, which is the amount of product predicted or obtained when the reaction is carried out, can be determined or predicted from the balanced equation. There are three distinct ways of reporting yields. The **theoretical yield** is the amount of product that can be predicted from a balanced equation, assuming that all of the limiting reagent has been used, that no competing side reactions have occurred, and all of the product has been collected. The theoretical yield is seldom obtained; therefore, chemists speak of the **actual yield,** which is the amount of product that is isolated from the reaction experimentally. There are a variety of reasons why the actual yield is less than the theoretical yield, even when the reaction is 100 percent complete. For example, many reactions are **reversible** (i.e., do not produce 100 percent from left to right). Another reason for the actual yield's being less than the theoretical yield is that some of the reactants may **interact** with one another to produce another end product.

The term **percent yield** is used to express the relationship between the actual yield and the theoretical yield and is given by the following equation:

$$\text{percent yield} = \frac{\text{actual yield}}{\text{theoretical yield}} \times 100\%$$

Example: What is the percent yield for a reaction in which 27 g of Cu is produced by reacting 32.5 g of Zn in excess $CuSO_4$ solution?

Solution: The balanced equation is as follows:

$$Zn \text{ (s)} + CuSO_4 \text{ (aq)} \rightarrow Cu \text{ (s)} + ZnSO_4 \text{ (aq)}$$

Calculate the theoretical yield for Cu.

$$32.5 \text{ g Zn} \times \frac{1 \text{ mol Zn}}{65 \text{ g}} = 0.5 \text{ mol Zn}$$

$$0.5 \text{ mol Zn} \times \frac{1 \text{ mol Cu}}{1 \text{ mol Zn}} = 0.5 \text{ mol Cu}$$

$$0.5 \text{ mol Cu} \times \frac{64 \text{ g}}{1 \text{ mol Cu}} = 32 \text{ g Cu} = \text{theoretical yield}$$

Finally, determine the percent yield.

$$\frac{27 \text{ g}}{32 \text{ g}} \times 100\% = 84\%$$

REVIEW PROBLEMS

1. What is the sum of the coefficients of the following equation when it is balanced?

$$C_6H_{12}O_6 + O_2 \rightarrow CO_2 + H_2O$$

   (A) 20
   (B) 38
   (C) 21
   (D) 19
   (E) 18

2. Determine the molecular formula and calculate the percent composition of each element present in nicotine, which has an empirical formula of C_5H_7N and a molecular weight of 162 g/mol.

3. Acetylene, used as a fuel in welding torches, is produced in a reaction between calcium carbide and water:

$$CaC_2 + 2\ H_2O \rightarrow Ca(OH)_2 + C_2H_2$$

   How many grams of C_2H_2 are formed from 0.400 moles of CaC_2?

   (A)   0.400
   (B)   0.800
   (C)   4.000
   (D) 10.400
   (E) 26.000

$$CH_3CO_2Na + HClO_4 \rightarrow CH_3CO_2H + NaClO_4$$

4. The above reaction is classified as a

   (A) double displacement reaction.
   (B) combination reaction.
   (C) decomposition reaction.
   (D) single displacement and decomposition reaction.
   (E) combination and decomposition reaction.

5. Aspirin ($C_9H_8O_4$) is prepared by reacting salicylic acid ($C_7H_6O_3$) and acetic anhydride ($C_4H_6O_3$).

   $$C_7H_6O_3 + C_4H_6O_3 \rightarrow C_9H_8O_4 + C_2H_4O_2$$

   How many moles of salicylic acid should be used to prepare six 5-grain aspirin tablets? (1 g = 15.5 grains)

   (A)   0.01
   (B)   0.10
   (C)   1.00
   (D)   2.00
   (E) 31.00

6. The percent composition of an unknown element X in CH_3X is 32 percent. Which of the following is element X?

    (A) H
    (B) F
    (C) Cl
    (D) Na
    (E) Li

7. Twenty-seven grams of silver was reacted with excess sulfur, according to the following equation:

    $2Ag + S \rightarrow Ag_2S$

    25.0 g of silver sulfide was collected. What are the theoretical yield, actual yield, and percent yield?

8. Which of the following represents the net ionic equation for the reaction given?

    $AgNO_3(aq) + Cu(s) \rightarrow CuNO_3(aq) + Ag(s)$

    (A) $AgNO_3(aq) + Cu(s) \rightarrow CuNO_3(aq) + Ag(s)$
    (B) $Ag^+(aq) + Cu(s) \rightarrow Cu^+(aq) + Ag(s)$
    (C) $AgNO_3(aq) + Cu(s) \rightarrow Cu^+(aq) + NO_3^-(aq) + Ag(s)$
    (D) $Ag^+(aq) + NO_3^-(aq) + Cu(s) \rightarrow CuNO_3(aq) + Ag(s)$
    (E) $Ag^+(aq) + Cu(s) \rightarrow Ag(s) + NO_3^-(aq)$

9. What is the mass in grams of a single chlorine atom? Of a single molecule of O_2?

The following reaction will be used to answer questions 10–12.

$$Ag(NH_3)_2^+ \rightarrow Ag^+ + 2NH_3$$

10. How many moles of $Ag(NH_3)_2^+$ are required for the production of 11 moles of ammonia?

11. If 5.8 g of $Ag(NH_3)_2^+$ yields 1.4 g of ammonia, how many moles of silver are produced?

    (A) 4.400
    (B) 5.800
    (C) 0.041
    (D) 0.054
    (E) 7.200

12. What are the percent compositions of Ag, N, and H in $Ag(NH_3)_2^+$?

13. A hydrocarbon (which by definition contains only C and H atoms) is heated in an excess of oxygen to produce 58.67 g of CO_2 and 27 g of H_2O. What is the empirical formula of the hydrocarbon?

14. Balance the following reaction:

$$NF_3 + H_2O \rightarrow HF + NO + NO_2$$

How many grams of HF are expected to form if 1.5 kg of a 5.2% NF_3 sample is used?

15. Balance the following reactions:

   (A) $I_2 + Cl_2 + H_2O \rightarrow HIO_3 + HCl$
   (B) $MnO_2 + HCl \rightarrow H_2O + MnCl_2 + Cl_2$
   (C) $BCl_3 + P_4 + H_2 \rightarrow BP + HCl$
   (D) $C_3H_5(NO_3)_3 \rightarrow CO_2 + H_2O + N_2 + O_2$
   (E) $HCl + Ba(OH)_2 \rightarrow BaCl_2 + H_2O$

SOLUTIONS TO REVIEW PROBLEMS

1. **D** To answer this question, the equation must first be balanced. Starting with carbon, it can be seen that there are 6 carbons on the reactant side and only one on the product side, so a coefficient of 6 should be placed in front of the carbon dioxide. For the hydrogen, there are 12 atoms on the left and only 2 on the right; thus, a coefficient of 6 should go in front of water. Now, for oxygen, there are 8 atoms on the left and 18 on the right. To balance the oxygen, 10 more atoms of oxygen must be added to the left side. The best way to do this is to put a coefficient of 6 in front of oxygen, since putting a stoichiometric coefficient in front of the glucose molecule would unbalance the equation in terms of carbon and hydrogen. Therefore, the final balanced equation is

$$C_6H_{12}O_6 + 6O_2 \rightarrow 6CO_2 + 6H_2O$$

Remember that $C_6H_{12}O_6$ has a coefficient of 1, and this must be added to the total number. So $1 + 6 + 6 + 6 = 19$.

2. $C_{10}H_{14}N_2$; 74.1% C, 8.6% H, 17.3% N

   To determine the molecular formula of nicotine, the empirical weight of the compound must be calculated.

   $5(C) + 7(H) + 1(N) =$ empirical weight

   $5(12 \text{ g/mol}) + 7(1 \text{ g/mol}) + 14 \text{ g/mol} = 81 \text{ g/mol}$

   The empirical weight (81 g/mol) is then divided into the molecular weight (162 g/mol) to determine the number by which each subscript in the empirical formula must be multiplied to obtain the molecular formula.

   $$\frac{162 \text{ g/mol}}{81 \text{ g/mol}} = 2$$

   $2(C_5H_7N) = C_{10}H_{14}N_2 =$ molecular formula

   To find the percent composition of each element, the following calculations are carried out.

   $$\% \text{ C} = \frac{120}{162} \times 100\% = 74.1\%$$

   $$\% \text{ H} = \frac{14}{162} \times 100\% = 74.1\%$$

   $$\% \text{ N} = \frac{28}{162} \times 100\% = 17.3\%$$

   The same percentages would be obtained if we use the empirical formula for this calculation.

3. **D** According to the balanced equation, one mole of CaC_2 yields one mole of C_2H_2. Therefore, if 0.400 moles of CaC_2 were used, 0.400 moles of C_2H_2 would be produced. Now the number of moles must be converted to grams by using the following formula:

   $$\text{mol} = \frac{\text{weight in g}}{\text{molecular weight}}$$

   The molecular weight of C_2H_2 is

   $2(12 \text{ g/mol}) + 2(1 \text{ g/mol}) = 26 \text{ g/mol}$

   Substituting into the above equation:

   $$0.400 \text{ mol} = \frac{x}{26 \text{ g/mol}}$$

   $x = 10.4 \text{g}$

4. **A** Because the only change is that the Na from CH_3CO_2Na exchanges with the H from $HClO_4$, this is a double displacement reaction. Alternately, this reaction could be classified as a neutralization, since it is an acid and a base which react.

5. **A** According to the balanced equation, one mole of salicylic acid will yield one mole of aspirin. Therefore, to solve this question, the number of moles of aspirin in six 5-grain tablets, or 30 *grains* of aspirin, must be determined, using the following relationship.

$$\frac{1 \text{ g}}{15.5 \text{ grains}} = \frac{x}{30 \text{ grains}}$$

$x \cong 2g$

Therefore, the weight of the aspirin produced is about 2 grams, which must be converted to moles. The molecular weight of aspirin is

$9(C) + 8(H) + 4(O) =$

$9(12 \text{ g/mol}) + 8(1 \text{ g/mol}) + 4(16 \text{ g/mol}) = 180 \text{ g/mol}$

Then, the number of moles in two grams of aspirin is calculated.

$$\frac{2 \text{ g}}{180 \text{ g / mol}} = 0.01 \text{ mol}$$

6. **E** The easiest way to solve this problem, short of trying every choice, is to work through the problem with slightly backwards logic. Because we know that element X comprises 32% of the compound, CH_3 must comprise 68% (100% – 32%). We must calculate the formula weight of CH_3 (12 + 3 = 15). The fact that 15 = 68% of the total weight can be restated as the equation 15 = 0.68 × total weight; we can solve this to show that the total molecular weight must be 22. The weight of X = total weight - 15 = 7. Choice (E), Li, has an atomic weight of 7.

7. **31 g, 25 g, 81%**
According to the balanced equation, two moles of silver should react with one mole of sulfur to form one mole of silver sulfide. The theoretical yield is the amount of product that would be collected if all of the limiting reagent reacts. Using a stoichiometric calculation, the theoretical yield of silver sulfide if 27.0 g of silver is used would be as follows:

$$27 \text{ g Ag} \times \frac{1 \text{ mol Ag}}{108 \text{ g Ag}} \times \frac{1 \text{ mol Ag}_2S}{2 \text{ mol Ag}} \times \frac{248 \text{ Ag}_2S}{1 \text{ mol Ag}_2S} = 31 \text{ Ag}_2S$$

The actual yield is the amount of product that is obtained from the experiment. It is usually less than the theoretical yield since the reagents may not react completely and the product may be difficult to collect. In this experiment, the actual yield is 25.0 g of silver sulfide. Finally, the percent yield represents the percentage of product actually collected in reference to the theoretical yield. Thus, the percent yield for this experiment would be

$$\frac{25.0 \text{ g}}{31.0 \text{ g}} \times 100\% = 81\%$$

8. **B** In displacement reactions, there are often ionic species that do not play a role in the overall reaction. Instead, they remain in solution throughout the entire reaction. Thus, displacement reactions can be written in terms of net ionic equations, which express the reactions of the participating species. In the reaction between aqueous silver nitrate and copper metal to form aqueous copper(I) nitrate and metallic silver, the nitrate ion does not participate in the reaction; thus, it is a spectator ion. Therefore, the only species that are involved in the reaction are copper metal and the Ag^+ ion, which react to form the Cu^+ ion and silver metal.

9. 5.81×10^{-23} **g/atom; 5.31×10^{-23} g/molecule**

   The mass of a single atom is determined by dividing the atomic weight by Avogadro's number. Therefore, the mass of a chlorine atom is

   $$\frac{32 \text{ g}}{6.022 \times 10^{-23} \text{ atoms}} = 5.81 \times 10^{-23} \text{ g/atom}$$

   The mass of an oxygen molecule (O_2) is similarly determined by dividing the molecular weight of oxygen by Avogadro's number.

   $$\frac{32 \text{ g}}{6.022 \times 10^{-23} \text{ molecules}} = 5.31 \times 10^{-23} \text{ g/molecule}$$

10. **5.5 mol**

    From the balanced equation, it can be seen that the ratio between $Ag(NH_3)_2^+$ and NH_3 is 1:2. Thus, to form 11 mol of ammonia, the following calculation must be performed.

    $$\frac{1 \text{ mol Ag } (H_3)_2^+}{2 \text{ mol NH}_3} = \frac{x \text{ mol Ag } (NH_3)_2^+}{11 \text{ mol NH}_3}$$

    $x = 5.5$ mol $Ag(NH3)_2^+$

11. **C** To answer this question, the law of conservation of mass, which says that the mass of the products must be equal to the mass of the reactants, is used. Therefore, if 5.8 g of $Ag(NH_3)_2^+$ are allowed to dissociate to form 1.4 g of ammonia, $5.8 - 1.4$ or 4.4 g of silver must be formed. The following calculation is used to determine the number of moles of silver that are formed.

    $$x \text{ mol} = \frac{4.4 \text{ g}}{108 \text{ g / mol}}$$

    $x = 0.041$ mol

12. **76.1%, 19.7%, 4.2%**

The percent composition of elements in a compound or formula is determined by dividing the mass of the element by the total formula weight of the compound. Therefore, in the complex ion $Ag(NH_3)_2^+$, which has a formula weight of 142 g/mol, the percent compositions of Ag, N, and H are as follows:

$$\% \ Ag = \frac{108 \text{ g/mol}}{142 \text{ g/mol}} \times 100\% = 76.1\%$$

$$\% \ N = \frac{2(14 \text{ g/mol})}{142 \text{ g/mol}} \times 100\% = 19.7\%$$

$$\% \ H = \frac{6(1 \text{ g/mol})}{142 \text{ g/mol}} \times 100\% = 4.2\%$$

13. **C_4H_9**

To answer this problem, several calculations must be performed. First, the number of moles of carbon and hydrogen present in the hydrocarbon must be determined using the assumption that the number of moles of atoms on the reactant side is equal to the number of moles of atoms on the product side. From this information, the empirical formula can be determined.

From the amounts of CO_2 and H_2O given, the mol of carbon and hydrogen are calculated.

$$\frac{58.67 \text{ g CO}_2}{44 \text{ g / mol}} = 1.33 \text{ mol of CO}_2$$

Since each mole of CO_2 contains 1 mole of carbon, 1.33 moles of CO_2 contains 1.33 moles of carbon. Therefore, the hydrocarbon contains 1.33 moles of carbon.

$$\frac{27 \text{ g H}_2O}{18 \text{ g / mol H}_2O} = 1.5 \text{ mol H}_2O$$

Since one mole of H_2O contains 2 moles of hydrogen atoms, 1.5 moles of H_2O contains 3.0 moles of hydrogen. Therefore, the hydrocarbon contains 3 moles of hydrogen.

Using these calculations, the simplest formula that can be written is $C_{1.33}H_3$. However, molecular formulas are not expressed with decimals or fractions, so these coefficients should be multiplied by their least common multiple to get whole number coefficients. Both 1.33 and 3 are multiplied by 3 to give an empirical formula of C_4H_9.

14. **66 g**

The balanced equation will be:

$$2NF_3 + 3H_2O \rightarrow 6HF + NO + NO_2$$

According to the balanced equation, 2 moles of NF_3 is needed to produce 6 moles of HF. To determine the number of grams of HF that will be formed, the amount of NF_3 used must first be calculated.

$$1,500 \text{ g} \times 0.052 = 78 \text{ g } NF_3 \text{ used}$$

Then a stoichiometric calculation can be set up to see what the theoretical yield of HF would be.

$$78 \text{ g } NF_3 \times \frac{1 \text{ mol } NF_3}{71 \text{ g } NF_3} \times \frac{6 \text{ mol HF}}{2 \text{ mol } NF_3} \times \frac{20 \text{ g HF}}{1 \text{ mol HF}} = 66 \text{ g HF}$$

Thus, 66 g of HF would be produced.

15. The following are the correct balanced equations:

(A) $I_2 + 5 Cl_2 + 6 H_2O \rightarrow 2 HIO_3 + 10 HCl$

(B) $MnO_2 + 4 HCl \rightarrow 2 H_2O + MnCl_2 + Cl_2$

(C) $4 BCl_3 + P_4 + 6 H_2 \rightarrow 4 BP + 12 HCl$

(D) $4 C_3H_5(NO_3)_3 \rightarrow 12 CO_2 + 10 H_2O + 6 N_2 + O_2$

(E) $2 HCl + Ba(OH)_2 \rightarrow BaCl_2 + 2 H_2O$

CHAPTER THIRTY-TWO

Chemical Kinetics and Equilibrium

When studying a chemical reaction, it is important to consider not only the chemical properties of the reactants but also the **conditions** under which the reaction occurs, the **mechanism** by which it takes place, the **rate** at which it occurs, and the **equilibrium** (or steady state) toward which it proceeds.

Chemical kinetics is the study of the rates (or speed) of reactions. The **reaction rate** is the change of concentration of reactant or finished product with respect to time. Any given chemical reaction can be represented by the following equation:

$$\text{Reactants} \rightarrow \text{Products}$$

This equation indicates that reactant molecules are decreasing or being consumed and the product molecules are increasing or being formed. The process of chemical kinetics is concerned with how "fast" the reactants are being transformed into products.

REACTION MECHANISMS

The **mechanism** of a chemical reaction is the actual series of steps through which it occurs. Knowing the accepted mechanism of a reaction often helps to explain the reaction's rate, position of equilibrium, and thermodynamic characteristics (see Chapter 33). Consider the reaction below:

$$\text{overall reaction: } A_2 + 2\,B \rightarrow 2\,AB$$

This equation seems to imply a mechanism in which two molecules of B collide with one molecule of A_2 to form two molecules of AB. But suppose instead that the reaction actually takes place in two steps.

Step 1: $A_2 + B \rightarrow A_2B$ (slow)

Step 2: $A_2B + B \rightarrow 2\,AB$ (fast)

Note that these two steps add up to the overall (net) reaction. A_2B, which does not appear in the overall reaction because it is neither a reactant nor a product, is called an **intermediate**. Reaction intermediates are often difficult to detect, but a proposed mechanism can be supported through kinetic experiments.

The slowest step in a proposed mechanism is called the **rate-determining step**, because the overall reaction cannot proceed faster than that step.

REACTION RATES

Definition of Rate

Consider a reaction $2A + B \rightarrow C$, in which one mole of C is produced from every two moles of A and one mole of B. The rate of this reaction may be described in terms of either the disappearance of reactants over time or the appearance of products over time.

$$\text{rate} = \frac{\text{decrease in concentration of reactants}}{\text{time}} = \frac{\text{increase in concentration of products}}{\text{time}}$$

Because the concentration of a reactant decreases during the reaction, a minus sign is placed before a rate that is expressed in terms of reactants. For the reaction above, the rate of reaction with respect to A is $-\Delta[A]/\Delta t$, with respect to B is $-\Delta[B]/\Delta t$, and with respect to C is $\Delta[C]/\Delta t$. In this particular reaction, the three rates are not equal. According to the stoichiometry of the reaction, A is used up twice as fast as B ($-\frac{1}{2}\Delta[A]/\Delta t = -\Delta[B]/\Delta t$), and A is consumed twice as fast as C is produced ($-\frac{1}{2}\Delta[A]/\Delta t = \Delta[C]/\Delta t$). To show a standard rate of reaction in which the rates with respect to all substances are equal, the rate for each substance should be divided by its stoichiometric coefficient.

$$\text{rate} = -\frac{1}{2}\frac{\Delta[A]}{\Delta t} = \frac{-\Delta[B]}{\Delta t} = \frac{\Delta[C]}{\Delta t}$$

In general, for the reaction $a\,A + b\,B \rightarrow c\,C + d\,D$;

$$\text{rate} = -\frac{1}{a}\frac{\Delta[A]}{\Delta t} = \frac{1}{b}\frac{-\Delta[B]}{\Delta t} = \frac{1}{c}\frac{\Delta[C]}{\Delta t} = \frac{1}{d}\frac{\Delta[D]}{\Delta t}$$

Rate is expressed in the units of moles per liter per second (mol/L $\times$ s) or molarity per second (molarity/s).

Rate Law

For nearly all forward, irreversible reactions, the rate is proportional to the product of the concentrations of the reactants, each raised to some power. For the general reaction

$$a\,A + b\,B \rightarrow c\,C + d\,D$$

the rate is proportional to $[A]^x[B]^y$, that is:

$$\text{rate} = k\,[A]^x[B]^y$$

This expression is the **rate law** for the general reaction above, where k is the **rate constant**. The rate constant is defined as a constant of proportionality between the chemical reaction rate and the concentration of the reactants. Multiplying the units of k by the concentration factors raised to the appropriate powers gives the rate in units of concentration/time. The exponents x and y are called the **orders of reaction**; x is the order with respect to A, and y is the order with respect to B. These exponents may be integers, fractions, or zero and must be determined experimentally.

It is important to note that the exponents of the rate law are **not** necessarily equal to the stoichiometric coefficients in the overall reaction equation. The exponents **are** equal to the stoichiometric coefficients of the rate-determining step. If one of the reactants or products in this step is an intermediate not included in the overall reaction, then calculating the rate law in terms of the original reactants is more complex.

The **overall order of a reaction** (or the **reaction order**) is defined as the sum of the exponents, here equal to x + y.

Experimental determination of rate law

The values of k, x, and y in the rate law equation (rate $= k[A]^x [B]^y$) must be determined experimentally for a given reaction at a given temperature. The rate is usually measured as a function of the initial concentrations of the reactants, A and B.

Example: Given the data below, find the rate law for the following reaction at 300 K.

$$A + B \rightarrow C + D$$

Trial	$[A]_{initial}(M)$	$[B]_{initial}(M)$	$r_{initial}(M/sec)$
1	1.00	1.00	2.0
2	1.00	2.00	8.1
3	2.00	2.00	15.9

Solution: First, look for two trials in which the concentrations of all but one of the substances are held constant.

a) In trials 1 and 2, the concentration of A is kept constant while the concentration of B is doubled. The rate increases by a factor of 8.1/2.0, or approximately 4. Write down the rate expression of the two trials.

Trial 1: $r_1 = k[A]^x [B]^y = k(1.00)^x (1.00)^y$

Trial 2: $r_2 = k[A]^x [B]^y = k(1.00)^x (2.00)^y$

Divide the second equation by the first:

$$\frac{r_2}{r_1} = \frac{8.1}{2.0} = \frac{k(1.00)^x (2.00)^y}{k(1.00)^x (1.00)^y} = (2.00)^y$$

$$4 = (2.00)^y$$

$$y = 2$$

b) In trials 2 and 3, the concentration of B is kept constant while the concentration of A is doubled; the rate is increased by a factor of 15.9/8.1, or approximately 2. The rate expressions of the two trials are:

Trial 2: $r_2 = k(1.00)^x (2.00)^y$

Trial 3: $r_3 = k(2.00)^x (2.00)^y$

Divide the second equation by the first:

$$\frac{r_3}{r_2} = \frac{15.9}{8.1} = \frac{k(2.00)^x (2.00)^y}{k(1.00)^x (2.00)^y} = (2.00)^x$$

$2 = (2.00)^x$

$x = 1$

So $r = k[A][B]^2$

The order of the reaction with respect to A is 1 and with respect to B is 2; the overall reaction order is $1 + 2 = 3$.

To calculate k, substitute the values from any one of the above trials into the rate law. For example:

$2.0 \text{ M/sec} = k \times 1.00 \text{ M} \times (1.00 \text{ M})^2$

$k = 2.0 \text{ M}^{-2} \text{ sec}^{-1}$

Therefore, the rate law is $r = 2.0 \text{ M}^{-2} \text{ sec}^{-1} [A][B]^2$

Reaction Orders

Chemical reactions are often classified on the basis of kinetics as zero-order, first-order, second-order, mixed-order, or higher-order reactions. The general reaction $aA + bB \rightarrow cC + dD$ will be used in the discussion below.

Zero-order reactions

A zero-order reaction has a constant rate, which is independent of the reactants' concentrations. Thus, the rate law is:

$$\text{rate} = k, \text{ where k has units of Msec}^{-1}$$

With respect to the administration of a medication, the amount of drug administered/eliminated remains constant over a given period of time. For example, 25 mg of a drug are administered/eliminated each hour.

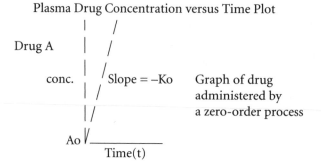

Plasma Drug Concentration versus Time Plot

Drug A

conc.

Slope = −Ko

Graph of drug administered by a zero-order process

Ao

Time(t)

The concentration of Drug A can be calculated at any given time with the equation:

A = Ao - (Ko)(t). Where: Ao = initial concentration of Drug A in the body
                            Ko = zero-order rate constant
                             t = Time

The zero-order half-life changes with time and is proportional to the initial drug concentration. It is inversely proportional to the zero-order rate constant and can be represented with the following equation: half-life = 0.5 Ao/Ko.

First-order reactions

A first-order reaction (order = 1) has a rate proportional to the concentration of one reactant.

$$\text{rate} = k[A] \text{ or } \text{rate} = k[B]$$

First-order rate constants have units of $\sec^{-1}$.

The classic example of a first-order reaction is the process of radioactive decay. The concentration of radioactive substance A at any time t can be expressed mathematically as:

$$[A_t] = [A_o] \, e^{-kt}$$

where $[A_o]$ = initial concentration of A

             $[A_t]$ = concentration of A at time t

             k = rate constant

             t = elapsed time

The half-life ($t_{1/2}$) of a reaction is the time needed for the concentration of the radioactive substance to decrease to one-half of its original value. Half-lives can be calculated from the rate law as follows:

$$t_{1/2} = \ln 2/k = 0.693/k$$

where k is the first order rate constant.

With respect to a first-order reaction in medicine, the percentage of drug administered/eliminated remains constant over a given period of time. In other words, the amount of drug administered/eliminated is proportional to the amount of drug remaining. For example, 25 percent of the drug is eliminated each hour.

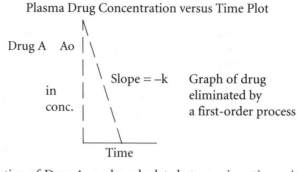

Plasma Drug Concentration versus Time Plot

- The concentration of Drug A can be calculated at any given time with the equation: Ln A = Ln Ao – Ke(t)
- Remember: $\ln x = (\log x)(2.3)$

Where Ao = initial concentration of Drug A in the body

Ke = first-order elimination rate constant

t = time

Regarding the first-order half-life, the time to decrease the remaining portion of the drug in the body by $\frac{1}{2}$ remains constant irrespective of the drug's concentration in the blood. The first-order half-life = 0.693 / K.

Now you can see how these chemical reaction equations can be related to the practice of Pharmacy.

Second-order reactions

A second-order reaction (order = 2) has a rate proportional to the product of the concentration of two reactants or to the square of the concentration of a single reactant. For example, rate = $k[A]^2$, rate = $k[B]^2$, or rate = $k[A][B]$. The units of second-order rate constants are $M^{-1} / \sec^{-1}$.

Higher-order reactions

A higher-order reaction has an order greater than 2.

Mixed-order reactions

A mixed-order reaction has a fractional order; e.g., rate = $k[A]^{1/3}$.

Efficiency of Reactions

Collision theory of chemical kinetics

For a reaction to occur, molecules must collide with each other. The collision theory of chemical kinetics states that the rate of a reaction is proportional to the **number of collisions per second** between the reacting molecules. It is important to note that reaction rates almost always increase with increasing temperatures. On the other hand, reaction rates decrease with decreasing temperatures.

Not all collisions, however, result in a chemical reaction. An **effective collision** (one that leads to the formation of products) occurs only if the molecules collide with correct orientation and sufficient force to break the existing bonds and form new ones. The minimum energy of collision necessary for a reaction to take place is called the **activation energy, E$_a$**, or the **energy barrier**. Only a fraction of colliding particles have enough kinetic energy to exceed the activation energy. This means that only a fraction of all collisions are effective. The rate of a reaction can therefore be expressed as:

$$\textbf{rate} = \textbf{fZ}$$

where Z is the total number of collisions occurring per second and f is the fraction of collisions that are effective.

Transition state theory

When molecules collide with sufficient energy, they form a **transition state**, in which the old bonds are weakened and the new bonds are beginning to form. The transition state then dissociates into products, and the new bonds are fully formed. For a reaction A$_2$ + B$_2$ → 2AB, the change along the **reaction coordinate** (a measure of the extent to which the reaction has progressed from reactants to products; see Figures 32.2 and 32.3) can be represented as follows:

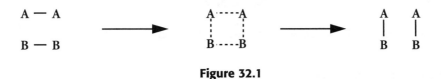

Figure 32.1

The **transition state**, also called the **activated complex**, has greater energy than either the reactants or the products and is denoted by the symbol ‡. The activation energy, as mentioned above, is the minimum amount of energy that is required to begin a given chemical reaction. The activation energy is required to bring the reactants to this particular energy level. Once an activated complex is formed, it can either dissociate into the products or revert to reactants without any additional energy input. Transition states are distinguished from intermediates in that, existing as they do at energy maxima, transition states do not have a finite lifetime.

A **potential energy diagram** illustrates the relationship between the activation energy, the heats of reaction, and the potential energy of the system. The most important factors in such diagrams are the **relative** energies of the products and reactants. The **enthalpy change** of the reaction (**ΔH**) is the difference between the potential energy of the products and the potential energy of the reactants (see Chapter 33). A negative enthalpy change indicates an **exothermic reaction** (where heat is given off) and a positive enthalpy change indicates an **endothermic reaction** (where heat is absorbed). The activated complex exists at the top of the energy barrier. The difference in potential energies between the activated complex and the reactants is the activation energy of the forward reaction; the difference in potential energies between the activated complex and the products is the activation energy of the reverse reaction.

For example, consider the formation of HCl from H$_2$ and Cl$_2$. The following figure gives the energy profile of the reaction:

$$H_2 + Cl_2 \rightleftarrows 2\,HCl$$

It shows that the reaction is exothermic. The potential energy of the products is less than the potential energy of the reactants; heat is evolved, and the heat of reaction is negative.

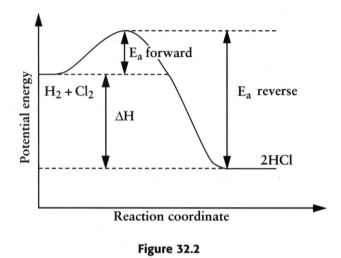

Figure 32.2

The thermodynamic properties of reactions are discussed further in Chapter 33.

Factors Affecting Reaction Rate

The rate of a chemical reaction depends upon the individual species undergoing reaction and upon the reaction environment. The rate of reaction will increase if either of the following occurs: an increase in the number of effective collisions or a stabilization of the activated complex compared to the reactants.

Reactant concentrations

The greater the concentrations of the reactants (the more particles per unit volume), the greater will be the number of effective collisions per unit time, and therefore the reaction rate will increase for all but zero-order reactions. For reactions occurring in the gaseous state, the partial pressures of the reactants can serve as a measure of concentration.

Temperature

For nearly all reactions, the reaction rate will increase as the temperature of the system increases. Since the temperature of a substance is a measure of the particles' average kinetic energy, increasing the temperature increases the average kinetic energy of the molecules. Consequently, the proportion of molecules having energies greater than E_a (thus capable of undergoing reaction) increases with higher temperature.

Medium

The rate of a reaction may also be affected by the medium in which it takes place. Certain reactions proceed more rapidly in aqueous solution, whereas other reactions may proceed more rapidly in benzene. The state of the medium (liquid, solid, or gas) can also have a significant effect.

Catalysts

Catalysts are substances that increase reaction rate without themselves being consumed; they do this by lowering the activation energy. Catalysts are important in biological systems and in industrial chemistry; **enzymes** are biological catalysts. Catalysts may increase the frequency of collision between the reactants, change the relative orientation of the reactants to make a higher percentage of collisions effective, donate electron density to the reactants, or reduce intramolecular bonding within reactant molecules. The following figure compares the energy profiles of catalyzed and uncatalyzed reactions.

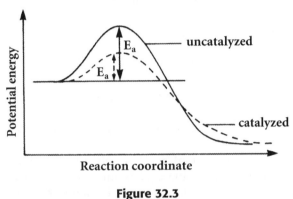

Figure 32.3

The energy barrier for the catalyzed reaction is much lower than the energy barrier for the uncatalyzed reaction. Note that the rates of both the forward and the reverse reactions are increased by catalysis, since E_a of the forward and reverse reactions are lowered by the same amount. Therefore, the presence of a catalyst causes the reaction to proceed more quickly toward equilibrium.

THE DYNAMIC CONCEPT OF EQUILIBRIUM

So far, reaction rates have been discussed under the assumption that the reactions were **irreversible** (i.e., only proceeded in one direction) and that the reactions proceeded to completion. However, a **reversible** reaction often does not proceed to completion because (by definition) the products can react to reform the reactants. This is particularly true of reactions occurring in closed systems, where products are not allowed to escape. When there is no **net** change in the concentrations of the products and reactants during a reversible chemical reaction, equilibrium exists. This is not to say that a reaction in equilibrium is static; change continues to occur in both the forward and reverse directions. Equilibrium can be thought of as a balance between the two reaction directions.

Consider the following reaction:

$$A \underset{\leftarrow}{\rightarrow} B$$

At equilibrium, the concentrations of A and B are constant, yet the reactions A → B and B → A continue to occur at equal rates.

LAW OF MASS ACTION

Consider the following **one-step** reaction:

$$2A \underset{\leftarrow}{\overset{\rightarrow}{}} B + C$$

Since the reaction occurs in one step, the rates of the forward and reverse reaction are given by:

$$\text{rate}_f = k_f[A]^2 \text{ and rate}_r = k_r[B] \, [C]$$

When $\text{rate}_f = \text{rate}_r$, equilibrium is achieved. Since the rates are equal, it can be stated that

$$k_f [A]^2 = k_r[B][C] \text{ or } \frac{k_f}{k_r} = \frac{[B][C]}{[A]^2}$$

Since k_f and k_r are both constants, this equation may be rewritten:

$$K_c = \frac{[B][C]}{[A]^2} \text{ (see below for the general equation)}$$

where K_c is called the **equilibrium constant**, and the subscript c indicates that it is in terms of concentration. (When dealing with gases, the equilibrium constant is referred to as K_p, and the subscript p indicates that it is in terms of pressure.) For dilute solutions, K_c and K_{eq} are used interchangeably; the symbol K is also often used, though it is not completely correct to do so.

While the forward and reverse reaction rates are equal at equilibrium, the **molar concentrations** of the reactants and products usually are not equal. This means that the forward and reverse rate constants, k_f and k_r, are also usually unequal. For the one-step reaction described above:

$$k_f [A]^2 = k_r[B][C]$$

$$k_f = k_r \left(\frac{[B][C]}{[A]^2} \right)$$

In a reaction of more than one step, the equilibrium constant for the overall reaction is found by multiplying together the equilibrium constants for each step of the reaction. When this is done, the equilibrium constant for the overall reaction is equal to the concentrations of products divided by reactants in the overall reaction, each raised to its stoichiometric coefficient. The forward and reverse rate constants for any step n are designated k_n and k_{-n} respectively. For example, if the reaction

$$a A + b B \underset{\leftarrow}{\overset{\rightarrow}{}} c C + d D$$

occurs in three steps, then

$$K_c = \frac{k_1 k_2 k_3}{k_{-1} k_{-2} k_{-3}} \text{ will equal } \frac{[C]^c[D]^d}{[A]^a[B]^b}$$

This expression is known as the **Law of Mass Action**.

Example: What is the expression for the equilibrium constant for the following reaction?

$$3 H_2 (g) + N_2 (g) \underset{\leftarrow}{\rightarrow} 2 NH_3 (g)$$

Solution: $K_c = \dfrac{[NH_3]2}{[H_2]^3[N_2]}$

The **reaction quotient**, Q, is a measure of the degree to which a reaction has gone to completion. Q_c is equal to

$$\frac{[C]^c[D]^d}{[A]^a[B]^b}$$

Q_c is a constant only at equilibrium, when it is equal to K_c.

PROPERTIES OF THE EQUILIBRIUM CONSTANT

The equilibrium constant, K_{eq}, has the following characteristics:
- Pure solids and liquids do not appear in the equilibrium constant expression.
- K_{eq} is characteristic of a given system at a given temperature.
- If the value of K_{eq} is very large compared to 1, an equilibrium mixture of reactants and products will contain very little of the reactants compared to the products.
- If the value of K_{eq} is very small compared to 1 (i.e., less than 0.1), an equilibrium mixture of reactants and products will contain very little of the products compared to the reactants.
- If the value of K_{eq} is close to 1, an equilibrium mixture of products and reactants will contain approximately equal amounts of reactants and products.

LE CHÂTELIER'S PRINCIPLE

The French chemist, Henry Louis Le Châtelier, indicated that if an external stress is applied to a system currently at equilibrium, the system will attempt to adjust itself to offset partially the stress. This rule, known as Le Châtelier's principle, is used to determine the direction in which a reaction at equilibrium will proceed when subjected to a stress, such as a change in concentration, pressure, temperature, or volume.

Changes in Concentration

Increasing the concentration of a species will tend to shift the equilibrium away from the species that is added to reestablish its equilibrium concentration, and vice versa. For example, in the reaction:

$$A + B \underset{\leftarrow}{\rightarrow} C + D$$

if the concentration of A and/or B is increased, the equilibrium will shift towards (or favor production of) C and D. Conversely, if the concentration of C and/or D is increased, the equilibrium will shift away from the production of C and D, favoring production of A and B. Similarly, decreasing the concentration of a species will tend to shift the equilibrium towards the production of that species. For example, if A and/or B is removed from the above reaction, the equilibrium will shift so as to favor increasing concentration of A and B.

This effect is often used in industry to increase the yield of a useful product or drive a reaction to completion. If D were constantly removed from the above reaction, the net reaction would produce more D and concurrently more C. Likewise, using an excess of the least expensive reactant helps to drive the reaction forward.

Change in Pressure or Volume

In a system at constant temperature, a change in pressure causes a change in volume, and vice versa. Since liquids and solids are practically incompressible, a change in the pressure or volume of systems involving only these phases has little or no effect on their equilibrium. Reactions involving gases, however, may be greatly affected by changes in pressure or volume, since gases are highly compressible.

Pressure and volume are inversely related. An increase in the pressure of a system will shift the equilibrium so as to decrease the number of moles of gas present. This reduces the volume of the system and relieves the stress of the increased pressure. Consider the following reaction:

$$N_2 \ (g) + 3 \ H_2 \ (g) \ \rightleftharpoons \ 2 \ NH_3 \ (g)$$

The left side of the reaction has four moles of gaseous molecules, whereas the right side has only two moles. When the pressure of this system is increased, the equilibrium will shift so that the side of the reaction producing fewer moles is favored. Since there are fewer moles on the right, the equilibrium will shift toward the right. Conversely, if the volume of the same system is increased, its pressure immediately decreases, which, according to Le Châtelier's principle, leads to a shift in the equilibrium to the left.

Change in Temperature

Changes in temperature also affect equilibrium. To predict this effect, heat may be considered as a product in an exothermic reaction and as a reactant in an endothermic reaction. Consider the following exothermic reaction:

$$A \ \rightleftharpoons \ B + heat$$

If this system were placed in an ice bath, its temperature would decrease, driving the reaction to the right to replace the heat lost. Conversely, if the system were placed in a boiling-water bath, the reaction equilibrium would shift to the left due to the increased "concentration" of heat.

Not only does a temperature change alter the position of the equilibrium, it also alters the numerical value of the equilibrium constant. In contrast, changes in the concentration of a species in the reaction, in the pressure, or in the volume will alter the position of the equilibrium without changing the numerical value of the equilibrium constant.

REVIEW PROBLEMS

1. All of the following are true statements concerning reaction orders EXCEPT
   - **(A)** The rate of a zero-order reaction is constant.
   - **(B)** After three half-lives, a sample will have one-ninth of its original activity.
   - **(C)** The units for the rate constant for first-order reactions are sec−1.
   - **(D)** Higher-order reactions are those with an order greater than two.

2. The half-life of radioactive sodium is 15.0 hours. How many hours would it take for a 64 g sample to decay to one-eighth of its original activity?
   - **(A)** 3
   - **(B)** 15
   - **(C)** 30
   - **(D)** 45

3. Consider the following hypothetical reaction and experimental data:

   $$A + B \rightarrow C + D \qquad\qquad T = 273 \text{ K}$$

	$[A]_o$ (mol/L)	$[B]_o$ (mol/L)	rate
Exp 1	0.10	1	0.035
Exp 2	0.10	4	0.070
Exp 3	0.20	1	0.140
Exp 4	0.10	16	0.140

   - **(A)** What is the order with respect to A?
   - **(B)** What is the order with respect to B?
   - **(C)** What is the rate equation?
   - **(D)** What is the overall order of the reaction?
   - **(E)** Calculate the rate constant.

4. Consider the following chemical reaction and experimental data:

   $$A\ (aq) \rightarrow B\ (aq) + C(g)$$

Trial 1		Trial 2	
[A] mol/L	rate	[A] mol/L	rate
0.10	0.6	0.10	0.9
0.20	0.6	0.20	0.9
0.30	0.6	0.30	0.9
0.40	0.6	0.40	0.9

   - **(A)** What is the rate expression for trial 1?
   - **(B)** What is the rate constant for trial 1?
   - **(C)** What is the most likely reason for the increased rate in trial 2?

5. Consider the following reaction and experimental data:

$$SO_3 + H_2O \rightarrow H_2SO_4$$

	[SO$_3$] (mol/L)	[H$_2$O] (mol/L)	rate
Trial 1	0.1	0.01	0.013
Trial 2	0.2	0.01	0.052
Trial 3	X	0.02	0.234
Trial 4	0.1	0.03	0.039

(A) What is the value of X?

(B) What is the order of the reaction?

(C) What is the rate constant?

(D) What would be the rate if [SO$_3$] in trial 4 were raised to 0.2?

6. In the following diagram, which labeled arrow represents the activation energy for the reverse reaction?

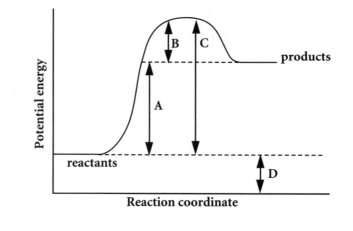

(A) A

(B) B

(C) C

(D) D

7. The activation energy for a reaction in the forward direction is 78 kJ. The activation energy for the same reaction in reverse is 300 kJ. If the energy of the products is 25 kJ, then:

(A) What is the energy of the reactants?

(B) Is the forward reaction endothermic or exothermic?

(C) Is the reverse reaction endothermic or exothermic?

(D) What is the enthalpy change for the forward reaction?

8. According to chemical kinetic theory, a reaction can occur

   (A) if the reactants collide with the proper orientation.

   (B) if the reactants possess sufficient energy of collision.

   (C) if the reactants are able to form a correct transition state.

   (D) all of the above

9. The number of undecayed nuclei in a sample of bromine-87 decreased by a factor of 4 over a period of 112 sec. What is the decay constant for bromine-87?

   (A) 56 sec

   (B) 6.93×10^{-1} sec^{-1}1

   (C) 1.24×10^{-2} sec^{-1}

   (D) 6.19×10^{-3} sec^{-1}

10. Which of the following is most likely to increase the rate of a reaction?

    (A) Decreasing the temperature

    (B) Increasing the volume of the reaction vessel

    (C) Reducing the activation energy

    (D) Decreasing the concentration of the reactant in the reaction vessel

11. All of the following are true statements concerning catalysts EXCEPT:

    (A) A catalyst will speed the rate-determining step.

    (B) A catalyst will be used up in a reaction.

    (C) A catalyst may induce steric strain in a molecule.

    (D) A catalyst will lower the activation energy of a reaction.

12. The equilibrium constant, $K_{eq,}$ of a certain single-reactant reaction is 0.16. Suppose an appropriate catalyst is added in twice the concentration of the reactant.

    (A) What will be the equilibrium constant?

    (B) Will the activation energy increase or decrease?

13. At equilibrium

    (A) the forward reaction will continue.

    (B) a change in reaction conditions will shift the equilibrium.

    (C) the reverse reaction will not continue.

    (D) both A and B will occur.

14. Given the following reaction

    $$2NO_2 (g) + 2H_2 (g) \times N_2 (g) + 2H_2O (g)$$

    what is the Law of Mass Action equation?

15. If $K_{eq} > 1$,

    (A) the equilibrium mixture will contain more product than reactant.
    (B) the equilibrium mixture will contain more reactant than product.
    (C) the equilibrium amounts of reactants and products are equal.
    (D) the reaction is irreversible.

16. Answer the following questions using the reaction given below.

    $$CH_3OH\ (l) + H_2\ (g) \rightarrow CH_4\ (g) + H_2O\ (l) \qquad \Delta H = -30\ kcal$$

    (A) In which direction would the reaction be shifted if the temperature were increased?
    (B) In which direction would the reaction be shifted if the volume were doubled?
    (C) In which direction would the reaction be shifted if methane were removed from the reaction vessel?

SOLUTIONS TO REVIEW PROBLEMS

1. **B** Discussed in the section on reaction orders.

2. **D** For a 64 g sample to decay to one-eighth of its original activity, or 8 g, the sample would have to go through three half-lives. Therefore, the amount of time needed for the decay is 3×15 hours.

3. First, the general rate equation must be written out. It is:

   rate $= k[A]^x[B]^y$

   where:

   k = the rate constant

   x = the order with respect to reactant A

   y = the order with respect to reactant B

   A $x = 2$

   To solve for x, it is necessary to find two trials in which B is held constant; here, experiments 1 and 3. The data shows that if the concentration of A is doubled, the rate increases by a factor of 4. Thus, the rate varies as the square of the concentration of A. The order, x, is therefore equal to 2.

   B $y = 0.5$

   To solve for y, follow the steps as in x. In experiments 1 and 2 (and 2 and 4) A is held constant, the concentration of B quadruples, and the rate doubles. The rate, therefore, varies as the square root of the concentration of B. The order, y, is therefore equal to 0.5.

   C rate $= k[A]^2 [B]^{0.5}$

   D order $= 2.5$

   The overall order is equal to $x + y = 2.5$.

   E **3.5**

   Given the rate expression, the rate constant can easily be calculated by substituting the rate and concentrations for any of the four trials into the rate expression; the rate constant will work out to 3.5 in each case.

   Trial 1: $0.035 = k[0.10]^2 [1]^{0.5}$: k = 3.5

   Trial 2: $0.070 = k[0.10]^2 [4]^{0.5}$: k = 3.5

   Trial 3: $0.140 = k[0.20]^2 [1]^{0.5}$: k = 3.5

   Trial 4: $0.140 = k[0.10]^2 [16]^{0.5}$: k = 3.5

4. **A** **rate = k[A]^0 = k**

This reaction has only one reactant. It is evident from the data that the rate of the reaction is not affected by reactant concentration. This is a zero-order reaction, and the rate is equal to its rate constant, k.

B **k = 0.6**

C The most likely reason for the increased rate in trial 2 is a change in temperature. We know that in a zero-order reaction, changing the concentration of the reactant will not cause a change in rate; the factor most likely to affect the rate is temperature.

5. **A** **X = 0.3**

To calculate X, first write the rate expression for this reaction. From the data, the rate expression is calculated as:

$$rate = k[SO_3]^2 [H_2O]$$

The order with respect to SO_3 is 2, since the rate quadruples when the concentration of SO_3 doubles (with the concentration of H_2O remaining constant) between trials 1 and 2. The order with respect to H_2O is 1, as the rate triples as the concentration of H_2O triples (with the concentration of SO_3 remaining constant) between trials 1 and 4.

X can be calculated by plugging the values from trial 3 into the rate expression. First, however, calculate the rate constant, k, by plugging in the known values from trial 1, 2, or 4. For instance:

Trial 4: $0.039 = k[0.1]^2 [0.03]$: $k = 130$

To calculate X, plug in the values of rate and $[H_2O]$ for trial 3, using $k = 130$.

$0.234 = 130[X]^2 [0.02]$

$X = 0.3$

B **3**

The order of the reaction is the sum of the exponents in the rate expression: in this case, $2 + 1 = 3$.

C **130**

For calculations see solution to part A.

D **0.156 units**

Substitute 0.2 instead of 0.1:

$$rate = (130)(0.2)^2(0.03) = 0.156$$

6. B The activation energy is the minimum amount of energy needed for a reaction to proceed. The activation energy for the reverse reaction is the change in potential energy between the products and the transition state indicated by arrow B.

7. A 247 kJ

The best way to visualize the solution to this set of problems is to draw a diagram.

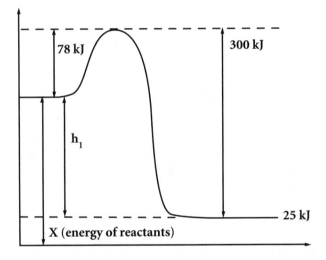

ΔH = Activation Energy$_{\text{forward}}$ − Activation Energy$_{\text{reverse}}$

= 78 kJ − 300 kJ = −222 kJ.

And because

ΔH = Energy$_{\text{products}}$ − Energy$_{\text{reactants}}$

−222 kJ = 25 kJ − X kJ,

X = 247 kJ= energy of reactants.

B The forward reaction is exothermic, because ΔH is negative.

C The reverse reaction is endothermic.

D The enthalpy change, ΔH, of the reaction is −222 kJ.

8. D Discussed in the section on the efficiency of reactions.

9. **C** If the number of nuclei decaying in a sample has decreased by a factor of 4, the sample has been through 2 half-lives, and the half-life will be

$$\frac{112 \text{ sec}}{2} = 56 \text{ sec} = t_{1/2}$$

The equation to determine the decay constant for the first-order reaction is

$$t_{1/2} = \frac{0.693}{k}$$

Thus, given that the half-life is 56 sec, the decay constant will be

$$56 \text{ sec} = \frac{0.693}{k}$$

$$k = 0.0124 \text{ sec}^{-1}$$

10. **C** Various conditions can affect the rate of reaction: increased temperature, increased concentration of reactants, and decreased volume or increased pressure (if any reactants are gases), or addition of a suitable catalyst. The effect of a catalyst is to decrease the activation energy, therefore choice C is correct.

11. **B** Discussed in the section on factors affecting reaction rate.

12. **A** K_{eq} remains constant at 0.16. Catalysts do not affect equilibrium position.

   B Addition of a catalyst decreases the activation energy.

13. **D** At equilibrium, both the forward and reverse reactions are proceeding. Any change in the equilibrium conditions will shift the equilibrium to alleviate the stress on the reaction.

14. $$K_{eq} = \frac{[N_2][H_2O]^2}{[NO_2]^2[H_2]^2}$$

15. **A** Discussed in the section on the equilibrium constant.

16. **A** The reaction shifts to the left. This is an exothermic reaction, as seen by the negative ΔH, and any increase in temperature will favor the reverse reaction.

   B The reaction will remain unchanged. Changing the volume constraints on a reaction that involves gases will affect the equilibrium only when one side of the reaction has a greater number of moles than the other.

   C The reaction would shift to the right. By removing methane gas from the reaction vessel, the reactant concentrations are effectively increased relative to the product concentrations, and the reaction will go to the right to correct for this.

CHAPTER THIRTY-THREE

Thermochemistry

All chemical reactions are accompanied by energy changes. Thermal, chemical, potential, and kinetic energies are all interconvertible, as they must obey the **Law of Conservation of Energy**. Energy changes determine whether reactions can occur and how easily they will do so; thus an understanding of thermodynamics is essential to an understanding of chemistry. In chemistry, **thermodynamics** help determine whether a chemical reaction is **spontaneous** (i.e., if under a given set of conditions it can occur, by itself, without outside assistance). A spontaneous reaction may or may not proceed to completion, depending upon the rate of the reaction, which is determined by chemical kinetics (see Chapter 32).

The application of thermodynamics to chemical reactions is called **thermochemistry**. Several thermodynamic definitions are very useful in thermochemistry. A **system** is the particular part of the universe being studied; everything outside the system is considered the **surroundings** or **environment**. A system may be:

- **Isolated**—It cannot exchange energy or matter with the surroundings, as with an insulated bomb reactor.

- **Closed**—It can exchange energy but not matter with the surroundings, as with a steam radiator.

- **Open**—It can exchange both matter and energy with the surroundings, as with a pot of boiling water.

A system undergoes a **process** when one or more of its properties changes. A process is associated with a change of state. An **isothermal** process occurs when the temperature of the system remains constant, an **adiabatic** process occurs when no heat exchange occurs, and an **isobaric** process occurs when the pressure of the system remains constant. Isothermal and isobaric processes are common since it is usually easy to control temperature and pressure.

HEAT

Definition

Heat is a form of energy that can easily transfer to or from a system as the result of a temperature difference between the system and its surroundings; this transfer will occur spontaneously from a warmer system to a cooler system. According to convention, heat absorbed by a system (from its surroundings) is considered positive, while heat lost by a system (to its surroundings) is considered negative.

A **system** is any given part of the universe that is of particular interest to chemists. The remaining portion of the universe outside of the system is described as **surroundings**. There are three general types of systems:

- **Open system**—This type of system can exchange both mass and energy with its surroundings. The energy is typically in the form of heat energy.

- **Closed system**—This type of system can exchange energy with the surroundings; however, it cannot exchange mass.

- **Isolated system**—This type of system will not allow the transfer of either mass or energy with the surroundings.

Heat change is the most common energy change in chemical processes. Reactions that absorb heat energy are said to be **endothermic**, while those that release heat energy are said to be **exothermic**. Heat is commonly measured in **calories (cal)**, or **Joules (J)**, and more commonly in **kcal or kJ** (1 cal = 4.184 J).

Calorimetry

Calorimetry measures heat changes. The terms **constant-volume calorimetry** and **constant-pressure calorimetry** are used to indicate the conditions under which the heat changes are measured. The heat (q) absorbed or released in a given process is calculated from the equation:

$$q = mc\Delta T$$

where m is the mass, c is the **specific heat**, and ΔT is the change in temperature.

When using the equation for specific heat, $q = mc\Delta T$, remember this only can be used when the phase remains the same. If there is a phase change (e.g., solid to liquid), you must calculate the heat during transformation using the equation $q = mL$, where L is either the heat of fusion or vaporization, depending on whether you are interchanging solid and liquid or liquid and gas, respectively.

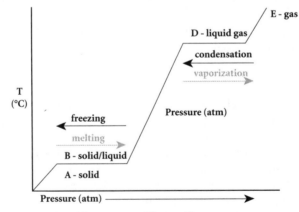

Figure 33.1, Phase Changes

Constant-volume calorimetry

In constant-volume calorimetry, the volume of the container holding the reacting mixture does not change during the course of the reaction. The heat of reaction is measured using a device called a **bomb calorimeter**. This apparatus consists of a steel bomb into which the reactants are placed. The bomb is immersed in an insulated container containing a known amount of water. The reactants are electrically ignited and heat is absorbed or evolved as the reaction proceeds. The heat of the reaction, q_{rxn}, can be determined as follows. Since no heat enters or leaves the system, the net heat change for the system is zero; therefore, the heat change for the reaction is compensated for by the heat change for the water and the bomb, which is easy to measure.

$$q_{system} = q_{rxn} + q_{water} + q_{steel} = 0$$
$$q_{rxn} = -(q_{water} + q_{steel})$$
$$= -(m_{water} \, c_{water} \, \Delta T + m_{steel} \, c_{steel} \, \Delta T)$$

Note that the overall system, as defined, is adiabatic, since no net heat gain or loss occurs. However, the heat exchange between the various components makes it possible to determine the heat of reaction.

STATES AND STATE FUNCTIONS

The state of a system is described by the macroscopic properties of the system. Examples of macroscopic properties include temperature (T), pressure (P), and volume (V). When the state of a system changes, the values of the properties also change. Properties whose magnitude depends only on the initial and final states of the system, not on the path of the change (how the change was accomplished), are known as **state functions**. Pressure, temperature, and volume are important state functions. Other examples are **enthalpy (H), entropy (S), free energy (G)** (all discussed below), and **internal energy (E or U)**. Although independent of path, state functions are not necessarily independent of one another.

A set of **standard conditions** (25°C and 1 atm) is normally used for measuring the enthalpy, entropy, and free energy of a reaction. A substance in its most stable form under standard conditions is said to be in its **standard state**. Examples of substances in their standard states include hydrogen as $H_2(g)$, water as $H_2O(l)$, and salt as $NaCl(s)$. The changes in enthalpy, entropy, and free energy that occur when a reaction takes place under standard conditions are called the **standard enthalpy, standard entropy**, and **standard free energy** changes respectively, and are symbolized by $\Delta H°$, $\Delta S°$, and $\Delta G°$.

Enthalpy

Most reactions in the lab occur under constant pressure (at 1 atm, in open containers). To express heat changes at constant pressure, chemists use the term *enthalpy* (H). The change in enthalpy (ΔH) of a process is equal to the heat absorbed or evolved by the system at constant pressure. The enthalpy of a process depends only on the enthalpies of the initial and final states, not on the path. Thus, to find the enthalpy change of a reaction, ΔH_{rxn}, one must subtract the enthalpy of the reactants from the enthalpy of the products:

$$\Delta H_{rxn} = H_{products} - H_{reactants}$$

A positive ΔH corresponds to an endothermic process, and a negative ΔH corresponds to an exothermic process.

Unfortunately, it is not possible to measure H directly; only ΔH can be measured, and even then, only for certain fast and spontaneous processes. Thus, several standard methods have been developed to calculate ΔH for any process.

Standard heat of formation

The enthalpy of formation of a compound, $\Delta H°_f$, is the enthalpy change that would occur if one mole of a compound were formed directly from its elements in their standard states. Note that $\Delta H°_f$ of an element in its standard state is zero. The $\Delta H°_f$'s of most known substances are tabulated.

Standard heat of reaction

The standard heat of a reaction, $\Delta H°_{rxn}$, is the hypothetical enthalpy change that would occur if the reaction were carried out under standard conditions; i.e., when reactants in their standard states are converted to products in their standard states at 298 K. It can be expressed as:

$$\Delta H°_{rxn} = (\text{sum of } \Delta H°_f \text{ of products}) - (\text{sum of } \Delta H°_f \text{ of reactants})$$

Hess's Law

Hess's Law states that enthalpies of reactions are additive. Specifically, Hess's Law states that when the reactants are transformed into products, the net change in enthalpy is the same irrespective if the reaction takes place in a series of steps or in a single step. When thermochemical equations (chemical equations for which energy changes are known) are added to give the net equation for a reaction, the corresponding heats of reaction are also added to give the net heat of reaction. Because enthalpy is a state function, the enthalpy of a reaction does not depend on the path taken, only on the initial and final states. For example, consider the reaction:

$$Br_2 \; (l) \rightarrow Br_2 \; (g) \quad \Delta H = (31 \text{ kJ/mol})(1 \text{ mol}) = 31 \text{ kJ}$$

The enthalpy change of the above reaction, called the **heat of vaporization**, $\Delta H°_{vap}$, will always be 31 kJ/mol provided that the same initial and final states, $Br_2(l)$ and $Br_2(g)$ respectively, exist at standard conditions. $Br_2(l)$ could instead be decomposed to Br atoms and then recombined to form $Br_2(g)$, but since the net reaction is the same, the change in enthalpy will always be the same.

$$
\begin{array}{lll}
Br_2 \; (l) & \rightarrow \; 2 \; Br \; (g) & \Delta H_1 \\
2 \; Br \; (g) & \rightarrow \; Br_2 \; (g) & \Delta H_2 \\
\hline
Br_2 \; (l) & \rightarrow \; Br_2 \; (g) & \Delta H = \Delta H_1 + \Delta H_2 = 31 \text{ kJ}
\end{array}
$$

Example: Given the following thermochemical equations:

a) $C_3H_8 \; (g) + 5 \; O_2 \; (g) \rightarrow 3 \; CO_2 \; (g) + 4 \; H_2O \; (l) \quad \Delta H_a = -2220.1 \text{ kJ}$
b) $C \; (graphite) + O_2 \; (g) \rightarrow CO_2 \; (g) \quad\quad\quad\quad\quad\quad \Delta H_b = -393.5 \text{ kJ}$
c) $H_2 \; (g) + 1/2 \; O_2 \; (g) \rightarrow H_2O \; (l) \quad\quad\quad\quad\quad\quad\;\; \Delta H_c = -285.8 \text{ kJ}$

   Calculate ΔH for the reaction:
d) $3 \; C \; (graphite) + 4 \; H_2 \; (g) \rightarrow C_3H_8 \; (g)$

Solution: Equations a, b, and c must be combined to obtain equation d. Since equation d contains only C, H_2, and C_3H_8, we must eliminate O_2, CO_2, and H_2O from the first three equations. Equation a is reversed to get C_3H_8 on the product side.

e) $3 \; CO_2 \; (g) + 4 \; H_2O \; (l) \rightarrow C_3H_8 \; (g) + 5 \; O_2 \; (g) \quad\quad \Delta He = 2,220.1 \text{ kJ}$

   Next, equation b is multiplied by 3 (this gives equation f) and c by 4 (this gives equation g). The following addition is done to obtain the required equation d: 3b + 4c + e.

e) $3 \; CO_2 \; (g) + 4 \; H_2O \; (l) \rightarrow C_3H_8 \; (g) + 5 \; O_2 \; (g) \quad \Delta He = 2,220.1 \text{ kJ}$
f) $3 \times [C \; (graphite) + O_2 \; (g) \rightarrow CO_2 \; (g)] \quad\quad\quad\quad \Delta H_f = 3 \times -393.5 \text{ kJ}$
g) $4 \times [H_2 \; (g) + \dfrac{1}{2} O_2 \; (g) \rightarrow H_2O \; (l)] \quad\quad\quad\quad \Delta H_g = 4 \times -285.8 \text{ kJ}$

$$
\begin{array}{ll}
\hline
3 \; C \; (graphite) + 4 \; H_2 \; (g) \rightarrow C_3H_8 \; (g) & \Delta H_d = -103.6 \text{ kJ}
\end{array}
$$

   where $\Delta H_d = \Delta H_e + \Delta H_f + \Delta H_g$.

It is important to note that the reverse of any reaction has an enthalpy of the same magnitude as that of the forward reaction, but its sign is opposite.

Bond dissociation energy

Heats of reaction are related to changes in energy associated with the breakdown and formation of chemical bonds. **Bond energy**, or bond dissociation energy, is an average of the energy required to break a particular type of bond in one mole of gaseous molecules. It is tabulated as the positive value of the energy absorbed as the bonds are broken. For example:

$$H_2 (g) \rightarrow 2H (g) \quad \Delta H = 436 \text{ kJ}$$

A molecule of H_2 gas is cleaved to produce two gaseous, unassociated hydrogen atoms. For each mole of H_2 gas cleaved, roughly 436 kJ of energy is absorbed by the system. The reaction is therefore endothermic. For bonds found in other than diatomic molecules, many compounds have been measured and the energy requirements averaged. For example, the C-H bond dissociation energy one would find in a table (415 kJ/mol) was compiled from measurements on thousands of different organic compounds.

Bond energies can be used to estimate enthalpies of reactions. The enthalpy change of a reaction is given by:

$$\Delta H_{rxn} = (\Delta H \text{ of bonds broken}) + (\Delta H \text{ of bonds formed})$$

$$= \text{total energy input} - \text{total energy released}$$

Note: Since energy is released when bonds are formed, the ΔH of bonds formed will be negative.

Example: Calculate the enthalpy change for the following reaction:

$$C (s) + 2 H_2 (g) \rightarrow CH_4 (g) \quad \Delta H = ?$$

Bond dissociation energies of H – H and C – H bonds are 436 kJ/mol and 415 kJ/mol, respectively.

ΔH_f of C (g) = 715 kJ/mol

Solution: CH_4 is formed from free elements in their standard states (C in solid and H_2 in gaseous state).

Thus here, $\Delta H_{rxn} = \Delta H_f$.

The reaction can be written as three steps:

     a) C $(s) \rightarrow$ C (g) ΔH_1
     b) 2 [$H_2 (g) \rightarrow$ 2 H (g)] $2\Delta H_2$
     c) C (g) + 4 H $(g) \rightarrow CH_4 (g)$ ΔH_3

and

$$\Delta H_f = [\Delta H_1 + 2\Delta H_2] + [\Delta H_3]$$

$$\Delta H_1 = \Delta H_f \, C(g) = 715 \text{ kJ/mol}$$

ΔH_2 is the energy required to break the H – H bond of one mole of H_2.

So:

$$\Delta H_2 = \text{bond energy of } H_2$$

$$= 436 \text{ kJ/mol}$$

ΔH_3 is the energy released when 4 C – H bonds are formed.

So:

$$\Delta H_3 = -(4 \times \text{bond energy of C} - \text{H})$$
$$= -(4 \times 415 \text{ kJ/mol})$$
$$= -1{,}660 \text{ kJ/mol}$$

Note: Since energy is released when bonds are formed, ΔH_3 is negative.

Therefore:

$$\Delta H_{rxn} = \Delta H_f = [715 + 2(436)] - (1{,}660) \text{ kJ/mol}$$
$$= -73 \text{ kJ/mol}$$

Heats of combustion

One more type of standard enthalpy change that is often used is the standard heat of combustion, ΔH°_{comb}. As stated earlier, a requirement for relatively easy measurement of ΔH is that the reaction be fast and spontaneous; combustion generally fits this description. The reactions used in the C_3H_8 (g) example above were combustion reactions, and the corresponding values ΔH_a, ΔH_b, and ΔH_c were thus heats of combustion.

Entropy

Entropy (**S**) is a measure of the disorder, or randomness, of a system. The units of entropy are energy/temperature, commonly J/K or cal/K. The greater the order in a system, the lower the entropy; the greater the disorder or randomness, the higher the entropy. At any given temperature, a solid will have lower entropy than a gas, because individual molecules in the gaseous state are moving randomly, while individual molecules in a solid are constrained in place. Entropy is a state function, so a change in entropy depends only on the initial and final states:

$$\Delta S = S_{final} - S_{initial}$$

A change in entropy is also given by:

$$\Delta S = \frac{q_{rev}}{T}$$

where q_{rev} is the heat added to the system undergoing a reversible process (a process that proceeds with infinitesimal changes in the system's conditions) and T is the absolute temperature.

A standard entropy change for a reaction, **ΔS°**, is calculated using the standard entropies of reactants and products:

$$\Delta S^\circ_{rxn} = (\text{sum of } S^\circ_{products}) - (\text{sum of } S^\circ_{reactants})$$

The Second Law of Thermodynamics states that all spontaneous processes proceed such that the entropy of the system plus its surroundings (i.e., the entropy of the universe) increases:

$$\Delta S_{universe} = \Delta S_{system} + \Delta S_{surroundings} > 0$$

A system reaches its maximum entropy at **equilibrium**, a state in which no observable change takes place as time goes on. For a reversible process, $\Delta S_{universe}$ is zero:

$$\Delta S_{universe} = \Delta S_{system} + \Delta S_{surroundings} = 0$$

A system will spontaneously tend toward an equilibrium state if left alone.

Gibbs Free Energy

Spontaneity of reaction

The thermodynamic state function, **G** (known as the Gibbs free energy), combines the two factors that affect the spontaneity of a reaction—changes in enthalpy, ΔH, and changes in entropy, ΔS. The change in the free energy of a system, ΔG, represents the maximum amount of energy released by a process, occurring at constant temperature and pressure, that is available to perform useful work. ΔG is defined by the equation:

$$\Delta G = \Delta H - T\Delta S$$

where T is the absolute temperature and $T\Delta S$ represents the total amount of heat absorbed by a system when its entropy increases reversibly.

In the equilibrium state, free energy is at a minimum. A process can occur spontaneously if the Gibbs function decreases (i.e., $\Delta G < 0$).

- If ΔG is negative, the reaction is spontaneous.
- If ΔG is positive, the reaction is not spontaneous.
- If ΔG is zero, the system is in a state of equilibrium; thus, $\Delta G = 0$ and $\Delta H = T\Delta S$.

Because the temperature is always positive (in Kelvins), the effects of the signs of ΔH and ΔS and the effect of temperature on spontaneity can be summarized as follows:

ΔH	ΔS	Outcome
−	+	spontaneous at all temperatures
+	−	nonspontaneous at all temperatures
+	+	spontaneous only at high temperatures
−	−	spontaneous only at low temperatures

It is very important to note that the **rate** of a reaction depends on the **activation energy**, not the ΔG.

Standard free energy

Standard free energy, $\Delta G°$, is defined as the ΔG of a process occurring at 25°C and 1 atm pressure and for which the concentrations of any solutions involved are 1 M. The **standard free energy of formation** of a compound, $\Delta G°_f$, is the free-energy change that occurs when one mol of a compound in its standard state is formed from its elements in their standard states under standard conditions. The standard free energy of formation of any element in its most stable form (and, therefore, its standard state) is zero. The standard free energy of a reaction, $\Delta G°_{rxn}$, is the free energy change that occurs when that reaction is carried out under standard state conditions; i.e., when the reactants in their standard states are converted to the products in their standard states, at standard conditions of T and P. For example, conversion of

C(*diamond*) to C(*graphite*) is spontaneous under standard conditions. However, its rate is so slow that the rxn is never observed.

$$\Delta G°_{rxn} = \text{(sum of } \Delta G°_f \text{ of products)} - \text{(sum of } \Delta G°_f \text{ of reactants)}$$

Reaction quotient

$\Delta G°_{rxn}$ can also be derived from the equilibrium constant for the equation:

$$\Delta G° = -RT \ln K_{eq}$$

where K_{eq} is the equilibrium constant, R is the gas constant, and T is the temperature in K.

Once a reaction commences, however, the standard state conditions no longer hold. K_{eq} must be replaced by another parameter, the **reaction quotient (Q)**. For the reaction, a A + b B $\rightleftarrows$ c C + d D:

$$Q = \frac{[C]^c [D]^d}{[A]^a [B]^b}$$

Likewise, ΔG must be used in place of $\Delta G°$. The relationship between the two is as follows:

$$\Delta G = \Delta G° + RT \ln Q$$

where R is the gas constant and T is the temperature in K.

Example:

Vaporization of water at one atmosphere pressure:

$$H_2O \ (l) + heat \rightarrow H_2O \ (g)$$

Discussion:

When water boils, hydrogen bonds (H-bonds) are broken. Energy is absorbed (the reaction is endothermic), and thus ΔH is positive. Entropy increases as the closely packed molecules of the liquid become the more randomly moving molecules of a gas; thus, $T\Delta S$ is also positive. Since ΔH and $T\Delta S$ are each positive, the reaction will proceed spontaneously only if $T\Delta S > \Delta H$. This is true only at temperatures above 100°C. Below 100°C, ΔG is positive and the water remains a liquid. At 100°C, $\Delta H = T\Delta S$ and $\Delta G = 0$: an equilibrium is established between water and water vapor. The opposite is true when water vapor condenses: H-bonds are formed, and energy is released; the reaction is exothermic (ΔH is negative) and entropy decreases, since a liquid is forming from a gas ($T\Delta S$ is negative). Condensation will be spontaneous only if $\Delta H < T\Delta S$. This is the case at temperatures below 100°C; above 100°C, $T\Delta S$ is more negative than H, ΔG is positive, and condensation is not spontaneous. Again, at 100°C, an equilibrium is established.

Example:

The combustion of C_6H_6 (benzene)

$$2 \ C_6H_6 \ (l) + 15 \ O_2 \ (g) \rightarrow 12 \ CO_2 \ (g) + 6 \ H_2O \ (g) + heat$$

Discussion:

In this case, heat is released (ΔH is negative) as the benzene burns and the entropy is increased ($T\Delta S$ is positive), because two gases (18 moles total) have greater entropy than a gas and a liquid (15 moles gas and 2 liquid). ΔG is negative and the reaction is spontaneous.

REVIEW PROBLEMS

1. A process involving no heat exchange is known as
   - (A) an isothermal process.
   - (B) an isobaric process.
   - (C) an adiabatic process.
   - (D) an isometric process.

2. What is the heat capacity of a 10 g sample that has absorbed 100 cal over a temperature change of 30°C and has not changed phases?
   - (A) 0.333 cal/g°C
   - (B) 0.666 cal/g°C
   - (C) 3 cal/g°C
   - (D) 300 cal/g°C

3. Calculate the enthalpy of formation of N (g) in the following reaction:

   $$N_2\ (g) \rightarrow 2N\ (g) \qquad \Delta H°_{rxn} = 945.2\ kJ$$

   - (A) −945.2 kJ/mol
   - (B) 0.0 kJ/mol
   - (C) 472.6 kJ/mol
   - (D) 945.2 kJ/mol

4. Calculate the amount of heat needed to bring 10 g of ice from −15°C to 110°C. Heat of fusion = 80 cal/g; heat of vaporization = 540 cal/g. The heat capacities of both ice and steam vary with temperature; for this problem, use the estimate of 0.5 cal/g · K for both.
   - (A) 7.325 cal
   - (B) 7.450 cal
   - (C) 7.325 kcal
   - (D) 7.450 kcal

5. Using the information given in the reaction equations below, calculate the heat of formation for one mole of carbon monoxide.

   $$2\ C\ (s) + 2\ O_2 \rightarrow 2\ CO_2 \qquad \Delta H_{rxn} = -787\ kJ$$
   $$2\ CO + O_2 \rightarrow 2\ CO_2 \qquad \Delta H_{rxn} = -566\ kJ$$

   - (A) −221 kJ/mol
   - (B) −110 kJ/mol
   - (C) 110 kJ/mol
   - (D) 221 kJ/mol

6. If the free energy change accompanying a reaction is negative,

   (A) the reaction can occur spontaneously.
   (B) the reaction can be used to do work by driving other reactions.
   (C) the entropy must always be negative.
   (D) both A and B are true.

7. All of the following are correct statements concerning entropy EXCEPT:

   (A) All spontaneous processes tend towards an increase in entropy.
   (B) The more highly ordered the system, the higher the entropy.
   (C) The entropy of a pure crystalline solid at 0 K is 0.
   (D) The change in entropy of an equilibrium process is 0.

8. A 50-g sample of metal was heated to 100°C and then dropped into a beaker containing 50 g of water at 25°C. If the specific heat capacity of the metal is 0.25 cal/g • °C, what is the final temperature of the water?

   (A) 27°C
   (B) 40°C
   (C) 60°C
   (D) 86°C

9. Calculate the maximum amount of work that can be done by the following reaction at 30°C ($\Delta H° = -125$ kJ, $\Delta S = -200$ J/K):

   $$FeCl_2 \ (aq) + 1/2 \ Cl_2 \ (g) \rightarrow FeCl_3 \ (aq)$$

   (A) 64.4 kJ
   (B) 119 kJ
   (C) 5,875 kJ
   (D) 60,475 kJ

10. Discuss the three different types of thermodynamic systems that can exist and give an example of each.

11. Calculate the bond energy of a BrF bond using the following reaction equation (ΔH_f of BrF_5 (g) $= -429$ kJ/mol, ΔH_f of Br (g) $= 112$ kJ/mol, ΔH_f of F (g) $= 79$ kJ/mol):

    $$Br \ (g) + 5 \ F \ (g) \rightarrow BrF_5 \ (g)$$

    (A) 936 kJ/mol
    (B) 187 kJ/mol
    (C) 86 kJ/mol
    (D) 47 kJ/mol

12. | Bond | Average Bond Energy |
|---|---|
| $C\equiv O$ | 1,075 kJ/mol |
| $C=O$ | 728 kJ/mol |
| $C–Cl$ | 326 kJ/mol |
| $Cl–Cl$ | 243 kJ/mol |

Calculate the heat of reaction for the following equation using the information given above:

$$CO + Cl_2 \rightarrow COCl_2$$

(A) 62 kJ

(B) −62 kJ

(C) −409 kJ

(D) 706 kJ

SOLUTIONS TO REVIEW PROBLEMS

1. **C** Discussed in the section on heat.

2. **A** In calorimetry, the amount of heat absorbed in a given process is calculated using the following equation:

$$q = mc\Delta T$$

Knowing that the heat absorbed is 100 cal, the mass is 10 g, and the temperature change is 30°C, the specific heat capacity can be calculated:

$$100 \text{ cal} = 10 \text{ g (c)}(30°C)$$

$$c = 0.333 \text{ cal/g°C}$$

3. **C** This problem uses the equation:

$$\Delta H_{rxn} = \Sigma\, \Delta H_{products} - \Sigma\, \Delta H_{reactants}$$

The equation for the enthalpy of formation of N is:

$$945.2 \text{ kJ} = 2(\Delta H_N)\ 2\ (\Delta H_{N_2})$$

where ΔH of N_2 is 0 kJ, because the heat of formation of any element in its elemental state is zero. Now solve for the enthalpy of formation of N.

$$\Delta H_N = \frac{924.2 \text{ kJ}}{2 \text{ mol}} = 472.6 \text{ kJ / mol}$$

4. **C** To answer this question, the ice must be imagined as passing through the following stages: ice from −15°C to ice at 0°C, ice at 0°C to water at 0°C, water from 0°C to water at 100°C, water at 100°C to steam at 100°C, and steam at 100°C to steam at 110°C. Once these steps have been outlined, the amount of heat needed to perform each of them must be calculated using the following equation:

$$
\begin{aligned}
\text{heat absorbed} = \ & (10g)\ (0.5 \text{ cal/g} \cdot K)\ (15 \text{ K}) \\
& +(10 \text{ g})\ (80 \text{ cal/g}) \\
& +(10 \text{ g})\ (1 \text{ cal/g} \cdot K)\ (100 \text{ K}) \\
& +(10 \text{ g})\ (540 \text{ cal/g}) \\
& +\underline{(10 \text{ g})\ (0.5 \text{ cal/g} \cdot K)\ (10 \text{ K})} \\
& =7{,}325 \text{ cal} \\
& =7.325 \text{ kcal}
\end{aligned}
$$

5. B This problem uses Hess's Law, which states that heats of reaction may be added to determine the enthalpy of another reaction. To calculate the heat of formation for one mole of carbon monoxide, the reaction equations must be manipulated as follows:

$$2\ C\ (s) + 2\ O_2 \rightarrow 2\ CO_2 \qquad \Delta H_{rxn} = -787\ kJ$$
$$2\ CO + O_2 \rightarrow 2\ CO_2 \qquad \Delta H_{rxn} = -566\ kJ$$

The second equation must be reversed:

$$2\ C\ (s) + 2O_2 \rightarrow 2\ CO_2 \qquad \Delta H_{rxn} = -787\ kJ$$
$$2\ CO_2 \rightarrow 2\ CO + O_2 \qquad \Delta H_{rxn} = 566\ kJ$$

If the two equations are added together, a third equation is obtained:

$$2\ C + O_2 \rightarrow 2\ CO \qquad \Delta H_{rxn} = -221\ kJ$$

However, the ΔH_f for one mol of CO will be:

$$\frac{-221\ kJ}{2\ mol} = -110\ kJ\ /\ mol$$

6. D A negative free energy change signifies that the reaction is spontaneous and that work can be done. If the energy that is released is coupled to less favorable reactions, they can be driven to completion.

7. B Discussed in the section on entropy.

8. B This problem uses the concept of conservation of energy. When the metal is put in the water, it will lose heat; that heat will be transferred to the water. Thus, the amount of heat released by the metal is the same as the amount of heat absorbed by the water. The following equation for heat transfer can be used:

$$q = mc\Delta T$$

The expressions for the heat released and absorbed by the metal and water respectively are:

$$q = 50\ g\ (0.25\ cal/g \cdot °C)(100°C - x)$$
$$q = 50\ g\ (1.0\ cal/g \cdot °C)(x - 25°C)$$

However, since q should be the same for both equations, the expression can be rewritten:

$$50\ g\ (0.25\ cal/g \cdot °C)\ (100°C - T_f) = 50\ g\ (1.0\ cal/g \cdot °C)(T_f - 25°C)$$

Canceling the 50 g from each side and solving for T_f, which is the final temperature, we get:

$$(0.25)(100°C - T_f) = (T_f - 25°C)$$
$$25°C - (0.25)T_f = (T_f - 25°C)$$
$$50°C = 1.25\ T_f \qquad \text{or, simply, } T_f = 40°C$$

9. A The maximum amount of work that can be done by a spontaneous reaction is the absolute value of its Gibbs free energy change, and the following equation can be used to solve for it:

$$\Delta G = \Delta H - T\Delta S$$

The free energy change due to the reaction can be calculated by substituting the information given for ΔH, T, and ΔS. Be sure that the units are consistent when solving the equation.

$$\Delta G = -125\ kJ - (30°C + 273)(-0.2\ kJ/K)$$
$$\Delta G = -125\ kJ - (303\ K)(-0.2\ kJ/K)$$
$$\Delta G = -64.4\ kJ$$

Thus, 64.4 kJ can be done by the system.

10. **Open, closed,** and **isolated.** Discussed in the introduction to this chapter.

11. **B** The enthalpy, or heat of reaction, for any reaction is the sum of the enthalpies of formation of the products minus the sum of the enthalpies of formation of the reactants:

$$\Delta H_{rxn} = \Sigma \Delta H_f \text{ products} - \Sigma \Delta H_f \text{ reactants}$$

Substituting the heats of formation of BrF_5 (g), Br (g), and F (g) into the equation, the heat of reaction can be calculated:

$$\Delta H_{rxn} = [(-429 \text{ kJ/mol})(1 \text{ mol})] - [(112 \text{ kJ/mol})(1 \text{ mol}) + (79 \text{ kJ/mol})(5 \text{ mol})]$$
$$= -936 \text{ kJ}$$

Because no bonds were broken in this reaction (i.e., the bond energies of the reactants are zero), the heat of formation here is equal to the sum of the bond energies of the product. As there are five equivalent Br—F bonds, each one would contribute to one-fifth of the total bond energy:

$$\frac{-936 \text{ kJ / mol}}{5} = -187 \Rightarrow 187 \text{ kJ / mole}$$

This means that for each bond formed, an average of 187 kJ/mol of energy was released (note the negative sign in front of the enthalpy). The bond energy is defined to be the energy required to *break* the bond, the reverse of the process we have just described. The Br—F bond energy is therefore 187 kJ/mol. As it always requires energy to break a bond, all bond enthalpies are positive.

12. **B** $\Delta H_{rxn} = \Delta H \text{ bonds broken} - \Delta H \text{ bonds formed} = 1{,}318 - 1{,}380 = -62$

$\Delta H \text{ bonds broken} = 1{,}075 \text{kJ/mole 1 mole}) + 243 \text{ kJ/mole (1 mole)} = 1{,}318 \text{ kL}$

$\Delta H \text{ bonds formed} = 728 \text{ kJ/mole (1 mole)} + 326 \text{ kJ/mole (2 moles)} = 1{,}380 \text{ kJ}$

CHAPTER THIRTY-FOUR

The Gas Phase

Matter can exist in three different physical forms, called **phases** or **states: gas**, **liquid**, and **solid**. Liquids and solids will be discussed in Chapter 35.

The gaseous phase, the subject of this chapter, is the simplest to understand, since all gases display similar behavior and follow similar laws regardless of their identity. The atoms or molecules in a gaseous sample move rapidly and are far apart from each other. In addition, only very weak intermolecular forces exist between gas particles; this results in certain characteristic physical properties, such as the ability to expand to fill any volume and to take on the shape of a container. Furthermore, gases are easily, though not infinitely, compressible.

The state of a gaseous sample is generally defined by four variables: **pressure (P), volume (V), temperature (T)**, and **number of moles (n)**. Gas pressures are usually expressed in units of atmospheres (atm) or millimeters of mercury (mm Hg or torr), which are related as follows:

$$1 \text{ atm} = 760 \text{ mm Hg} = 760 \text{ torr}$$

Volume is generally expressed in liters (L) or milliliters (mL). The temperature of a gas is usually given in Kelvin (K, *not* °K). Gases are often discussed in terms of **standard temperature and pressure (STP)**, which refers to conditions of 273.15 K (0°C) and 1 atm.

Note: It is important not to confuse STP with **standard conditions**—the two standards involve different temperatures and are used for different purposes. STP (0°C or 273 K) is generally used for gas law calculations; standard conditions (25°C or 298 K) is used when measuring standard enthalpy, entropy, Gibbs free energy, and voltage.

IDEAL GASES

When examining the behavior of gases under varying conditions of temperature and pressure, scientists speak of ideal gases. An ideal gas represents a hypothetical gas whose molecules have no intermolecular forces and occupy no volume. Although gases actually deviate from this idealized behavior, at relatively low pressures (atmospheric pressure) and high temperatures, many gases behave in a nearly ideal fashion. Therefore, the assumptions used for ideal gases can be applied to real gases with reasonable accuracy.

Boyle's Law

Experimental studies performed by Robert Boyle in 1660 led to the formulation of Boyle's Law. His work showed that for a given gaseous sample held at constant temperature (isothermal conditions), the volume of the gas is inversely proportional to its pressure: $PV = k$.

It is important to note that the individual values of pressure and volume can vary greatly for a given sample of gas. However, as long as the temperature remains constant and the amount of gas does not change, both P and V will equal the same constant (k). Subsequently, for a given sample of gas under two sets of conditions, the following equation can be derived:

$$P_1V_1 = k_1 = P_2V_2 \quad \text{or simply} \quad P_1V_1 = P_2V_2$$

$$PV = k \text{ or } P_1V_1 = P_2V_2$$

where k is a proportionality constant and the subscripts 1 and 2 represent two different sets of conditions. A plot of pressure versus volume for a gas is shown in Figure 34.1.

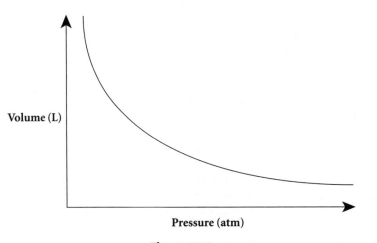

Figure 34.1

Example: Under isothermal conditions, what would be the volume of a 1 L sample of helium after its pressure is changed from 12 atm to 4 atm?

Solution:

$$P_1 = 12 \text{ atm} \qquad P_2 = 4 \text{ atm}$$
$$V_1 = 1 \text{ L} \qquad V_2 = X$$
$$P_1V_1 = P_2V_2$$
$$12 \text{ atm } (1 \text{ L}) = 4 \text{ atm } (X)$$
$$\frac{12}{4}L = X$$
$$X = 3 \text{ L}$$

Law of Charles and Gay-Lussac

The Law of Charles and Gay-Lussac, or simply Charles's Law, was developed during the early 19th century. The law states that at constant pressure, the volume of a gas is directly proportional to its absolute temperature. The absolute temperature is the temperature expressed in Kelvin, which can be calculated from the expression $T_K = T_{°C} + 273.15$.

$$\frac{V}{T} = k \ \text{ or } \ \frac{V_1}{T_1} = \frac{V_2}{T_2}$$

where k is a constant and the subscripts 1 and 2 represent two different sets of conditions. It is important to note that the temperature $-273.15°C$ is the theoretical lowest attainable temperature, known as **absolute zero**. Below is a summary to help understand this principle:

absolute zero	0 K	−273.15°C
water freezes	273.15 K	0°C
water boils	373.15 K	100°C

A plot of temperature versus volume is shown in Figure 34.2.

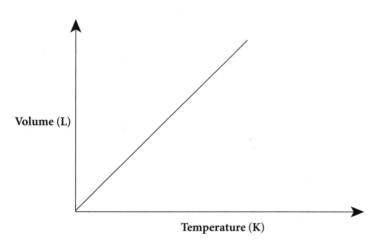

Figure 34.2

Example: If the absolute temperature of 2 L of gas at constant pressure is changed from 283.15 K to 566.30 K, what would be the final volume?

Solution:

$$T_1 = 283.15 \text{ K} \qquad V_1 = 2 \text{ L}$$

$$T_2 = 566.30 \text{ K} \qquad V_2 = X$$

$$\frac{V_1}{T_1} = \frac{V_2}{T_2}$$

$$\frac{2\text{L}}{28,315 \text{ K}} = \frac{X}{56,630 \text{ K}}$$

$$X = \frac{2 \text{ L}(56,630 \text{ K})}{28,315 \text{ K}}$$

$$X = 4 \text{ L}$$

Avogadro's Principle

In 1811, Amedeo Avogadro proposed that for all gases at a constant temperature and pressure, the volume of the gas will be directly proportional to the number of moles of gas present; therefore, all gases have the same number of moles in the same volume.

$$\frac{n}{V} = k \text{ or } \frac{n_1}{V_1} = \frac{n_2}{V_2}$$

The subscripts 1 and 2 once again apply to two different sets of conditions with the same temperature and pressure.

Ideal Gas Law

A theoretical gas whose volume-pressure-temperature behavior can be completely understood by the ideal gas equation is known as an "ideal gas." The ideal gas law combines the relationships outlined in Boyle's Law, Charles's Law, and Avogadro's Principle to yield an expression which can be used to predict the behavior of a gas. The ideal gas law shows the relationship between four variables that define a sample of gas—pressure (P), volume (V), temperature (T), and number of moles (n)—and is represented by the equation

$$PV = nRT$$

The constant R is known as the **gas constant.** Under STP conditions (273.15 K and 1 atmosphere), one mole of gas was shown to have a volume of 22.4 L. Substituting these values into the ideal gas equation gave $R = 8.21 \times 10^{-2}$ L $\cdot$ atm/(mol $\cdot$ K).

The gas constant may be expressed in many other units: another common value is 8.314 J/(K $\cdot$ mol), which is derived when SI units of Pascals (for pressure) and cubic meters (for volume) are substituted into the ideal gas law.

Note: When carrying out calculations based on the ideal gas law, it is important to choose a value of R that matches the units of the variables.

Example: What volume would 12 g of helium occupy at 20°C and a pressure of 380 mmHg?

Solution: The ideal gas law can be used, but first, all of the variables must be converted to yield units that will correspond to the expression of the gas constant as 0.0821 L $\cdot$ atm/(mol $\cdot$ K).

$$P = 380 \text{ mmHg} \times \frac{1 \text{ atm}}{760 \text{ mmHg}} = 0.5 \text{ atm}$$

$$T = 20°C + 273.15 = 293.15K$$

$$n = 12g \text{ He} \times \frac{1 \text{ mol He}}{4.0 \text{ g}} = 3 \text{ mol He}$$

Substituting into the ideal gas equation:

PV = nRT

(0.5 atm)(V) = (3 mol)(0.0821 L $\cdot$ atm/(mol $\cdot$ K)(293.15K)

V = 144.4 L

In addition to standard calculations to determine the pressure, volume, or temperature of a gas, the ideal gas law may be used to determine the **density** and **molar mass** of the gas.

Density

Density is defined as the mass per unit volume of a substance and, for gases, is usually expressed in units of g/L. By rearrangement, the ideal gas equation can be used to calculate the density of a gas.

$$PV = nRT$$

where $\quad n = \dfrac{m}{MM} \quad \dfrac{\text{(mass in g)}}{\text{(molar mass)}}$

therefore $\quad PV = \dfrac{m}{MM} RT$

and $\quad d = \dfrac{m}{v} = \dfrac{P(MM)}{RT}$

Another way to find the density of a gas is to start with the volume of a mole of gas at STP, 22.4 L, calculate the effect of pressure and temperature on the volume, and finally calculate the density by dividing the mass by the new volume. The following equation, derived from Boyle's and Charles's Laws, is used to relate changes in the temperature, volume, and pressure of a gas:

$$\frac{P_1 V_1}{T_1} = \frac{P_2 V_2}{T_2}$$

where the subscripts 1 and 2 refer to the two states of the gas (at STP and under the actual conditions). To calculate a change in volume, the equation is rearranged as follows:

$$V_2 = V_1 \left(\frac{P_1}{P_2}\right)\left(\frac{T_2}{T_1}\right)$$

V_2 is then used to find the density of the gas under nonstandard conditions:

$$d = \frac{m}{V_2}$$

If you **visualize** how the changes in pressure and temperature affect the volume of the gas, this can serve as a check to be sure you have not accidentally confused the pressure or temperature value that belongs in the numerator with the one that belongs in the denominator.

Example: What is the density of HCl gas at 2 atm and 45°C?

Solution: At STP, a mole of gas occupies 22.4 liters. Since the increase in pressure to 2 atm decreases volume, 22.4 L must be multiplied by $\left(\dfrac{1 \text{ atm}}{2 \text{ atm}}\right)$. And since the increase in temperature increases volume, the temperature factor will be $\left(\dfrac{318 \text{ K}}{273 \text{ K}}\right)$.

$$V2 = \left(\frac{22.4 \text{ L}}{\text{mol}}\right)\left(\frac{1 \text{ atm}}{2 \text{ atm}}\right)\left(\frac{318 \text{ K}}{273 \text{ K}}\right) = \frac{13.0 \text{ l}}{\text{mol}}$$

$$d = \left(\frac{36 \text{ g/mol}}{13.0 \text{ L/mol}}\right) = 2.77 \text{ g/L}$$

Molar mass

Sometimes the identity of a gas is unknown, and the molar mass must be determined to identify it. Using the equation for density derived from the ideal gas law, the molar mass of a gas can be determined experimentally as follows. The pressure and temperature of a gas contained in a bulb of a given volume are measured, and the weight of the bulb plus sample is found. Then the bulb is evacuated, and the empty bulb is weighed. The weight of the bulb plus sample minus the weight of the bulb yields the weight of the sample. Finally, the density of the sample is determined by dividing the weight of the sample by the volume of the bulb. The density at STP is calculated. The molecular weight is then found by multiplying the number of grams per liter by 22.4 liters per mole.

Example: What is the molar mass of a 2 L sample of gas that weighs 8 g at a temperature of 15°C and a pressure of 1.5 atm?

Solution: $d = \dfrac{8g}{2L}$ at 15° and 1.5 atm

$$V_{STP} = (2 \text{ L}) \left(\frac{273 \text{ K}}{288 \text{ K}} \right) \left(\frac{1.5 \text{ atm}}{1 \text{ atm}} \right) = 2.84 \text{ L}$$

$$\frac{8 \text{ g}}{2.84 \text{ L}} = 2.82 \text{ g / L at STP}$$

$$\left(\frac{2.82 \text{ g}}{L} \right) \left(\frac{22.4 \text{ L}}{\text{mol}} \right) = 63.2 \text{ g / mol}$$

REAL GASES

In general, the ideal gas law is a good approximation of the behavior of real gases, but all real gases deviate from ideal gas behavior to some extent, particularly when the gas atoms or molecules are forced into close proximity under high pressure and at low temperature, so that molecular volume and intermolecular attractions become significant.

Deviations Due to Pressure

As the pressure of a gas increases, the particles are pushed closer and closer together. As the condensation pressure for a given temperature is approached, intermolecular attraction forces become more and more significant until the gas condenses into the liquid state (see gas-liquid equilibrium in Chapter 35).

At moderately high pressure (a few hundred atmospheres) a gas' volume is less than would be predicted by the ideal gas law, due to intermolecular attraction. At extremely high pressure the size of the particles becomes relatively large compared to the distance between them, and this causes the gas to take up a larger volume than would be predicted by the ideal gas law.

Deviations Due to Temperature

As the temperature of a gas is decreased, the average velocity of the gas molecules decreases, and the attractive intermolecular forces become increasingly significant. As the condensation temperature is approached for a given pressure, intermolecular attractions eventually cause the gas to condense to a liquid state (see gas-liquid equilibrium in Chapter 35).

As the temperature of a gas is reduced toward its condensation point (which is the same as its boiling point), intermolecular attraction causes the gas to have a smaller volume than would be predicted by the ideal gas law. The closer the temperature of a gas is to its boiling point, the less ideal is its behavior.

DALTON'S LAW OF PARTIAL PRESSURES

When two or more gases are found in one vessel without chemical interaction, each gas will behave independently of the other(s). Therefore, the pressure exerted by each gas in the mixture will be equal to the pressure that gas would exert if it were the only one in the container. The pressure exerted by each individual gas is called the **partial pressure** of that gas. In 1801, John Dalton derived an expression, now known as Dalton's Law of Partial Pressures, which states that the total pressure of a gaseous mixture is equal to the sum of the partial pressures of the individual components. The equation is:

$$P_T = P_A + P_B + P_C + \ldots$$

The partial pressure of a gas is related to its mole fraction and can be determined using the following equations:

$$P_A = P_T X_A$$

$$X_A = \frac{n_A \text{ (moles of A)}}{n_T \text{ (total moles)}}$$

Example: A vessel contains 0.75 mol of nitrogen, 0.20 mol of hydrogen, and 0.05 mol of fluorine at a total pressure of 2.5 atm. What is the partial pressure of each gas?

First calculate the mole fraction of each gas.

$$X_{N2} = \frac{0.75 \text{ mol}}{1.0 \text{ mol}} = 0.75 \quad X_{H2} = \frac{0.20 \text{ mol}}{1.0 \text{ mol}} = 0.20 \quad X_{F2} = \frac{0.05 \text{ mol}}{1.0 \text{ mol}} = 0.05$$

Then calculate the partial pressure.

$$P_A = X_A P_T$$

$$P_{N_2} = (2.5 \text{ atm})(0.75) \qquad P_{H_2} = (2.5 \text{ atm})(0.20) \qquad P_{F_2} = (2.5 \text{ atm})(0.05)$$

$$= 1.875 \text{ atm} \qquad\qquad = 0.5 \text{ atm} \qquad\qquad = 0.125 \text{ atm}$$

KINETIC MOLECULAR THEORY OF GASES

As indicated by the gas laws, all gases show similar physical characteristics and behavior. A theoretical model to explain the behavior of gases was developed during the second half of the 19th century. The combined efforts of Boltzmann, Maxwell, and others led to a simple explanation of gaseous molecular behavior based on the motion of individual molecules. This model is called the kinetic molecular theory of gases. Like the gas laws, this theory was developed in reference to ideal gases, although it can be applied with reasonable accuracy to real gases as well.

Assumptions of the Kinetic Molecular Theory

- Gases are made up of particles whose volumes are negligible compared to the container volume.

- Gas atoms or molecules exhibit no intermolecular attractions or repulsions.

- Gas particles are in continuous, random motion, undergoing collisions with other particles and the container walls.

- Collisions between any two gas particles are elastic, meaning that there is no overall gain or loss of energy.

- The average kinetic energy of gas particles is proportional to the absolute temperature of the gas and is the same for all gases at a given temperature.

Applications of the Kinetic Molecular Theory of Gases

Average molecular speeds

According to the kinetic molecular theory of gases, the average kinetic energy of a gas particle is proportional to the absolute temperature of the gas:

$$KE = \frac{1}{2} mv^2 = 3/2\ kT$$

where k is the Boltzmann constant. This equation also shows that the speed of a gas molecule is related to its absolute temperature. However, because of the large number of rapidly and randomly moving gas particles, the speed of an individual gas molecule is nearly impossible to define. Instead, it is the **average speed** of all the gas particles that can be related exactly to the temperature. Some particles will be moving at higher speeds and some at lower speeds.

A **Maxwell-Boltzmann distribution curve** shows the distribution of speeds of gas particles at a given temperature. Figure 34.3 shows a distribution curve of molecular speeds at two temperatures, T1 and T2, where T2 > T1. Notice that the bell-shaped curve flattens and shifts to the right as the temperature increases, indicating that at higher temperatures, more molecules are moving at high speeds.

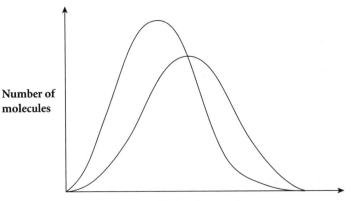

Figure 34.3

Graham's Law of diffusion and effusion

Diffusion of gases can provide a demonstration of random motion when the molecules of these gases mix with one another by virtue of their individual kinetic properties. Diffusion occurs when gas molecules diffuse through a mixture. Diffusion accounts for the fact that an open bottle of perfume can quickly be smelled across a room. The kinetic molecular theory of gases predicted that heavier gas molecules diffuse more slowly than lighter ones because of their differing average speeds. In 1832, Thomas Graham showed mathematically that under isothermal and isobaric conditions, the rates at which two gases diffuse are inversely proportional to the square root of their molar masses. Thus:

$$\frac{r_1}{r_2} = \left(\frac{MM_2}{MM_1}\right)^{\frac{1}{2}} = \sqrt{\frac{MM_2}{MM_1}}$$

where r1 and MM1 represent the diffusion rate and molar mass of gas 1, and r2 and MM2 represent the diffusion rate and molar mass of gas 2.

Effusion is the flow of gas particles under pressure from one compartment to another through a small opening. Graham used the kinetic molecular theory of gases to show that for two gases at the same temperature, the rates of effusion are proportional to the average speeds. He then expressed the rates of effusion in terms of molar mass and found that the relationship is the same as that for diffusion:

$$\frac{r_1}{r_2} = \left(\frac{MM_2}{MM_1}\right)^{\frac{1}{2}}$$

REVIEW PROBLEMS

1. Boyle's Law can be used for which of the following?

   (A) Predicting the expected volumes of two party balloons
   (B) Predicting the relative pressures inside a hot air balloon
   (C) Predicting the change in volume of an inflatable toy from summer to winter
   (D) Predicting the height of a mercury barometer column in a low-pressure system
   (E) Predicting the change in volume of a party balloon inside a bell jar as a vacuum is being drawn

2. The word *kinetic* appears in the kinetic molecular theory of gases because

   (A) the properties of a gas are dependent primarily on the motion of its component particles.
   (B) gases possess kinetic energy.
   (C) gases possess more kinetic than potential energy.
   (D) collisions in real gases do not dissipate kinetic energy.
   (E) collisions in real gases dissipate kinetic energy.

3. A sample of argon occupies 50 L at standard temperature. Assuming constant pressure, what volume will the gas occupy if the temperature is doubled?

   (A) 25 L
   (B) 50 L
   (C) 100 L
   (D) 200 L
   (E) 2,500 L

4. What is the molecular weight of an unknown gas if 2.5 g of it occupies 2 L at 630 torr and a temperature of 600 K?

5. Explain the conditions that define an ideal gas.

6. If a 360 mL sample of helium contains 0.25 mol of the gas, how many molecules of chlorine gas would occupy the same volume at the same temperature and pressure?

   (A) 1.2×10^{24}
   (B) 6.022×10^{23}
   (C) 3.01×10^{23}
   (D) 1.51×10^{23}
   (E) 7.55×10^{22}

7. In the kinetic molecular theory of gases, the speed of molecules is most often discussed in terms of the average speed. Which of the following statements concerning average speeds is TRUE?

   (A) Most of the molecules are moving at the average speed.
   (B) Any given molecule moves at the average speed most of the time.
   (C) When the temperature increases, more of the molecules will move at the new average speed.
   (D) When the temperature increases, fewer molecules will move at the new average speed.
   (E) When the temperature increases, the average speed decreases.

8. What is the density of a gas at 76 torr and 37°C (MM = 25 g/mol)?

   (A) 0.1 g/L
   (B) 0.8 g/L
   (C) 22.4 g/L
   (D) 75 g/L
   (E) 633 g/L

9. The following reaction represents the production of hydrogen chloride gas:

$$H_2 + Cl_2 \rightarrow 2\ HCl$$

   How many grams of chlorine gas are needed to produce 3 L of HCl gas at a pressure of 2 atm and a temperature of 19°C?

10. Dalton's Law of partial pressures says that the total pressure of all the gases in a system

    (A) is less than the sum of the partial pressures of the gases.
    (B) is more than the sum of the partial pressures of the gases.
    (C) is equal to the sum of the partial pressures of the gases.
    (D) is not related to the partial pressures of the gases.
    (E) cannot be calculated.

11. A student performing an experiment has a bulb containing 14 g of N_2, 64 g of O_2, 8 g of He, and 35 g of Cl_2 at a total pressure of 380 torr. What are the partial pressures of each gas?

12. A 1.74-g sample of gas is found to occupy 1 L at 10°C and 2 atm. What is the molar mass of the gas?

13. All of the following statements underlie the kinetic molecular theory of gases EXCEPT:

    (A) Gas molecules have no intermolecular forces.
    (B) Gas particles are in random motion.
    (C) The collisions between gas particles are elastic.
    (D) Gas particles have no volume.
    (E) The average kinetic energy is proportional to the temperature (°C) of the gas.

14. What will be the final pressure of a gas that expands from 1 L at 10°C to 10 L at 100°C, if the original pressure was 3 atm?

15. In the reaction $N_2 + 2O_2 \rightarrow 2\ NO_2$, what volume of NO_2 is produced from 7 g of nitrogen gas at 27°C and 0.9 atm?

SOLUTIONS TO REVIEW PROBLEMS

1. **E** Boyle's Law states that when a gas is held at constant temperature, its pressure and volume are inversely proportional. This means that as the pressure increases, the volume decreases, and vice versa. Of the answer choices, the only one that involves both pressure and volume—in addition to a controlled variation of one of the variables—is (E). When a balloon is placed in a bell jar, the volume of the balloon will increase as a vacuum is being drawn in the jar. Boyle's Law can be used to predict this behavior.

2. **A** In developing the kinetic molecular theory of gases, it was found that the properties of a gas sample, such as pressure, volume, and temperature, can be explained in terms of the motion of the individual gas molecules. Because *kinetic* is defined as "relating to motion," the theory of gases was called the kinetic molecular theory.

3. **C** This question is an application of Charles's Law, which states that at constant pressure, the volume and temperature of a gas will vary in direct proportion to each other. If a 50-L volume of gas is heated from standard temperature, which is 273 K, to two times standard temperature, 576 K, the volume will double as well. Therefore, the volume of the gas will increase from 50 L to 100 L. The answer can be calculated using proportions.

$$\frac{V_1}{V_2} = \frac{T_1}{T_2}$$

$$\frac{50\ L}{x} = \frac{273\ K}{546\ L}$$

$$x = (2)(50\ L)$$

$$x = (100\ L)$$

4. **74.1 g/mol**

   The molecular weight of a gas is the number of grams that occupy 22.4 L at STP. At 630 torr and 600 K, the density of this gas is 2.5 g/2 L. First, find the volume at STP.

   $$(2L)\ \left(\frac{630\ torr}{760\ torr}\right)\left(\frac{273\ K}{600\ K}\right) = 0.754\ L\ at\ STP$$

   Next, find the density at STP.

   $$\frac{2.5\ g}{0.754\ L} = \frac{3.31\ g}{L}\ at\ STP$$

   Finally, find the gram molecular weight of 22.4 L of gas.

   $$\left(\frac{3.31\ g}{L}\right)\left(\frac{22.4\ L}{mol}\right) = \frac{74.1\ g}{mol}$$

5. The conditions that define an ideal gas are low pressure and high temperature. Under these conditions, the gas molecules are assumed to have no intermolecular forces and to occupy no volume. Therefore, it is possible to predict their behavior.

6. **D** This question is an application of Avogadro's Principle, which states that at a constant temperature and pressure, all gases will have the same number of moles in the same volume. This is true regardless of the identity of the gas. Thus, to answer the question, the

number of particles in 0.25 mol of helium must be calculated; that value will represent the number of molecules of chlorine gas in the same volume. The number of helium atoms is $(0.25 \text{ mol}) (6.022 \times 10^{23} \text{ atoms/mol}) = 1.51 \times 10^{23}$ atoms. Thus, (D) is correct.

7. **D** The average speed of a gas is defined as the mathematical average of all the speeds of the gas particles in a sample. To answer this question, you must understand the Maxwell-Boltzmann distribution curve, which shows the distribution of speeds of all the gas particles in a sample at a given temperature. The distribution curve is a bell-shaped curve that flattens and shifts to the right as the temperature increases. The flattening of the curve means that gas particles within the sample are traveling at a greater range of speeds. As a result, a smaller proportion of the molecules will move at exactly the new average speed.

8. **A** A gas weighing 25 g/mol will have a density of 25 g/22.4 L at STP. The density at 76 torr and 37°C is found by calculating the change in volume of a mole of gas under these conditions.

$$\frac{P_1 V_1}{T_1} = \frac{P_2 V_2}{T_2}$$

$$\frac{P_1 V_1 T_2}{T_1 P_2} = V_2$$

$$\left(\frac{22.4 \text{ L}}{\text{mol}}\right) \left(\frac{760 \text{ torr}}{76 \text{ torr}}\right) \left(\frac{310 \text{ K}}{273 \text{ K}}\right) = 254 \text{ L/mol}$$

$$\frac{25 \text{ g/mol}}{254 \text{ L/mol}} = 0.098 \text{ g / L} \cong 0.1 \text{ g / L}$$

9. **8.88 g**

First, let's find out how many moles of HCl would occupy 3 L at the pressure and temperature given.

$$\left(\frac{22.4 \text{ L}}{\text{mol at STP}}\right) \left(\frac{1 \text{ atm}}{2 \text{ atm}}\right) \left(\frac{293 \text{ K}}{273 \text{ K}}\right) = 12.0 \text{ L/mol}$$

If one mole of HCl occupies 12 L at this temperature and pressure, then 3 L of HCl = 0.25 mol. Because 2 mol of HCl are produced from each mol of Cl_2, 0.25 mol HCl would be produced from 0.125 mol of Cl_2. The molecular weight of Cl_2 is 71, so the answer is $(71 \text{ g } Cl_2/\text{mol}) (0.125 \text{ mol}) = 8.88 \text{ g } Cl_2$.

10. **C** Discussed in the section on Dalton's Law of partial pressures.

11. **38 torr, 152 torr, 152 torr, 38 torr**

According to Dalton's Law of partial pressures, the sum of the partial pressures of the gases in a mixture is equal to the total pressure of the mixture. Therefore, the partial pressures of nitrogen, oxygen, helium, and chlorine will add up to 380 torr. The partial pressure of a gas is calculated as follows:

$$P_p = XP_t$$

where X is the mole fraction of the gas. Thus, the mole fractions of each of the gases must be determined.

$$X = \frac{n_i}{n_t}$$

$$X_{N_2} = \frac{0.5 \text{ mol}}{5 \text{ mol}} = 0.1$$

$$X_{O_2} = \frac{2 \text{ mol}}{5 \text{ mol}} = 0.4$$

$$X_{He} = \frac{2 \text{ mol}}{5 \text{ mol}} = 0.4$$

$$X_{Cl_2} = \frac{0.5 \text{ mol}}{5 \text{ mol}} = 0.1$$

Now the partial pressures may be calculated.

$P_{N_2} = (380 \text{ torr})(0.1) = 38 \text{ torr}$
$P_{O_2} = (380 \text{ torr})(0.4) = 152 \text{ torr}$
$P_{He} = (380 \text{ torr})(0.4) = 152 \text{ torr}$
$P_{Cl_2} = (380 \text{ torr})(0.1) = 38 \text{ torr}$

12. **20.2 g/mol**

Convert the density given to the density at STP.

$$(1L) \left(\frac{273 \text{ K}}{283 \text{ K}} \right) \left(\frac{2 \text{ atm}}{1 \text{ atm}} \right) = 1.93 \text{ L at STP}$$

$$1.74 \text{ g} / 1.93 \text{ L} = 0.902 \text{ g} / \text{L at STP}$$

Now find the molar mass by multiplying by 22.4.

MM = (0.902 g/L) (22.4 L/mol) = 20.2 g/mol

13. **E** K temperature, not °C.

14. **0.4 atm**

This question is different from the previous ones in that the new volume is given and you are looking for the final pressure. Rearranging the equation

$$\frac{P_1 V_1}{T_1} = \frac{P_2 V_2}{T_2}$$

gives

$$P_2 = P_1 \left(\frac{V_1}{V_2}\right)\left(\frac{T_2}{T_1}\right)$$

$$= (3 \text{ atm})\left(\frac{1 \text{ L}}{10 \text{ L}}\right)\left(\frac{373 \text{ K}}{283 \text{ K}}\right)$$

$$= 0.40 \text{ atm}$$

15. **13.7 L**

$$\frac{7 \text{ g N}_2}{28 \text{ g N}_2 / \text{mol}} = 0.25 \text{ mol N}_2$$

From the balanced reaction equation, 2 mol of NO_2 are produced from each mol of N_2, so 0.50 mol of NO_2 will be produced from 0.25 mol of N_2. Therefore, the volume at STP will be (0.5 mol NO_2) (22.4 L/mol at STP) = 11.2 L NO_2

Now find the volume under the conditions given.

$$(11.2 \text{ L at STP})\left(\frac{300}{273 \text{ K}}\right)\left(\frac{1 \text{ atm}}{0.9 \text{ atm}}\right) = 13.7 \text{ L NO}_2$$

CHAPTER THIRTY-FIVE

Phases and Phase Changes

In the last chapter, we discussed gases. In and this chapter, we will focus on principles of liquids and solids as well as gases. To help grasp the concepts of all three, below is a summary table describing the properties of each.

Phase	Volume and shape relationship	Motion principles	Density	Ability to be compressed
Gas	Conforms to the volume and shape of the container it is in	Continual motion	Low	Easily compressed to smaller volume
Liquid	Conforms to the shape of the container; however, has definite volume	Sliding motion of particles past one another	Moderate	Small ability to be compressed
Solid	Defined volume and shape	Particles in a fixed position	High	Difficult to compress

When the attractive forces between molecules (i.e., van der Waals forces) overcome the kinetic energy that keeps them apart, the molecules move closer together such that they can no longer move about freely, entering the **liquid** or **solid** phase. Because of their smaller volume relative to gases, liquids and solids are often referred to as the **condensed phases**.

LIQUIDS

In a liquid, atoms or molecules are held close together with little space between them. As a result, liquids have definite volumes and cannot easily be expanded or compressed. However, the molecules can still move around and are in a state of relative disorder. Consequently, the liquid can change shape to fit its container, and its molecules are able to **diffuse** and **evaporate**.

One of the most important properties of liquids is their ability to mix, both with each other and with other phases, to form **solutions** (see Chapter 36). The degree to which two liquids can mix is called their **miscibility**. Oil and water are almost completely **immiscible**; that is, their molecules tend to repel each other due to their polarity difference. Oil and water normally form separate layers when mixed, with oil on top because it is less dense. Under extreme conditions, such as violent shaking, two immiscible liquids can form a fairly homogeneous mixture called an **emulsion**. Although they look like solutions, emulsions are actually mixtures of discrete particles too small to be seen distinctly.

SOLIDS

In a solid, the attractive forces between atoms, ions, or molecules are strong enough to hold them rigidly together; thus the particles' only motion is vibration about fixed positions, and the kinetic energy of solids is predominantly **vibrational energy**. As a result, solids have definite shapes and volumes.

A solid may be **crystalline** or **amorphous**. A crystalline solid, such as NaCl, possesses an ordered structure; its atoms exist in a specific, three-dimensional geometric arrangement with repeating patterns of atoms, ions, or molecules. An amorphous solid, such as glass, has no ordered three-dimensional arrangement, although the molecules are also fixed in place.

Most solids are crystalline in structure. The two most common forms of crystals are **metallic** and **ionic** crystals.

Ionic solids are aggregates of positively and negatively charged ions; there are no discrete molecules. The physical properties of ionic solids include high melting points, high boiling points, and poor electrical conductivity in the solid phase. These properties are due to the compounds' strong electrostatic interactions, which also cause the ions to be relatively immobile. Ionic structures are given by empirical formulas that describe the ratio of atoms in the lowest possible whole numbers. For example, the empirical formula $BaCl_2$ gives the ratio of barium to chloride within the crystal.

Metallic solids consist of metal atoms packed together as closely as possible. Metallic solids have high melting and boiling points as a result of their strong covalent attractions. Pure metallic structures (consisting of a single element) are usually described as layers of spheres of roughly similar radii.

The repeating units of crystals (both ionic and metallic) are represented by **unit cells**. There are many types of unit cells. We will now consider only the three cubic unit cells: **simple cubic**, **body-centered cubic**, and **face-centered cubic**.

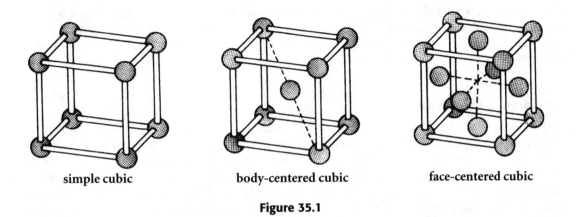

simple cubic body-centered cubic face-centered cubic

Figure 35.1

Atoms are represented as points, but are actually adjoining spheres. Each unit cell is surrounded by similar units. In the ionic unit cell, the spaces between points (anions) are filled with other ions (cations).

 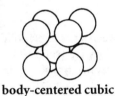 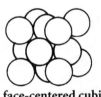

simple cubic body-centered cubic face-centered cubic

Figure 35.2

PHASE EQUILIBRIA

In an isolated system, phase changes (solid to liquid to gas) are reversible, and an equilibrium exists between phases. For example, at 1 atm and 0°C in an isolated system, an ice cube floating in water is in equilibrium. Some of the ice may absorb heat and melt, but an equal amount of water will release heat and freeze. Thus, the relative amounts of ice and water remain constant.

Gas-Liquid Equilibrium

The temperature of a liquid is related to the average kinetic energy of the liquid molecules; however, the kinetic energy of the molecules will vary. A few molecules near the surface of the liquid may have enough energy to leave the liquid phase and escape into the gaseous phase. This process is known as **evaporation** (or **vaporization**). Each time the liquid loses a high-energy particle, the temperature of the remaining liquid decreases; thus, evaporation is a cooling process. Given enough kinetic energy, the liquid will completely evaporate.

If a cover is placed on a beaker of liquid, the escaping molecules are trapped above the solution. These molecules exert a countering pressure, which forces some of the gas back into the liquid phase; this process is called **condensation**. Atmospheric pressure acts on a liquid in a similar fashion as a solid lid. As evaporation and condensation proceed, an equilibrium is reached in which the rates of the two processes become equal. Once this equilibrium is reached, the pressure that the gas exerts over the liquid is called the **vapor pressure** of the liquid. Vapor pressure increases as temperature increases, since more molecules have sufficient kinetic energy to escape into the gas phase. The temperature at which the vapor pressure of the liquid equals the external pressure is called the **boiling point**.

Liquid-Solid Equilibrium

The liquid and solid phases can also coexist in equilibrium (e.g., the ice water mixture discussed above). Even though the atoms or molecules of a solid are confined to definite locations, each atom or molecule can undergo motions about some equilibrium position. These motions (vibrations) increase when heat is applied. If atoms or molecules in the solid phase absorb enough energy in this fashion, the solid's three-dimensional structure breaks down, and the liquid phase begins. The transition from solid to liquid is called **fusion** or **melting**. The reverse process, from liquid to solid, is called **solidification**, **crystallization**, or **freezing**. The temperature at which these processes occur is called the **melting point** or **freezing point**, depending on the direction of the transition. Whereas pure crystals have distinct, very sharp melting points, amorphous solids, such as glass, tend to melt over a larger range of temperatures due to their less-ordered molecular distribution.

Gas-Solid Equilibrium

A third type of phase equilibrium is that between a gas and a solid. When a solid goes directly into the gas phase, the process is called **sublimation**. Dry ice (solid CO_2) sublimes; the absence of the liquid phase makes it a convenient refrigerant. The reverse transition, from the gaseous to the solid phase, is called **deposition**.

The Gibbs Function

The thermodynamic criterion for each of the above equilibria is that the change in Gibbs free energy must equal zero; $\Delta G = 0$. For an equilibrium between a gas and a solid:

$$\Delta G = G \; (g) - G \; (s),$$
$$\text{so } G \; (g) = G \; (s) \text{ at equilibrium}$$

The same is true of the Gibbs functions for the other two equilibria.

PHASE DIAGRAMS

Single Component

A standard **phase diagram** depicts the phases and phase equilibria of a substance at defined temperatures and pressures. In general, the gas phase is found at high temperature and low pressure; the solid phase is found at low temperature and high pressure; and the liquid phase is found at high temperature and high pressure. A typical phase diagram is shown in Figure 35.3.

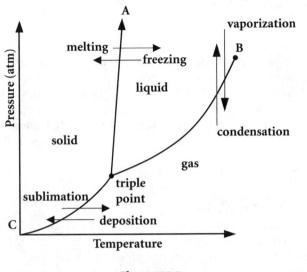

Figure 35.3

The three phases are demarcated by lines indicating the temperatures and pressures at which two phases are in equilibrium. Line A represents freezing/melting, line B evaporation/condensation, and line C sublimation/deposition. The intersection of the three lines is called the **triple point**. At this temperature and pressure, unique for a given substance, all three phases are in equilibrium. The point at B is known as the **critical point**, the temperature and pressure above which no distinction between liquid and gas is possible.

Multiple Components

The phase diagram for a mixture of two or more components is complicated by the requirement that the composition of the mixture, as well as the temperature and pressure, must be specified. Consider a solution of two liquids, A and B. The vapor above the solution is a mixture of the vapors of A and B. The pressures exerted by vapor A and vapor B on the solution are the vapor pressures that each exerts above its individual liquid phase. **Raoult's Law** (described below) enables one to determine the relationship between the vapor pressure of vapor A and the concentration of liquid A in the solution.

COLLIGATIVE PROPERTIES

Colligative properties are physical properties derived solely from the number of particles present, not the nature of those particles. These properties are usually associated with dilute solutions (see Chapter 36).

Freezing-Point Depression

Pure water (H_2O) freezes at 0°C; however, for every mole of solute particles dissolved in 1 L of water, the freezing point is lowered by 1.86°C. This is because the solute particles interfere with the process of crystal formation that occurs during freezing; the solute particles lower the temperature at which the molecules can align themselves into a crystalline structure.

The formula for calculating this freezing-point depression is:

$$\Delta T_f = K_f m$$

where ΔT_f is the freezing-point depression, K_f is a proportionality constant characteristic of a particular solvent, and m is the molality of the solution (mol solute/kg solvent; see Chapter 36). The K_f for water—which you do not need to memorize—is $1.86°Cm^{-1}$. Each solvent has its own characteristic K_f.

One of the best examples of this principle is seen when there is ice on a highway and salt is sprinkled on the road to make the ice melt. This thawing occurs because the salt depresses the freezing point of the water.

Boiling-Point Elevation

A liquid boils when its vapor pressure equals the atmospheric pressure. If the vapor pressure of a solution is lower than that of the pure solvent, more energy (and consequently a higher temperature) will be required before its vapor pressure equals atmospheric pressure. The extent to which the boiling point of a solution is raised relative to that of the pure solvent is given by the following formula:

$$\Delta T_b = K_b m$$

where ΔT_b is the boiling-point elevation, K_b is a proportionality constant characteristic of a particular solvent, and m is the molality of the solution. The K_b for water is $0.51°Cm^{-1}$.

One of the best examples of this principle is seen when there is a boiling pot of water on the stove and spaghetti is added to the pot of water. Once the spaghetti is added, the water almost immediately stops boiling. This occurs because the spaghetti raises the boiling point elevation for the water.

Osmotic Pressure

Consider a container separated into two compartments by a semipermeable membrane (which, by definition, selectively permits the passage of certain molecules). One compartment contains pure water, while the other contains water with dissolved solute. The membrane allows water but not solute to pass through. Because substances tend to flow, or **diffuse**, from higher to lower concentrations (which increases entropy), water will diffuse from the compartment containing pure water to the compartment containing the water-solute mixture. This net flow will cause the water level in the compartment containing the solution to rise above the level in the compartment containing pure water.

Because the solute cannot pass through the membrane, the concentrations of solute in the two compartments can never be equal. However, the pressure exerted by the water level in the solute-containing compartment will eventually oppose the influx of water; thus, the water level will rise only to the point at which it exerts a sufficient pressure to counterbalance the tendency of water to flow across the membrane. This pressure is defined as the **osmotic pressure** (Π) of the solution and is given by the formula:

$$\Pi = MRT$$

where M is the molarity of the solution (see Chapter 36), R is the ideal gas constant, and T is the temperature on the Kelvin scale. This equation clearly shows that molarity and osmotic pressure are directly proportional (i.e., as the concentration of the solution increases, the osmotic pressure also increases). Thus, the osmotic pressure depends only on the amount of solute, not its identity.

Vapor-Pressure Lowering (Raoult's Law)

When solute B is added to pure solvent A, the vapor pressure of A above the solvent decreases. If the vapor pressure of A above pure solvent A is designated by P°_A and the vapor pressure of A above the solution containing B is P_A, the vapor pressure decreases as follows:

$$\Delta P = P^\circ_A - P_A$$

In the late 1800s, the French chemist François Marie Raoult determined that this vapor pressure decrease is also equivalent to:

$$\Delta P = X_B P^\circ_A$$

where X_B is the mole fraction of the solute B in solvent A. Because $X_B = 1 - X_A$ and $\Delta P = P^\circ_A - P_A$, substitution into the above equation leads to the common form of Raoult's Law:

$$P_A = X_A P^\circ_A$$

Similarly, the expression for the vapor pressure of the solute in solution (assuming it is volatile) is given by:

$$P_B = X_B P^\circ_B$$

Raoult's Law holds only when the attraction between molecules of the different components of the mixture is equal to the attraction between the molecules of any one component in its pure state. When this condition does not hold, the relationship between mole fraction and vapor pressure will deviate from Raoult's Law. Solutions that obey Raoult's Law are called **ideal solutions**.

REVIEW PROBLEMS

1. Which of the following indicates the relative randomness of molecules in the three states of matter?

    (A) solid > liquid > gas

    (B) liquid < solid < gas

    (C) liquid > gas > solid

    (D) gas > liquid > solid

    (E) none of the above

2. What factors determine whether or not two liquids are miscible?

    (A) Molecular size

    (B) Molecular polarity

    (C) Density

    (D) Both B and C

3. Discuss the physical properties of ionic crystals.

4. Alloys are mixtures of pure metals in either the liquid or solid phase. Which of the following is usually true of alloys?

    (A) The melting/freezing point of an alloy will be lower than that of either of the component metals, because the new bonds are stronger.

    (B) The melting/freezing point of an alloy will be lower than that of either of the component metals, because the new bonds are weaker.

    (C) The melting/freezing point of an alloy will be greater than that of either of the component metals, because the new bonds are weaker.

    (D) The melting/freezing point of an alloy will be greater than that of either of the component metals, because the new bonds are stronger.

Refer to the phase diagram below for questions 5–8.

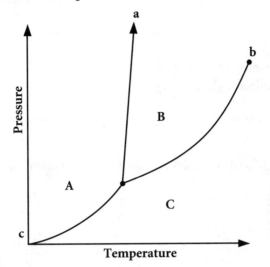

5. What is the typical form of a substance in state B?

   (A) Pure crystalline solid
   (B) Amorphous solid
   (C) Gas
   (D) Liquid

6. What is the typical form of a substance in state C?

   (A) Pure crystalline solid
   (B) Amorphous solid
   (C) Gas
   (D) Liquid

7. If line a were widened to cover a range of temperatures, what would state A have to be?

   (A) Pure crystalline solid
   (B) Amorphous solid
   (C) Gas
   (D) Liquid

8. What is the triple point?

9. A semipermeable membrane separates a container of freshwater from one of saltwater. If the volume of freshwater decreases significantly, what must be true of the semipermeable membrane? Assume that evaporation is negligible.

10. Once equilibrium is reached, if the temperature in Question 9 is suddenly increased, the osmotic pressure

    (A) will decrease.
    (B) will increase.
    (C) will remain the same.
    (D) cannot be determined.

11. What is the freezing point of a solution containing 0.5 mol of glucose dissolved in 200 g of H_2O? (The K_f for water is $1.86°$ Cm^{-1}.)

12. The osmotic pressure at STP of a solution made from 1 L of NaCl (*aq*) containing 117 g of NaCl is

    (A) 44.77 atm.
    (B) 48.87 atm.
    (C) 89.54 atm.
    (D) 117 atm.

13. At 18°C and 1 atm, the vapor pressure of pure water is 0.02 atm, and the vapor pressure of pure ethyl alcohol (MW = 46) is 0.50 atm. For a water-alcohol mixture with the alcohol present in a mole fraction of 0.2, find the vapor pressure due to the alcohol and the vapor pressure due to the water.

SOLUTIONS TO REVIEW PROBLEMS

1. **D** Because gas molecules have the greatest freedom to move around, gases have the greatest disorder. Liquids are denser than gases, and therefore the molecules are less free to move around. The arrangement of molecules in solids is the least random. Thus, melting and boiling are accompanied by an increase in entropy (i.e., $\Delta S > 0$).

2. **B** The miscibility of two liquids strongly depends on their polarities. In general, polar and nonpolar liquids are not miscible, while a polar liquid can usually be mixed with another polar liquid and a nonpolar liquid with another nonpolar liquid. (A), molecular size, and (C), the density of a liquid, do not directly affect the miscibility. However, (C) should remind you that two immiscible liquids will form separate layers, with the denser liquid on the bottom. Thus, (B) is the only correct choice.

3. Ionic crystals contain repeating units of cations and anions. Because of the strong electrostatic attraction between the ions, these crystals have high melting points. Since the charges in these crystals are tightly fixed in the lattice, ionic solids are poor conductors of electricity. In the liquid or solution phase, the charged particles can move around, and thus liquid ionic compounds will conduct electricity, as do solutions of such salts.

4. **B** The bonds between different metal atoms in an alloy are much weaker than those between the atoms in pure metals. Therefore, breaking these bonds requires less energy than does breaking the bonds in pure metals. Since melting and freezing points are inversely proportional to the stability of bonds, they tend to be lower for alloys than for pure metals. Alternately, an alloy can be looked at as a solid solution; impurities lower the melting point.

5. **D** Discussed in the section on phase diagrams.

6. **C** Discussed in the section on phase diagrams.

7. **B** Discussed in the section on phase diagrams.

8. The unique combination of temperature and pressure at which the solid, liquid, and gas phases coexist at equilibrium.

9. The membrane must be permeable to water but not to salt. If it were permeable to salt, the salt would diffuse across the membrane into the freshwater container (down its concentration gradient) until the molarities of the two containers were the same. However, the volume of the salt water container increased, indicating that fresh water diffused across the membrane from a region of low solute concentration to one of high solute concentration. The water level rose until it exerted enough pressure to counterbalance the tendency to diffuse; this pressure is known as the osmotic pressure.

10. **B** Using the formula $\Pi = MRT$, we see that osmotic pressure and temperature are directly proportional (i.e., if temperature increases, osmotic pressure will also increase). Thus, (B) is the correct answer.

11. **−4.65°C**

This question applies the concept of freezing-point depression. If 0.5 mol of a nonelectrolyte solute such as glucose is dissolved in 200 g of H_2O, then the molality of the solution is

$$\frac{0.5 \text{ mol}}{0.200 \text{ kg } H_2O} = 2.5 \text{ mol solute / kg } H_2O$$

Using the equation $\Delta T_f = K_f m$, the freezing point depression is $2.5 \times 1.86°C$, or $4.65°C$, and the new freezing point is $−4.65°C$. Note that ΔT_f is the change in freezing point and not the freezing point itself.

12. **C** The osmotic pressure (Π) of a solution is given by $\Pi = MRT$. At STP, $T = 273K$; R, the ideal gas constant, equals 8.2×10^{-2} L·atm/K·mol. To determine the molarity, find the formula weight of NaCl from the periodic table; FW = 58.5. The number of moles in the solution described is:

$$\frac{117 g/L}{58.5 \text{ g/mol}} = 2 \text{ moles of undissociated NaCl/L}$$

But since NaCl is a strong electrolyte, it dissociates in aqueous solution, and there are actually 4 moles of **particles** per liter of solution (i.e., 2 moles of Na^+ and 2 moles of Cl^-). Thus:

$$\Pi = \quad (4 \text{ mol/L})(8.2 \times 10^{-2} \text{ L·atm/(K·mol)})(273 \text{ K})$$
$$= \quad 89.54 \text{ atm}$$

Remember that colligative properties depend on the number of particles, not their identity.

13. Use Raoult's Law to answer this question, with A = H_2O and B = ethyl alcohol.

$$P_A = \quad X_A P°_A$$
$$P_B = \quad X_B P°_B$$

Because we are given that $X_B = 0.2$, then $X_A = 1 - X_B = 1 - 0.2 = 0.8$.

$$P°_A = \quad 0.02 \text{ atm}$$
$$P°_B = \quad 0.50 \text{ atm}$$
$$P_A = \quad (0.8)(0.02 \text{ atm}) = 0.016 \text{ atm}$$
$$P_B = \quad (0.2)(0.50 \text{ atm}) = 0.10 \text{ atm}$$

Thus, the vapor pressure due to water is 0.016 atm, and the vapor pressure due to alcohol is 0.10 atm.

CHAPTER THIRTY-SIX

Solutions

Solutions are **homogeneous** (everywhere the same) mixtures of substances that combine to form a single phase, generally the liquid phase. Many important chemical reactions, both in the laboratory and in nature, take place in solution (including almost all reactions in living organisms).

NATURE OF SOLUTIONS

A solution consists of a **solute** (e.g., NaCl, NH_3, or $C_{12}H_{22}O_{11}$) dispersed (dissolved) in a solvent (e.g., H_2O or benzene). The solvent is the component of the solution whose phase remains the same after mixing. If the two substances are already in the same phase, the solvent is the component present in greater quantity. Solute molecules move about freely in the solvent and can interact with other molecules or ions; consequently, chemical reactions occur easily in solution.

Solvation

The interaction between solute and solvent molecules is known as solvation or **dissolution**; when water is the solvent, it is called **hydration**, and the resulting solution is known as an **aqueous solution**. Solvation is possible when the attractive forces between solute and solvent are stronger than those between the solute particles. For example, when NaCl dissolves in water, its component ions dissociate from one another and become surrounded by water molecules. Because water is polar, ion-dipole interactions can occur between the Na^+ and Cl^- ions and the water molecules. For nonionic solutes, solvation involves van der Waals forces between the solute and solvent molecules. The general rule is that like dissolves like: ionic and polar solutes are soluble in polar solvents, and nonpolar solutes are soluble in nonpolar solvents.

Solubility

The solubility of a substance is the maximum amount of that substance that can be dissolved in a particular solvent at a particular temperature. When this maximum amount of solute has been added, the solution is in equilibrium and is said to be **saturated**; if more solute is added, it will not dissolve. For example, at 18°C, a maximum of 83 g of glucose ($C_6H_{12}O_6$) will dissolve in 100 mL of H_2O. Thus the solubility of glucose is 83 g/100 mL. If more glucose is added, it will remain in solid form, precipitating to the bottom of the container. A solution in which the proportion of solute to solvent is small is said to be **dilute**, and one in which the proportion is large is said to be **concentrated**.

When a dissolved solute comes out of solution and forms crystals, this process is known as **crystallization**. It is also important to note that some substances can form **supersaturated** solutions, which are solutions that contain more solute than found in a saturated solution. In a supersaturated solution, the addition of additional solute will cause the excess solute in the supersaturated solution to separate, and a saturated solution will subsequently form.

Aqueous Solutions

The most common class of solutions are the aqueous solutions, in which the solvent is water. The aqueous state is denoted by the symbol *aq*. In discussing the chemistry of aqueous solutions, it is useful to know how soluble various salts are in water; this information is given by the solubility rules below.

- All salts of alkali metals are water soluble.
- All salts of the ammonium ion (NH_4^+) are water soluble.
- All chlorides, bromides, and iodides are water soluble, with the exceptions of Ag^+, Pb^{2+}, and Hg_2^{2+}.
- All salts of the sulfate ion (SO_4^{2-}) are water soluble, with the exceptions of Ca^{2+}, Sr^{2+}, Ba^{2+}, and Pb^{2+}.
- All metal oxides are insoluble, with the exception of the alkali metals and CaO , SrO , and BaO, all of which hydrolyze to form solutions of the corresponding metal hydroxides.
- All hydroxides are insoluble, with the exception of the alkali metals and Ca^{2+}, Sr^{2+}, and Ba^{2+}.
- All carbonates (CO_3^{2-}), phosphates (PO_4^{3-}), sulfides (S^{2-}), and sulfites (SO_3^{2-}) are insoluble, with the exception of the alkali metals and ammonium.

IONS

Ionic solutions are of particular interest to chemists because certain important types of chemical interactions—acid-base reactions and oxidation-reduction reactions, for instance—take place in ionic solutions. Ions and their properties in solution will be introduced here; the chemical reactions mentioned are discussed in detail in Chapter 37, Acids and Bases, and Chapter 38, Redox Reactions and Electrochemistry.

Catons and Anions

Ionic compounds are made up of cations and anions, where a cation is a positive ion and an anion is a negative ion. The nomenclature of ionic compounds is based on the names of the component ions.

- For elements (usually metals) that can form more than one positive ion, the charge is indicated by a Roman numeral in parentheses following the name of the element.

Fe^{2+} Iron (II)	Cu^+ Copper (I)
Fe^{3+} Iron (III)	Cu^{2+} Copper (II)

- An older but still commonly used method is to add the endings **-ous** or **-ic** to the root of the Latin name of the element to represent the ions with lesser or greater charge respectively.

Fe^{2+} Ferrous Cu^+ Cuprous

Fe^{3+} Ferric Cu^{2+} Cupric

- Monatomic anions are named by dropping the ending of the name of the element and adding **-ide.**

H^- Hydride S^{2-} Sulfide

F^- Fluoride N^{3-} Nitride

O^{2-} Oxide P^{3-} Phosphide

- Many polyatomic anions contain oxygen and are therefore called **oxyanions**. When an element forms two oxyanions, the name of the one with less oxygen ends in -ite and the one with more oxygen ends in -ate.

NO_2^- Nitrite SO_3^{2-} Sulfite

NO_3^- Nitrate SO_4^{2-} Sulfate

- When the series of oxyanions contains four oxyanions, prefixes are also used. **Hypo-** and **per-** are used to indicate less oxygen and more oxygen, respectively.

ClO^- Hypochlorite

ClO_2^- Chlorite

ClO_3^- Chlorate

ClO_4^- Perchlorate

- Polyatomic anions often gain one or more H+ ions to form anions of lower charge. The resulting ions are named by adding the word *hydrogen* or *dihydrogen* to the front of the anion's name. An older method uses the prefix **bi-** to indicate the addition of a single hydrogen ion.

HCO_3^- Hydrogen carbonate or bicarbonate

HSO_4^- Hydrogen sulfate or bisulfate

$H_2PO_4^-$ Dihydrogen phosphate

Ion Charges

Metals, which are found in the left part of the periodic table, generally form positive ions, whereas nonmetals, which are found in the right part of the periodic table, generally form negative ions. Note, however, the existence of anions that contain metallic elements; e.g., MnO_4^- (permanganate) and CrO_4^{2-} (chromate). All elements in a given group tend to form monatomic ions with the same charge. Thus ions of alkali metals (Group I) usually form cations with a single positive charge, the alkaline earth metals (Group II) form cations with a double positive charge, and the halides (Group VII) form anions with a single negative charge. Though other main group elements follow this trend, the intermediate electronegativity of such elements (making them less likely to form ionic compounds) and the transition from metallic to nonmetallic character complicates the picture.

Electrolytes

The electrical conductivity of aqueous solutions is governed by the presence and concentration of ions in solution. Therefore, pure water does not conduct an electrical current well since the concentrations of hydrogen and hydroxide ions are very small. Solutes whose solutions are conductive are called electrolytes. A solute is considered a strong electrolyte if it dissociates completely into its constituent ions. Examples of **strong electrolytes** include ionic compounds, such as NaCl and KI, and molecular compounds with highly polar covalent bonds that dissociate into ions when dissolved, such as HCl in water. A **weak electrolyte**, on the other hand, ionizes or hydrolyzes incompletely in aqueous solution, and only some of the solute is present in ionic form. Examples include acetic acid and other weak acids, ammonia and other weak bases, and $HgCl_2$. Many compounds do not ionize at all in aqueous solution, retaining their molecular structure in solution, which usually limits their solubility. These compounds are called **nonelectrolytes** and include many nonpolar gases and organic compounds, such as oxygen and sugar.

CONCENTRATION

Units of Concentration

Concentration denotes the amount of solute dissolved in a solvent. The concentration of a solution is most commonly expressed as **percent composition by mass, mole fraction, molarity, molality,** or **normality.**

Percent composition by mass

The percent composition by mass (%) of a solution is the mass of the solute divided by the mass of the solution (solute plus solvent), multiplied by 100.

Example: What is the percent composition by mass of a salt water solution if 100 g of the solution contains 20 g of NaCl?

Solution:

$$\frac{20 \text{ g NaCl}}{100 \text{ g}} \times 100 = 20\% \text{ NaCl solution}$$

Mole fraction

The mole fraction (X) of a compound is equal to the number of moles of the compound divided by the total number of moles of all species within the system. The sum of the mole fractions in a system will always equal 1.

The mole fraction can be calculated with the following equation:

$$X_B = \text{moles of B/sum of moles of all components}$$

where X_B is the mole fraction of component B.

Example: If 92 g of glycerol is mixed with 90 g of water, what will be the mole fractions of the two components? (MW of H_2O = 18; MW of $C_3H_8O_3$ = 92)

Solution:

$$90 \text{ g water} = 90 \text{ g} \times \frac{1 \text{ mol}}{18 \text{ g}} = 5 \text{ mol}$$

$$92 \text{ g glycerol} = 92 \text{ g} \times \frac{1 \text{ mol}}{92 \text{ g}} = 1 \text{ mol}$$

$$\text{Total mol} = 5 + 1 = 6 \text{ mol}$$

$$X_{water} = \frac{5 \text{ mol}}{6 \text{ mol}} = 0.833$$

$$X_{glycerol} = \frac{1 \text{ mol}}{6 \text{ mol}} = 0.167$$

$$X_{water} + X_{glycerol} = 0.833 + 0.167 = 1.000$$

Molarity

The molarity (M) of a solution is the number of moles of solute per liter of solution. Solution concentrations are usually expressed in terms of molarity. Molarity depends on the volume of the solution, not on the volume of solvent used to prepare the solution.

Example: If enough water is added to 11 g of $CaCl_2$ to make 100 mL of solution, what is the molarity of the solution?

Solution:

$$\frac{11 \text{ g } CaCl_2}{110 \text{ g } CaCl_2 \text{ / mol } CaCl_2} = 0.10 \text{ mol } CaCl_2$$

$$100 \text{ mL} \times \frac{1 \text{ L}}{1,000 \text{ mL}} = 0.10 \text{ L}$$

$$\text{molarity} = \frac{0.10 \text{ mol}}{0.10 \text{ L}} = 1.0 \text{ M}$$

Molality

The molality (m) of a solution is the number of moles of solute per kilogram of solvent. For dilute aqueous solutions at 25°C, the molality is approximately equal to the molarity, because the density of water at this temperature is 1 kilogram per liter. But note that this is an approximation and true only for dilute aqueous solutions.

Example: If 10 g of NaOH are dissolved in 500 g of water, what is the molality of the solution?

Solution:

$$\frac{10 \text{ g NaOH}}{40 \text{ g NaOH / mol NaOH}} = 0.25 \text{ mol NaOH}$$

$$500 \text{ g} \times \frac{1 \text{ kg}}{1,000 \text{ g}} = 0.50 \text{ kg}$$

$$\text{molality} = \frac{0.25 \text{ mol}}{0.50 \text{ kg}} = 0.50 \text{ mol / kg} = 0.50 \text{ m}$$

Normality

The normality (N) of a solution is equal to the number of gram equivalent weights of solute per liter of solution. A gram equivalent weight, or **equivalent**, is a measure of the reactive capacity of a molecule (see Chapter 31, Compounds and Stoichiometry).

To calculate the normality of a solution, we must know for what purpose the solution is being used, because it is the concentration of the reactive species with which we are concerned. Normality is unique among concentration units in that it is reaction dependent. For example, a 1-molar solution of sulfuric acid would be 2 normal for acid-base reactions (because each mole of sulfuric acid provides 2 moles of H^+ ions) but is only 1 normal for a sulfate precipitation reaction (because each mole of sulfuric acid only provides 1 mole of sulfate ions).

Dilution

A solution is **diluted** when solvent is added to a solution of high concentration to produce a solution of lower concentration. The concentration of a solution after dilution can be conveniently determined using the equation below:

$$M_i V_i = M_f V_f$$

where M is molarity, V is volume, and the subscripts i and f refer to initial and final values, respectively.

Example: How many mL of a 5.5 M NaOH solution must be used to prepare 300 mL of a 1.2 M NaOH solution?

Solution:

$$5.5 \text{ M} \times v_i = 1.2 \text{ M} \times 0.3 \text{ l}$$

$$V_i = \frac{1.2 \text{ m} \times 0.3 \text{ L}}{5.5 \text{ M}}$$

$$V_i = 0.065 \text{ L} = 65 \text{ mL}$$

SOLUTION EQUILIBRIA

The process of solvation, like other reversible chemical and physical changes, tends toward an **equilibrium**. Immediately after solute has been introduced into a solvent, most of the change taking place is dissociation, because no dissolved solute is initially present. However, according to Le Châtelier's principle, as solute dissociates, the reverse reaction (precipitation of the solute) also begins to occur. Eventually an equilibrium is reached, with the rate of solute dissociation equal to the rate of precipitation, and the net concentration of the dissociated solute remains unchanged regardless of the amount of solute added.

An ionic solid introduced into a polar solvent dissociates into its component ions. The dissociation of such a solute in solution may be represented by

$$A_mB_n \ (s) \rightleftharpoons mA^{n+} \ (aq) + nB^{m-} \ (aq)$$

$$AgCl \ (s) \rightleftharpoons Ag^+ \ (aq) + Cl^- \ (aq)$$

THE SOLUBILITY PRODUCT CONSTANT

A slightly soluble ionic solid exists in equilibrium with its saturated solution. In the case of AgCl, for example, the solution equilibrium is as follows:

$$AgCl \ (s) \rightleftharpoons Ag+ \ (aq) + Cl- \ (aq)$$

The **ion product** (**I.P.**) of a compound in solution is defined as follows:

$$\text{I.P.} = [A^{n+}]m[B^{m-}]n$$

The same expression for a saturated solution at equilibrium defines the **solubility product constant (Ksp)**.

$$K_{sp} = [A^{n+}]m[B^{m-}]n \text{ in a saturated solution}$$

However, I.P. is defined with respect to initial concentrations and does not necessarily represent either an equilibrium or a saturated solution, while K_{sp} does; at any point other than at equilibrium, the ion product is often referred to as Q_{sp}.

Each salt has its own distinct K_{sp} at a given temperature. If at a given temperature a salt's I.P. is equal to its K_{sp}, the solution is saturated, and the rate at which the salt dissolves equals the rate at which it precipitates out of solution. If a salt's I.P. exceeds its K_{sp}, the solution is supersaturated (holding more salt than it should be able to at a given temperature) and unstable. If the supersaturated solution is disturbed by adding more salt, other solid particles, or jarring the solution by a sudden decrease in temperature, the solid salt will precipitate until I.P. equals the K_{sp}. If I.P. is less than K_{sp}, the solution is unsaturated and no precipitate will form.

Example: The solubility of $Fe(OH)_3$ in an aqueous solution was determined to be 4.5×10^{-10} mol/L. What is the value of the K_{sp} for $Fe(OH)_3$?

Solution: The molar solubility (the solubility of the compound in mol/L) is given as 4.5×10^{-10} M. The equilibrium concentration of each ion can be determined from the molar solubility and the balanced dissociation reaction of $Fe(OH)_3$. The dissociation reaction is:

$$Fe(OH)^3 \ (s) \rightleftarrows Fe^{3+} \ (aq) + 3OH^- \ (aq)$$

Thus, for every mol of $Fe(OH)_3$ that dissociates, one mol of Fe^{3+} and three mol of OH– are produced. Since the solubility is 4.5×10^{-10} M, the Ksp can be determined as follows:

$$K_{sp} = [Fe^{3+}][OH^-]^3$$

$$[OH^-] = 3[Fe^{3+}]; \qquad [Fe^{3+}] = 4.5 \times 10^{-10} M$$

$$K_{sp} = [Fe^{3+}](3[Fe^{3+}])^3 = 27[Fe^{3+}]^4$$

$$K_{sp} = (4.5 \times 10^{-10})[3(4.5 \times 10^{-10})]^3 = 27(4.5 \times 10^{-10})^4$$

$$K_{sp} = 1.1 \times 10^{-36}$$

Example: What are the concentrations of each of the ions in a saturated solution of $PbBr_2$, given that the K_{sp} of $PbBr_2$ is 2.1×10^{-6}? If 5 g of $PbBr_2$ are dissolved in water to make 1 L of solution at 25°C, would the solution be saturated, unsaturated, or supersaturated?

Solution: The first step is to write out the dissociation reaction:

$$PbBr_2 \ (s) \rightleftarrows Pb^{2+} \ (aq) + 2Br^- \ (aq)$$

$$K_{sp} = [Pb^{2+}][Br^-]^2$$

Let x = the concentration of Pb^{2+} , then $2x$ = the concentration of Br^- in the saturated solution at equilibrium (since $[Br^-]$ is two times $[Pb^{2+}]$).

$$(x)(2x)^2 = 4x^3$$

$$2.1 \times 10^{-6} = 4x^3$$

Solving for x, the concentration of Pb^{2+} in a saturated solution is 8.07×10^{-3} M, and the concentration of Br^- $(2x)$ is 1.61×10–2 M.

Next, we convert 5 g of $PbBr_2$ into moles:

$$5 \ g \ \frac{1 \ mol \ PbBr_2}{367 \ g} = 1.36 \times 10^{-2} \ mol$$

1.36×10^{-2} mol of $PbBr_2$ is dissolved in 1 L of solution, so the concentration of the solution 1.36×10^{-2} M. Since this is higher than the concentration of a saturated solution, this solution would be supersaturated.

Factors Affecting Solubility

The solubility of a substance varies depending on the temperature of the solution, the solvent, and, in the case of a gas-phase solute, the pressure. Solubility is also affected by the addition of other substances to the solution.

The solubility of a salt is considerably reduced when it is dissolved in a solution that already contains one of its ions, rather than in a pure solvent. For example, if a salt such as CaF_2 is dissolved in a solution already containing Ca^{2+} ions, the dissociation equilibrium will shift toward the production of the solid salt. This reduction in solubility, called the **common ion effect**, is another example of Le Châtelier's principle.

Example: The K_{sp} of AgI in aqueous solution is 1×10^{-16} mol/L. If a 1×10^{-5} M solution of $AgNO_3$ is saturated with AgI, what will be the final concentration of the iodide ion?

Solution: The concentration of Ag^+ in the original $AgNO_3$ solution will be 1×10^{-5} mol/L. After AgI is added to saturation, the iodide concentration can be found by the formula:

$$1 \times 10^{-16} = [Ag^+][I^-]$$

$$= (1 \times 10^{-5})[I^-]$$

$$[I^-] = 1 \times 10^{-11} \text{ mol/L.}$$

If the AgI had been dissolved in pure water, the concentration of both Ag^+ and I^- would have been 1×10^{-8} mol/L. The presence of the common ion, silver, at a concentration one thousand times higher than what it would normally be in a silver iodide solution, has reduced the iodide concentration to one thousandth of what it would have been otherwise. An additional 1×10^{-11} mol/L of silver will, of course, dissolve in solution along with the iodide ion, but this will not significantly affect the final silver concentration, which is much higher.

REVIEW PROBLEMS

1. Which of the following choices correctly describes the solubility behavior of potassium chloride (KCl)?

   (A) Solubility in CCl_4 > Solubility in CH_3CH_2OH > Solubility in H_2O
   (B) Solubility in H_2O > Solubility in CH_3CH_2OH > Solubility in CCl_4
   (C) Solubility in CH_3CH_2OH > Solubility in CCl_4 > Solubility in H_2O
   (D) Solubility in H_2O > Solubility in CCl_4 > Solubility in CH_3CH_2OH

2. A simple cake icing can be made by dissolving a large quantity of sugar (sucrose) in boiling water, cooling the mixture, and applying it to the cake before it reaches room temperature. The mixture hardens as it cools because

   (A) the sugar molecules freeze from liquid to solid.
   (B) the sugar concentration increases as water boils off.
   (C) the solubility of sugar in water decreases as the solution cools.
   (D) the sugar concentration increases as water boils off, and the solubility of sugar in water decreases as the solution cools.

3. How much NaOH must be added to 200 mL of water to make a 1 M of NaOH solution?

   (A) 8 g
   (B) 16 g
   (C) 40 g
   (D) 80 g

4. To what volume must 10.0 mL of 5.00 M of HCl be diluted to make a 0.500 M of HCl solution?

   (A) 1 mL
   (B) 50 mL
   (C) 100 mL
   (D) 500 mL
   (E) 1,000 mL

5. What is the normality of a 2 M solution of phosphoric acid, H_3PO_4, for an acid-base titration?

   (A) 0.67
   (B) 2
   (C) 3
   (D) 6

6. Given that the molecular weight of ethyl alcohol, CH_3CH_2OH, is 46, and that of water is 18, how many grams of ethyl alcohol must be mixed with 100 mL of water for the mole fraction (X) of ethyl alcohol to be 0.2?

7. What is the concentration of the Ag^+ ion in a saturated solution of AgCl? (K_{sp} for AgCl = 1.7×10^{-10})

$$AgCl\ (s) \rightleftarrows Ag^+\ (aq) + Cl^-\ (aq)$$

(A) 1.7×10^{-10}

(B) 3.4×10^{-10}

(C) 1.3×10^{-5}

(D) 2.6×10^{-5}

8. Explain the common ion effect in terms of Ksp.

9. Name the following ionic compounds

(A) $NaClO_4$

(B) $NaClO$

(C) $NaNO_3$

(D) KNO_2

(E) Li_2SO_4

(F) $MgSO_3$

10. Which of the following will be the most electrically conductive?

(A) Sugar dissolved in water

(B) Saltwater

(C) Salt dissolved in an organic solvent

(D) An oil and water mixture

SOLUTIONS TO REVIEW PROBLEMS

1. B KCl is an ionic salt and, therefore, should be soluble in polar solvents and insoluble in nonpolar solvents. Water, H_2O, is a highly polar liquid. The carbon atom in carbon tetrachloride, CCl_4, is bonded to four atoms, so the molecule is tetrahedral. This geometry means that the individual dipole moments of the bonds cancel and CCl_4 is nonpolar. Ethanol (CH_3CH_2OH) has two carbon atoms in tetrahedral arrangement; most of the dipole moments associated with the bonds are the same, but the C—C and C—OH bonds are different, so ethanol is somewhat polar. Thus, the polarities of the three solvents decrease in the following sequence: $H_2O > CH_3CH_2OH > CCl_4$, with the solubility of KCl decreasing along that sequence.

2. D Both B and C contribute to the hardening of cake icing. The sugar-water solution hardens because it becomes supersaturated as it cools, since the solubility of sucrose in water decreases significantly with temperature (C). Evaporation of water during boiling (B) also contributes to the solution's supersaturated state by reducing the amount of solvent present. However, this makes a smaller contribution to the supersaturation of the solution. (A) is wrong: in this example the sugar is dissolved, not melted (sucrose melts at 185–86°C, well above the boiling point of even sucrose-saturated water).

3. A To answer this question, first find the formula weight of NaOH from the periodic table. Rounding to whole numbers, the atomic mass of Na is 23, the atomic mass of O is 16, and the atomic mass of H is 1, so the formula weight of NaOH is 40. Thus, 40 g of NaOH is 1 mol, and 40 g of NaOH dissolved in 1 L of water is a 1M solution of NaOH. To determine how much of the solute is needed to make 200 mL of such a solution, set up the following ratio:

$$\frac{X \text{ g}}{200 \text{ mL}} = \frac{40 \text{ g}}{1 \text{ L}} \times \frac{1 \text{ L}}{1,000 \text{ mL}}$$

$$\frac{X \text{ g}}{200 \text{ mL}} = \frac{40 \text{ g}}{1,000 \text{ mL}}$$

$$X \text{ g} = \frac{(40 \text{ g})(200 \text{ mL})}{1,000 \text{ mL}} = 8 \text{ g}$$

4. C When a solution is diluted, more solvent is added, yet the number of moles of solute remains the same. To solve a dilution problem, the following equation is used:

$$M_i V_i = M_f V_f$$

where i represents the initial conditions and f represents the final conditions. Therefore, the calculation to solve for the final volume is

$$(5.0 \text{ M})(0.01 \text{ L}) = (0.50 \text{ M})(V_f)$$

$$V_f = 0.100 \text{ L} = 100 \text{ mL}$$

and the correct answer is (C).

5. **D** Each mole of H_3PO_4 contains 3 moles of hydrogen and (since this is an acid) three mole equivalents. A 2 M of solution of this acid is thus

$$2\,M \times \frac{3\,N}{M} = 6N$$

6. **64.4 g**

The number of moles of water is found by estimating the density of water to be 1 g/mL.

$$\text{mol } H_2O = (100 \text{ mL } H_2O)(1 \text{ g/mL})/(18 \text{ g/mol}) = 5.6 \text{ mol}$$

If the mole fraction of ethyl alcohol is to be 0.2, then the mole fraction of water must be 0.8. If X equals the total number of moles:

$$5.6 = 0.8X$$
$$X = 7 \text{ moles}$$

Then

$$\text{mol ethyl alcohol} = (0.2)(7) = 1.4 \text{ mol,}$$

and

$$(1.4 \text{ mol ethyl alcohol})(46 \text{ g/mol}) = 64.4 \text{ g ethyl alcohol.}$$

7. **C** 1.3×10^{-5}

$$\begin{aligned} K_{sp} &= [Ag^+][Cl^-] \\ \text{Let } x &= [Ag^+] \\ \text{Since } [Ag^+] &= [Cl^-],\ 1.7 \times 10^{-10} = x^2 \\ x &= 1.3 \times 10^{-5} \end{aligned}$$

8. Consider as an example a dilute solution of AgCl. The K_{sp} of AgCl at 25°C is 1.7×10^{-10}. If the original concentration of AgCl is 1×10^{-6}, then I.P. $= (1 \times 10^{-6})2 = 1 \times 10^{-12}$, which is lower than the K_{sp}; thus, all the salt is dissolved.

Now suppose NaCl is added to this solution until the NaCl concentration is 1×10^{-2}. $[Cl^-]$ will now be the sum of $[Cl^-]$ due to AgCl and $[Cl^-]$ due to NaCl; $[Cl^-] = 1 \times 10^{-2} + 1 \times 10^{-6}$ $= 1.0001 \times 10^{-2}$, or approximately 1×10^{-2}.

Thus, the Q_{sp} for AgCl is $(1 \times 10{-6})(1 \times 10{-2}) = 1 \times 10^{-8}$, which is greater than the K_{sp}. AgCl will therefore precipitate until I.P. is reduced to the K_{sp}. Because of the high concentration of Cl^-, the final concentration of Ag^+ will be lower than it would have been otherwise.

9. (Oxidation numbers have been placed in parentheses for additional practice.)

   A Sodium perchlorate (Cl^{7+})
   B Sodium hypochlorite (Cl^{1+})
   C Sodium nitrate (N^{5+})
   D Potassium nitrite (N^{3+})
   E Lithium sulfate (S^{6+})
   F Magnesium sulfite (S^{4+})

10. **B** Only ionic compounds (electrolytes) dissolved in polar solvents will conduct electricity. Sugar is a covalent solid and therefore is not an electrolyte even when dissolved in water. Answers (C) and (D) are incorrect because salt will not dissolve appreciably in an organic solvent and oil and water are immiscible. NaCl is an ionic compound, so (B) is correct.

CHAPTER THIRTY-SEVEN

Acids and Bases

Many important reactions in chemical and biological systems involve two classes of compounds called **acids** and **bases.** Acids and bases cause color changes in certain compounds called **indicators,** which may be in solution or on paper. A particularly common indicator is **litmus paper**, which turns red in acidic solution and blue in basic solution. A more extensive discussion of the chemical properties of acids and bases is outlined below.

Acids	Bases
• Have a sour taste.	• Have a bitter taste.
• Aqueous solutions can conduct electricity.	• Feel slippery to the touch.
• React with bases to form water and a "salt."	• Cause color changes in plant dyes—turn litmus paper blue.
• Nonoxidizing acids react with metals to produce hydrogen gas.	• React with acids to form water and a "salt."
• Cause color changes in plant dyes—turn litmus paper red.	• Aqueous solutions can conduct electricity.

DEFINITIONS

Arrhenius Definition

The first definitions of acids and bases were formulated by Svante Arrhenius toward the end of the 19th century. Arrhenius defined an acid as a species that produces H^+ (a proton) in an aqueous solution and a base as a species that produces OH^- (a hydroxide ion) in an aqueous solution. These definitions, though useful, fail to describe acidic and basic behavior in nonaqueous media.

An example of an Arrhenius acid (HCl), base (NaOH), and acid-base reactions, respectively, are as follows:

$$HCl\ (aq) \rightarrow H^+(aq) + Cl^-(aq)$$
$$NaOH\ (aq) \rightarrow Na^+(aq) + OH^-(aq)$$
$$HCl\ (aq) + NaOH(aq) \rightarrow NaCl(aq) + H_2O(l)$$

Brønsted-Lowry Definition

A more general definition of acids and bases was proposed independently by Johannes Brønsted and Thomas Lowry in 1923. A Brønsted-Lowry acid is a species that donates protons, while a Brønsted-Lowry base is a species that accepts protons. For example, NH_3 and Cl^- are both Brønsted-Lowry bases because they accept protons. However, they cannot be called Arrhenius bases since in aqueous solution they do not dissociate to form OH^-. The advantage of the Brønsted-Lowry concept of acids and bases is that it is not limited to aqueous solutions.

Brønsted-Lowry acids and bases always occur in pairs, called **conjugate acid-base pairs.** The two members of a conjugate pair are related by the transfer of a proton. For example, H_3O^+ is the conjugate acid of the base H_2O, and NO_2^- is the conjugate base of HNO_2:

$$H_3O^+ (aq) \rightleftarrows H_2O (aq) + H^+ (aq)$$
$$HNO_2 (aq) \rightleftarrows NO_2^- (aq) + H^+ (aq)$$

Lewis Definition

At approximately the same time as Brønsted and Lowry, Gilbert Lewis also proposed definitions of acids and bases. Lewis defined an acid as an electron-pair acceptor and a base as an electron-pair donor. Lewis's are the most inclusive definitions. Just as every Arrhenius acid is a Brønsted-Lowry acid, every Brønsted-Lowry acid is also a Lewis acid (and likewise for bases). However, the Lewis definition encompasses some species not included within the Brønsted-Lowry definition. For example, BCl_3 and $AlCl_3$ can each accept an electron pair and are therefore Lewis acids, despite their inability to donate protons.

NOMENCLATURE OF ARRHENIUS ACIDS

The name of an acid is related to the name of the parent anion (the anion that combines with H^+ to form the acid). Acids formed from anions whose names end in **-ide** have the prefix **hydro-** and the ending **-ic.**

F^-	Fluoride	HF	Hydrofluoric acid
Br^-	Bromide	HBr	Hydrobromic acid

Acids formed from oxyanions are called **oxyacids.** If the anion ends in **-ite** (less oxygen), then the acid will end with **-ous acid.** If the anion ends in **-ate** (more oxygen), then the acid will end with **-ic acid.** Prefixes in the names of the anions are retained. Some examples:

ClO^-	Hypochlorite	HClO	Hypochlorous acid
ClO_2^-	Chlorite	$HClO_2$	Chlorous acid
ClO_3^-	Chlorate	$HClO_3$	Chloric acid
ClO_4^-	Perchlorate	$HClO_4$	Perchloric acid
NO_2^-	Nitrite	HNO_2	Nitrous acid
NO_3^-	Nitrate	HNO_3	Nitric acid

PROPERTIES OF ACIDS AND BASES

Hydrogen Ion Equilibria (pH AND pOH)

Hydrogen ion concentration, $[H^+]$, is generally measured as **pH,** where:

$$pH = -\log[H^+] = \log(1/[H^+])$$

Likewise, hydroxide ion concentration, $[OH^-]$, is measured as **pOH** where:

$$pOH = -\log[OH^-] = \log(1/[OH^-])$$

In any aqueous solution, the H_2O solvent dissociates slightly:

$$H_2O(l) \underset{\rightarrow}{\leftarrow} H^+\,(aq) + OH^-\,(aq)$$

This dissociation is an equilibrium reaction and is therefore described by a constant, K_w, the water dissociation constant:

$$K_w = [H^+][OH^-] = 10^{-14}$$

Rewriting this equation in logarithmic form gives:

$$pH + pOH = 14$$

In pure H_2O, $[H^+]$ is equal to $[OH^-]$ because for every mole of H_2O that dissociates, one mole of H^+ and one mole of OH^- are formed. A solution with equal concentrations of H^+ and OH^- is neutral and has a pH of 7($-\log 10^{-7} = 7$). A pH below 7 indicates a relative excess of H^+ ions and, therefore, an acidic solution; a pH above 7 indicates a relative excess of OH^- ions and, therefore, a basic solution.

Math note: Estimating p-scale values

A useful skill for various problems involving acids and bases, as well as their corresponding buffer solutions, is the ability to quickly convert pH, pOH, pK_a, and pK_b into nonlogarithmic form and vice versa.

When the original value is a power of 10, the operation is relatively simple; changing the sign on the exponent gives the corresponding p-scale value directly. For example:

   If $[H^+] = 0.001$, or 10^{-3}, then pH = 3.

   If $K_b = 1.0 \times 10^{-7}$, then $pK_b = 7$.

More difficulty arises (in the absence of a calculator) when the original value is not an exact power of 10; exact calculation would be excessively onerous, but a simple method of approximation exists. If the nonlogarithmic value is written in proper scientific notation, it will look like: $n \times 10^{-m}$, where n is a number between 1 and 10. The log of this product can be written as: $\log(n \times 10^{-m}) = -m + \log n$, and the negative log is thus $m - \log n$. Now, since n is a number between 1 and 10, its logarithm will be a fraction between 0 and 1, thus, $m - \log n$ will be between $m - 1$ and m. Further, the larger n is, the larger the fraction $\log n$ will be, and therefore the closer to $m - 1$ our answer will be.

Example: If Ka = 1.8×10^{-5}, then pKa = $5 - \log 1.8$. Because 1.8 is small, its log will be small, and the answer will be closer to 5 than to 4. (The actual answer is 4.74.)

Relative Strengths of Acids and Bases

The strength of an acid or base will depend largely upon its ability to ionize. The strength of an acid, for example, can be measured by the fraction of the molecules of that acid undergoing ionization. Subsequently, the acid strength can be expressed by the following equation:

$$\text{Percent ionization} = \frac{\text{ionized acid concentration at equilibrium}}{} \times 100\%$$

When an acid or base is strong, its conjugate base and acid will have no measurable strength, respectively. For example, the stronger the acid, the weaker the conjugate base. Furthermore, within a series of weak acids, the stronger the acid, the weaker its conjugate base for all acids and bases included.

Example: HF is a stronger acid than HCN; therefore, F^- would be expected to be a weaker bases than CN^-.

Strong Acids and Bases

Strong acids and bases are those that completely dissociate into their component ions in aqueous solution. For example, when NaOH is added to water, it dissociates completely:

$$NaOH(s) + \text{excess } H_2O(l) \rightarrow Na^+ (aq) + OH^- (aq)$$

Hence, in a 1-M solution of NaOH, complete dissociation gives 1 mole of OH^- ions per liter of solution.

$$pH = 14 - (-\log[OH^-]) = 14 + \log[1] = 14$$

Virtually no undissociated NaOH remains. Note that the $[OH^-]$ contributed by the dissociation of H_2O is considered to be negligible in this case. The contribution of OH^- and H^+ ions from the dissociation of H_2O can be neglected only if the concentration of the acid or base is greater than 10^{-7} M. For example, the pH of a 1×10^{-8} M HCl solution (HCl is a strong acid) might appear to be 8 because $\{-\log (1 \times 10^{-8})\} = 8$. However, a pH of 8 is in the basic pH range, and an HCl solution is not basic. The discrepancy arises from the fact that at low HCl concentrations, H^+ from the dissociation of water does contribute significantly to the total $[H^+]$. The $[H^+]$ from the dissociation of water is less than 1×10^{-7}M due to the common ion effect. The total concentration of H^+ can be calculated from

$K_w = (x + 1 \times 10^{-8})(x) = 1.0 \times 10^{-14}$, where x = $[H^+]$ = $[OH^-]$ (both from the dissociation of water molecules).

Solving for x gives x = 9.5×10^{-8} M, so $[H^+]_{total}$ = $(9.5 \times 10^{-8} + 1 \times 10^{-8})$ M = 1.05×10^{-7} M, and pH = $-\log (1.05 \times 10^{-7})$ = 6.98, slightly less than 7, as should be expected for a very dilute, yet acidic solution.

Strong acids commonly encountered in the laboratory include $HClO_4$ (perchloric acid), HNO_3 (nitric acid), H_2SO_4 (sulfuric acid), and HCl (hydrochloric acid). Commonly encountered strong bases include NaOH (sodium hydroxide), KOH (potassium hydroxide), and other soluble hydroxides of Group IA and IIA metals. Calculation of the pH and pOH of strong acids and bases assumes complete dissociation of the acid or base in solution: $[H^+]$ = normality of strong acid and $[OH^-]$ = normality of strong base.

Weak Acids and Bases

Weak acids and bases are those that only partially dissociate in aqueous solution. A **weak monoprotic acid (HA)** in aqueous solution will achieve the following equilibrium after dissociation (H_3O^+ is equivalent to H^+ in aqueous solution):

$$HA\ (aq) + H_2O\ (l) \underset{\rightarrow}{\leftarrow} H_3O^+\ (aq) + A^-\ (aq)$$

The **acid dissociation constant, K_a,** is a measure of the degree to which an acid dissociates.

$$K_a = \frac{[H_3O+][A-]}{[HA]}$$

The weaker the acid, the smaller the K_a. Note that K_a does not contain an expression for the pure liquid, water.

A **weak monovalent base (BOH)** undergoes dissociation to give B^+ and OH^-. The **base dissociation constant, K_b,** is a measure of the degree to which a base dissociates. The weaker the base, the smaller its K_b. For a monovalent base, K_b is defined as follows:

$$Kb = \frac{[B+][OH-]}{[BOH]}$$

A **conjugate acid** is defined as the acid formed when a base gains a proton. Similarly, a **conjugate base** is formed when an acid loses a proton. For example, in the HCO_3^-/CO_3^{2-} conjugate acid/base pair, CO_3^{2-} is the conjugate base and HCO_3^- is the conjugate acid:

$$HCO_3^-\ (aq) \underset{\rightarrow}{\leftarrow} H^+\ (aq) + CO_3^{2-}\ (aq)$$

To find the K_a of the conjugate acid HCO_3^-, the reaction with water must be considered.

$$HCO_3^-\ (aq) + H_2O\ (l) \underset{\rightarrow}{\leftarrow} H_3O^+\ (aq) + CO_3^{2-}\ (aq)$$

Likewise, for the K_b of CO_3^{2-}:

$$CO_3^{2-}\ (aq) + H_2O\ (l) \underset{\rightarrow}{\leftarrow} HCO_3^-\ (aq) + OH^-\ (aq)$$

In a conjugate acid/base pair formed from a weak acid, the conjugate base is generally stronger than the conjugate acid. Thus, for HCO_3^- and CO_3^{2-}, the reaction of CO_3^{2-} (the conjugate base) in water to produce HCO_3^- (the conjugate acid) and OH^- occurs to a great extent (i.e., is more favorable) than the reverse reaction.

The equilibrium constants for these reactions are as follows:

$$K_a = \frac{[H+][CO_3^{2-}]}{[HCO_3^-]} \text{ and } K_b = \frac{[HCO_3^-][OH^-]}{[CO_3^{2-}]}$$

Adding the two reactions shows that the net reaction is simply the dissociation of water:

$$H_2O\ (l) \underset{\rightarrow}{\leftarrow} H^+\ (aq) + OH^-\ (aq)$$

The **equilibrium constant** for this net reaction is $K_w = [H^+][OH^-]$, which is the product of K_a and K_b. Thus, if the dissociation constant either for an acid or for its conjugate base is known, then the **dissociation constant** for the other can be determined, using the equation:

$$K_a \times K_b = K_w = 1 \times 10^{-14}$$

Thus, K_a and K_b are inversely related. In other words, if K_a is large (the acid is strong), then K_b will be small (the conjugate base will be weak), and vice versa.

Applications of K_a and K_b

To calculate the concentration of H^+ in a 2.0 M aqueous solution of acetic acid, CH_3COOH ($Ka = 1.8 \times 10^{-5}$), first write the equilibrium reaction:

$$CH_3COOH\ (aq) \underset{\rightarrow}{\leftarrow} H^+\ (aq) + CH_3COO^-\ (aq)$$

Next, write the expression for the acid dissociation constant:

$$K_a = \frac{[H+][CH_3COOO-]}{[CH_3COOH]} = 1.8 \times 10^{-5}$$

Because acetic acid is a weak acid, the concentration of CH_3COOH at equilibrium is equal to its initial concentration, 2.0 M, less the amount dissociated, x. Likewise $[H^+] = [CH_3COO^-] = x$, since each molecule of CH_3COOH dissociates into one H^+ ion and one CH_3COO^- ion. Thus, the equation can be rewritten as follows:

$$K_a = \frac{[x][x]}{[2.0 - x]} = 1.8 \times 10^{-5}$$

We can approximate that $2.0 - x \approx 2.0$ since acetic acid is a weak acid, and only slightly dissociates in water. This simplifies the calculation of x:

$$K_a = \frac{[x][x]}{[2.0]} = 1.8 \times 10^{-5}$$

$$x = 6.0 \times 10^{-3} M$$

The fact that $[x]$ is so much less than the initial concentration of acetic acid (2.0 M) validates the approximation; otherwise, it would have been necessary to solve for x using the quadratic formula. (A rule of thumb is that the approximation is valid as long as x is less than 5 percent of the initial concentration.)

SALT FORMATION

Acids and bases may react with each other, forming a salt and (often, but not always) water, in what is termed a **neutralization reaction** (see Chapter 31). For example:

$$HA + BOH \rightarrow BA + H_2O$$

The salt may precipitate out or remain ionized in solution, depending on its solubility and the amount produced. Neutralization reactions generally go to completion. The reverse reaction, in which the salt ions react with water to give back the acid or base, is known as **hydrolysis.**

Four combinations of strong and weak acids and bases are possible:

1. strong acid + strong base: e.g., $HCl + NaOH \rightarrow NaCl + H_2O$
2. strong acid + weak base: e.g., $HCl + NH_3 \rightarrow NH_4Cl$
3. weak acid + strong base: e.g., $HClO + NaOH \rightarrow NaClO + H_2O$
4. weak acid + weak base: e.g., $HClO + NH_3 \underset{\rightarrow}{\leftarrow} NH_4ClO$

The products of a reaction between equal concentrations of a strong acid and a strong base are a salt and water. The acid and base neutralize each other, so the resulting solution is neutral (pH = 7), and the ions formed in the reaction do not react with water. The product of a reaction between a strong acid and a weak base is also a salt, but usually no water is formed since weak bases are usually not hydroxides; however, in this case, the cation of the salt will react with the water solvent, reforming the weak base. This reaction constitutes hydrolysis. For example:

$$HCl\ (aq) + NH_3\ (aq) \underset{\rightarrow}{\leftarrow} NH_4^+\ (aq) + Cl^-\ (aq)\ \text{Reaction I}$$
$$NH_4^+\ (aq) + H_2O\ (aq) \underset{\rightarrow}{\leftarrow} NH_3\ (aq) + H_3O^+\ (aq)\ \text{Reaction II}$$

NH_4^+ is the conjugate acid of a weak base (NH_3) and is, therefore, stronger than the conjugate base (Cl^-) of the strong acid HCl. NH_4^+ will thus react with OH^-, reducing the concentration of OH^-. There will thus be an excess of H^+, which will lower the pH of the solution.

On the other hand, when a weak acid reacts with a strong base, the solution is basic due to the hydrolysis of the salt to reform the acid with the concurrent formation of hydroxide ion from the hydrolyzed water molecules. The pH of a solution containing a weak acid and a weak base depends on the relative strengths of the reactants. For example, the acid HClO has a $K_a = 3.2 \times 10^{-8}$, and the base NH_3 has a $K_b = 1.8 \times 10^{-5}$. Thus an aqueous solution of HClO and NH_3 is basic since K_a for HClO is less than K_b for NH_3.

POLYVALENCE AND NORMALITY

The relative acidity or basicity of an aqueous solution is determined by the relative concentrations of **acid** and **base equivalents.** An acid equivalent is equal to one mole of H^+ (or H_3O^+) ions; a base equivalent is equal to one mole of OH^- ions. Some acids and bases are polyvalent, that is, each mole of the acid or base liberates more than one acid or base equivalent. For example, the diprotic acid H_2SO_4 undergoes the following dissociation in water:

$$H_2SO_4(aq) \rightarrow H^+(aq) + HSO_4^-(aq)$$
$$HSO_4^-(aq) \underset{\rightarrow}{\leftarrow} H^+(aq) + SO_4^{2-}(aq)$$

One mole of H_2SO_4 can thus produce two acid equivalents (two moles of H^+). The acidity or basicity of a solution depends upon the concentration of acidic or basic equivalents that can be liberated. The quantity of acidic or basic capacity is directly indicated by the solution's normality (see Chapter 36, Solutions). Because each mole of H_3PO_4 can liberate three moles (equivalents) of H^+, a 2 M H_3PO_4 solution would be 6 N (6 normal).

Another useful measurement is **equivalent weight.** For example, the gram molecular weight of H_2SO_4 is 98 g/mol. Because each mole liberates two acid equivalents, the gram equivalent weight of H_2SO_4 would be $\frac{98}{2} = 49g$; that is, the dissociation of 49 g of H_2SO_4 would release one acid equivalent. Common polyvalent acids include H_2SO_4, H_3PO_4, and H_2CO_3.

AMPHOTERIC SPECIES

An amphoteric, or **amphiprotic,** species is one that can act either as an acid or a base, depending on its chemical environment. In the Brønsted–Lowry sense, an amphoteric species can either gain or lose a proton. **Water** is the most common example. When water reacts with a base, it behaves as an acid:

$$H_2O + B^- \underset{\rightarrow}{\leftarrow} HB + OH^-$$

When water reacts with an acid, it behaves as a base:

$$HA + H_2O \underset{\rightarrow}{\leftarrow} H_3O^+ + A^-$$

The partially dissociated conjugate base of a polyprotic acid is usually amphoteric (e.g., HSO_4^- can either gain an H^+ to form H_2SO_4 or lose an H^+ to form SO_4^{2-}). The hydroxides of certain metals (e.g., Al, Zn, Pb, and Cr) are also amphoteric. Furthermore, species that can act as either oxidizing or reducing agents (see Chapter 38) are considered to be amphoteric as well, since by accepting or donating electron pairs they act as Lewis acids or bases, respectively.

TITRATION AND BUFFERS

Titration is a procedure used to determine the molarity of an acid or base. This is accomplished by reacting a known volume of a solution of unknown concentration with a known volume of a solution of known concentration. When the number of acid equivalents equals the number of base equivalents added, or vice versa, the **equivalence point** is reached. It is important to emphasize that, while a strong acid/strong base titration will have an equivalence point at pH 7, the equivalence point need *not* always occur at pH 7. Also, when titrating polyprotic acids or bases, there are several equivalence points, as each different acidic or basic species is titrated separately (see Polyprotic Acids and Bases later in this chapter).

The equivalence point in a titration is estimated in two common ways: either by using a graphical method, plotting the pH of the solution as a function of added titrant by using a **pH meter** (e.g., Figure 37.1 below), or by watching for a color change of an added **indicator.** Indicators are weak organic acids or bases that have different colors in their undissociated and dissociated states. Indicators are used in low concentrations and therefore do not significantly alter the equivalence point. The point at which the indicator actually changes color is not the equivalence point but is called the **end point**. If the titration is performed well, the volume difference (and therefore the error) between the end point and the equivalence point is usually small and may be corrected for or ignored.

Strong Acid and Strong Base

Consider the titration of 10 mL of a 0.1 N solution of HCl with a 0.1 N solution of NaOH. Plotting the pH of the reaction solution versus the quantity of NaOH added gives the curve shown in Figure 37.1

Because HCl is a strong acid and NaOH is a strong base, the equivalence point of the titration will be at pH 7, and the solution will be neutral. Note that the endpoint shown is close to, but not exactly equal to, the equivalence point; selection of a better indicator, say one that changes colors at pH 8, would have given a better approximation.

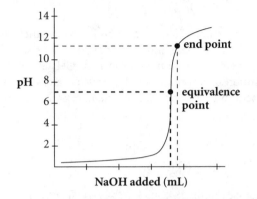

Figure 37.1 Titration of HCl with NaOH

In the early part of the curve (when little base has been added), the acidic species predominates, and so the addition of small amounts of base will not appreciably change either the [OH⁻] or the pH. Similarly, in the last part of the titration curve (when an excess of base has been added), the addition of small amounts of base will not change the [OH⁻] significantly, and the pH remains relatively constant. The addition of base most alters the concentrations of H^+ and OH^- near the equivalence point, and thus the pH changes most drastically in that region.

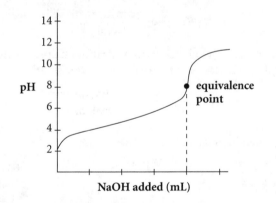

Figure 37.2 Titration of a Weak Acid, HA, with NaOH

Weak Acid and Strong Base

Titration of a weak acid, HA, with a strong base produces the titration curve shown in Figure 37.2.

Comparing Figure 37.2 with Figure 37.1 shows that the initial pH of the weak acid solution is greater than the initial pH of the strong acid solution. The pH changes most significantly early on in the titration, and the equivalence point is in the basic range.

Buffers

A **buffer solution** consists of a mixture of a weak acid and its salt (which consists of its conjugate base and a cation) or a mixture of a weak base and its salt (which consists of its conjugate acid and an anion). Two examples of buffers are a solution of acetic acid (CH_3COOH) and its salt, sodium acetate ($CH_3COO^-Na^+$), and a solution of ammonia (NH_3) and its salt, ammonium chloride ($NH_4^+Cl^-$). Buffer solutions have the useful property of resisting changes in pH when small amounts of acid or base are added.

Consider a buffer solution of acetic acid and sodium acetate:

$$CH_3COOH \rightleftharpoons H^+ + CH_3COO^-$$

When a small amount of NaOH is added to the buffer, the OH^- ions from the NaOH react with the H^+ ions present in the solution; subsequently, more acetic acid dissociates (equilibrium shifts to the right), restoring the $[H^+]$. Thus, an increase in $[OH^-]$ does not appreciably change pH. Likewise, when a small amount of HCl is added to the buffer, H^+ ions from the HCl react with the acetate ions to form acetic acid. Thus, $[H^+]$ is kept relatively constant, and the pH of the solution is relatively unchanged.

The **Henderson-Hasselbalch equation** is used to estimate the pH of a solution in the buffer region where the concentrations of the species and its conjugate are present in approximately equal concentrations. For a weak acid buffer solution:

$$pH = pKa + \log \frac{[\text{conjugate base}]}{[\text{weak acid}]}$$

Note that when [conjugate base] = [weak acid] (in a titration, halfway to the equivalent point), the pH = pK_a because the log 1 = 0. Likewise, for a weak base buffer solution:

$$pOH = pK_b + \log \frac{[\text{conjugate acid}]}{[\text{weak base}]}$$

$pOH = pK_b$ when [conjugate acid] = [weak base].

Polyprotic Acids and Bases

The titration curve for a polyprotic acid or base looks different from that for a monoprotic acid or base. Figure 37.3 shows the titration of Na_2CO_3 with HCl in which the polyprotic acid H_2CO_3 is the ultimate product.

In region I, little acid has been added, and the predominant species is CO_3^{2-}. In region II, more acid has been added, and the predominant species are CO_3^{2-} and HCO_3^-, in relatively equal concentrations. The flat part of the curve is the first buffer region, corresponding to the pK_a of HCO_3^- ($K_a = 5.6 \times 10^{-11}$ implies $pK_a = 10.25$).

Region III contains the equivalence point, at which all of the CO_3^{2-} is titrated to HCO_3^-. As the curve illustrates, a rapid change in pH occurs at the equivalence point; in the latter part of region III, the predominant species is HCO_3^-.

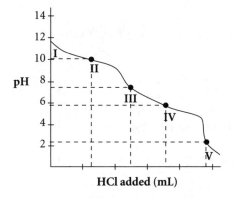

Figure 37.3 Titration of Na2CO3 with HCl

In region IV, the acid has neutralized approximately half of the HCO_3^-, and now H_2CO_3 and HCO_3^- are in roughly equal concentrations. This flat region is the second buffer region of the titration curve, corresponding to the pK_a of H_2CO_3 ($K_a = 4.3 \times 10^{-7}$ implies $pK_a = 6.37$). In region V, the equivalence point for the entire titration is reached, as all of the HCO_3^-, is converted to H_2CO_3. Again, a rapid change in pH is observed near the equivalence point as acid is added.

REVIEW PROBLEMS

1. A certain aqueous solution has $[OH^-] = 6.2 \times 10^{-5}$ M.

   (A) Calculate $[H^+]$.
   (B) Calculate the pH of the solution.
   (C) Is the solution acidic or basic?

2. What is the ratio of $[H^+]$ of a solution of pH = 4 to the $[H^+]$ of a solution of pH = 7?

3. Write equations expressing what happens to each of the following bases in aqueous solutions:

   (A) LiOH
   (B) $Ba(OH)_2$
   (C) NH_3
   (D) NO_2^-

4. What volume of a 3-M solution of NaOH is required to titrate 0.05 L of a 4-M solution of HCl to the equivalence point?

5. If 10 mL of 1-M NaOH is titrated with 1 M of HCl to a pH of 2, what volume of HCl was added?

6. Identify the conjugate acids and bases in the following equation:
$$NH_3 + H_2O \overset{\leftarrow}{\rightarrow} NH_4^+ + OH^-$$

7. Identify each of the following as an Arrhenius acid or base, Brønsted-Lowry acid or base, or Lewis acid or base.

   (A) NaOH, in $NaOH \rightarrow Na^+ + OH^-$
   (B) HCl, in $HCl \rightarrow H^+ + Cl^-$
   (C) NH_3, in $NH_3 + H^+ \rightarrow NH_4^+$
   (D) NH_4^+, in $NH_4^+ \rightarrow NH_3 + H^+$
   (E) $(CH_3)_3N:$, in $(CH_3)_3N: + BF_3 \rightarrow (CH_3)_3N:BF_3$
   (F) BF_3 in the above equation

8. At equilibrium, a certain acid, HA, in solution yields 0.94 M [HA] and 0.060 M [A⁻].

   (A) Calculate K_a.
   (B) Is this acid stronger or weaker than sulfurous acid ($K_a = 1.7 \times 10^{-2}$)?
   (C) Calculate K_b.
   (D) Calculate pH.
   (E) Calculate the pK_a.

9. For each of the following choices, choose that which describes the weaker acid:

   (A) $K_a = X$, $K_a = 3X$
   (B) $[H^+] = X$, $[H^+] = 3X$
   (C) $pK_a = X$, $pK_a = 3X$
   (D) $pH = X$, $pH = 3X$

10. For a certain acid, HA, $K_b(A^-) = 2.22 \times 10^{-11}$, calculate the pH of a 0.5 M solution of HA.

11. Which of the following sets of materials would make the best buffer solution?
    (A) H_2O, 1 M NaOH, 1 M H_2SO_4
    (B) H_2O, 1 M $HC_2H_3O_2$, 1 M $NaC_2H_3O_2$
    (C) H_2O, 1 M $HC_2H_3O_2$, 6 M $NaC_2H_3O_2$
    (D) H_2O, 1 M $HC_2H_3O_2$, 1 M NaOH

12. A certain buffer solution is 3 M in HF and 2 M in NaF. Calculate the pH of this buffer given that the K_a of HF = 7.0×10^{-4}.

13. Which of the following combinations would produce a buffer solution of pH = 4?
    (K_a HNO_2 = 4.5×10^{-4})
    (A) 0.30 M HNO_2, 0.22 M $NaNO_2$
    (B) 0.22 M HNO_2, 0.30 M $NaNO_2$
    (C) 0.11 M HNO_2, 0.50 M $NaNO_2$
    (D) 0.50 M HNO_2, 0.11 M $NaNO_2$

14. Write out chemical equations describing the buffer activity that prevents drastic pH changes when 1) a strong acid 2) a strong base is added.

SOLUTIONS TO REVIEW PROBLEMS

1. **A** 1.6×10^{-10} M

   The concentration of H^+ (in mol/L of hydronium ion) is 1.6×10^{-10} M. Water is composed of hydronium and hydroxide ions, and the dissociation constant of water, K_w, is defined as $[H^+][OH^-] = 1.0 \times 10^{-14}$ M.

   If $[OH^-] = 6.2 \times 10^{-5}$, then $[H^+] = K_w/[OH^-] = \dfrac{1.0 \times 10^{-14}}{6.2 \times 10^{-5}} = 1.6 \times 10^{-10}$ M.

   B 9.79

   The pH of a solution is a logarithmic measurement of $[H^+]$, which expresses the degree of acidity.

   pH is defined as $-\log[H^+]$. In this case, pH $= -\log(1.6 \times 10^{-10}) = 9.79$.

   C A pH of 9.79 indicates a basic solution, as does any $[OH^-] > 1.0 \times 10^{-7}$ M.

2. **1,000:1**

   This problem can be solved by calculating the $[H^+]$ of the pH = 4 solution and the $[H^+]$ of the pH = 7 solution. Then divide the former by the latter: because pH $= -\log[H^+]$, $[H^+]$ = antilog $(-$pH$)$. For pH = 4, antilog $(-4) = 1.0 \times 10^{-4}$. For pH = 7, antilog $(-7) = 1.0 \times 10^{-7}$. 1×10^{-4}: $1 \times 10^{-7} = 1,000:1$. Alternately, we could subtract the pH's first, and then antilog: $7 - 4 = 3$ implies 10^3, or 1,000:1.

3. **A** $LiOH \rightarrow Li^+ + OH^-$

   B $Ba(OH)_2 \rightarrow Ba^{2+} + 2OH^-$

   C $NH_3 + H_2O \rightarrow NH_4^+ + OH^-$

   D $NO_2^- + H_2O \rightarrow HNO_2 + OH^-$

4. **0.067 L**

   At the equivalence point,

   $(Normality)_{acid}(Volume)_{acid} = (Normality)_{base}(Volume)_{base}$

   4 M HCl = 4 N HCl

   3 M NaOH = 3 N NaOH

   Plugging into the formula,

   $(4)(0.05) = (3)(V)$

   $V_B = 0.067$ L

5. **10.2 mL**

   First, add enough HCl to neutralize the solution. Because both the acid and the base are 1 M, 10 mL of HCl will neutralize 10 mL of NaOH, from $N_A V_A = N_B V_B$. This produces 20 mL of 0.5 M NaCl solution.

   Next calculate how much more HCl must be added to produce a $[H^+]$ of 1×10^{-2}. Let x be the amount of HCl to be added. The total volume of the solution will be $(20 + x)$ mL. Since this is now a dilution problem, the amount of HCl to be added can be found by using the formula:

   $M_1 V_1 = M_2 V_2$

   $(1\ M)(x\ mL) = (0.01\ M)[(20 + x)mL]$

   When this equation is solved, x is found to have the value of 0.2. The final volume is 20.2 mL, so 10.2 mL of HCl was added to the original NaOH solution.

6. NH_4^+ is the conjugate acid of the weak base, NH_3; OH^- is the conjugate base of the weak acid H_2O.

The reaction in question is:

$NH_3 + H_2O \underset{\rightarrow}{\leftarrow} NH_4^+ + OH^-$

According to the Brønsted-Lowry theory of acids and bases, an acid releases a proton, whereas a base accepts a proton. In the case of weak acids and bases, an equilibrium is established whereby a weak acid, in this case H_2O, dissociates partially, donating a proton to a weak base, which is NH_3. The weak acid, H_2O, loses a proton and becomes a relatively stronger conjugate base, OH^-. This is one conjugate acid-base pair (H_2O, OH^-). Meanwhile, the weak base, NH_3, picks up a proton to become a relatively stronger conjugate acid, NH_4^+. This is the second conjugate acid-base pair (NH_4^+, NH_3).

7. **A**   NaOH is an Arrhenius base

    B   HCl is an Arrhenius acid and a Brønsted-Lowry acid

    C NH_3 is a Brønsted-Lowry base and a Lewis base

    D NH_4^+ is an Arrhenius acid and a Brønsted-Lowry acid

    E $(CH_3)_3N$: acts only as a Lewis base

    F BF_3 acts only as a Lewis acid

8. **A** $\mathbf{3.8 \times 10^{-3}}$

K_a is the equilibrium constant for an acid, also called the dissociation constant for the particular equilibrium state that is achieved by the dissociation of an acid. We are told that, at equilibrium $[HA]$ is 0.94 M, whereas $[A^-]$ is 0.060 M. The dissociation of HA can be written as follows:

$HA \rightarrow H^+ + A^-$

The molar ratio of A^- to H^+ is 1:1, so $[H^+]$ must also be 0.060 M at equilibrium. It follows, then, that:

$K_a = [A^-][H^+]/[HA] = (0.060)(0.060)/(0.94) = 3.8 \times 10^{-3}$

    B   **Weaker**

K_a is a measure of the strength of an acid. An acid with a high K_a is a strong acid because its equilibrium position lies further to the right (more product increases numerator and makes K_a larger), meaning that dissociation is more complete. Greater dissociation means a stronger acid. The K_a of sulfurous acid is 1.7×10^{-2} and the K_a of HA is 3.8×10^{-3}. The K_a of HA is less than that of sulfurous acid; therefore, HA is a weaker acid.

    C $\mathbf{2.6 \times 10^{-12}}$

Just as K_a is the dissociation constant for an acid, K_b is the dissociation constant of a base. Whereas K_a measures the degree to which H^+ is liberated, K_b measures the degree to which OH^- is liberated. Because H^+ and OH^- are related by $K_w = 1.0 \times 10^{-14}$, K_b can be easily calculated. In this case,

$$K_b = \frac{1.0 \times 10^{14}}{3.8 \times 10^{-3}} = 2.6 \times 10^{-12}$$

    D $pH = -\log[H^+] = -\log(0.060) = 1.22$

    E $pK_a = -\log K_a = -\log(3.8 \times 10^{-3}) = 2.42$

9. **A** K_a is a measure of the dissociation of an acid and, therefore, the strength of an acid. A higher K_a indicates a stronger acid; a lower K_a indicates a weaker acid. X is one-third the value of 3X and, therefore, a weaker acid.

B [H^+] is a direct measure of the strength of an acid. The greater the concentration of H^+ in solution, the stronger the acid. An acid that liberates X moles of H^+ per liter is weaker, therefore, than an acid that liberates 3X moles of H^+ per liter.

C $pK_a = -\log K_a$; therefore, a pK_a of 3X corresponds to a K_a lower in value than that of a pK_a of X. A lower K_a means a weaker acid, and a lower pK_a means a stronger acid. 3X is greater than X, so the acid whose pK_a is 3X is weaker than the acid whose pK_a is X.

D The acid with a pH of 3X is the weaker acid, using the same reasoning as for C.

10.   **1.82**

If $K_b = 2.22 \times 10^{-11}$, then

$$K_a = \frac{1.0 \times 10^{14}}{2.22 \times 10^{-11}}$$

$K_a = 4.5 \times 10^{-4}$

If HA dissociates according to the following expression,

$HA \underset{\rightarrow}{\leftarrow} H^+ + A^-$,

then the equilibrium expression for this dissociation is:

$K_a = [H^+][A^-]/[HA]$.

We can let [H^+] = x at equilibrium and, since [H^+]:[A^-] = 1:1, [A^-] = x.

If the original [HA] was 0.5M, and x mol/L are dissociated, then at equilibrium, [HA] = 0.5 – x.

Thus the equilibrium expression becomes:

$4.5 \times 10^{-4} = ([x][x])/(0.5 - x)$

We can approximate that $0.5 - x = \approx 0.5$ since HA has a small K_a, which indicates it is a weak acid.

$4.5 \times 10^{-4} = x^2/0.5$

$x^2 = 2.25 \times 10^{-4}$

$x = 0.015 = [H^+]$

$pH = -\log [H^+] = -\log [0.015] = 1.82$

11. **B** A buffer solution is prepared from a weak acid and its conjugate base, preferably in near-equal quantities. Choices (A) and (D) are wrong because they do not show conjugate acid/base pairs. (C) is wrong because it shows a weak acid and its conjugate base, where the concentrations of the acid and the base are quite different. Thus, the best buffer solution would be that prepared from (B), which shows a conjugate acid/base pair, both present in 1 M concentrations.

12. **2.98**

$$K_a = \frac{[H^+][F^-]}{[HF]}$$

$$7 \times 10^{-4} = \frac{[H^+](2)}{3}$$

$[H^+] = 1.05 \times 10^{-3}$

$pH = -\log[H^+] = 2.98$

Another way to solve this problem is by using the Henderson-Hasselbalch equation:

$pH = pK_a + \log$ [conjugate base]/[weak acid]. Using the Henderson-Hasselbalch equation for this problem:

$pH = -\log K_a + \log [F^-]/[HF]$

$pH = -\log (7.0 \times 10^{-4}) + \log 2/3$

$pH = 3.155 - 0.176 = 2.98$

13. **C** The Henderson-Hasselbalch equation may again be used here:

$pH = pK_a + \log [A^-]/[HA]$

$4 = 3.35 + \log [A^-]/[HA]$

$0.65 = \log [A^-]/[HA]$

$[A^-]/[HA] = 4.5$

Only Choice (C) fulfills this criterion as $0.50/0.11 = 4.5$.

14. 1) Strong acid:

Salt in buffer dissociates completely:

$NaX \underset{\rightarrow}{\leftarrow} Na^+ + X^-$

Added strong acid dissociates completely:

$HCl \underset{\rightarrow}{\leftarrow} H^+ + Cl^-$

Protons from the acid are absorbed by the strong conjugate base of the salt:

$H^+ + X^- \underset{\rightarrow}{\leftarrow} HX$

2) Strong base:

Weak acid in buffer hardly dissociates:

$HX \underset{\rightarrow}{\leftarrow} HX$

Added strong base dissociates completely:

$NaOH \underset{\rightarrow}{\leftarrow} Na^+ + OH^-$

OH^- is a strong base, which abstracts protons from the weak acid:

$OH^- + HX \underset{\rightarrow}{\leftarrow} H_2O + X^-$

CHAPTER THIRTY-EIGHT

Redox Reactions and Electrochemistry

Electrochemistry is the study of the relationships between chemical reactions and electrical energy. **Electrochemical reactions** include **spontaneous** reactions that produce electrical energy and **nonspontaneous** reactions that use electrical energy to produce a chemical change. Both types of reactions always involve a **transfer of electrons** with conservation of charge and mass.

OXIDATION-REDUCTION REACTIONS

Oxidation and Reduction

The law of conservation of charge states that an electrical charge can be neither created nor destroyed. Thus, an isolated loss or gain of electrons cannot occur; oxidation (loss of electrons) and reduction (gain of electrons) must occur simultaneously, resulting in an electron transfer called a **redox reaction**. An **oxidizing agent** causes another atom in a redox reaction to undergo oxidation, and is itself reduced. A **reducing agent** causes the other atom to be reduced, and is itself oxidized.

Assigning Oxidation Numbers

It is important, of course, to know which atom is oxidized and which is reduced. **Oxidation numbers** are assigned to atoms to keep track of the redistribution of electrons during a chemical reaction. From the oxidation numbers of the reactants and products, it is possible to determine how many electrons are gained or lost by each atom. The oxidation number is specifically the number of charges an atom would have in a molecule if electrons were completely transferred in the direction that is indicated by the difference in electronegativity. Along the same lines, an element is said to be oxidized if its oxidation number is increased in a given reaction. An element is said to be reduced if the oxidation number of the element decreases in a given reaction. The oxidation number of an atom in a compound is assigned according to the following rules:

- The oxidation number of a free element (an element in its elemental state) is zero, irrespective of how complex the molecule is.
- The oxidation number for a monatomic ion is equal to the charge of the ion. For example, the oxidation numbers for Na^+, Cu^{2+}, Fe^{3+}, Cl^-, and N^{3-} are +1, +2, +3, −1, and −3, respectively.

- The oxidation number of each Group IA element in a compound is +1. The oxidation number of each Group IIA element in a compound is +2.

- The oxidation number of each Group VIIA element in a compound is –1, except when combined with an element of higher electronegativity. For example, in HCl, the oxidation number of Cl is –1; in HOCl, however, the oxidation number of Cl is +1.

- The oxidation number of hydrogen is + 1. However, the oxidation number is of hydrogen is –1 in compounds with less electronegative elements than hydrogen (Groups IA and IIA). Examples include NaH and CaH_2. The more common oxidation number of hydrogen is +1.

- In most compounds, the oxidation number of oxygen is –2. This is not the case, however, in molecules such as OF_2. Here, because F is more electronegative than O, the oxidation number of oxygen is +2. Also, in peroxides such as BaO_2, the oxidation number of O is –1 instead of –2 because of the structure of the peroxide ion, $[O–O]^{2-}$. (Note that Ba, a group IIA element, can not be a +4 cation.)

- The sum of the oxidation numbers of all the atoms present in a neutral compound is zero. The sum of the oxidation numbers of the atoms present in a polyatomic ion is equal to the charge of the ion. Thus, for SO_4^{2-}, the sum of the oxidation numbers must be –2.

- Fluorine has an oxidation number of –1 in all compounds because it has the highest electronegativity of all the elements.

- Metallic elements have only positive oxidation numbers; however, nonmetallic elements may have a positive or negative oxidation number.

Example: Assign oxidation numbers to the atoms in the following reaction to determine the oxidized and reduced species and the oxidizing and reducing agents:

$$SnCl_2 + PbCl_4 \rightarrow SnCl_4 + PbCl_2$$

Solution: All these species are neutral, so the oxidation numbers of each compound must add up to zero. In $SnCl_2$, since there are two chlorines present and chlorine has an oxidation number of –1, Sn must have an oxidation number of +2. Similarly, the oxidation number of Sn in $SnCl_4$ is +4; the oxidation number of Pb is +4 in $PbCl_4$ and +2 in $PbCl_2$. Notice that the oxidation number of Sn goes from +2 to +4; it loses electrons and thus is oxidized, making it the reducing agent. Since the oxidation number of Pb has decreased from +4 to +2, it has gained electrons and been reduced. Pb is the oxidizing agent. The sum of the charges on both sides of the reaction is equal to zero, so charge has been conserved.

Balancing Redox Reactions

By assigning oxidation numbers to the reactants and products, one can determine how many moles of each species are required for conservation of charge and mass, which is necessary to balance the equation. To balance a redox reaction, both the net charge and the number of atoms must be equal on both sides of the equation. The most common method for balancing redox equations is the **half-reaction method**, also known as the **ion-electron method**, in which the equation is separated into two half-reactions—the oxidation part and the reduction part. Each half-reaction is balanced separately, and they are then added to give a balanced overall reaction. Consider a redox reaction between $KMnO_4$ and HI in an acidic solution.

$$MnO_4^- + I^- \rightarrow I_2 + Mn^{2+}$$

Step 1: Separate the two half-reactions.

$$I^- \rightarrow I_2$$
$$MnO_4^- \rightarrow Mn^{2+}$$

Step 2: Balance the atoms of each half-reaction. First, balance all atoms except H and O. Next, in an acidic solution, add H_2O to balance the O atoms and then add H^+ to balance the H atoms. (In a basic solution, use OH^- and H_2O to balance the O's and H's.)

To balance the iodine atoms, place a coefficient of two before the I^- ion.

$$2\,I^- \rightarrow I_2$$

For the permanganate half-reaction, Mn is already balanced. Next, balance the oxygens by adding $4H_2O$ to the right side.

$$MnO_4^- \rightarrow Mn^{2+} + 4H_2O$$

Finally, add H^+ to the left side to balance the 4 H_2Os. These two half-reactions are now balanced.

$$MnO_4^- + 8\,H^+ \rightarrow Mn^{2+} + 4H_2O$$

Step 3: Balance the charges of each half-reaction. The reduction half-reaction must consume the same number of electrons as are supplied by the oxidation half. For the oxidation reaction, add 2 electrons to the right side of the reaction:

$$2\,I^- \rightarrow I_2 + 2e^-$$

For the reduction reaction, a charge of +2 must exist on both sides. Add 5 electrons to the left side of the reaction to accomplish this:

$$5\,e^- + 8\,H^+ + MnO_4^- \rightarrow Mn^{2+} + 4\,H_2O$$

Next, both half-reactions must have the same number of electrons so that they will cancel. Multiply the oxidation half by 5 and the reduction half by 2.

$$5(2I^- \rightarrow I_2 + 2e^-)$$
$$2(5e^- + 8H^+ + MnO_4^- \rightarrow Mn^{2+} + 4\,H_2O)$$

Step 4: Add the half-reactions:

$$10\,I^- \rightarrow 5\,I_2 + 10\,e^-$$
$$16\,H^+ + 2\,MnO_4^- + 10\,e^- \rightarrow 2\,Mn^{2+} + 8\,H_2O$$

The final equation is:

$$10\,I^- + 10\,e^- + 16\,H^+ + 2\,MnO_4^- \rightarrow 5\,I_2 + 2\,Mn^{2+} + 10\,e^- + 8\,H_2O$$

To get the overall equation, cancel out the electrons and any H_2Os, H^+s, or OH^-s that appear on both sides of the equation.

$$10\,I^- + 16\,H^+ + 2\,MnO_4^- \rightarrow 5\,I_2 + 2\,Mn^{2+} + 8\,H_2O$$

Step 5: Finally, confirm that mass and charge are balanced. There is a +4 net charge on each side of the reaction equation, and the atoms are stoichiometrically balanced.

Oxidation Reduction Reactions

There are three major types of redox reactions: combination, decomposition, and displacement.

1. **Combination reactions**—These types of reactions occur with one or more free elements.

    Example: Equation $N_2(g) + 3H_2(g) \rightarrow 2NH_3(g)$
                Redox #'s   0   0   -3 +1

2. **Decomposition reactions**—These types of reactions lead to the production of one or more free elements.

    Example: Equation $2H_2O(l) \rightarrow H_2(g) + O2(g)$
                Redox #'s   +1 -2   0   0

3. **Displacement reactions**—In this type of reaction, an atom or an ion of one element is displaced from a given compound by an atom from a totally different element.

    Example: Equation $2Na(s) + 2H_2O(l) \rightarrow 2NaOH + H_2(g)$
                Redox #'s   0   +1   +1 +1   O

ELECTROCHEMICAL CELLS

Electrochemical cells are contained systems in which a redox reaction occurs. There are two types of electrochemical cells, **galvanic cells** (also known as **voltaic cells**) and **electrolytic cells**. Spontaneous reactions occur in galvanic cells, and nonspontaneous reactions in electrolytic cells. Both types contain **electrodes** at which oxidation and reduction occur. For all electrochemical cells, the electrode at which oxidation occurs is called the **anode**, and the electrode where reduction occurs is called the **cathode.**

Galvanic Cells

A redox reaction occurring in a galvanic cell has a negative ΔG and is, therefore, a **spontaneous reaction**. Galvanic cell reactions supply energy and are used to do work. This energy can be harnessed by placing the oxidation and reduction half-reactions in separate containers called **half-cells**. The half-cells are then connected by an apparatus that allows for the flow of electrons.

A common example of a galvanic cell is the **Daniell cell**.

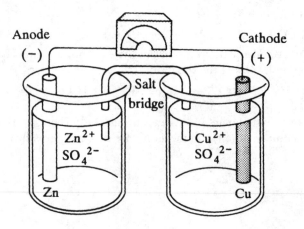

Figure 38.1

In the Daniell cell, a zinc bar is placed in an aqueous $ZnSO_4$ solution, and a copper bar is placed in an aqueous $CuSO_4$ solution. The anode of this cell is the zinc bar where Zn (s) is oxidized to $Zn^{2+}(aq)$. The cathode is the copper bar, and it is the site of the reduction of $Cu^{2+}(aq)$ to Cu (s). The half-cell reactions are written as follows:

$$Zn\ (s) \rightarrow Zn^{2+}\ (aq) + 2e^- \rightarrow (anode)$$
$$Cu^{2+}\ (aq) + 2e \rightarrow Cu\ (s) \rightarrow (cathode)$$

If the two half-cells were not separated, the Cu^{2+} ions would react directly with the zinc bar, and no useful electrical work would be obtained. To complete the circuit, the two solutions must be connected. Without connection, the electrons from the zinc oxidation half-reaction would not be able to get to the copper ions, thus a wire (or other conductor) is necessary. If only a wire were provided for this electron flow, however, the reaction would soon cease anyway because an excess negative charge would build up in the solution surrounding the cathode and an excess positive charge would build up in the solution surrounding the anode. This charge gradient is dissipated by the presence of a **salt bridge**, which permits the exchange of cations and anions. The salt bridge contains an inert electrolyte, usually KCl or NH_4NO_3, whose ions will not react with the electrodes or with the ions in solution. At the same time, the anions from the salt bridge (e.g., Cl^-) diffuse from the salt bridge of the Daniell cell into the $ZnSO_4$ solution to balance out the charge of the newly created Zn^{2+} ions, and the cations of the salt bridge (e.g. K^+) flow into the $CuSO_4$ solution to balance out the charge of the SO_4^{2-} ions left in solution when the Cu^{2+} ions deposit as copper metal.

During the course of the reaction, electrons flow from the zinc bar (anode) through the wire and the voltmeter, toward the copper bar (cathode). The anions (Cl^-) flow externally (via the salt bridge) into the $ZnSO_4$, and the cations (K^+) flow into the $CuSO_4$. This flow depletes the salt bridge and, along with the finite quantity of Cu^{2+} in the solution, accounts for the relatively short lifetime of the cell.

A **cell diagram** is a shorthand notation representing the reactions in an electrochemical cell. A cell diagram for the Daniell cell is as follows:

$$Zn\ (s)\ |\ Zn^{2+}(xM\ SO_4^{2-})\ ||\ Cu^{2+}(yM\ SO_4^{2-})\ |\ Cu\ (s)$$

The following rules are used in constructing a cell diagram:

- The reactants and products are always listed from left to right in the form:
  anode | anode solution || cathode solution | cathode
- A single vertical line indicates a phase boundary.
- A double vertical line indicates the presence of a salt bridge or some other type of barrier.

Ecectrolytic Cells

A redox reaction occurring in an electrolytic cell has a positive ΔG and is therefore **nonspontaneous**. In **electrolysis**, electrical energy is required to induce reaction. The oxidation and reduction half-reactions are usually placed in one container.

Michael Faraday was the first to define certain quantitative principles governing the behavior of electrolytic cells. He theorized that the amount of chemical change induced in an electrolytic cell is directly proportional to the number of moles of electrons that are exchanged during a redox reaction. The number of moles exchanged can be determined from the balanced half-reaction. In general, for a reaction which involves the transfer of n electrons per atom:

$$\mathbf{M^{n+} + n\ e^- \rightarrow M(s)}$$

One mole of M(s) will be produced if n moles of electrons are supplied.

The number of moles of electrons needed to produce a certain amount of M(s) can now be related to a measurable electrical property. One electron carries a charge of 1.6×10^{-19} coulombs (C). The charge carried by one mole of electrons can be calculated by multiplying this number by Avogadro's number, as follows:

$$(1.6 \times 10^{-19})(6.022 \times 10^{23}) = 96{,}487 \text{ C/mol } e^-$$

This number is called **Faraday's constant**, and one **Faraday (F)** is equivalent to the amount of charge contained in one mole of electrons (1 F = 96,487 coulombs, or J/V).

An example of an electrolytic cell, in which molten NaCl is electrolyzed to form Cl_2 (g) and Na (l), is shown in Figure 38.2

In this cell, Na^+ ions migrate towards the cathode, where they are reduced to Na (l). Similarly, Cl^- ions migrate towards the anode, where they are oxidized to Cl_2 (g). This cell is used in industry as the major means of sodium and chlorine production. Note that sodium is a liquid at the temperature of molten NaCl; it is also less dense than the molten salt and thus is easily removed as it floats to the top of the reaction vessel.

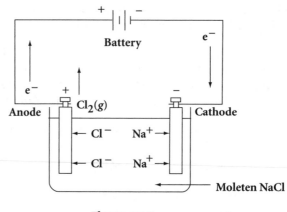

Figure 38.2

Electrode Charge Designations

The anode of an **electrolytic cell** is considered positive, since it is attached to the positive pole of the battery and so attracts anions from the solution. The anode of a **galvanic cell,** on the other hand, is considered negative because the spontaneous oxidation reaction that takes place at the galvanic cell's anode is the original source of that cell's negative charge (i.e., it is the source of electrons). In spite of this difference in designating charge, oxidation takes place at the anode in both types of cells, and electrons always flow through the wire from the anode to the cathode.

In a galvanic cell, charge is spontaneously created as electrons are released by the oxidizing species at the anode; since this is the source of electrons, the anode of a galvanic cell is considered the negative electrode.

In an electrolytic cell, electrons are forced through the cathode where they encounter the species which is to be reduced. Here it is the cathode which is providing electrons, and thus the cathode of an electrolytic cell is considered the negative electrode. Alternatively, one can think of the cathode as the electrode attached to the negative pole of the battery (or other power source) used for the electrolysis.

In either case, a simple mnemonic is that the **CAThode attracts the CATions**. In the Daniell Cell, for example, the electrons created at the anode as the zinc oxidizes travel through the wire to the copper half-cell where they attract copper(II) cations to the cathode.

One common topic in which this distinction arises is **electrophoresis**, a technique often used to separate amino acids based on their isoelectronic points, or pI's. The positively charged amino acids (i.e., those are protonated at the pH of the solution) will migrate toward the cathode; negatively charged amino acids (i.e., those that are deprotonated at the solution pH) migrate instead toward the anode.

REDUCTION POTENTIALS AND THE ELECTROMOTIVE FORCE

Reduction Potentials

Sometimes when electrolysis is carried out in an aqueous solution, water rather than the solute is oxidized or reduced. For example, if an aqueous solution of NaCl is electrolyzed, water may be reduced at the cathode to produce H_2 (g) and OH^- ions, instead of Na^+ being reduced to Na (s), as occurs in the absence of water. The species in a reaction that will be oxidized or reduced can be determined from the **reduction potential** of each species, defined as the tendency of a species to acquire electrons and be reduced. Each species has its own intrinsic reduction potential; the more positive the potential, the greater the species' tendency to be reduced.

A reduction potential is measured in volts (V) and is defined relative to the **standard hydrogen electrode (SHE)**, which is arbitrarily given a potential of 0.00 volts. **Standard reduction potential, (E°)**, is measured under **standard conditions**: 25°C, a 1 M concentration for each ion participating in the reaction, a partial pressure of 1 atm for each gas that is part of the reaction, and metals in their pure state. The relative reactivities of different half-cells can be compared to predict the direction of electron flow. A higher E° means a greater tendency for reduction to occur, while a lower E° means a greater tendency for oxidation to occur.

Example: Given the following half-reactions and E° values, determine which species would be oxidized and which would be reduced.

$Ag^+ + e- \rightarrow Ag$ (s)   E° = +0.80 V

$Tl^+ + e- \rightarrow Tl(s)$ E° = –0.34 V

Solution: Ag^+ would be reduced to Ag (s), and Tl (s) would be oxidized to Tl^+ since Ag^+ has the higher E°. Therefore, the reaction equation would be:

$Ag^+ + Tl$ (s) $\rightarrow Tl^+ + Ag$ (s)

which is the sum of the two spontaneous half-reactions.

It should be noted that reduction and oxidation are opposite processes. Therefore, to obtain the oxidation potential of a given half-reaction, the reduction half-reaction and the sign of the reduction potential are both reversed. For instance, from the example above, the oxidation half-reaction and oxidation potential of Tl(s) are:

$Tl(s) \rightarrow Tl^+ + e^-$ E° = +0.34 V

The Electromotive Force

Standard reduction potentials are also used to calculate the **standard electromotive force** (**EMF or E°$_{cell}$**) of a reaction, the difference in potential between two half-cells. The EMF of a reaction is determined by adding the standard reduction potential of the reduced species and the standard oxidation potential of the oxidized species. When adding standard potentials, *do not* multiply by the number of moles oxidized or reduced.

$$EMF = E^\circ_{red} + E^\circ_{ox} \qquad \text{(Equation 1)}$$

The standard EMF of a galvanic cell is positive, while the standard EMF of an electrolytic cell is negative.

Example: Given that the standard reduction potentials for Sm^{3+} and $[RhCl_6]^{3-}$ are -2.41 V and $+0.44$ V respectively, calculate the EMF of the following reaction:

$Sm^{3+} + Rh + 6\ Cl^- \rightarrow [RhCl_6]^{3-} + Sm$

Solution: First, determine the oxidation and reduction half-reactions. As written, the Rh is oxidized and the Sm^{3+} is reduced. Thus the Sm^{3+} reduction potential is used as is, while the reverse reaction for Rh, $[RhCl_6]^{3-} \rightarrow Rh + 6\ Cl^-$, applies and the oxidation potential of $[RhCl_6]^{3-}$ must be used. Then, using Equation 1, the EMF can be calculated to be $(-2.41$ V$) + (-0.44$ V$) = -2.85$ V. The cell is thus electrolytic as written. From this result, it is evident that the reaction would proceed spontaneously to the left, in which case the Sm would be oxidized while $[RhCl_6]^{3-}$ would be reduced.

THERMODYNAMICS OF REDOX REACTIONS

EMF and Gibbs Free Energy

The thermodynamic criterion for determining the spontaneity of a reaction is ΔG, Gibbs free energy, the maximum amount of useful work produced by a chemical reaction. In an electrochemical cell, the work done is dependent on the number of coulombs and the energy available. Thus, ΔG and EMF are related as follows:

$$\Delta G = -nFE_{cell} \qquad \text{(Equation 2)}$$

where n is the number of moles of electrons exchanged, F is Faraday's constant, and E_{cell} is the EMF of the cell.

Note: Keep in mind that if Faraday's constant is expressed in coulombs (J/V), then ΔG must be expressed in J, not kJ.

If the reaction takes place under standard conditions (25°C, 1 atm pressure, and all solutions at 1M concentration), then the ΔG is the standard Gibbs free energy and E_{cell} is the standard cell potential. The above equation then becomes:

$$\Delta G = -nFE^\circ_{cell} \qquad \text{(Equation 3)}$$

The Effect of Concentration on EMF

Thus far, only the calculations for the EMF of cells in unit concentrations (all the ionic species present have a molarity of 1 and all gases are at a pressure of 1 atm) have been discussed. However, concentration does have an effect on the EMF of a cell: EMF varies with the changing concentrations of the species involved. It can also be determined by the use of the **Nernst equation:**

$$E_{cell} = E^\circ_{cell} - (RT/nF)(\ln Q)$$

Q is the reaction quotient for a given reaction. For example, in the following reaction:

$$a\,A + b\,B \rightarrow c\,C + d\,D$$

the reaction quotient would be:

$$Q = \frac{[C]^c[D]^d}{[A]^a[B]^b}$$

The EMF of a cell can be measured by a **voltmeter**. A **potentiometer** is a kind of voltmeter that draws no current and gives a more accurate reading of the difference in potential between two electrodes.

EMF and the Equilibrium Constant (Keq)

For reactions in solution, ΔG° can determined in another manner, as follows:

$$\Delta G^\circ = -RT \ln K_{eq} \quad \textbf{(Equation 4)}$$

where R is the gas constant 8.314 J/(K•mol), T is the temperature in K, and Keq is the equilibrium constant for the reaction.

If Equations 3 and 4 are combined, then:

$$\Delta G^\circ = -nFE^\circ_{cell} = -RT \ln K_{eq}$$

or simply:

$$nFE^\circ_{cell} = RT \ln Keq \quad \textbf{(Equation 5)}$$

If the values for n, T, and K_{eq} are known, then the E°_{cell} for the redox reaction can be readily calculated.

REVIEW PROBLEMS

1. If one F is equivalent to 96,487 C/mol e⁻, what is the charge on an individual electron?

   (A) 5.76×10^{28} C/e⁻
   (B) 6.022×10^{23} C/e⁻
   (C) 1.6×10^{19} C/e⁻
   (D) 1.6×10^{-19} C/e⁻

2. How many F are required for the reduction of 1 mole of Ni^{2+} to Ni (s)?

   (A) 1 F
   (B) 2 F
   (C) 96,487 F
   (D) 6.022×10^{23} F

3. The gold-plating process involves the following reaction:

   Au^{3+} (aq) + 3e⁻ → Au (s). If 0.600 g of Au is plated onto a metal, how many coulombs are used?

   (A) 298.5 C
   (B) 868.4 C
   (C) 2,985 C
   (D) 8,684 C

4. If a current of 3 amps (1 A = 1 C/s) is used, how long will the process in Question 3 take?

   (A) 48 minutes
   (B) 4.8 minutes
   (C) 2.6 minutes
   (D) 1.7 minutes

5. If the plating process in Question 3 is done for 35 minutes with a 7 A current, how many grams of Au will be plated?

   (A) 88.7 g Au
   (B) 29.6 g Au
   (C) 9.85 g Au
   (D) 4.27 g Au

6. The standard reduction potential of Cr^{3+} (aq) + 3 e⁻ → Cr (s) is –0.74 V. The standard reduction potential of Cl_2 (g) + 2 e⁻ → 2 Cl⁻ (aq) is 1.36 V.

   Based on the information given, it must be true that:

   (A) Cl_2 is more easily oxidized than Cr^{3+}, and Cl_2 is thus a better oxidizing agent than Cr^{3+}.
   (B) Cl_2 is more easily oxidized than Cr^{3+}, and Cl_2 is thus a better reducing agent than Cr^{3+}.
   (C) Cl_2 is more easily reduced than Cr^{3+}, and Cl_2 is thus a better reducing agent than Cr^{3+}.
   (D) Cl_2 is more easily reduced than Cr^{3+}, and Cl_2 is thus a better oxidizing agent than Cr^{3+}.

7. The standard reduction potential of Cu^{2+} (aq) is +0.34 V. What is the oxidation potential of $Cu(s)$?

   (A) +0.68 V
   (B) +0.34 V
   (C) -0.34 V
   (D) -0.68 V

8. (Equation 1) $F_2 + 2 e^- \rightarrow 2 F^-$ (aq) $E° = +2.87$ V

   (Equation 2) $Ca^{2+} + 2 e^- \rightarrow Ca$ (s) $E° = -2.76$ V

   When the above half-reactions are combined in a galvanic cell, which species will be reduced and which will be oxidized?

   (A) F^- will be oxidized and Ca^{2+} will be reduced.
   (B) Ca^{2+} will be oxidized and F_2 will be reduced.
   (C) $Ca(s)$ will be oxidized and F_2 will be reduced.
   (D) F_2 will be oxidized and $Ca(s)$ will be reduced.

9. What is the standard EMF if the following half-reactions are combined in a galvanic cell?

   (Equation 1) $Co^{3+}(aq) + e^- \rightarrow Co^{2+}$ (aq) $E° = 1.82$ V

   (Equation 2) Na^+ (aq) $+ e^- \rightarrow Na$ (s) $E° = -2.71$

   (A) 4.53 V
   (B) 0.89 V
   (C) −0.89 V
   (D) −4.53V

10. In a galvanic cell, the anode is _____, and the cathode is _____.

    In an electrolytic cell, the anode is _____, and the cathode is _____.

    (A) positive, negative; positive, negative
    (B) negative, positive; positive, negative
    (C) negative, positive; negative, positive
    (D) positive, negative; negative, positive

11. What is $E°_{cell}$ for a reaction where the $\Delta G° = -553.91$ kJ and 2 electrons are transferred?

    (A) −2.87 V
    (B) −0.00287 V
    (C) 0.00287 V
    (D) 2.87 V

12. What is the $\Delta G°$ for the following reaction equation?

    $Ti^{2+} (aq) + Mg (s) \rightarrow Ti (s) + Mg^{2+} (aq)$

    $Ti^{2+} (aq) + 2 e^- \rightarrow Ti (s) \qquad E° = -1.63$ V

    $Mg^{2+} (aq) + 2 e^- \rightarrow Mg (s) \qquad E° = -2.38$ V

    (A) 144.73 kJ
    (B) 144.73 J
    (C) −144.73 J
    (D) −144.73 kJ

13. Given that the $E°$ for Au^{3+}/Au is 1.50 V and the $E°$ for Li^+/Li is −3.05 V, what is E_{cell} for the reaction:

    $Au3+ (aq) + 3 Li (s) \rightarrow Au (s) + 3Li+ (aq)$

    (A) if $[Li^+] = 10$ M and $[Au^{3+}] = 0.01$ M?
    (B) if $[Li^+] = 0.1$ M and $[Au^{3+}] = 0.001$ M?
    (C) if $[Li^+] = 1$ M and $[Au^{3+}] = 1$ M?

14. If E_{cell} for the reaction in Question 13 is 4.4909 V and $[Li^+] = 10$ M, what is the concentration of Au^{3+}?

15. What is $\Delta G°$ for the reaction in Question 13?

16. Assign oxidation numbers to each atom of the following reaction equation:

    $2 Fe (s) + O_2 (g) + 2 H_2O (l) \rightarrow 2 Fe(OH)_2 (s)$

17. Using the ion-electron method, balance the following equation of a reaction taking place in an acidic solution:

    $ClO_3^- + AsO_2^- \rightarrow AsO_4^{3-} + Cl^-$

18. Write out the anode and cathode half-reactions from the following cell diagram:

    $Al \mid Al^{3+}(1.00$ M$) \parallel Co^{2+}(1.00$ M$) \mid Co$

19. Given the standard reduction potentials for the following half-reactions,

    $ClO_4^- (aq) + 2H^+ (aq) + 2e^- \rightarrow ClO_3^- (aq) + H_2O (l) \qquad E° = +1.19$ V

    $Ag^+ (aq) + e^- \rightarrow Ag (s) \qquad\qquad\qquad\qquad\qquad E° = +0.799$ V

    predict which half-reaction would occur at the anode and which would occur at the cathode in a galvanic cell.

SOLUTIONS TO REVIEW PROBLEMS

1. **D** Avogadro's number (6.022×10^{23}) defines the number of particles present in one mole of anything. Electrons are particles, so there are 6.022×10^{23} electrons in one mole of electrons.

    $$1\ F = 96{,}487\ \frac{C}{mol\ e^-} \times \frac{1\ mol\ e^-}{6.022 \times 10^{23}\ e^-} = 1.602 \times 10^{-19}\ \frac{C}{e^-}$$

2. **B** The reduction of one mole of Ni^{2+} to one mole of Ni (*s*) requires two moles of electrons. The transfer of one mole of electrons is equivalent to the transfer of 1 F of charge. Therefore, since two moles of electrons are required to reduces one mole of Ni^{2+}, 2 F are required as well.

3. **B** To solve this problem, first determine the number of moles of Au present in 0.6 g.

    $$0.600\ g\ Au \times \frac{mol\ Au}{197.0\ g} = 0.0030\ mol\ Au$$

    Next, determine the number of moles of electrons used to reduce $Au^{3+}(aq)$ to 0.0030 mol of Au (*s*). From the given reduction half-reaction of Au, it is evident that for every mole of Au^{3+}, three moles of electrons are transferred to produce one mole of Au (*s*); therefore:

    $$0.0030\ mol\ Au \times \frac{3\ mol\ e^-}{1\ mol\ Au} = 0.0090\ mol\ e^-$$

    Finally, convert 0.0090 mol e^- to its equivalent in C:

    $$0.0090\ mol\ e^- \times \frac{96{,}487\ C}{1\ mol\ e^-} = 868.4\ C$$

4. **B** A 3 A source supplies a current of 3 C/sec. From the answer to the previous question, 868.4 C are needed to plate out 0.600 g of Au from solution; therefore:

    $$868.4\ C \times \frac{1\ sec}{3C} = 289.5\ sec = 4.8\ min$$

5. **C** First, convert minutes to seconds:

    $$35\ min \times \frac{60\ sec}{min} = 2{,}100\ sec$$

    Next, determine how many Coloumbs a 7 A source can provide in 2,100 sec:

    $$2{,}100\ sec \times \frac{7\ C}{sec} = 14{,}700\ C$$

    Now determine the number of moles of electrons equivalent to 14,700 C:

    $$14{,}700\ C \times \frac{1\ mol\ e^-}{96{,}487\ C} = 0.15\ mol\ e^-$$

    Then convert 0.15 moles of e^- into an equivalent amount of moles of Au, and then to grams of Au:

    $$0.15\ mol\ e^- \times \frac{1\ mol\ Au}{3\ mol\ e^-} \times \frac{197.0\ g\ Au}{1\ mol\ Au} = 9.85\ g\ Au$$

6. **D** Discussed in the section on reduction potentials.

7. **C** Discussed in the section on reduction potentials.

8. **C** The half-reaction with the greater reduction potential will proceed forward as written, while the half-reaction with the smaller reduction potential will proceed in the opposite direction. F_2 has a greater tendency to be reduced than Ca^{2+} because it has the greater reduction potential. Therefore, Equation 1 will proceed as written, while Equation 2 will proceed in the opposite direction. As a result, F_2 is reduced to $2 F^-$ and $Ca(s)$ is oxidized to Ca^{2+}.

9. **A** 4.53 V is the correct answer. From the values of the reduction potentials, it is evident that Equation 1 will be the reduction half-reaction, since it has the larger reduction potential, and Equation 2 will be reversed for the oxidation half-reaction. The EMF of a reaction is determined by adding the standard potentials of the reduced and oxidized species. The standard reduction potential for of Co^{3+} is +1.82 V. The standard oxidation potential of $Na(s)$ is +2.71 V, which is equivalent, but opposite in sign, to the standard reduction potential of $Na^+ (aq)$

    EMF = 1.82 V + 2.71 V = 4.53 V

10. **B** Discussed in the section on electrode charge designations.

11. **D** Use the relationship $\Delta G° = -nFE°$, which can be rearranged to $E° = -\Delta G°/(nF)$. $\Delta G° = -553.91$ kJ, n = 2, and F = 96,487 C/mol e^-. The next step is to convert the value of $\Delta G°$ from kJ to J. When this is done, $\Delta G°$ is equal to −553,910 J. The final step is to substitute the values into the formula $E° = \dfrac{\Delta G°}{(nF)}$ to get the final answer of $E_0 = 2.87$ V.

12. **D** First, determine the EMF (also called E°) by adding the potentials of the reduced and oxidized species.
    $$-1.63 \text{ V} + (+2.38 \text{ V}) = 0.75 \text{ V} = 0.75 \frac{J}{C}$$

    By inspection, two moles of electrons are transferred to produce one mole of product; therefore, n = 2. Now determine $\Delta G°$:

    $$\Delta G° = -nFE°$$

    $$\Delta G° = -(2 \text{ mol } e^-) \left(\frac{96,487 \text{ C}}{1 \text{ mol } e-} \right) \left(0.75 \frac{J}{C} \right)$$

    $$\Delta G° = -144,730 \text{ J} = -144.73 \text{ kJ}$$

13. The Nernst Equation can be used to calculate the voltage of a reaction under nonstandard conditions. Remember that reduction potentials as listed are standard reduction potentials, which implies standard conditions of concentration of reactants (1M). Concentrations, however, are not always standard, and so the voltage of a given reaction with varying concentration may vary from the voltage under standard concentration conditions. The Nernst Equation is:

$E_{cell} = E°_{cell} - (0.0591/n)(\log Q)$

where E_{cell} = voltage under nonstandard concentrations,

$E°_{cell}$ = standard voltage for the reaction,

n = number of moles of electrons transferred in the reaction,

Q = reaction quotient,

and 0.0591 is a constant equal to 2.303 RT/F at 298K.

To solve this problem, plug the values given into the equation. Remember that any solid reactants or products should not appear in the Q expression.

Using the standard reduction potentials, $E°_{cell}$ for the reaction can be calculated to be +4.55 V. It is evident from the reaction that n = 3 electrons and $Q = [Li^+]^3/[Au^{3+}]$ (solid products and reactants are excluded). Plugging into the Nernst Equation:

A $E_{cell} = 4.55 - (0.0591/3)\log(10^3/0.01)$

  = 4.45 V

B $E_{cell} = 4.55 - (0.0591/3)\log((0.1)^3/0.001)$

  = 4.55 V

C Calculation is not really necessary since 1-M solutions are the standard, but for verification:

  $E_{cell} = 4.55 - (0.0591/3)\log(1^3/1)$

  = 4.55 V

14. **1 M**

Again, we can use the Nernst Equation to solve this problem.

$E_{cell} = E°_{cell} - (0.0591/n)\log([Li^+]^3/[Au^{3+}])$ rearranges to
$(E_{cell} - E°_{cell})(n/0.0591) + \log 10^3 = \log [Au^{3+}]$.

Now substitute the numbers into the equation:
$(4.4909 - 4.55)(3/0.0591) + \log 10^3 = \log [Au^{3+}]$
$-3.0 + 3.0 = 0 = \log [Au^{3+}]$, therefore $[Au^{3+}] = 1$ M

15. **−1,317 kJ**

Substitute the values given into the equation $\Delta G° = -nFE°_{cell}$:

n = 3

F = 96,487 C/mol e^-

$E°_{cell}$ = +4.55 V

So $\Delta G° = -1,317$ kJ

16. $2 \text{ Fe } (s) + \text{O}_2 (g) + \text{H}_2\text{O } (l) \rightarrow \text{Fe(OH)}_2 (s)$

To assign oxidation numbers, use the rules given in the text. Fe (s) and O_2 (g) have oxidation numbers of zero because they are free elements. Hydrogen in H_2O (l) has an oxidation number of $+1$ because oxygen is more electronegative than hydrogen; likewise, oxygen in H_2O (l) has an oxidation number of -2. Oxygen and hydrogen in Fe(OH)_2 (s) have the same oxidation numbers as in H_2O (l). Each OH group contributes a charge of -1 to Fe(OH)_2, and since there are 2 OH groups, their overall contribution to the compound is -2. Since Fe(OH)_2 (s) is a neutral compound and thus has no overall charge, the sum of all the oxidation numbers of the atoms in this compound is zero. Consequently, the Fe in Fe(OH)_2 (s) must possess a charge of $+2$ to make the overall charge on the compound zero.

17. The balanced equation is:

$\text{ClO}_3^- + 3\text{H}_2\text{O} + 3\text{AsO}_2^- \rightarrow 3\text{AsO}_4^{3-} + \text{Cl}^- + 6\text{H}^+$

18. In a cell diagram, the anode half-reaction is always written first and is followed by the cathode half-reaction. Oxidation occurs at the anode and reduction occurs at the cathode, as discussed in the notes. Therefore, the anode half-reaction is:

$\text{Al } (s) \rightarrow \text{Al}^{3+}(aq) + 3 \text{ e}^-$

The cathode half-reaction is:

$\text{Co}^{2+}(aq) + 2\text{e}^- \rightarrow \text{Co } (s)$

19. The rule is that the half-reaction with the greater reduction potential will be the reduction reaction and the reverse of the other will be the oxidation reaction. Since the first reaction (reduction of ClO_4^-) has the greater reduction potential, this will proceed as a forward reaction, and ClO_4^- will be reduced. The second reaction (reduction of Ag^+), which has the lower reduction potential, will proceed as a reverse reaction, and Ag (s) will be oxidized to Ag^+. As mentioned in the solution to the previous question, oxidation occurs at the anode and reduction at the cathode. Thus, the reduction of ClO_4^- to ClO_3^- will occur at the cathode, and the oxidation of Ag (s) to Ag^+ will occur at the anode.

CHAPTER THIRTY-NINE

Nuclear Phenomena

The subject of this chapter is the nucleus and nuclear phenomena. It begins with a review of some of the standard terminology used in nuclear chemistry and physics. The concept of binding energy and the equivalent concept of the mass defect are then introduced. Briefly, an amount of energy, called the **binding energy**, is required to break up a given nucleus into its constituent protons and neutrons. That energy is converted to mass via Einstein's $E = mc^2$, resulting in a larger mass for the constituent protons and neutrons than that of the original nucleus, the difference being called the **mass defect**. The remainder of the chapter is concerned with a brief discussion of nuclear reactions (**fission** and **fusion**) and an extended treatment of radioactive decay, which itself is presented in two distinct parts. The first deals with the four different types of **radioactive decay** and a discussion of the reaction equations that describe them. The second covers the general problem of determining the number of nuclei that have not decayed as a function of time, along with the associated concept of the half-life of a decay process.

NUCLEI

At the center of an atom lies its nucleus, consisting of one or more **nucleons** (protons or neutrons) held together with considerably more energy than the energy needed to hold electrons in orbit around the nucleus. The radius of the nucleus is about 100,000 times smaller than the radius of the atom. Following are some common nuclear properties.

Atomic Number

Z is always an integer and is equal to the **number of protons** in the nucleus. Each element has a unique number of protons; therefore the atomic number Z identifies the element. Z is used as a presubscript to the chemical symbol in **isotopic notation**. The chemical symbols and the atomic numbers of all the elements are given in the periodic table.

Atomic numbers of the chemical elements		
Atomic number Z	Chemical symbol	Element name
1	H	hydrogen
2	He	helium
3	Li	lithium
.	.	.
.	.	.
92	U	uranium
.	.	.
.	.	.
.	.	.

Figure 39.1

Mass Number

A is an integer equal to the total **number of nucleons** (neutrons and protons) in a nucleus. Let N represent the number of neutrons in a nucleus. The equation relating A, N, and Z is simply:

$$A = N + Z$$

In isotopic notation, A appears as a presuperscript to the chemical symbol.

Examples: $^{1}_{1}H$ is a single proton; the nucleus of ordinary hydrogen.

$^{4}_{2}He$ is the nucleus of ordinary helium, consisting of two protons and two neutrons. It is also known as an alpha particle (*a*-particle).

$^{235}_{92}U$ is a fissionable form of uranium, consisting of 92 protons and 143 neutrons.

Isotope

The nucleus of a given element can have different numbers of neutrons, hence different mass numbers. For a nucleus of a given element with a given number of protons (atomic number Z), the various nuclei with different numbers of neutrons are called **isotopes** of that element. The term *isotope* is also used in a generic sense to refer to any nucleus. The term **radionuclide** is another generic term used to refer to any radioactive isotope, especially those used in **nuclear medicine.**

Example: The three isotopes of hydrogen are:

1. $^{1}_{1}H$—A single proton; the nucleus of ordinary **hydrogen**

2. $^{2}_{1}H$—A proton and a neutron together often called a **deuteron;** the nucleus of one type of heavy hydrogen called **deuterium**

3. $^{3}_{1}H$—A proton and two neutrons together often called a **triton;** the nucleus of a heavier type of heavy hydrogen called **tritium**

Atomic Mass and Atomic Mass Unit

Atomic mass is most commonly measured in atomic mass units (abbreviated amu or simply u). By definition, 1 amu is exactly one-twelfth the mass of the neutral carbon-12 atom (not just the nucleus—the atom includes the nucleus and all six electrons). In terms of more familiar mass units:

$$1 \text{ amu} = 1.66 \times 10^{-27} \text{ kg} = 1.66 \times 10^{-24} \text{ g}$$

Atomic Weight

Because isotopes exist, atoms of a given element can have different masses. The atomic weight refers to a weighted average of the **masses** (not the weights) of an element. The average is weighted according to the natural abundances of the various isotopic species of an element. The atomic weight can be measured in amu.

Example: 99.985499% of hydrogen occurs in the common 1H isotope with a mass of 1.00782504 u. About 0.0142972% occurs as deuterium with a mass (including the electron) of 2.01410 u, and about 0.0003027% occurs as tritium with a mass of 3.01605 u. The atomic weight of hydrogen $A_r(H)$ is the sum of the mass of each isotope multiplied by its natural abundance (x):

$$A_r(H) = m_{1H}x_{1H} + m_{2H}x_{2H} + m_{3H}x_{3H}$$
$$= (1.00782504)(0.99985499)$$
$$+ (2.01410)(0.000142972)$$
$$+ (3.01605)(0.000003027)$$
$$= 1.00797 \text{ amu}$$

Nuclear versus Chemical Reactions

All nuclei of atoms, with the exception of hydrogen, contain protons and neutrons. When the nucleus of an atom is unstable, it may spontaneously emit particles or electromagnetic radiation otherwise known as radioactivity. Nuclei may also "change" when nuclear transmutation occurs. This process involves the bombardment of the nucleus by electrons, neutrons, as well as other nuclei. This is a specific type of nuclear reaction. Below is a summary of the major differences between nuclear and chemical reactions.

Nuclear reactions	Chemical reactions
• Elements or isotopes are changed from one to another.	• Atoms can be rearranged by the formation or breaking of chemical bonds.
• Reactions result in the release or absorption of large amounts of energy.	• Reactions generally result in the release or absorption of small amounts of energy.
• Reaction rates are generally not affected by catalysts, temperature, or pressure.	• Reaction rates are generally affected by catalysts, temperature, or pressure.
• Protons, neutrons, or electrons can be involved.	• Only electrons in the affected orbital of the atom are involved in the formation and breaking of bonds.

NUCLEAR BINDING ENERGY AND MASS DEFECT

Every nucleus (other than $^1_1$H) has a smaller mass than the combined mass of its constituent protons and neutrons. The difference is called the **mass defect.** Scientists had difficulty explaining why this mass defect occurred until Einstein discovered the equivalence of matter and energy, embodied by the equation $E = mc^2$. The mass defect is a result of matter that has been converted to energy. This energy, called **binding energy,** holds the nucleons together in the nucleus.

Note: The binding energy per nucleon peaks at iron, which implies that iron is the most stable atom. In general, intermediate-sized nuclei are more stable than large and small nuclei.

The mass defect and binding energy of ^{4}He are calculated in the following example.

Example: Measurements of the atomic mass of a neutron and a proton yield these results:

proton = 1.00728 amu

neutron = 1.00867 amu

A measurement of the atomic mass of a ^{4}He nucleus yields:

^{4}He = 4.00260 amu

4He consists of two protons and two neutrons which should theoretically give a ^{4}He mass of:

$Z(m_p) + N(m_n) = 2(1.00728) + 2(1.00867)$

$= 4.03190$ amu

What is the mass defect and binding energy of this nucleus?

Solution: The difference $4.03190 - 4.00260 = 0.02930$ amu is the mass defect for ^{4}He and is interpreted as the conversion of mass into the binding energy of the nucleus. The rest energy of 1 amu is 932 MeV, so using $E = mc^2$, we find that $c^2 = 932$ MeV/amu. Therefore, the binding energy of ^{4}He is:

B.E. $= \Delta m\, c^2$

$= (0.02930)(932)$

$= 27.3$ MeV

NUCLEAR REACTIONS AND DECAY

Nuclear reactions such as fusion, fission, and radioactive decay involve either combining or splitting the nuclei of atoms. Since the binding energy per nucleon is greatest for intermediate-sized atoms, when small atoms combine or large atoms splits a great amount of energy is released.

Fusion

Fusion occurs when small nuclei combine into a larger nucleus. As an example, many stars, including the sun, power themselves by fusing four hydrogen nuclei to make one helium nucleus. By this method, the sun produces 4×10^{26} J every second. Here on earth, researchers are trying to find ways to use fusion as an alternative energy source. Because these fusion reactions can only take place at extremely high temperatures, they are generally referred to as **thermonuclear reactions**.

Fission

Fission is a process in which a large, heavy (mass number > 200) atom splits to form smaller nuclei and one or more neutrons. It is important to note that because a large nucleus is more unstable than its products, there is the release of a large amount of energy. Spontaneous fission rarely occurs. However, by the absorption of a low-energy neutron, fission can be induced in certain nuclei. Of special interest are those fission reactions that release more neutrons, since these other neutrons will cause other atoms to undergo fission. This in turn releases more neutrons, creating a **chain reaction**. Such induced fission reactions power commercial nuclear electric-generating plants.

Example: A fission reaction occurs when uranium-235 (U-235) absorbs a low-energy neutron, briefly forming an excited state of U-236, which then splits into xenon-140, strontium-94, and x more neutrons. In isotopic notation form the reactions are:

$$^{235}_{92}U + {}^{1}_{0}n \rightarrow {}^{236}_{92}U \rightarrow {}^{140}_{54}Xe\ 1\ {}^{94}_{38}Sr + x{}^{1}_{0}n$$

How many neutrons are produced in the last reaction?

Solution: The question is asking "What is x?" By treating each arrow as an equal sign, the problem is simply asking to balance the last "equation." The mass numbers (A) on either side of each arrow must be equal. This is an application of **nucleon** or **baryon number conservation,** which says that the total number of neutrons plus protons remains the same, even if neutrons are converted to protons and vice versa, as they are in some decays. Because $235 + 1 = 236$, the first arrow is indeed balanced. To find the number of neutrons, solve for x in the last equation (arrow):

$$236 = 140 + 94 + x$$
$$x = 236 - 140 - 94$$
$$= 2$$

So two neutrons are produced in this reaction. These neutrons are free to go on and be absorbed by more ^{235}U and cause more fissioning, and the process continues in a chain reaction. Note that it really was not necessary to know that the intermediate state $^{236}_{92}U$ was formed.

Some radioactive nuclei may be induced to fission via more than one **decay channel** or **decay mode.** For example, a different fission reaction may occur when uranium-235 absorbs a slow neutron and then immediately splits into barium-139, krypton-94, and three more neutrons with no intermediate state:

$$^{235}_{92}U + {}^{1}_{0}n \rightarrow {}^{139}_{56}Ba + {}^{94}_{36}Kr + 3{}^{1}_{0}n$$

Radioactive Decay

Radioactive decay is a naturally occurring spontaneous decay of certain nuclei accompanied by the emission of specific particles. It could be classified as a certain type of fission. Radioactive decay problems are of three general types:

1. The integer arithmetic of particle and isotope species
2. Radioactive half-life problems
3. The use of exponential decay curves and decay constants

Isotope decay arithmetic and nucleon conservation

Let the letters X and Y represent nuclear isotopes, and let us further consider the three types of decay particles and how they affect the mass number and atomic number of the **parent isotope** $^A_Z X$ and the resulting **daughter isotope** $^{A'}_{Z'} Y$ in the decay:

$$^A_Z X \longrightarrow {}^{A'}_{Z'} Y + \text{emitted decay particle}$$

Alpha decay is the emission of an a-particle, which is a $^4_2 He$ nucleus that consists of two protons and two neutrons. The alpha particle is very massive (compared to a beta particle) and doubly charged. Alpha particles interact with matter very easily; hence they do not penetrate shielding (such as lead sheets) very far.

The emission of an a-particle means that the daughter's atomic number Z will be 2 less than the parent's atomic number and the daughter's mass number will be 4 less than the parent's mass number. This can be expressed in two simple equations:

$$\alpha \text{ decay}$$
$$Z_{\text{daughter}} = Z_{\text{parent}} - 2$$
$$A_{\text{daughter}} = A_{\text{parent}} - 4$$

The generic alpha decay reaction is then:

$$^A_Z X \rightarrow Z\, {}^{A-4}_{Z-2} Y + \alpha$$

Example: Suppose a parent X alpha decays into a daughter Y such that:
$$^{238}_{92} X \rightarrow {}^{A'}_{Z'} Y + \alpha$$

What are the mass number (A') and atomic number (Z') of the daughter isotope Y?

Solution: Since $\alpha = {}^4_2 He$, balancing the mass numbers and atomic numbers is all that needs to be done:

$238 = A' + 4$

$A' = 234$

$92 = Z' + 2$

$Z' = 90$

So A' = 234 and Z' = 90. Note that it was not necessary to know the chemical species of the isotopes to do this problem. However, it would have been possible to look at the periodic table and see that Z = 92 means X is uranium-238 ($^{238}_{92} U$) and that Z = 90 means Y is thorium-234 ($^{234}_{90} Th$).

Beta decay is the emission of a β-particle, which is an electron given the symbol e– or β⁻. Electrons do not reside in the nucleus but are emitted by the nucleus when a neutron in the nucleus decays into a proton and a β⁻ (and an antineutrino). Since an electron is singly charged and about 1,836 times lighter than a proton, the beta radiation from radioactive decay is more penetrating than alpha radiation. In some cases of induced decay, a positively charged antielectron known as a **positron** is emitted. The positron is given the symbol e⁺ or β⁺.

β⁻ decay means that a neutron disappears and a proton takes its place. Hence, the parent's mass number is unchanged, and the parent's atomic number is increased by 1. In other words, the daughter's A is the same as the parent's, and the daughter's Z is one more than the parent's.

In positron decay, a proton (instead of a neutron as in β⁻ decay) splits into a positron and a neutron. Therefore, a β⁺ decay means that the parent's mass number is unchanged and the parent's atomic number is decreased by 1. In other words, the daughter's A is the same as the parent's, and the daughter's Z is one less than the parent's. In equation form:

$$\beta^- \text{ decay}$$
$$Z_{\text{daughter}} = Z_{\text{parent}} + 1$$
$$A_{\text{daughter}} = A_{\text{parent}}$$

$$\beta^+ \text{ decay}$$
$$Z_{\text{daughter}} = Z_{\text{parent}} - 1$$
$$A_{\text{daughter}} = A_{\text{parent}}$$

The generic negative beta decay reaction is:

$$^A_Z X \rightarrow\; ^A_{Z+1} Y + \beta-$$

The generic positive beta decay reaction is:

$$^A_Z X \rightarrow\; ^A_{Z-1} Y + \beta+$$

Example: Suppose a cobalt-60 nucleus beta-decays:

$$^{60}_{27}\text{Co} \rightarrow\; ^A_{Z+1} Y + e-$$

What is the element Y, and what are A' and Z'?

Solution: Again, balance mass numbers:

$60 = A' + 0$

$A' = 601$

Now balance the atomic numbers, taking into account that cobalt has 27 protons (you learn this by consulting the periodic table) and that there is one more proton on the right-hand side:

$Z' = Z + 1$

$28 = 27 + 1$

By looking at the periodic table, one finds that Z' = 28 is nickel:

$Y = {}^{60}_{28}\text{Ni}$

Gamma decay is the emission of γ–particles, which are high-energy photons. They carry no charge and simply lower the energy of the emitting (parent) nucleus without changing the mass number or the atomic number. In other words, the daughter's A is the same as the parent's and the daughter's Z is the same as the parent's.

$$\gamma \text{ decay}$$

$$Z_{parent} = Z_{daughter}$$

$$A_{parent} = A_{daughter}$$

The generic gamma decay reaction is thus:

$$_Z^A X^* \rightarrow {}_Z^A X + \gamma$$

Example: Suppose a parent isotope $_Z^A X$ emits a β+ and turns into an excited state of the isotope $_{Z'}^{A'} Y^*$, which then γ decays to $_{Z''}^{A''} Y$, which in turn α decays to $_{Z'''}^{A'''} W$. If W is ^{60}Fe, what is $_Z^A X$?

Solution: Since the final daughter in this chain of decay is given, it will be necessary to work backward through the reactions. By looking at the periodic table, one finds that W = Fe means Z''' = 26; hence the last reaction is the following α decay:

$$_{Z''}^{A''} Y \rightarrow {}_{26}^{60} Fe + {}_2^4 He$$

By balancing the atomic numbers you find:

Z'' = 26 + 2 = 28

A balancing of the mass numbers implies:

A'' = 60 + 4 = 64

The second-to-last reaction is a γ decay that simply releases energy from the nucleus but does not alter the atomic number or the mass number of the parent. That is: Z' = Z'' = 28 and A' = A'' = 64. So the second reaction is:

$$_{28}^{64} Y^* \rightarrow {}_{28}^{64} Y + \gamma$$

The first reaction was a b$^+$ decay that must have looked like:

$$_Z^A X \rightarrow {}_{28}^{64} Y^* + e+$$

Again, balance the atomic numbers:

Z = 28 + 1 = 29

You carry out a balancing of mass numbers by taking into account that a proton has disappeared on the left and reappeared as a neutron on the right, leaving the mass number unchanged:

A = 64 + 0 = 64

By looking at the periodic table, you find that Z = 29 means that X is Cu. Since A = 64, that means that the solution is:

$$_Z^A X \rightarrow {}_{29}^{64} Cu$$

While the problem did not ask for it, it is possible again to look at the periodic table to find that Z' = Z" = 28 means Y* = Y = Ni. The total chain of decays can be written as:

$$^{64}_{29}\text{Cu} \rightarrow {}^{64}_{28}\text{Ni}^* + \beta+$$

$$^{64}_{28}\text{Ni}^* \rightarrow {}^{64}_{28}\text{Ni} + \gamma$$

$$^{64}_{28}\text{Ni} \rightarrow {}^{60}_{26}\text{Fe} + \alpha$$

Electron capture—Certain unstable radionuclides are capable of capturing an inner (K or L shell) electron that combines with a proton to form a neutron. The atomic number is now one less than the original, but the mass number remains the same. Electron capture is a rare process that is perhaps best thought of as an inverse β^- decay.

Radioactive decay half-life ($T_{1/2}$)

In a collection of a great many identical radioactive isotopes, the **half-life** ($T_{1/2}$) of the sample is the time it takes for half of the sample to decay.

Example: If the half-life of a certain isotope is 4 years, what fraction of a sample of that isotope will remain after 12 years?

Solution: If 4 years is one half-life, then 12 years is three half-lives. During the first half-life—the first 4 years—half of the sample will have decayed. During the second half-life (years 4 to 8), half of the remaining half will decay, leaving one-fourth of the original. During the third and final period (years 8 to 12), half of the remaining fourth will decay, leaving one-eighth of the original sample. Thus the fraction remaining after 3 half-lives is $(1/2)^3$ or $(1/8)$.

Exponential decay

Let n be the number of radioactive nuclei that have not yet decayed in a sample. It turns out that the **rate** at which the nuclei decay (Dn/Dt) is proportional to the number that remain (n). This suggests the equation:

$$\frac{\Delta n}{\Delta t} = -\lambda n$$

where λ is known as the **decay constant.** The solution of this equation tells us how the number of radioactive nuclei changes with time.

The solution is known as an **exponential decay:**

$$n = n_0 e^{-\lambda \tau}$$

where n_0 is the number of undecayed nuclei at time t = 0. (The decay constant is related to the half-life by $\lambda = \dfrac{\ln 2}{T_{1/2}} = \dfrac{0.693}{T_{1/2}}$.)

Example: If at time t = 0 there is a two mole sample of radioactive isotopes of decay constant 2 (hour)$^{-1}$, how many nuclei remain after 45 minutes?

Solution: Because 45 minutes is 3/4 of an hour, the exponent is

$$\lambda t = 2\left(\frac{3}{4}\right) = \frac{6}{4} = \frac{3}{2}$$

The exponential factor will be a number smaller than 1:

$$e^{-\lambda t} = e^{-3/2} = 0.22$$

So only 0.22 or 22% of the original two-mole sample will remain. To find n_0, we can multiply the number of moles we have by the number of particles per mole (Avogadro's number):

$$n_0 = 2(6.02 \times 10^{23}) = 1.2 \times 10^{24}$$

From the equation that describes exponential decay, you can calculate the number that remain after 45 minutes

$$n = n_0 e^{-\lambda t}$$
$$= (1.2 \times 10^{24})(0.22)$$
$$= 2.6 \times 10^{23} \text{ particles}$$

REVIEW PROBLEMS

1. Element $^{102}_{20}\varsigma$ is formed as a result of 3 α and 2 $\beta-$ decays. Which of the following is the parent element?

   (A) $^{90}_{16}\Gamma$

   (B) $^{114}_{24}\Phi$

   (C) $^{114}_{28}\Theta$

   (D) $^{12}_{8}\Delta + ^{90}_{12}\vartheta$

2. Element X is radioactive and decays via α-decay with a half-life of 4 days. If 12.5% of an original sample of element X remains after N days, then determine N.

3. A patient undergoing treatment for thyroid cancer receives a dose of radioactive iodine (^{131}I), which has a half-life of 8.05 days. If the original dose contained 12 mg of ^{131}I, what mass of ^{131}I remains after 16.1 days?

4. In an exponential decay, if the natural logarithm of the ratio of intact nuclei (n) at time t to the intact nuclei at time t = 0 (n_0) is plotted against time, what does the slope of the graph correspond to?

SOLUTIONS TO REVIEW PROBLEMS

1. **B** Emission of three alpha particles by the (as yet unknown) parent results in the following changes:

   Mass number: decreases by 3×4 or 12 units

   Atomic number: decreases by 3×2 or 6 units

   Emission of two negative betas results in the following changes:

   Mass number: no change

   Atomic number: increases by 2×1 or 2 units

   So the net change is: mass number decreases by 12 units; atomic number decreases by 4 units. Therefore, the mass number of the parent is 12 greater than 102, or 114; the atomic number of the parent is 4 greater than 20, or 24. The only choice given with these numbers is (B).

2. **N = 12 days**

   Because the half-life of element X is 4 days, then 50% of an original sample remains after 4 days, 25% of an original sample remains after 8 days, and 12.5% of an original sample remains after 12 days. Thus, N = 12 days. A different approach is to set $(1/2)^n = 0.125$, where n is the number of half-lives that have elapsed. Solving for n gives $n = 3$. Thus, 3 half-lives have elapsed, so given the half-life is 4 days, we have that N = 12 days.

3. **3 mg**

   Given that the half-life of ^{131}I is 8.05 days, we have that two half-lives have elapsed after 16.1 days, which means that 25% of the original amount of ^{131}I is still present. Thus, only 25% of the original number of ^{131}I nuclei remains, which also means that only 25% of the original mass of ^{131}I remains. Because the original dose contained 12 mg of ^{131}I, only 3 mg remain after 16.1 days.

4. **$-\lambda$**

   The expression $n = n_0 e^{-\lambda \tau}$ is equivalent to $n/n_0 = e^{-\lambda \tau}$. Taking the natural logarithm of both sides of the latter expression you find $\ln(n/n0) = -\lambda \tau$.

   From this expression it is clear that plotting $\ln(n/n0)$ versus t will give a straight line of slope $-\lambda$.

CHAPTER FORTY

Organic Chemistry

As discussed in Chapter 3, there are two types of chemical bonds: **ionic**, in which an electron is transferred from one atom to another, and **covalent**, in which pairs of electrons are shared between two atoms. In organic chemistry, it is important to understand the details of covalent bonding, as these play a crucial role in determining the properties and reactions of organic compounds.

ATOMIC ORBITALS

The first three quantum numbers, n, l, and m_ℓ, describe the size, shape, and number of the atomic orbitals an element possesses. The number n, which can equal $1, 2, 3, \ldots$, corresponds to the energy levels in an atom and is essentially a measure of size. Within each electron shell, there can be several types of orbitals ($s, p, d, f, g, \ldots$ corresponding to the quantum numbers $l = 0, 1, 2, 3, 4, \ldots$). Each type of atomic orbital has a specific shape. An s orbital is spherical and symmetrical, centered around the nucleus. A p orbital is composed of two lobes located symmetrically about the nucleus and contains a **node** (an area where the probability of finding an electron is zero). A d orbital is composed of four symmetrical lobes and contains two nodes. Both d and f orbitals are complex in shape and are rarely encountered in organic chemistry.

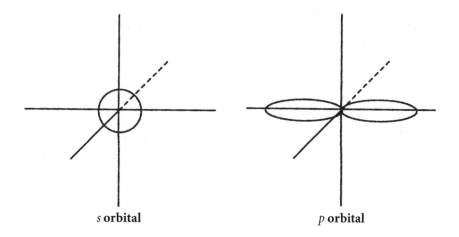

s orbital   *p* orbital

Figure 40.1

MOLECULAR ORBITALS

Single Bonds

Two atomic orbitals can be combined to form what is called a **molecular orbital (MO)**. Molecular orbitals are obtained mathematically by adding the wave functions of the atomic orbitals. If the signs of the wave functions are the same, a lower-energy **bonding orbital** is produced. If the signs are different, a higher-energy **antibonding orbital** is produced. This is represented schematically by the addition of two *s* orbitals. Two *p* orbitals or one *p* and one *s* orbital can also be combined in a similar fashion.

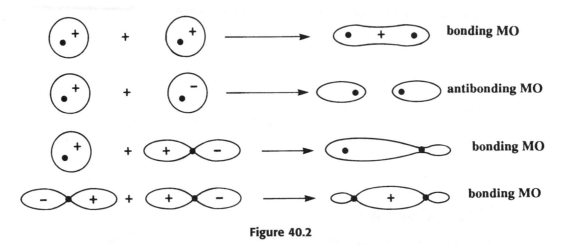

Figure 40.2

When a molecular orbital is formed by head-to-head overlap as in Figure 40.2, the resulting bond is called a **sigma (σ) bond**. All single bonds are sigma bonds, accommodating two electrons. Shorter single bonds are stronger than longer single bonds.

Double and Triple Bonds

When two *p* orbitals overlap in a parallel fashion, a bonding MO is formed called a **pi (π) bond**. When both a sigma and a pi bond exist between two atoms, a **double bond** is formed. When a sigma bond and two pi bonds exist, a **triple bond** is formed. As can be seen in Figure 40.3, the overlap of the *p* orbitals involved in a *p* bond hinder rotation about double and triple bonds.

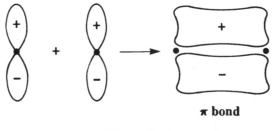

π bond

Figure 40.3

A pi bond cannot exist independently of a sigma bond. Only after the formation of a sigma bond will the *p* orbitals of adjacent carbons be parallel, because without the bond, the three *p* orbitals are orthogonal to one another.

In general, pi bonds are weaker than sigma bonds; it is possible to break one bond of a double bond, leaving a single bond intact.

HYBRIDIZATION

The carbon atom has the electron configuration $1s^2 2s^2 2p^2$ and, therefore, needs four electrons to complete its octet. A typical molecule formed by carbon is methane, CH_4. Experimentation shows that the four sigma bonds in methane are equal. This is inconsistent with the unsymmetrical distribution of valence electrons: two electrons in the $2s$ orbital, one in the p_x orbital, one in the p_y orbital, and none in the p_z orbital.

sp^3

The theory of **orbital hybridization** was developed to account for this discrepancy. Hybrid orbitals are formed by mixing different types of atomic orbitals. If one s orbital and three p orbitals are mathematically combined, the result is four sp^3 hybrid orbitals that have a new shape.

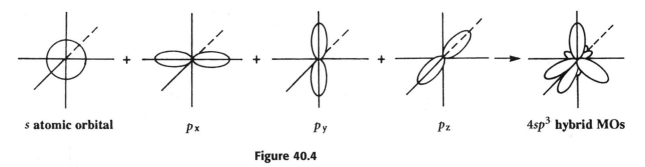

s **atomic orbital** p_x p_y p_z $4sp^3$ **hybrid MOs**

Figure 40.4

These four orbitals will point toward the vertices of a tetrahedron, minimizing repulsion. This explains the preferred tetrahedral geometry adopted by carbon.

The hybridization is accomplished by promoting one of the $2s$ electrons into the $2p_z$ orbital (see Figure 40.5). This produces four valence orbitals, each with one electron, which can be mathematically mixed to provide the hybrids.

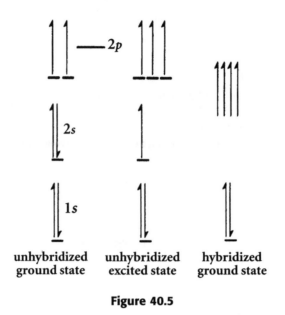

Figure 40.5

sp²

Although carbon is most often found with sp^3 hybridization, there are other possibilities. If one s orbital and two p orbitals are mixed, three sp^2 hybrid orbitals are obtained.

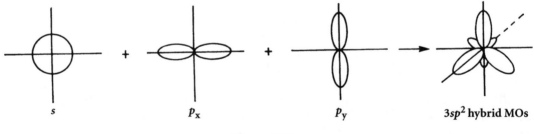

Figure 40.6

This occurs, for example, in ethylene. The third p orbital of each carbon atom is left unhybridized and participates in the pi bond. The three sp^2 orbitals are 120° apart, allowing maximum separation. These orbitals participate in the formation of the C=C and C–H single bonds.

sp

If two p orbitals are used to form a triple bond and the remaining p orbital is mixed with an s orbital, two sp hybrid orbitals are obtained. They are oriented 180° apart, explaining the linear structure of molecules like acetylene.

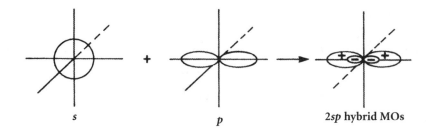

Figure 40.7

BONDING SUMMARY

The following table summarizes the major features of bonding in organic molecules.

Bond order	Component bonds	Hybridization	Angles	Examples
single	sigma	sp^3	109.5°	C–C; C–H
double	sigma	sp^2	120°	C=C; C=O
	pi			
triple	sigma	sp	180°	C≡C; C≡N
	pi			
	pi			

HYDROCARBONS

Hydrocarbons are compounds that contain only carbon and hydrogen atoms. Depending on the kinds of bonds found between the carbon atoms (only single bonds can exist between carbon and hydrogen), hydrocarbons can be classified into one of four classes: alkanes, alkenes, alkynes, and aromatics.

Alkanes

Alkanes are hydrocarbons that contain only single bonds. They all have a molecular formula of the general form C_nH_{2n+2}, where n is some positive integer. They are all named by attaching the suffix **-ane** to a prefix that indicates the number of carbon atoms.

These prefixes will be used again in the naming of other hydrocarbons, and it is therefore worth knowing at least a few:

# of C atoms	Prefix	Name of Alkane	Molecular Formula
1	*meth-*	methane	CH_4
2	*eth-*	ethane	C_2H_6
3	*prop-*	propane	C_3H_8
4	*but-*	butane	C_4H_{10}
5	*pent-*	pentane	C_5H_{12}
6	*hex-*	hexane	C_6H_{14}

The simplest alkane is methane, CH_4. Ethane, the next in the series, has the molecular formula C_2H_6, but this does not convey its structure:

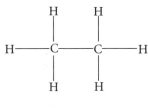

Figure 40.8

(Keep in mind the convention about drawing the Lewis structures of sp^3 hybridized carbon atoms discussed above.) The formula for ethane is more informatively (and frequently) written as CH_3CH_3. This tells us unambiguously that each carbon atom is attached to three hydrogen atoms. This kind of notation is known as a **condensed structural formula**. Similarly, the condensed structural formula for the next alkane, propane, is $CH_3CH_2CH_3$.

For alkanes with four or more carbons, there are different ways that the carbon atoms can be connected to each other, which makes the condensed structural formula all that more useful. Butane, for example, can have either one of the following structures:

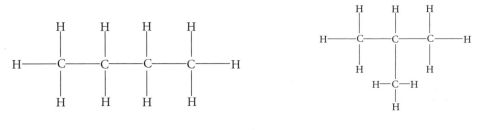

Figure 40.9

These two structures have the same molecular formula, C_4H_{10} (and hence the same molecular weight), but have different physical properties, such as boiling point and melting point. They are known as isomers (more specifically **structural isomers**) of each other. One can also say that the compound butane has two isomers: the top one is known as a straight-chain alkane for obvious reasons and is given the name n-butane, and the bottom one is a branched alkane and is known as isobutane.

The number of isomers increases for each alkane as the number of carbon atoms increases. Pentane, for example, has 3 isomers, while hexane has 5 and decane, with 10 carbon atoms, has 75.

Alkanes, especially straight-chain or n-alkanes, are the major constituents of petroleum. Since different alkanes, not to mention their respective isomers, have different boiling and melting points, the different alkane components in petroleum can be separated by distillation. Those compounds with the lowest boiling points would vaporize first; one can trap these vapors and condense them and thus achieve a separation of the more volatile from the less volatile components.

Alkenes

Alkenes are hydrocarbons involving carbon-carbon double bonds. They possess a molecular formula of the form C_nH_{2n}. They are named using the same scheme as alkanes, except that the suffix used is **-ene**. Also, since it takes at least two carbon atoms to form a double bond, the smallest alkene is ethene, C_2H_4, which contains two carbon atoms.

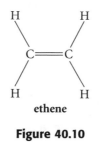

ethene

Figure 40.10

Alkynes

Alkynes are hydrocarbons involving carbon-carbon triple bonds. They follow the same naming scheme as alkanes and alkenes but use the suffix **-yne**. Alkenes and alkynes are said to be **unsaturated**, while alkanes are said to be **saturated**.

We have only considered noncyclic compounds so far. Alkanes, alkenes, or alkynes can also be **cyclic**: the carbon atoms form a ring. Such compounds are named exactly as they would normally be but with the additional prefix **cyclo-** attached at the beginning. The smallest number of carbon atoms that is needed to form a ring is three; the smallest cyclic alkane is therefore cyclopropane. The structures of cyclohexane, cyclohexene, and cyclohexyne are shown below.

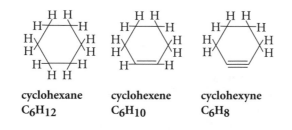

cyclohexane
C_6H_{12}

cyclohexene
C_6H_{10}

cyclohexyne
C_6H_8

Figure 40.11

The carbon atoms are not explicitly drawn but occupy the positions where the bonds join together. This is a common convention in organic chemistry. Notice how the molecular formulas for cyclic compounds do not follow the generic formulas given above for alkanes, alkenes, and alkynes: the extra carbon-carbon bond formed in making a ring upsets the ratio of carbon to hydrogen atoms. One final warning is that as Lewis structures, the drawings do not accurately reflect the three-dimensional appearance of the compounds; cyclohexane, for example, is not a planar hexagon but instead adopts a "chairlike" conformation in its most stable state.

Aromatics

Certain unsaturated cyclic hydrocarbons are known as aromatics. We need not concern ourselves with exactly what makes a compound aromatic, but all such compounds have in common a cyclic, planar structure and possess a higher degree of stability (a lower enthalpy of formation) than expected. This extra stability comes from the effects of resonance. The prime example of an aromatic compound is benzene, C_6H_6, which in a Lewis structure is represented as having alternating double and single bonds that can switch their positions to give an equivalent resonance structure:

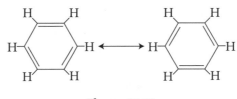

Figure 40.12

It is important, however, to keep in mind what resonance structures such as these really mean: benzene does *not* exist as an equilibrium mixture of the two Lewis structures, nor does it flip back and forth between the two structures as time passes. Instead, a benzene molecule is always in a state that is intermediate between the two structures that cannot be accurately captured by a normal Lewis structure. Every carbon-carbon bond in the molecule has characteristics intermediate between those of a single and those of a double bond. If we have to try to depict this using a Lewis structure, we would draw the following:

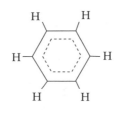

Figure 40.13

where the dashed lines indicate a partial π bond. Each of the six carbon atoms is sp^2 hybridized, and therefore each has an unhybridized p orbital that is coming out of (and going into) the plane of the paper. These orbitals interact through π bonding and form the partial π bonds—partial because six electrons total are part of this "π cloud" (one from each carbon atom) and, therefore, there are enough electrons to form only three such bonds that need to be shared among six atoms.

OXYGEN-CONTAINING COMPOUNDS

Organic compounds that include oxygen in addition to carbon and hydrogen include alcohols, ethers, carbohydrates, and carbonyl compounds such as aldehydes, ketones, esters, and carboxylic acids.

Alcohols

Alcohols contain the functional group –OH, sometimes called the hydroxyl group. Ethanol, for example, can be considered a derivative of ethane, with the hydroxyl group in the place of a hydrogen atom:

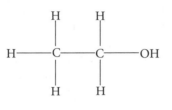

Figure 40.14

Because oxygen has such high electronegativity, the hydrogen attached to it (the hydrogen of the hydroxyl group) can participate in hydrogen bonding. The diagram below illustrates how this can occur; the R represents the organic group to which the alcohol functionality is attached (e.g., for ethanol, R = CH_3CH_2-).

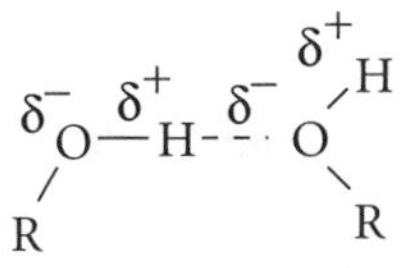

$$\delta^-_O \overset{\delta^+}{-} H \overset{\delta^-}{-\cdot\cdot} \overset{\delta^+}{O}\underset{R}{\overset{H}{\diagup}}$$

Figure 40.15

Hydrogen bonding is a strong intermolecular attractive force, and this causes alcohols to have boiling points that are significantly higher than those of the analogous hydrocarbons. The boiling point of propane ($CH_3CH_2CH_3$), for example, is –42.1 °C, whereas that of propanol ($CH_3CH_2CH_2OH$) is 97.4 °C. Ethylene glycol, which is ethane with two hydroxyl groups attached (one to each carbon atom) is used as antifreeze because its high boiling point makes it a good nonvolatile solute when exploiting the colligative property of freezing-point depression.

Ethers

Ethers are compounds containing a C-O-C bond. Following the same convention as above where R is used to designate some organic group, the generic formula for an ether is ROR'.

Examples of ethers include:

methoxyethane
(ethyl methyl ether)

ethoxybenzene
(ethyl phenyl ether)

Figure 40.16

In the diagrams above, we have extended the common practice in organic chemistry where the carbon atoms are not explicitly depicted but are assumed to occupy the positions where there is a "kink" in the structure drawn. (Previously we have only done this in cyclic compounds.)

Ethers are not capable of hydrogen bonding and, therefore, have low boiling points. They are also relatively inert and are frequently used as solvents in organic chemistry reactions.

Carbonyl Compounds

Carbonyl compounds are those containing a carbon-oxygen double bond, the carbonyl bond. The generic structure for such a compound is:

Figure 40.17

Depending on what exactly the two other groups attached to the carbon atom are, one can be more specific in naming the class of compounds to which the molecule belongs. Below are some examples.

Aldehydes

The carbon atom is attached to a hydrogen atom on one side and an R group (which may be another H atom in the case of formaldehyde) on the other.

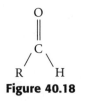

Figure 40.18

Ketones

The carbon atom is attached to two R groups that are not hydrogen atoms. It is important to note that the major difference between an aldehyde and a ketone is that in aldehydes, at least one hydrogen atom is bound to the carbon atom in the carbonyl group. However, in ketones, no hydrogen atoms are bound to the carbon atom.

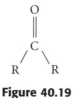

Figure 40.19

Esters

The carbonyl carbon atom in an ester is bonded to an R group on one side and an OR' group (that is not OH) on the other. Specifically, the R1 can either be an H, aryl group, or alkyl group, and the R can be an aryl group or an alkyl group.

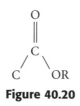

Figure 40.20

Carboxylic acids

The carbon atom is attached to an R group and a hydroxyl (–OH) group. Like alcohols that also contain the hydroxyl group, carboxylic acids can participate in hydrogen bonding. These compounds are weak acids (weak compared to inorganic acids like HCl) because the hydroxyl hydrogen can be donated as a proton. Fatty acids, for example, are carboxylic acids with a long hydrocarbon chain (the R group attached to the carbonyl carbon is a long hydrocarbon). After the donation of a proton, the carboxylic group left behind has a negative charge and is thus attracted to polar medium. The hydrocarbon chain, on the other hand, is nonpolar. In aqueous solution, therefore, these long carboxylate molecules (conjugate bases of carboxylic acids) arrange themselves into spherical structures known as **micelles**, in which the charged "heads" (the –COO⁻ groups) are exposed to the water while the organic chains are inside the sphere. Nonpolar molecules such as grease can dissolve in the hydrocarbon interior of the spherical micelle. This is why these molecules, which are salts of long-chain carboxylic acids, are called **soaps**.

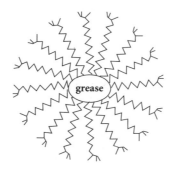

Figure 40.21

Summary of Functional Groups

Functional Group	Structure	Functional Group	Structure
Carboxylic acid	R—C(=O)—OR	Alkane	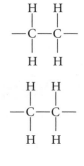
Ester	R—C(=O)—OR	Alkene	
Amide	R—C(=O)—NH₂	Alkyne	—C≡C—
Aldehyde	R—C(=O)—H	Phenyl	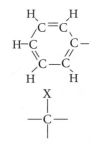
Ketone	R—C(=O)—R	Alkyl halide	
Amine	—C(NH₂)—	Alcohol	—C(OH)—
Ether	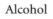—C—O—C—		

Table 40.22

BIOLOGICAL MOLECULES

Carbohydrates

Carbohydrates are so named because they are "hydrates of carbon." They have the general formula $C_n(H_2O)_m$, where n is not necessarily the same as m. They serve as chemical sources of energy for most organisms.

Simple sugars or monosaccharides are carbohydrates and can be classified according to the number of carbons they possess. They have the general formula $C_n(H_2O)_n$ or $C_nH_{2n}O_n$. Trioses, tetroses, pentoses, and hexoses have three, four, five, and six carbon atoms respectively. Glucose and fructose are the two most common examples of hexoses.

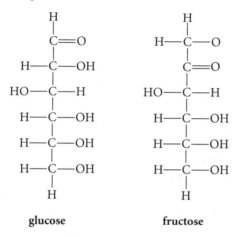

glucose   fructose

Figure 40.23

As you can see, then, these compounds also contain the carbonyl group. In particular, glucose has an aldehyde functionality, while fructose contains a ketone functionality. In solution, however, the straight-chain forms of these sugars (structures shown above) exist in equilibrium with a cyclic form. In fact, it is in this cyclic form that most of the interesting chemistry occurs. Linking of monosaccharides to form disaccharides and polysaccharides, for example, takes place between cyclic sugars. An example of such a reaction is shown below:

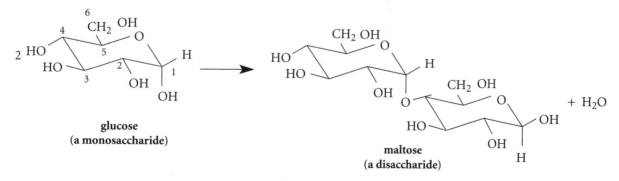

glucose
(a monosaccharide)

maltose
(a disaccharide)

Figure 40.24

The cyclic form of the five-carbon sugar ribose is a component of nucleotides, the building blocks of nucleic acids in DNA and RNA.

Amino Acids

Nitrogen-containing compounds are another large class of organic compounds. The most important nitrogen-containing functional group is the amine group, $-NH_2$, which is found in amino acids, the basic building blocks of proteins.

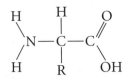

Figure 40.25

An amino acid contains an amine group, a carboxyl group, and a **side group R** that is different for different amino acids. In fact, R essentially defines what amino acid it is. It can be as simple as just another hydrogen atom (in which case the amino acid is glycine), or it can be more complex, with distinctive functional groups of its own. It may even contain atoms other than carbon, oxygen, and nitrogen: cysteine and methionine are two amino acids that contain sulfur atoms in their side chains.

There are 20 naturally occurring amino acids, and these amino acids can be joined together by bonds called **peptide bonds** to form small chains of amino acids known as peptides. Two amino acids joined together form a **dipeptide**, three form a **tripeptide**, and many amino acids linked together form a **polypeptide**. At some point (the exact boundary is not well defined), the polypeptide becomes long enough and we call it a **protein**. Proteins serve many diverse functions in biological systems, acting as enzymes, hormones, elements of cell structure, etc. The protein's amino acid sequence—the precise ordering and identity of each amino acid in the protein—is called its primary structure and determines the shape and function of the protein. The actual prediction of a protein's shape from its primary sequence is an active area of research.

REVIEW PROBLEMS

For questions 1–5, use the following diagram:

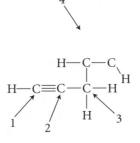

1. What is the hybridization of the carbon atom labeled 1?

2. What is the hybridization of the carbon atom labeled 2?

3. What is the hybridization of the carbon atom labeled 3?

4. What is the hybridization of the carbon atom labeled 4?

5. How many *s* and π bonds are there total in the molecule?

6. Which of the following statements is TRUE of ethene?

    (A) Both carbon atoms are sp^2 hybridized, and the molecule is planar.
    (B) Both carbon atoms are sp^2 hybridized, and all bond angles are approximately 109.5°.
    (C) One carbon atom is sp hybridized, whereas the other is sp^2.
    (D) Both carbon atoms are sp^3 hybridized, and all bond angles are approximately 109.5°.
    (E) Both carbon atoms are sp hybridized, and the molecule is planar.

SOLUTIONS TO REVIEW PROBLEMS

1. *sp*: The carbon forms a single bond and a triple bond.

2. *sp*: The carbon forms a single bond and a triple bond.

3. sp^3: The carbon forms four single bonds.

4. sp^2: The carbon forms a double and two single bonds.

5. There are eight single bonds, one double bond, and one triple bond. Each single bond gives one *s* bond, a double bond gives one *s* and one π bond, and a triple bond gives one *s* and two π bonds. So there is a total of $8 + 1 + 1 = 10$ *s* bonds, and 1 (from double bond) + 2 (from triple bond) = 3 π bonds in the molecule.

6. **A** The two carbon atoms in ethene are bonded to each other via a double bond. They are thus both sp^2 hybridized, and the three attached groups each has will be arranged in a planar configuration roughly 120° apart, since that will minimize the electron-pair repulsion. (B) is wrong because of the bond angle. The other choices are wrong because both carbons are sp^2 hybridized; *sp* hybridization is found on carbon atoms with two adjacent double bonds (allenes) or, more commonly, a triple bond and a single bond (alkynes), while sp^3 hybridization is found on saturated carbon atoms.

CHAPTER FORTY-ONE

The PCAT Essay

The Writing sections of the test are your chance to demonstrate how adept you are at conveying a point clearly and concisely in essay form. In this chapter we will walk you through Kaplan's Five-Step Method for success on the writing samples. Even if you do not consider yourself a "writer," it's easy to master the basic skills that the Writing sections test. If you are willing to work and practice, practice… you can score a 5.

Each of the two PCAT Writing tests will require that you write a **problem-solving essay** in 30 minutes. A problem-solving topic will present a problem and ask you to write about a possible solution.

When writing a problem-solving essay, you will need to perform three tasks: 1) explain the problem and state a possible solution, 2) provide a counterexample where your solution runs into problems, and 3) reconcile the counterexample with your solution. These three tasks should be accomplished in a unified essay that flows well, remains focused, and has minimal mistakes. Your essay will be assessed for its ability to:

- Suggest a solution to the problem
- State a clear solution with relevant supporting evidence
- Evaluate alternative solutions
- Use correct grammar, punctuation, and style

Kaplan's Five-Step Method, if followed correctly, will help you prepare an essay that meets, if not exceeds, expectations. Following is a table that outlines the purpose of each step, as well as the amount of time you should spend on each step or group of steps.

KAPLAN'S FIVE-STEP METHOD FOR PREPARING AND WRITING A SUCCESSFUL ESSAY:

Step 1: Read and Annotate Purpose: Clarify what the given statement or problem means.	5 minutes
Step 2: Prewrite Each Task Purpose: Sketch out a sensible solution, counterexample, and resolution—essential for success!	
Step 3: Clarify Main Idea and Plan Purpose: Make sure the main idea is stated concisely, and that it is the centerpiece of your essay, for which support will be developed in the body.	
Step 4: Write! Purpose: Build a unified essay based on your prewritten tasks.	23 minutes
Step 5: Proofread Purpose: Detect errors that affect clarity: an error-free essay will score better!	2 minutes
Total Time:	30 minutes

Below is an example of a problem-solving writing topic. We will refer to this topic as we navigate through the Kaplan Five-Step Method.

> *Discuss a solution to the problem of increased levels of greenhouse gases, such as carbon dioxide, and the possibility of global warming.*

Step 1: Read and Annotate

This first step may seem obvious, but it is essential. You should not simply read the topic and immediately begin writing. It is important to take a moment to digest the topic in full, considering each word as a possible source of ideas. Note any key words and phrases. Remember that certain words can be interpreted differently. Consider how you interpret each word in the context of the given topic, and remember that you must support your interpretation with concrete examples. Think of counterexamples. Look at the topic from all possible angles and jot down as many notes as you can in a couple of minutes.

Step 2: Prewrite Each Task

After you have a clear idea of what the statement means and of how you would begin to explain it, you are ready to prewrite each implied task. This will help you solidify your interpretation of the statement, and it is the key to using your writing time effectively and to writing efficiently and clearly.

Prewrite Task 1: Explanation

Explain the elements of the problem, making sure to define key concepts and words in the statement of the problem. For example, it would be important to explain the relationship between greenhouse gases and global warming, what is meant by global warming, and the sources of greenhouse gases. You also want to explain the key elements of your solution at this point. Here, for example, we can state that other sources of energy need to be more widely employed to reduce the sources of greenhouse gases and that uses for greenhouse gases need to be implemented. Mention the cost of implementation without getting into great detail. It would be a bonus to provide a *brief* example that demonstrates your solution.

Prewrite Task 2: Counterexample

Here provide a counterexample where your solution runs into obstacles. This example should take advantage of weaknesses in your solution. Generally at this point, you will choose an example that weakens one of the elements of your solution as discussed in task 1.

Prewrite Task 3: Resolution

Here you need to reconcile the differences between the counterexample and your solution. For example, this paragraph may start as follows:

> Decreasing emissions of greenhouse gases is a significant part of the solution to greenhouse gas buildup and the possibility of global warming. While we have seen that the cost of implementation is a limiting factor, this cost may be distributed over many years. Tax credits (e.g., to industry for exploring alternate fuel sources) may make the reduction of greenhouse gases more attractive, assuming a healthy domestic economy.

Step 3: Clarify Main Idea and Plan

If you have budgeted your time wisely in the first two tasks, you should have about a minute left to clarify your main idea and to discard ideas that do not belong or that may detract from the cohesiveness of your essay plan. As you review your notes, make sure that your ideas work together and that the three primary tasks of explanation, counterexample, and resolution are balanced. This is your final chance to envision how all the major points will work together.

Step 4: Write!

You are now ready to begin writing. Use the ideas written down in your prewrite as the outline for your essay. Stay with the prewrite and be careful not to veer off track. Introducing a new idea, no matter how good, is a surefire way to start digressing from the central focus of the paragraphs. It's also important to avoid language that's too complex and that could detract from unity. Use a basic three-paragraph structure that covers the three implied tasks, and use simple, straightforward language and strong reasoning. We recommend that you *do not* double-space your essay, as this can be distracting to the reader.

> Success is up to you! If you're not confident in your grammar and syntax skills, pick up a book and study the rules or sign up for a writing workshop.

Step 5: Proofread

Use your last couple of minutes to correct any errors that may obfuscate the key point you are making. Look out for critical word omissions, run-on sentences, and subject-verb agreement. As you go, correct spelling errors and common misuses of words such as *their/there* and *affect/effect*. Avoid any changes that make your essay harder to read! Cross out deletions with a single line and insert new words with a caret symbol.

A LOOK AT HOW YOUR SCORE IS DETERMINED

The following scoring rubric demonstrates how PCAT judges your writing skills.

Scores don't start at perfect, with points taken off for errors. Each level has to be earned. You can't get a 5 if you haven't earned a 4. Scores 1–2 are about what an essay failed to do. A score of 3 is adequate in all categories. Above 3 is how well the tasks were completed.

Difference Between a 2 and a 3:

Essays that score a 3 address each task and are clear and logical. They follow the directions. An essay that receives a 2 lacks at least one of these qualities. The difference is objective: tasks completed versus not completed. The other criteria are more subjective, but there's no reason ever to be in the 1–2 range; simply following the directions prevents that from happening.

	5—Superior	4—Effective	3—Adequate	2—Marginal	1—Weak
Argument	Superior reasoning and argument; strong composition	Strong essay and effective composition; some lapses in reasoning	Adequate composition	Writing digresses from the task	Weak argument and ineffective writing
Solution	Clearly relevant and developed with strong evidence	Clearly relevant and developed with evidence	Relevant but evidence is very general	Present but not explicit	Unclear how solution relates
Explanation	Strong, integrated explanation of problem and solution	Clear explanation of problem and solution	Clearly discussed but lacks specifics	Support unclear or partially irrelevant	Support lacking or irrelevant
Alternate solutions	More than one solution evaluated	More than one solution mentioned	None	None	None
Organization	Logical, focused, and coherent	Logically organized in general	Coherent but has digressions and repetition	Weak organization	Lacks organization

Table 41.1

Practice makes perfect!

The best way to learn is to practice writing an essay, then to score your essay yourself based on the scoring rubric or to have a friend score it.

Good luck!

Final Exam
Answer Sheet

Remove (or photocopy) this answer sheet and use it to complete the practice test.

If a section has fewer questions than answer spaces, leave the extra spaces blank.

Verbal Ability

1 (A) (B) (C) (D)   12 (A) (B) (C) (D)   23 (A) (B) (C) (D)   34 (A) (B) (C) (D)   45 (A) (B) (C) (D)
2 (A) (B) (C) (D)   13 (A) (B) (C) (D)   24 (A) (B) (C) (D)   35 (A) (B) (C) (D)   46 (A) (B) (C) (D)
3 (A) (B) (C) (D)   14 (A) (B) (C) (D)   25 (A) (B) (C) (D)   36 (A) (B) (C) (D)   47 (A) (B) (C) (D)
4 (A) (B) (C) (D)   15 (A) (B) (C) (D)   26 (A) (B) (C) (D)   37 (A) (B) (C) (D)   48 (A) (B) (C) (D)
5 (A) (B) (C) (D)   16 (A) (B) (C) (D)   27 (A) (B) (C) (D)   38 (A) (B) (C) (D)
6 (A) (B) (C) (D)   17 (A) (B) (C) (D)   28 (A) (B) (C) (D)   39 (A) (B) (C) (D)
7 (A) (B) (C) (D)   18 (A) (B) (C) (D)   29 (A) (B) (C) (D)   40 (A) (B) (C) (D)
8 (A) (B) (C) (D)   19 (A) (B) (C) (D)   30 (A) (B) (C) (D)   41 (A) (B) (C) (D)
9 (A) (B) (C) (D)   20 (A) (B) (C) (D)   31 (A) (B) (C) (D)   42 (A) (B) (C) (D)
10 (A) (B) (C) (D)   21 (A) (B) (C) (D)   32 (A) (B) (C) (D)   43 (A) (B) (C) (D)
11 (A) (B) (C) (D)   22 (A) (B) (C) (D)   33 (A) (B) (C) (D)   44 (A) (B) (C) (D)

Biology

1 (A) (B) (C) (D)   12 (A) (B) (C) (D)   23 (A) (B) (C) (D)   34 (A) (B) (C) (D)   45 (A) (B) (C) (D)
2 (A) (B) (C) (D)   13 (A) (B) (C) (D)   24 (A) (B) (C) (D)   35 (A) (B) (C) (D)   46 (A) (B) (C) (D)
3 (A) (B) (C) (D)   14 (A) (B) (C) (D)   25 (A) (B) (C) (D)   36 (A) (B) (C) (D)   47 (A) (B) (C) (D)
4 (A) (B) (C) (D)   15 (A) (B) (C) (D)   26 (A) (B) (C) (D)   37 (A) (B) (C) (D)   48 (A) (B) (C) (D)
5 (A) (B) (C) (D)   16 (A) (B) (C) (D)   27 (A) (B) (C) (D)   38 (A) (B) (C) (D)
6 (A) (B) (C) (D)   17 (A) (B) (C) (D)   28 (A) (B) (C) (D)   39 (A) (B) (C) (D)
7 (A) (B) (C) (D)   18 (A) (B) (C) (D)   29 (A) (B) (C) (D)   40 (A) (B) (C) (D)
8 (A) (B) (C) (D)   19 (A) (B) (C) (D)   30 (A) (B) (C) (D)   41 (A) (B) (C) (D)
9 (A) (B) (C) (D)   20 (A) (B) (C) (D)   31 (A) (B) (C) (D)   42 (A) (B) (C) (D)
10 (A) (B) (C) (D)   21 (A) (B) (C) (D)   32 (A) (B) (C) (D)   43 (A) (B) (C) (D)
11 (A) (B) (C) (D)   22 (A) (B) (C) (D)   33 (A) (B) (C) (D)   44 (A) (B) (C) (D)

Chemistry

1 (A) (B) (C) (D)   11 (A) (B) (C) (D)   21 (A) (B) (C) (D)   31 (A) (B) (C) (D)   41 (A) (B) (C) (D)
2 (A) (B) (C) (D)   12 (A) (B) (C) (D)   22 (A) (B) (C) (D)   32 (A) (B) (C) (D)   42 (A) (B) (C) (D)
3 (A) (B) (C) (D)   13 (A) (B) (C) (D)   23 (A) (B) (C) (D)   33 (A) (B) (C) (D)   43 (A) (B) (C) (D)
4 (A) (B) (C) (D)   14 (A) (B) (C) (D)   24 (A) (B) (C) (D)   34 (A) (B) (C) (D)   44 (A) (B) (C) (D)
5 (A) (B) (C) (D)   15 (A) (B) (C) (D)   25 (A) (B) (C) (D)   35 (A) (B) (C) (D)   45 (A) (B) (C) (D)
6 (A) (B) (C) (D)   16 (A) (B) (C) (D)   26 (A) (B) (C) (D)   36 (A) (B) (C) (D)   46 (A) (B) (C) (D)
7 (A) (B) (C) (D)   17 (A) (B) (C) (D)   27 (A) (B) (C) (D)   37 (A) (B) (C) (D)   47 (A) (B) (C) (D)
8 (A) (B) (C) (D)   18 (A) (B) (C) (D)   28 (A) (B) (C) (D)   38 (A) (B) (C) (D)   48 (A) (B) (C) (D)
9 (A) (B) (C) (D)   19 (A) (B) (C) (D)   29 (A) (B) (C) (D)   39 (A) (B) (C) (D)
10 (A) (B) (C) (D)   20 (A) (B) (C) (D)   30 (A) (B) (C) (D)   40 (A) (B) (C) (D)

Reading Comprehension

1 (A) (B) (C) (D) 11 (A) (B) (C) (D) 21 (A) (B) (C) (D) 31 (A) (B) (C) (D) 41 (A) (B) (C) (D)
2 (A) (B) (C) (D) 12 (A) (B) (C) (D) 22 (A) (B) (C) (D) 32 (A) (B) (C) (D) 42 (A) (B) (C) (D)
3 (A) (B) (C) (D) 13 (A) (B) (C) (D) 23 (A) (B) (C) (D) 33 (A) (B) (C) (D) 43 (A) (B) (C) (D)
4 (A) (B) (C) (D) 14 (A) (B) (C) (D) 24 (A) (B) (C) (D) 34 (A) (B) (C) (D) 44 (A) (B) (C) (D)
5 (A) (B) (C) (D) 15 (A) (B) (C) (D) 25 (A) (B) (C) (D) 35 (A) (B) (C) (D) 45 (A) (B) (C) (D)
6 (A) (B) (C) (D) 16 (A) (B) (C) (D) 26 (A) (B) (C) (D) 36 (A) (B) (C) (D) 46 (A) (B) (C) (D)
7 (A) (B) (C) (D) 17 (A) (B) (C) (D) 27 (A) (B) (C) (D) 37 (A) (B) (C) (D) 47 (A) (B) (C) (D)
8 (A) (B) (C) (D) 18 (A) (B) (C) (D) 28 (A) (B) (C) (D) 38 (A) (B) (C) (D) 48 (A) (B) (C) (D)
9 (A) (B) (C) (D) 19 (A) (B) (C) (D) 29 (A) (B) (C) (D) 39 (A) (B) (C) (D)
10 (A) (B) (C) (D) 20 (A) (B) (C) (D) 30 (A) (B) (C) (D) 40 (A) (B) (C) (D)

Quantitative Ability

1 (A) (B) (C) (D) 11 (A) (B) (C) (D) 21 (A) (B) (C) (D) 31 (A) (B) (C) (D) 41 (A) (B) (C) (D)
2 (A) (B) (C) (D) 12 (A) (B) (C) (D) 22 (A) (B) (C) (D) 32 (A) (B) (C) (D) 42 (A) (B) (C) (D)
3 (A) (B) (C) (D) 13 (A) (B) (C) (D) 23 (A) (B) (C) (D) 33 (A) (B) (C) (D) 43 (A) (B) (C) (D)
4 (A) (B) (C) (D) 14 (A) (B) (C) (D) 24 (A) (B) (C) (D) 34 (A) (B) (C) (D) 44 (A) (B) (C) (D)
5 (A) (B) (C) (D) 15 (A) (B) (C) (D) 25 (A) (B) (C) (D) 35 (A) (B) (C) (D) 45 (A) (B) (C) (D)
6 (A) (B) (C) (D) 16 (A) (B) (C) (D) 26 (A) (B) (C) (D) 36 (A) (B) (C) (D) 46 (A) (B) (C) (D)
7 (A) (B) (C) (D) 17 (A) (B) (C) (D) 27 (A) (B) (C) (D) 37 (A) (B) (C) (D) 47 (A) (B) (C) (D)
8 (A) (B) (C) (D) 18 (A) (B) (C) (D) 28 (A) (B) (C) (D) 38 (A) (B) (C) (D) 48 (A) (B) (C) (D)
9 (A) (B) (C) (D) 19 (A) (B) (C) (D) 29 (A) (B) (C) (D) 39 (A) (B) (C) (D)
10 (A) (B) (C) (D) 20 (A) (B) (C) (D) 30 (A) (B) (C) (D) 40 (A) (B) (C) (D)

CHAPTER FORTY-TWO

Final Exam

WRITING

1 Topic
Time: 30 minutes

Discuss a solution to the problem of heightened levels of eating disorders among preteen and teen girls and boys.

_____

_____

_____

_____

_____

_____

_____

_____

_____

_____

_____

_____

_____

_____

_____

_____

_____

_____

_____

****Please note***: Due to the variable and subjective nature of the possible answers, an explanation is not available for this section of the exam.

STOP

VERBAL ABILITY

Questions: 48
Time: 30 minutes

Sentence Completion

Directions: Each sentence below has one or two blanks, each blank indicating that something has been omitted. Beneath the sentence are five lettered words or sets of words. Choose the word or set of words for each blank that best fit the meaning of the sentence as a whole.

1. Many believe that jazz improvisation is a creation of the 20th century, but it is _____ that improvisation has its _____ in the figured-bass techniques of the 17th and 18th centuries.

    (A) unlikely ... roots
    (B) possible ... past
    (C) arguable ... origin
    (D) proven ... future
    (E) interesting ... unity

2. Whales hurt nothing and no one in their peaceful migrations through the earth's seas, yet they are savagely hunted by man, who _____ superior need.

    (A) assumes
    (B) perpetuates
    (C) retains
    (D) assimilates
    (E) manifests

3. His unbridled curiosity led him to explore every field of _____ , yet his _____ stances kept him at odds with the devout society he so wanted to be acknowledged by.

    (A) science ... interesting
    (B) interest ... common
    (C) thought ... unorthodox
    (D) hope ... heretical
    (E) study ... optimistic

4. Because of his inherent _____ , Harry steered clear of any job that he suspected could turn out to be a travail.

    (A) impudence
    (B) insolence
    (C) eminence
    (D) indolence
    (E) integrity

5. First published in 1649, Pacheco's _____ treatise contains not only chapters outlining iconography and technique but also commentary on contemporary painters that now _____ our most comprehensive information on these artists, as well as the most thorough discussion available on Baroque aesthetics.

    (A) inconsequential ... comprises
    (B) invaluable ... constitutes
    (C) historical ... lacks
    (D) superficial ... supports
    (E) important ... excludes

6. Very little is known of the writer Theophilus; however, from his eclectic writings, we can _____ that he was well _____ .

    (A) assume ... educated
    (B) understand ... disciplined
    (C) appreciate ... respected
    (D) expect ... exposed
    (E) acknowledge ... received

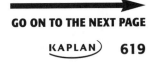

GO ON TO THE NEXT PAGE

7. Her systematic approach to scientific research was often rewarded in her _____ life, but it proved disastrous when her _____ mind examined every flaw in her friends and family, preventing her from truly appreciating others.

   (A) career ... disorganized
   (B) private ... analytical
   (C) public ... fragile
   (D) professional ... methodical
   (E) family ... orderly

8. Personal correspondence is often a marvelous reflection of the spirit of an age; the subtle _____ of Swift's epistles mirrored the 18th century's delight in elegant _____ .

   (A) profundity ... ditties
   (B) poignancy ... pejoratives
   (C) contempt ... anachronisms
   (D) provinciality ... pomposity
   (E) vitriol ... disparagement

9. Our spokesperson seems to be uncertain of our eventual victory but _____ facing the alternative, as if merely admitting the possibility of defeat would lead to the dread thing itself.

   (A) unsure of
   (B) complacent when
   (C) fearful of
   (D) certain of
   (E) helped by

10. Victorien Sardou's play *La Tosca* was originally written as a _____ for Sarah Bernhardt and later _____ into the famous Puccini opera.

    (A) role ... reincarnated
    (B) biography ... changed
    (C) metaphor ... edited
    (D) present ... fictionalized
    (E) vehicle ... adapted

11. Because the law and custom require that a definite determination be made, the judge is forced to behave as if the verdict is _____, when in fact the evidence may not be _____.

    (A) negotiable ... persuasive
    (B) justified ... accessible
    (C) unassailable ... insubstantial
    (D) incontrovertible ... admissible
    (E) self-evident ... conclusive

12. The author presumably believes that all businesspeople are _____, for her main characters, whatever qualities they may lack, are virtual paragons of _____.

    (A) clever ... ingenuity
    (B) covetous ... greed
    (C) virtuous ... deceit
    (D) successful ... ambition
    (E) cautious ... achievement

13. Filmed on a ludicrously _____ budget and edited at breakneck speed, Melotti's documentary nonetheless _____ the Cannes critics with its ingenuity and verve.

    (A) low...disappointed
    (B) inflated...distracted
    (C) uneven...amused
    (D) disproportionate...appalled
    (E) inadequate...surprised

14. Ginnie expects her every submission to be published or selected for performance, and this time her _____ is likely to be _____.

    (A) candor ... dispelled
    (B) anticipation ... piqued
    (C) enthusiasm ... dampened
    (D) optimism ... vindicated
    (E) awareness ... clouded

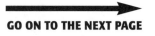

GO ON TO THE NEXT PAGE

15. His opponent found it extremely frustrating that the governor's solid support from the voting public was not eroded by his _____ of significant issues.

    (A) exaggeration
    (B) misapprehension
    (C) discussion
    (D) selection
    (E) acknowledgment

16. The fundamental _____ between dogs and cats is for the most part a myth; members of these species often coexist _____.

    (A) antipathy … amiably
    (B) disharmony … uneasily
    (C) compatibility … together
    (D) relationship … peacefully
    (E) difference … placidly

17. His desire to state his case completely was certainly reasonable; however, his lengthy technical explanations were monotonous and tended to _____ rather than _____ the jury.

    (A) enlighten … inform
    (B) interest … persuade
    (C) provoke … influence
    (D) allay … pacify
    (E) bore … convince

18. In some countries, government restrictions are so _____ that businesses operate with nearly complete impunity.

    (A) traditional
    (B) judicious
    (C) ambiguous
    (D) exacting
    (E) lax

Analogies

Directions: Choose the word that **best** completes the analogy.

19. CONDUCTOR : COMPOSER :: DIRECTOR :

    (A) agent
    (B) screenwriter
    (C) producer
    (D) musician

20. FLUSTER : COMPOSURE :: CORRUPT :

    (A) cleanliness
    (B) study
    (C) integrity
    (D) eminence

21. SCABBARD : SWORD :: HOLSTER :

    (A) spade
    (B) dagger
    (C) knife
    (D) gun

22. NOD : ASSENT :: SHRUG :

    (A) beneficence
    (B) capriciousness
    (C) kindliness
    (D) indifference

23. CROWD : PERSON :: GALAXY :

    (A) moon
    (B) asteroid
    (C) supernova
    (D) star

24. AMNESIA : MEMORY :: BLINDNESS :

    (A) insight
    (B) perception
    (C) lamentation
    (D) vision

GO ON TO THE NEXT PAGE

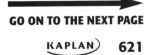

25. PAIN : WINCE :: EMBARRASSMENT :
    (A) dream
    (B) writhe
    (C) leer
    (D) blush

26. INFLAMMABLE : IGNITED :: FRAGILE :
    (A) magnified
    (B) flexible
    (C) shattered
    (D) plagiarized

27. SHARD : GLASS :: SPLINTER :
    (A) sand
    (B) morsel
    (C) wood
    (D) rope

28. DESICCATE : MOISTURE :: DEBILITATE :
    (A) strength
    (B) augur
    (C) exonerate
    (D) pain

29. ANODYNE : RELIEF :: SOPORIFIC :
    (A) illusion
    (B) balm
    (C) confusion
    (D) sleep

30. FLOOD : DILUVIAL :: HEART :
    (A) cardiac
    (B) biological
    (C) judicial
    (D) pulmonary

31. ATTENTIVE : RAPT :: CRITICAL :
    (A) unscrupulous
    (B) derisive
    (C) polite
    (D) jealous

32. SPHINX : PERPLEX :: SIREN :
    (A) oracle
    (B) anger
    (C) lure
    (D) astound

33. PIG : STY :: HORSE :
    (A) field
    (B) forest
    (C) dune
    (D) stable

34. BASEBALL : DIAMOND :: BASKETBALL :
    (A) referee
    (B) player
    (C) game
    (D) court

35. SHACKLE : PRISONER :: CHARGE :
    (A) suspect
    (B) sentence
    (C) judge
    (D) credit card

36. MAP : ATLAS :: RECIPE :
    (A) food
    (B) cookbook
    (C) kitchen
    (D) oven

37. HOWL : WIND :: RUMBLE :
    (A) rain
    (B) thunder
    (C) snow
    (D) wave

38. BRIGAND : BAND :: PERFORMER :
    (A) crew
    (B) retinue
    (C) troupe
    (D) bureaucracy

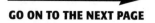

GO ON TO THE NEXT PAGE

39. PENNILESS : MONEY :: CALLOUS :
    - (A) innocent
    - (B) haughty
    - (C) compassion
    - (D) power

40. ASYMMETRICAL : BALANCE :: CHAOTIC :
    - (A) alluring
    - (B) confident
    - (C) order
    - (D) intelligence

41. NUPTIAL : WEDDING :: NATAL :
    - (A) election
    - (B) national
    - (C) graduation
    - (D) birth

42. FILTER : IMPURITY :: EXPURGATE :
    - (A) obscenity
    - (B) whitewash
    - (C) perjury
    - (D) explanation

43. PARAPHRASE : VERBATIM :: ESTIMATE :
    - (A) description
    - (B) precise
    - (C) apt
    - (D) valid

44. OSTRICH : FLY :: ELEPHANT
    - (A) bird
    - (B) walk
    - (C) jump
    - (D) masticate

45. SHARPEN : HONE :: WIPE
    - (A) dust
    - (B) burnish
    - (C) cleanse
    - (D) neaten

46. HEPATITIS : LIVER :: ENCEPHALITIS
    - (A) skull
    - (B) pharynx
    - (C) brain
    - (D) endometrium

47. MINIMALIST : SPARTAN :: MANNERIST
    - (A) ostentatious
    - (B) dour
    - (C) saturnine
    - (D) titan

48. RELIGIOUS : HIERATIC :: SECULAR
    - (A) commercial
    - (B) demotic
    - (C) dorian
    - (D) seraphic

STOP

BIOLOGY

Questions: 48
Time: 30 minutes

Directions: Choose the **best** answer to each of the following questions.

1. Which of the following aspects of cellular respiration is correctly paired with the location in the cell where it occurs?

   (A) Glycolysis – outer mitochondrial membrane
   (B) Krebs cycle enzymes and intermediates – mitochondrial matrix
   (C) Coenzyme A formation – inner mitochondrial membrane
   (D) ATP synthesis – cytoplasm

2. Which of the following statements about the heart is TRUE?

   (A) Both the superior and inferior vena cava route blood into the right atrium.
   (B) In adults, blood can flow between the right and left atria.
   (C) The valve between the left atrium and left ventricle is known as the tricuspid valve.
   (D) The pericardium is the network of blood vessels that supplies nourishment to the heart.

3. According to the endosymbiotic hypothesis, chloroplasts are believed to have been descended from free-living

   (A) eukaryotic autotrophs.
   (B) prokaryotic autotrophs.
   (C) eukaryotic heterotrophs.
   (D) prokaryotic heterotrophs.

4. Which of the following is TRUE of both a prokaryotic cell and a eukaryotic cell?

   (A) Both contain membrane-bound organelles.
   (B) Both contain plasmids.
   (C) Both have cell walls made of peptidoglycan.
   (D) Both contain DNA.

5. Which of the following statements concerning the kidney is CORRECT?

   (A) The kidney keeps the relative concentrations of inorganic ions in the body's blood plasma at a constant level.
   (B) Active transport is directly involved in movement of water.
   (C) The descending limb of the loop of Henle is impermeable to water.
   (D) Glucose is primarily reabsorbed in the distal convoluted tubule.

6. If a DNA molecule were to replicate itself three times, what percent of the total DNA present would be composed of the original DNA molecule?

   (A) 0%
   (B) 3.125%
   (C) 6.25%
   (D) 12.5%

7. Which of the following paths does oxygen follow when traveling through the respiratory structures?

   (A) external nares → internal nares → larynx → pharynx → trachea → bronchi → bronchioles → alveoli
   (B) external nares → nasal cavity → internal nares → trachea → pharynx → larynx → bronchi → bronchioles → alveoli
   (C) external nares → nasal cavity → internal nares → larynx → pharynx → trachea → pleura → alveoli
   (D) external nares → nasal cavity → internal nares → pharynx → larynx → trachea → bronchi → bronchioles → alveoli

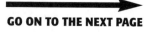

GO ON TO THE NEXT PAGE

8. Enzymes are responsible for which of the following?

    (A) Catalysis of a wide range of chemical reactions

    (B) Making a reaction proceed that would not have been able to proceed without the enzyme

    (C) Increasing the rate of a spontaneous reaction

    (D) Increasing the activation energy of a reaction

9. Which of the following statements agrees with modern evolutionary theory?

    (A) Species only produce the exact amount of progeny that can survive to reproductive maturity.

    (B) Genetically, all offspring are exactly alike.

    (C) Individuals with favorable characteristics are more likely to survive.

    (D) All heritable variation arises ultimately from mutations.

10. Which of the following cellular substituents is made within the nucleus?

    (A) Lysosome

    (B) Golgi apparatus

    (C) Ribosome

    (D) Smooth endoplasmic reticulum

11. A capillary has

    (A) a higher hydrostatic pressure at the arteriole end and a lower hydrostatic pressure at the venule end.

    (B) a lower hydrostatic pressure at the arteriole end and a higher hydrostatic pressure at the venule end.

    (C) a hydrostatic pressure that results from the contraction of skeletal muscles.

    (D) a lower osmotic pressure in its blood plasma than the osmotic pressure of the interstitial fluid bathing the tissues.

12. Which of the following statements about the glycolytic pathway is TRUE?

    (A) Oxygen serves as a major reactant in glycolysis.

    (B) During glycolysis, glucose is partially reduced.

    (C) For each molecule of glucose that undergoes glycolysis, two net molecules of ATP and two molecules of reduced NADH are produced.

    (D) For each molecule of glucose that undergoes glycolysis, one molecule of pyruvic acid is formed.

13. Which of the following statements about fertilization is CORRECT?

    (A) The sex of an individual is determined after the zygote has implanted in the uterus.

    (B) The sex of an individual is determined by the egg, not the sperm.

    (C) After fertilization, a special membrane forms around the zygote to protect it from penetration by additional sperm.

    (D) Once fertilized, the zygote decreases its rate of oxygen consumption.

14. Which of the following is NOT reabsorbed from the tubules of the nephron?

    (A) Water

    (B) Glucose

    (C) Amino acids

    (D) Proteins

15. Which of the following statements is TRUE regarding lambda phage, a virus that infects bacteria?

    (A) In the lytic cycle, the bacterial host replicates viral DNA, passing it on to daughter cells during binary fission.

    (B) In the lysogenic cycle, the bacterial host replicates viral DNA, passing it on to daughter cells during binary fission.

    (C) In the lytic cycle, viral DNA is integrated into the host genome.

    (D) In the lysogenic cycle, the host bacterial cell bursts, releasing phages.

16. What is the probability of a tall child with blue eyes being born to a heterozygous tall, heterozygous brown-eyed mother and a homozygous tall, homozygous blue-eyed father if tall height, and brown eye color are dominant? (Note: the genes for eye color and height are unlinked.)

    (A) $\frac{1}{4}$

    (B) $\frac{1}{2}$

    (C) $\frac{3}{4}$

    (D) $\frac{1}{8}$

17. Lymph vessels eventually return fluid to systemic circulation via the

    (A) lymph veins.
    (B) lymph arteries.
    (C) lymph nodes.
    (D) thoracic duct.

18. The light reactions of photosynthesis

    (A) break down water into hydrogen ions and oxygen gas molecules.
    (B) involve only one class of pigments, the chlorophylls.
    (C) form ATP and NADP.
    (D) result in the release of carbon dioxide.

19. During what stage of meiosis are tetrads present within a single nucleus?

    (A) Metaphase I
    (B) Interkinesis
    (C) Prophase II
    (D) Metaphase II

20. Which of the following is responsible for hydrolyzing disaccharides into monosaccharides?

    (A) Pancreatic amylase
    (B) Carboxypeptidase
    (C) Maltose
    (D) Lactase

21. Which of the following statements about cellular respiration is TRUE?

    (A) The Krebs cycle must turn once to completely oxidize each molecule of glucose that enters the glycolytic pathway.
    (B) All of the reactions of the Krebs cycle are catalyzed by the same enzyme.
    (C) Two acetyl coenzyme A molecules are produced from the pyruvate decarboxylation of one pyruvic acid molecule.
    (D) Two pyruvic acid molecules are produced for each glucose molecule that undergoes respiration.

22. A scientist developing a drug that specifically targets fungal cells rather than prokaryotic cells might choose which of the following cellular components to target?

    (A) DNA
    (B) RNA
    (C) Chitin
    (D) Peptidoglycan

23. Which of the following statements concerning nucleic acids is CORRECT?

    (A) Adenine and thymine are purines; guanine and cytosine are pyrimidines.
    (B) RNA is similar to DNA except that its sugar is ribose, it contains uracil instead of thymine, and it is usually double stranded.
    (C) The total amount of purines must equal the total amount of pyrimidines in a sample of double-stranded DNA.
    (D) Thymine always forms three hydrogen bonds with adenine; guanine always forms two hydrogen bonds with cytosine.

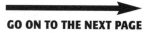

GO ON TO THE NEXT PAGE

24. Match the letter in the diagram with the appropriate region of the sarcomere.

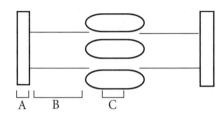

- **(A)** (A) Z-line   (B) H-band   (C) actin
- **(B)** (A) Z-line   (B) I-band   (C) myosin
- **(C)** (A) Z-line   (B) H-band   (C) I-band
- **(D)** (A) Z-line   (B) I-band   (C) H-band

25. Which of the following crosses of ABO blood types CANNOT produce type O offspring?

- **(A)** A × O
- **(B)** AB × O
- **(C)** A × B
- **(D)** A × A

26. Red-green color blindness is a sex-linked recessive trait. What is the probability that a boy born to a normal man and a carrier woman will be color-blind?

- **(A)** $\frac{1}{4}$
- **(B)** $\frac{1}{2}$
- **(C)** $\frac{3}{4}$
- **(D)** 1

27. The role of cholecystokinin in the digestive system is to

- **(A)** stimulate the gall bladder to release bile.
- **(B)** stimulate the pancreas to secrete lactase.
- **(C)** stimulate the gastric glands to release gastric juices.
- **(D)** break down protein molecules into amino acids.

28. Which of the following nutrients would yield the MOST energy per unit weight?

- **(A)** Carbohydrate
- **(B)** Fat
- **(C)** Protein
- **(D)** Cellulose

29. In a certain species of flower, a gene at a single locus codes for flower color. A homozygous red flower is crossed with a homozygous white flower, and the offspring are heterozygous pink flowers. The principle exemplified best by this example is

- **(A)** segregation.
- **(B)** a testcross.
- **(C)** nondisjunction.
- **(D)** incomplete dominance.

30. Which of the following statements is TRUE concerning the electron transport system?

- **(A)** Oxygen does not participate.
- **(B)** Most of the ATP generated in cellular oxidation is produced by the electron transport system.
- **(C)** The electrons carried by each molecule of reduced FAD yield more ATP molecules than the electrons carried by each molecule of reduced NAD.
- **(D)** The enzymes of the electron transport system lie in the outer mitochondrial membrane.

31. Which of the following most accurately describes one of the distinct muscle types found in the human body?

		Number of nuclei per fiber	Cross striations	Type of control
(A)	Skeletal:	many	present	voluntary
(B)	Smooth:	one	present	involuntary
(C)	Cardiac:	many	present	involuntary
(D)	Cannot be determined			

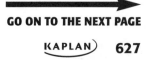

32. Which of the following is derived from the mesoderm?

    (A) Intestinal mucosa
    (B) Lung epithelium
    (C) Heart
    (D) Peripheral nerves

33. Which organelle is chiefly responsible for digestive breakdown of the cell during autolysis?

    (A) Golgi apparatus
    (B) Ribosome
    (C) Mitochondrion
    (D) Lysosome

34. A laboratory has discovered a new organism hypothesized to be a prokaryote. The presence of which of the following structures would contradict this hypothesis?

    (A) Ribosome
    (B) Nuclear membrane
    (C) Cell wall
    (D) DNA

35. Which of the following cannot cross the plasma membrane without assistance?

    (A) Water
    (B) Oxygen molecules
    (C) Calcium ions
    (D) Carbon dioxide molecules

36. The tRNA anticodon for the amino acid valine is AAC. What is the mRNA codon for valine?

    (A) UUG
    (B) TTG
    (C) GGU
    (D) CCA

37. The major site of action for the hormone ADH is the

    (A) collecting tubule.
    (B) Bowman's capsule.
    (C) proximal convoluted tubule.
    (D) loop of Henle.

38. Which of the following associations of brain structure and function is correct?

    (A) Hypothalamus – higher intellectual function
    (B) Medulla oblongata – basic emotional drives
    (C) Cerebellum – motor coordination
    (D) Cerebral cortex – appetite

39. Which of the following cells does NOT have a nucleus?

    (A) Leukocyte
    (B) Epithelial cell
    (C) Erythrocyte
    (D) Sperm

40. All viruses

    (A) carry DNA.
    (B) carry RNA.
    (C) lack protein.
    (D) cannot reproduce outside of cells.

41. Tetracycline is toxic to prokaryotes but harmless to eukaryotes. Which of the following cellular components would most likely be a target of tetracycline?

    (A) Ribosomal subunits
    (B) Endoplasmic reticulum
    (C) Lysosomes
    (D) Amino acids

42. Which of the following demonstrates the correct order of developmental events?

    (A) Blastula, implantation, gastrula, neurulation
    (B) Morula, blastula, gastrula, implantation
    (C) Gastrula, implantation, blastula
    (D) Morula, neurulation, implantation, gastrula

GO ON TO THE NEXT PAGE

43. In humans, most digestion occurs in the

    (A) mouth.
    (B) small intestine.
    (C) liver.
    (D) large intestine.

44. Which of the following is TRUE concerning the human respiratory system?

    (A) Ventilation is controlled by the cerebellum.
    (B) Gas exchange occurs across the alveolar-capillary membrane.
    (C) The rate of breathing is increased by parasympathetic stimulation.
    (D) Contraction of the diaphragm contracts the thoracic cavity and permits the lungs to fill.

45. Which of the following statements is TRUE regarding retroviruses?

    (A) Retroviruses contain reverse transcriptase, which transcribes RNA from DNA.
    (B) Retroviruses contain reverse transcriptase, which transcribes DNA from RNA.
    (C) Retroviruses immediately lyse their host cells.
    (D) Retroviruses are capable of reproducing outside of a host cell.

46. Which of the following processes utilizes ATP?

    (A) Diffusion
    (B) Facilitated diffusion
    (C) Active transport
    (D) Osmosis

47. The genetic code is considered degenerate because

    (A) more than one codon can code for a single amino acid.
    (B) one codon can code for multiple amino acids.
    (C) more than one anticodon can bind to a given codon.
    (D) only one anticodon can bind to a given codon.

48. Which of the following would be LEAST able to make bacteria more virulent and infectious?

    (A) The ability to evade nonspecific and specific body defenses
    (B) The secretion of lipoteichoic acid, which contributes to septic shock
    (C) Increasing the rate of bacterial replication
    (D) Increasing the production of proteins allowing bacterial pili to extend and contact other pili
    (E) The sudden ability of the bacteria to infect several different kinds of species rather than only one

STOP

CHEMISTRY

Questions: 48
Time: 30 minutes

Directions: Choose the **best** answer to each of the following questions.

1. If an acid has a pK_a of 7, what is the value of the acid dissociation constant K_a?

    (A) −7
    (B) 7
    (C) 10^{-7}
    (D) 10^7

2. The boiling point of a liquid is the temperature at which the vapor pressure of the liquid is

    (A) less than the atmospheric pressure.
    (B) equal to the atmospheric pressure.
    (C) greater than the atmospheric pressure.
    (D) unaffected by atmospheric pressure.

3. Gas A is at 30°C, and gas B is at 20°C. Both gases are at 1 atmosphere. What is the ratio of the volume of 1 mole of gas A to 1 mole of gas B?

    (A) 2:3
    (B) 3:2
    (C) 303:293
    (D) 606:293

4. When 1 mole of sulfur burns to form SO_2, 1,300 calories are released. When 1 mole of sulfur burns to form SO_3, 3,600 calories are released. What is ΔH when 1 mole of SO_2 is burned to form SO_3?

    (A) −1,950 calories
    (B) +1,000 calories
    (C) −500 calories
    (D) −2,300 calories

5. What is the number of half-filled orbitals in one ground-state atom of atomic number 16?

    (A) 2
    (B) 3
    (C) 4
    (D) 6

6. Which of the following is the formula for a noncyclic, saturated hydrocarbon?

    (A) C_7H_{12}
    (B) C_7H_{14}
    (C) C_7H_{16}
    (D) C_7H_{18}

7. One liter of 0.01 M aqueous acetic acid solution is titrated with 0.10 M $Ca(OH)2(aq)$. What volume of the basic solution must be added to reach the equivalence point of the titration?

    (A) 25 mL
    (B) 50 mL
    (C) 75 mL
    (D) 100 mL

8. What is the percent composition by mass of oxygen in NaOH? (atomic weights: Na = 23, O = 16, H = 1)

    (A) 2.5%
    (B) 10%
    (C) 40%
    (D) 60%

9. What is the empirical formula of glucose $(C_6H_{12}O_6)$?

    (A) CHO
    (B) CH_2O
    (C) $C_3H_6O_3$
    (D) $C_6H_{12}O_6$

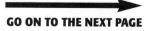

GO ON TO THE NEXT PAGE

10. What functional groups are present in the compound below?

    (A) Eter and ether
    (B) Ester and amine
    (C) Ester and carboxylic acid
    (D) Ether and carboxylic acid

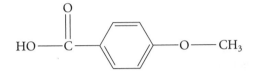

11. What is product X in the following reaction?

    HCl(*aq*) + NaOH(*aq*) → NaCl + X

    (A) $H_2(g)$
    (B) $H_2O(l)$
    (C) $O_2(g)$
    (D) $H_2O_2(aq)$

12. How much energy is needed to heat 100 g of water from 5°C to 75°C? (The specific heat of water is 4.184 J/g•°C.)

    (A) 293 J
    (B) 418 J
    (C) 29.3 kJ
    (D) 31.4 kJ

13. Which of the following is the most accurate representation of benzene?

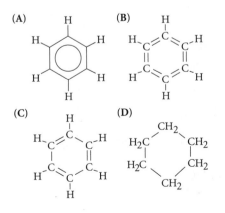

14. At constant temperature, the volume of a gas is inversely proportional to its pressure. This is known as

    (A) Charles's Law
    (B) Boyle's Law
    (C) Avogadro's Law
    (D) Gay-Lussac's Law

15. Five hundred milliliters of an ideal gas is placed in a sealed container at a pressure of 700 mmHg. If the volume is decreased to 100 mL at constant temperature, what is the final pressure of the gas?

    (A) 1,500 mmHg
    (B) 2,500 mmHg
    (C) 3,500 mmHg
    (D) 4,500 mmHg

16. A physicist starts out with 320 grams of a radioactive element Z. After 20 minutes, he has only 20 grams of element Z left. What is the half-life of element Z?

    (A) 2 minutes
    (B) 3 minutes
    (C) 4 minutes
    (D) 5 minutes

17. What is the name of the following compound?

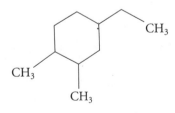

    (A) 1-ethyl-3,4-dimethylcycloheptane
    (B) 2-ethyl-4,5-dimethylcyclohexane
    (C) 1-ethyl-3,4-dimethylcyclohexane
    (D) 4-ethyl-1,2-dimethylcyclohexane

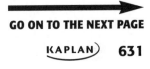

18. What is the electron configuration of chlorine (atomic number 17)?

    (A) $1s^2 2s^2 2p^6 3s^2 3p^6$
    (B) $1s^2 2s^2 2p^6 4s^2 3p^5$
    (C) $1s^2 2s^2 2p^6 3s^1 3p^6$
    (D) $1s^2 2s^2 2p^6 3s^2 3p^5$

19. Which of the following compounds has the lowest boiling point?

    (A) Ethanoic acid
    (B) Ethanal
    (C) Ethanol
    (D) Ethane

20. The Ksp for AgI is 8.5×10^{-17}. What is the solubility of AgI in water?

    (A) 9.2×10^{-9}
    (B) 2.9×10^{-17}
    (C) 4.3×10^{-17}
    (D) 8.5×10^{-17}

21. Within one principal quantum level of a many-electron atom, which orbital has the minimum energy?

    (A) s
    (B) p
    (C) d
    (D) f

Questions 22 and 23 refer to the following hypothetical reaction

$$2\,X(g) + Y(g) \rightarrow Z(g)$$

22. If stoichiometric quantities of X(g) and Y(g) are introduced into a sealed, rigid container at constant temperature with a total initial pressure of 12 atmospheres, what will the pressure in the container be when the reaction is complete?

    (A) 12 atm
    (B) 6 atm
    (C) 4 atm
    (D) 3 atm

23. If stoichiometric quantities of X(g) and Y(g) are placed in a sealed, flexible container with an initial volume of 30 liters at STP, what volume of Z(g) will be produced?

    (A) 10 L
    (B) 30 L
    (C) 90 L
    (D) 3.5 L

24. Which of the following ionization reactions requires the greatest energy input?

    (A) $X(g) + \text{energy} \rightarrow X^+(g) + e^-$
    (B) $X^+(g) + \text{energy} \rightarrow X^{2+}(g) + e^-$
    (C) $X^{2+}(g) + \text{energy} \rightarrow X^{3+}(g) + e^-$
    (D) $X^{3+}(g) + \text{energy} \rightarrow X^{4+}(g) + e^-$

25. The molecule below is an example of a(n)

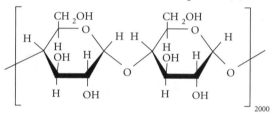

    (A) polysaccharide.
    (B) monosaccharide.
    (C) disaccharide.
    (D) oligosaccharide.

26. Which of the following possesses a trigonal planar geometry?

    (A) NH_3
    (B) BF_3
    (C) $AlCl_{4-}$
    (D) AsH_3

27. What is the Cl-C-Cl bond angle in CCl_4?

    (A) 90°
    (B) 109.5°
    (C) 120°
    (D) 180°

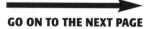

GO ON TO THE NEXT PAGE

28. Diamond and graphite are both composed of carbon, but they have different properties. What is the best explanation for this?

    (A) They are composed of different isotopes of carbon.

    (B) The arrangement of carbon atoms in the crystal structure of diamond is different from that in graphite.

    (C) Graphite contains impurities that make it black.

    (D) Graphite contains macromolecules at the lattice points.

29. Which of the following contributes to the primary structure of a protein?

    (A) Dipole-dipole interactions

    (B) Hydrogen bonds

    (C) Peptide bonds

    (D) Dispersion forces

30. In the phase diagram below, which letter represents the solid phase of a substance?

    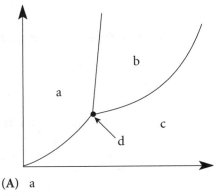

    (A) a

    (B) b

    (C) c

    (D) d

31. In a double-bonded carbon atom:

    (A) hybridization between the *s* orbital and one *p* orbital occurs.

    (B) hybridization between the *s* orbital and two *p* orbitals occurs.

    (C) hybridization between the *s* orbital and three *p* orbitals occurs.

    (D) no hybridization occurs between the *s* and *p* orbitals.

32. In the equation below, what is the value of X?

    $3Ag(s) + XH^+(aq) + NO_3^-(aq) \rightarrow 3Ag^+(aq) + NO(g) + 2H_2O(l)$

    (A) 1

    (B) 2

    (C) 3

    (D) 4

33. The hybridization of the carbon atom and the nitrogen atom in the ion CN^- are

    (A) sp^3 and sp^3, respectively.

    (B) sp^3 and sp, respectively.

    (C) sp and sp^3, respectively.

    (D) sp and sp, respectively.

34. What is the overall order of a reaction where rate = $k[A][B]^2$?

    (A) 0

    (B) 1

    (C) 2

    (D) 3

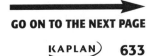

35. The reaction profile for the process A + B →
C + D is shown below. Which of the following
graphs represents the same reaction when a
catalyst is added?

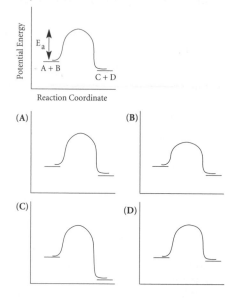

36. The unbalanced redox reaction shown below
occurs in a solution of aqueous base. Which
species is the reducing agent?

$$K_2Cr_2O_{7(aq)} + KClO_{(aq)} \rightarrow Cr(OH)_{3(s)} + KClO_{3(aq)}$$

(A) Cr in $Cr_2O_7^{2-}$
(B) Cl in ClO^-
(C) Cr in $Cr(OH)_3$
(D) Cl in ClO_3^-

37. Molecular orbitals can contain a maximum of

(A) one electron.
(B) two electrons.
(C) four electrons.
(D) $2n^2$ electrons, where n is the principal
quantum number of the combining atomic
orbitals.

38. If the pOH of a solution is equal to 4, what is the
[H+] concentration?

(A) 10^{-14} M
(B) 10^{-10} M
(C) 10^{-7} M
(D) 10^{-4} M

39. Boron found in nature has an atomic weight of
10.811 and is made up of the isotopes ^{10}B (mass
10.013 amu) and ^{11}B (mass 11.0093 amu). What
percentage of naturally occurring boron is made
up of ^{10}B and ^{11}B, respectively?

(A) 30%, 70%
(B) 25%, 75%
(C) 20%, 80%
(D) 10%, 90%

40. Which of the following is the strongest acid?

(A) HI
(B) HBr
(C) HCl
(D) HF

Questions 41–42 refer to the following kinetic rates:

Trial 1	$[A]_o$ (M)	$[B]_o$ (M)	rate (M/min)
1	1×10^{-2}	3×10^{-3}	2×10^{-3}
2	1×10^{-2}	6×10^{-3}	8×10^{-23}
3	2×10^{-2}	1.2×10^{-2}	3.2×10^{-2}

41. What is the reaction order with respect to A?

(A) 0
(B) 1
(C) 2
(D) 3

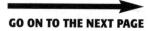

GO ON TO THE NEXT PAGE

42. What would be the initial rate of the reaction in a fourth trial if $[A]_o = 4 \times 10^{-2}$ M and $[B]_o = 3 \times 10^{-3}$ M?

    (A) 1×10^{-3} M/min
    (B) 2×10^{-3} M/min
    (C) 8×10^{-3} M/min
    (D) 8×10^{-2} M/min

43. How many σ bonds and π bonds are present in the following compound?

    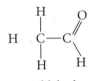

    acetaldehyde

    (A) 6 σ bonds and 1 π bond
    (B) 6 σ bonds and 2 π bonds
    (C) 7 σ bonds and 1 π bond
    (D) 7 σ bonds and 2 π bonds

44. Which of the following will possess the lowest freezing point?

    (A) 0.1 m Na_3PO_4
    (B) 0.1 m H_2SO_4
    (C) 0.1 m $C_6H_{12}O_6$
    (D) 0.1 m NaCl

45. The compound below is classed as a(n)

    $$CH_3CH_2C \overset{O}{\underset{N(CH_3)_2}{\diagup}}$$

    (A) aldehyde.
    (B) quaternary ammonium salt.
    (C) amine.
    (D) amide.

46. How many sigma and pi bonds are found in ethyne, CH≡CH?

    (A) $2\sigma, 2\pi$
    (B) $3\sigma, 2\pi$
    (C) $1\sigma, 2\pi$
    (D) $4\sigma, 1\pi$

47. Which of the reactions below is an example of β^- decay?

    (A) $^{60}_{27}C^{\ddagger} \rightarrow\ ^{60}_{27}C + \gamma$
    (B) $^{32}_{15}P \rightarrow\ ^{32}_{16}S + e^-$
    (C) $^{238}_{92}U \rightarrow\ ^{248}_{90}Th + ^4_2He$
    (D) $^{64}_{29}Cu \rightarrow\ ^{64}_{28}Ni + e^+$

48. Which of the compounds below has the shortest carbon-carbon bond length?

    (A) Ethane
    (B) Ethyne
    (C) Ethene
    (D) Benzene

READING COMPREHENSION

Questions: 48
Time: 50 minutes

Directions: Each of the following sets of questions is preceded by descriptive material. After reading the material, select the best answer to each question.

Despite the falling popularity of smoking in the United States, the increase in smoking among young women continues. Whereas older teenage boys appear to have reached a plateau in the early 1970s, with approximately 19 percent smoking, over 26 percent of older teenage girls are now regular smokers.

A 1989 study examined smoking habits among young women as reported by approximately 600 undergraduate women at four Maryland colleges. Researcher Mary Smith and colleagues examined the respondents' description of parental and peer smoking behavior to determine whether these factors were correlated with their smoking behavior.

The researchers first analyzed the effects of parental smoking on the initiation of smoking. Smith views the initiation of smoking as a function of psychosocial rather than physiological influences because the physical effects of nicotine are not felt until later in life. Smoking behavior of the respondents' mothers was significantly associated with the college women's own early smoking behavior. Among respondents with mothers who smoked, 56.9 percent of the daughters had smoked or did smoke, whereas 43.1 percent had never smoked; 46.5 percent of respondents with nonsmoking mothers had smoked or did smoke, whereas 53.3 percent of such respondents had never smoked. The smoking behavior of the father during the initiation stage appears to have little or no effect upon the respondents' smoking behavior.

The next stage of the smoking career, the maintenance of smoking habits, was less significantly related to the smoking behavior of the primary socialization agents. The smoking behavior of the respondents' fathers seemed to have no effect on their smoking maintenance, whereas the smoking behavior of the mother was related only to the frequency of smoking, not the duration of the habit. Of much greater importance to the maintenance of smoking

habits of respondents was the smoking behavior of particular members of her proximal social environment—her closest female friends.

Interestingly, smoking habits of even the closest male members of the respondent's social network seemed to have no bearing upon the frequency and duration of the respondents' smoking behavior. According to Smith, cessation constitutes the third stage of an individual's smoking career; in the Maryland study, cessation was measured by the respondents' categorizations of perceived or actual difficulties associated with giving up cigarettes. Her parents' smoking behavior was not taken into consideration, but the relationship between cessation of smoking and the smoking behavior of members of the respondent's social network was similar to that cited above: only the smoking behavior of female friends was significantly correlated with the respondent's perceived or actual difficulty in breaking her own habit. Smith and her associates concluded that same-sex relationships are important in every phase of a woman's smoking career.

1. According to the passage, a young woman's closest female friends

    (A) have little effect on her smoking habits.
    (B) encourage her to smoke heavily.
    (C) determine whether she will start smoking.
    (D) influence the duration of her smoking habit.

2. The passage suggests that male smoking behavior

    (A) helps to explain female smoking behavior.
    (B) influences the smoking habits of other males.
    (C) affects women's decisions to stop smoking.
    (D) does not account for female smoking habits.

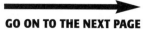

GO ON TO THE NEXT PAGE

3. Which of the following would most seriously weaken Smith's basic argument?

(A) Mothers have influence over the earliest stages of their daughters' smoking careers.

(B) Close female friends influence the duration, but not the frequency, of young women's smoking.

(C) The maintenance of one's smoking habits is heavily influenced by one's economic status.

(D) The smoking habits of both parents significantly influence a daughter's initial decision to smoke.

4. Which of the following most accurately describes the passage?

(A) A refutation of an earlier hypothesis

(B) An explanation of a popular theory

(C) A summary of recent research findings

(D) A description of a controversial study

5. According to the passage, in the early 1970s, the percentage of male smokers

(A) leveled off at 26%.

(B) decreased to 19%.

(C) increased to 26%.

(D) leveled off at 19%.

6. The passage suggests that nicotine

(A) has no effect on smoking behavior.

(B) has less effect than maternal influence on the initiation of smoking.

(C) affects female smokers more than male smokers.

(D) encourages young women to begin smoking.

7. The author's tone is best described as

(A) interested.

(B) emotional.

(C) dismissive.

(D) flippant.

GO ON TO THE NEXT PAGE

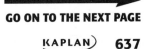

Stress ulceration, a medical condition generally associated with critical illness, is not uncommon for patients in the intensive care setting. It is important to note that physical stressors experienced in intensive care make the patient more susceptible toward contracting an ulcer. However, ulceration can be prevented with the removal of the ulcer-provoking stressors or with the proper prophylactic treatments. In the intensive care setting, stress-related ulceration is commonly seen in patients on respiratory ventilators or in patients with severe burns.

When an individual experiences severe mental or physical stress, the body naturally responds by increasing the production of hydrochloric acid in the stomach and decreasing the production of the protective substances that make up the stomach lining. Healthy individuals possess a thick mucuslike layer that protects the stomach from hydrochloric acid. However, in situations that cause acid hypersecretion or a decreased production of mucoprotective factors, ulceration can occur. Ulcers form when the stomach acid burns through the protective layer of the stomach. Substantial ulceration can cause potentially life-threatening bleeds. Therefore, individuals at risk for developing ulceration should take the appropriate prophylactic measures.

Stress ulceration prophylaxis includes both nonpharmacologic and pharmacologic methods. The most important nonpharmacologic method for the prevention of stress ulceration is removing the patient from the stressful environment. For example, individuals who are on a respiratory ventilator have a dramatically increased chance of contracting an ulcer. The faster the patient is weaned from the ventilator, the better their chances for not developing an ulcer. Unfortunately, the stressor (a respiratory ventilator) cannot always be removed, making pharmacologic ulcer prophylaxis necessary.

Pharmacologic interventions work by neutralizing stomach acid and by inhibiting the production of acid. Frequent administration of antacids is effective in the neutralization of hydrochloric acid in the stomach. Unfortunately, antacids only provide effective ulcer prophylaxis for short periods of time, and they do not prevent acid production. However, acid production can be inhibited by a class of drugs called H2-receptor antagonists. These agents bind to their histamine-2 receptor of parietal cells, the acid-producing cells of the stomach, thereby inhibiting further production of hydrochloric acid.

Both antacids and H2-blockers are effective because they increase stomach pH to the desired level of 3.5. However, both classes of drugs can raise the stomach pH to a much higher level, causing problems for certain individuals. When alkaline levels in the stomach become very high, bacteria may colonize. Aspiration of these bacteria into the lungs can cause pneumonia. Fortunately, the incidence of pneumonia secondary to ulcer prophylaxis is not high. But if it is determined that the individual is at a serious risk for developing pneumonia, a cytoprotective agent may be a better choice because it does not alter stomach pH. Sulcrafate, a cytoprotective drug, is another pharmacologic treatment used in the prevention and treatment of stomach ulceration. Its acts by binding to the ulcerated area in the stomach, providing a protective barrier. Studies show that sulcrafate is less effective than H2-antagonists for the prevention of ulceration.

8. What is the main idea of the passage.
   - (A) Stress ulceration can cause a life-threatening gastrointestinal bleed.
   - (B) Stress ulcer prophylaxis should be instituted for high-risk patients.
   - (C) H2-blockers are more effective than antacids in preventing a stress ulcer.
   - (D) All patients in the intensive care setting need ulcer prophylaxis.

9. Based on the passage, the BEST way to treat gastric ulceration is to
   - (A) maintain a stomach pH greater than > 3.5.
   - (B) remove the patient from the stressful environment.
   - (C) totally inhibit gastric acid secretion.
   - (D) administer sulcrafate.

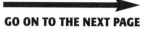

GO ON TO THE NEXT PAGE

10. It can be inferred from the passage that the author

    (A) believes every patient in the intensive care setting should receive ulcer prophylaxis.

    (B) favors the use of sulcrafate over H2-antagonists.

    (C) feels ulcer prophylaxis may harm certain individuals.

    (D) feels that the severe stressors imposed upon people in the intensive care setting can usually be resolved.

11. Suppose an individual who has just experienced a severe heart attack is put into an intensive care unit and becomes severely agitated. The patient has a history of gastrointestinal problems and is at a risk for developing pneumonia. Based on this information and the information in the passage, what would be the best thing to do? Assume the patient is not on a ventilator.

    (A) Nothing should be done because the individual is not on a ventilator.

    (B) Treat the patient with large doses of antacids and monitor the patient.

    (C) Treat the patient only if an ulcer develops.

    (D) Treat the patient with a cytoprotective agent, and monitor the patient.

12. It can be inferred from the passage that the author

    (A) feels that a cytoprotective agent may be more beneficial than an H2-blocker for patients at risk of developing pneumonia.

    (B) believes everyone in an intensive care setting will develop an ulcer; therefore, ulcer prophylaxis should be instituted in all intensive care patients.

    (C) will never recommend the use of antacids over H2-blockers.

    (D) would recommend the use of a pharmacologic method of treatment over the use of a nonpharmacologic method of treatment.

13. Based on the passage, which of the following is NOT true concerning H$_2$-antagonists?

    (A) They may be used for stress ulcer prophylaxis.

    (B) They inhibit cellular activity.

    (C) They may contribute to an aspiration pneumonia.

    (D) They prevent bacterial colonization in the stomach.

14. The author mentions that "antacids only provide effective ulcer prophylaxis for short periods of time, and they do not prevent acid production" for all of the following reasons EXCEPT:

    (A) They are ineffective for long-term treatment.

    (B) To be effective, they must be administered frequently.

    (C) They are less effective than H2-blockers for raising the stomach pH.

    (D) They are often used in conjunction with another agent in order to be effective.

15. It can be inferred that the author regards stress ulceration as

    (A) a serious condition, but it is not fatal.

    (B) an interesting condition that needs further research.

    (C) a condition that should not occur when the patient is treated appropriately.

    (D) a condition that is not serious because there are many medications that can effectively treat ulcers.

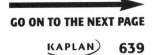

The deadly nightshade is one of the most potent and dangerous botanicals found in nature. Pharmaceuticals derived from the plant are of great importance to modern medicine and are widely used as antispasmodics, antidiuretics, sedatives, cardiostimulants, and opthamological treatments. However, if the extracts of the deadly nightshade are administered in excessively large doses, they can cause hallucinations and even convulsions.

The scientific name of the deadly nightshade (*Atropa belladonna*) has quite an interesting etymology. *Atropa* comes from the Greek term *atropos*, which means "inflexible," referring to the irreversibly poisonous nature of the drug. *Belladonna*, on the other hand, comes from a more historical reference. In Italy, during the Renaissance, women administered the extract of the deadly nightshade to their eyes, which caused mydriasis. It was thought that dilated pupils were striking and seductive; therefore, this plant was used by fashionable women of the period in their attempt to become *belladonnas*, Italian for "beautiful women."

The extracts of the deadly nightshade have anticholinergic effects, acting as antagonists to the parasympathetic nervous system. Products derived from the plant act as cardiostimulants, and they also inhibit salivation, lacrimation, urination, defecation, and digestion. These anticholinergic drugs are commonly used in many cold and cough preparations because of their "drying effect." Anticholinergic medications relieve the symptoms of sinus drainage by drying up the nasal passage. However, a patient taking anticholinergic medication may also experience adverse effects, such as a dry mouth or possibly even urinary hesitancy or constipation.

Two of the most common drugs extracted from the deadly nightshade are atropine and scopolamine. Because dilated pupils aren't considered desirable in modern society, atropine is no longer used to enhance beauty. Now opthamologists use atropine to view the retina of the human eye. When the pupil fully dilates, any excessive light can damage the retina; thus, doctors need to protect patients' eyes. Atropine is also used to treat inflammatory conditions of the iris. Ironically, scopolamine, once used by witches to cause the delusion of flying, is now used to prevent motion sickness.

16. Atropine in large doses can cause all of the following physiologic effects EXCEPT
    (A) pupillary dilation.
    (B) hallucination.
    (C) lacrimation.
    (D) convulsions.

17. Belladonna extract causes the iris to
    (A) increase in size.
    (B) decrease in size.
    (C) maintain a constant size.
    (D) become inflammated.

18. Which part of the botanical name refers to the toxic nature of the plant?
    (A) *Bella*
    (B) *Atropos*
    (C) *Donna*
    (D) *Atropa*

19. Which of the following does not demonstrate atropine's effect on the parasympathetic nervous system?
    (A) Constipation
    (B) Urinary hesitancy
    (C) Dry eyes
    (D) Congestion

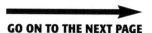

GO ON TO THE NEXT PAGE

20. Based on the passage, the parasympathetic nervous system normally causes the heart rate to

    (A) increase.
    (B) decrease.
    (C) not change.
    (D) increase then decrease.

21. What condition could best be treated with an extract of the deadly nightshade?

    (A) Fast heart rate
    (B) Diarrhea
    (C) Xerostomia (dry mouth)
    (D) Hallucinogenic overdose

22. It can be inferred from the passage that the author

    (A) doubts the folklore stories of the belladonna plant.
    (B) underestimates the pharmacological effects of the plant.
    (C) would promote cautious use of belladonna products.
    (D) believes that alternative medications would be better to use.

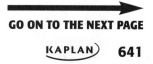

Hypercalcemia, an electrolyte abnormality, can cause various systems in the body to malfunction, such as the cardiovascular, central nervous, renal, neuromuscular, and gastrointestinal. High calcium levels can cause serious, even fatal, consequences. Normal blood calcium levels range between 8.5 and 10.5 mg/dL. Severe hypercalcemia is defined by a blood calcium level greater than 13 mg/dL. At this blood concentration, the individual is generally symptomatic, and the most appropriate medical treatment needs to be instituted because of the risk of fatality. High-risk individuals, those with either cancer or hyper-parathyroidism, need their blood calcium levels closely monitored. Physical assessment of the hypercalcemic individual is crucial in determining the severity of the hypercalcemia because an overly aggressive treatment can be just as harmful as no treatment.

The method of treatment depends on many factors, including blood levels as well as the hypercalcemic patient's clinical presentation. For example, if the concentration of calcium in the blood is near 13 mg/dL and the patient is not showing any severe clinical signs or any symptoms of toxicity, then a mild form of treatment should be instituted. When treating hypercalcemia, it is very important to not "overtreat" the patient because of the risk of hypocalcemia. Ultimately, the objective of treatment is to obtain a normal blood calcium level.

Hydration, supplemented with sodium and potassium, is the primary treatment for non-life-threatening hypercalcemia. This increases blood volume, thereby lowering calcium levels via a dilution-like effect. This treatment produces a healthy calcium output in the urine because when sodium is excreted in the urine, it will take calcium with it. If the hydration treatment alone fails, forced diuresis may be implemented, along with continued hydration. Forced diuresis is generally achieved with the use of "loop diuretics," effective in lowering calcium levels. However, they also lower blood potassium levels, sometimes producing hypokalemia. Ironically, a rebound hypercalcemia may result. Therefore, potassium needs to be supplemented during forced diuresis treatment. If forced diuresis is unable to lower calcium levels, a more aggressive approach needs to be chosen.

Biphosphonates, such as pamidronate, are considered to be the drugs of choice for treating severe hypercalcemia because they quickly lower calcium levels by exerting an antiosteoclastic activity without causing any severe side effects. Plicamycin, an antineoplastic agent primarily used in the treatment of testicular cancer, can also be used to treat hypercalcemia because of its ability to induce hypocalcemia. Plicamycin is particularly useful for treating cases of hypercalcemia that are secondary to cancer.

In the event that all of the previously mentioned therapies fail or in a severely emergent situation, calcium levels can be quickly lowered with dialysis, either hemodialysis or peritoneal dialysis. Dialysis physically removes the calcium from the body by mechanical means. Another way to quickly lower blood calcium levels is via the administration of EDTA. The EDTA binds free calcium, forming an EDTA/calcium complex that is eliminated renally. EDTA is not a firstline agent in treatment of hypercalcemia because of its unfavorable, and even toxic, side effect profile.

23. The author would agree with all of the following statements concerning hypercalcemia EXCEPT:

    (A) An individual with a blood calcium level greater than 13 mg/dL will generally be symptomatic for hypercalcemia.

    (B) There are many ways to effectively treat hypercalcemia, and the condition of the individual will aid in choosing the proper treatment.

    (C) Overtreatment of hypercalcemia can be just as harmful as no treatment at all.

    (D) The blood calcium level is the most important factor in choosing the most appropriate method of treatment.

24. Based on the passage, what can loop diuretics do to blood calcium levels?

    (A) Decrease only

    (B) Increase only

    (C) Decrease and increase

    (D) No change in calcium levels

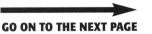

GO ON TO THE NEXT PAGE

25. Based on the information in the passage, what should be done to an individual who has a calcium blood level of 13 mg/dL?

    (A) Nothing should be done.
    (B) Start administering biphosphonates.
    (C) Start dialysis.
    (D) Determine the symptomatology of the individual and treat based on results.

26. If EDTA lowers blood calcium by binding to calcium ions in the blood, which of the following statements must be true?

    (A) Calcium bound to EDTA may still be toxic.
    (B) EDTA is a nontoxic substance.
    (C) Calcium is more likely to be eliminated when it is bound to EDTA.
    (D) As the concentration of EDTA is increased, the free calcium will increase.

27. In paragraph 2, the author states that hydration and forced diuresis should not be used in individuals with renal failure. The author most likely mentioned this point because

    (A) individuals in renal failure should not receive any medical treatment.
    (B) individuals in renal failure will not be able to properly excrete the fluid that is added.
    (C) hydration and forced diuresis is an ineffective treatment for hypercalcemia and should not be used in any patient.
    (D) forced diuresis generally leads to hypokalemia.

28. Which of the following would most weaken the idea that asymptomatic individuals with hypercalcemia should not receive the urgent treatment received by symptomatic individuals?

    (A) Nonurgent medical treatment for asymptomatic individuals causes more side effects.
    (B) The incidence of mortality in the untreated asymptomatic population is greater than that of the symptomatic population.
    (C) Urgent treatment has a greater cost associated with it, and most people cannot afford the treatment.
    (D) When treating either an asymptomatic or symptomatic individual, both will leave the hospital at the same time.

29. Calcitonin is a hormone that lowers blood calcium levels by prohibiting calcium release from bones. It can be inferred in the passage that

    (A) calcitonin release is suppressed in testicular cancer patients.
    (B) calcitonin ceases to operate at blood calcium levels above 13 mg/dL.
    (C) patients suffering from hypercalcemia lack sufficient levels of calcitonin.
    (D) calcitonin is unable to prohibit all calcium release from bones in hypercalcemic patients.

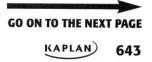

GO ON TO THE NEXT PAGE

There are approximately 300 species of the aloe plant, most of which are indigenous to Africa. The aloe plant, a member of the Liliaceae family, has been used for thousands of years in the treatment of many different conditions. The species most commonly used for medicinal purposes, *Aloe barbadensis*, has fleshy gel-filled leaves with spiny protrusions at the margins. Aloe vera, a gel-like substance obtained from the fleshy leaves of the plant, is typically used to provide medicinal benefit. The name *aloe vera* comes from the Arabic word *alloeh* meaning "shining, bitter substance" and from the Latin word *verus*, which means "true."

The aqueous, gum-like juice of the *Aloe barbadensis* has been used for many years in the treatment of burns, abrasions, and other skin irritations by the native people of the countries where the plant is indigenous. For example, Native Americans would split the leaves and apply them directly to wounds and other skin irritations to promote the healing process. Today, aloe vera is primarily recommended for the topical treatment of minor burns, such as sunburns, thermal burns, and even radiation burns. Commercial preparation of aloe vera for medicinal purposes consists of blending the gel contained inside the leaf with a lanolin base. Lanolin functions as a buffer, preventing any skin irritation caused by the acidic pH of the crude gel-like substance derived from the aloe plant. The commercial product has a cool and soothing effect on the skin. It is also recommended for topical use in other skin conditions, such as general skin irritations, hemorrhoids, eczema, and minor skin ulcerations.

Aloe is effective in these conditions because it is believed to have antiinflammatory, bacteriostatic, and anesthetic properties. The proposed mechanism for aloe's antiinflammatory property involves a substance found in the aloe gel called bradykininase. It appears that bradykininase decreases levels of thromboxane B_2 and prostaglandin F_2 alpha. Under normal conditions, these substances increase the inflammatory response. The antimicrobial action of aloe gel is not yet understood. However, in the presence of the aloe gel, many of the bacteria that commonly cause skin infections, such as the staphylococci and streptococci species, tend to grow at a slower rate. Aloe gel has also been shown to decrease the growth rates of several different fungi species, such as candida and trichophyton. It appears that aloe vera gel is able to weakly stunt bacterial and fungal growth. The weak anesthetic properties of the aloe vera gel are believed to be because of its ability to penetrate and moisturize the skin, which decreases irritation of the nerve endings.

In addition to aloe's healing power on the skin, it produces a cathartic effect when taken orally. The latexlike derivative of the plant provides a laxative effect by acting primarily in the large intestine. However, aloe tends to elicit a rather dramatic cathartic effect, producing profound irritation on the large intestines, which in turn leads to other gastrointestinal problems. When used for cathartic purposes, aloe generally causes the user great discomfort. Consequently, many authorities advocate the use of better-tolerated cathartic substances.

Aloe vera possesses many different medicinal properties and has been referred to as "nature's miracle plant" because of its many uses and minimal side effects. It generally ensures the patient relief from pain and itching while also minimizing skin ulceration. Aloe vera has been used for many years and will probably continue to be used for many more in the treatment of minor skin ailments.

30. Which of the following statements is FALSE?

   (A) *Aloe barbadensis* is a member of the Liliaceae family.
   (B) Aloe may be effectively used as a laxative.
   (C) Aloe may be used in the treatment of minor skin ulcerations.
   (D) Aloe does not prevent bacterial growth.

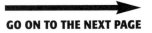

GO ON TO THE NEXT PAGE

31. According to the passage, all of the following statements are true EXCEPT:

    (A) Aloe vera is not generally recommended for use as a laxative.

    (B) Aloe vera may effectively treat many minor skin conditions.

    (C) Traditional Native American use of aloe vera is similar to use of aloe vera today.

    (D) Aloe vera may be used effectively to treat skin infections.

32. Based on the passage, it can be inferred that the author would disagree with which of the following statements?

    (A) Aloe vera should be used in the treatment of human ailments.

    (B) Aloe vera may provide therapeutic benefits that have not yet been discovered.

    (C) Aloe vera should not be used to treat skin infections.

    (D) Aloe vera can be used for the treatment of burns.

33 Based on the passage, which of the following would aloe vera treat LEAST effectively?

    (A) Skin burns caused by radiation

    (B) Inflammation of the skin caused by a bug bite

    (C) Wind burn

    (D) Inflammation of the colon

34 Drug X inhibits the production of prostaglandins; therefore, it possesses what kind of property?

    (A) Bacteriocidal

    (B) Bacteriostatic

    (C) Antiinflammatory

    (D) Anesthetic

35. It can be inferred from the passage that when Native Americans placed pure aloe gel on a wound it

    (A) killed any bacteria instantly.

    (B) caused a burning sensation because of a lack of lanolin.

    (C) caused the entire area around the wound to go numb.

    (D) stopped bacterial growth.

36. The author probably mentioned that "aloe produces a dramatic cathartic effect...which, in turn, leads to other gastrointestinal problems" in order to

    (A) prevent possible death caused by aloe vera toxicity.

    (B) promote the use of aloe as a laxative.

    (C) emphasize the fact that aloe is preferably used as a topical agent.

    (D) prevent someone from killing all the "good bacteria" that normally grow in the intestinal tract.

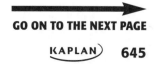

A behavior as complex as sleep—with its highly differentiated component non-REM and REM phases—is unlikely to be dedicated to any one particular function, yet folk wisdom has tended to collaborate with scientific reductionism in supposing that one, and only one, function is served by sleep. The universal favorite candidate for this function is rest. This is probably the carryover of the naive notion that in sleep, our brains are at a low and monotonous level of activity. Yet in spite of years of research, science has not definitely established even one function for sleep.

It is at least logically appropriate to assume, as our mothers did, that sleep is necessary for health since we subjectively experience sleep as restful and restorative. So overwhelmingly clear is the sense of restoration following a good night of sleep that no one in his or her right mind would abandon the rest theory despite the deafening silence of physiology on this question. In this sense, the subjective experience of sleep should more powerfully motivate us to seek physiological or behavioral explanations, just as the experience of dreaming should have motivated scientists to look for evidence of brain activation during sleep.

But the rest theory is likely to require a more specialized answer in the case of the kind of sleep we humans share with our fellow mammals. The reason is that rest does not require sleep. Inactivity alone should suffice to provide us with rest. And many organisms already spend a good deal of their wake-state time at rest.

The rest function may well be further elaborated in higher animals with complex brains so as specifically to restore efficiency to such crucial wake-state functions as attention and memory. Such rest is likely to be associated with more active processes than the simple passive one the rest theory would imply. For example, while the brain-mind is freed of the task of monitoring and remembering new information in sleep, it can review and reorganize its own already acquired data. It is in this sense that most of the new hypotheses arising from modern sleep research distinguish themselves from Freud's contributions and those of his contemporaries and predecessors.

The reason it has been difficult to establish convincing functional hypotheses is, as usual, methodological. The most obvious experimental approach to functional questions is to deprive people of sleep and then observe any behavioral deficits. But anyone who has undergone a night of self-imposed sleep deprivation will know that this approach is not only painful but difficult. So many things need to be done to keep oneself awake that it is virtually impossible to control for nonspecific and unintentional effects of the deprivation procedure itself. These nonspecific procedural factors may cause the deficits in performance. And despite all efforts to stay awake, we doze off anyway!

Preferable to sleep deprivation would be some measure of brain function (or behavioral capability, or psychological process) that could be tested around the clock and be found to (1) deteriorate as the wake period is prolonged and (2) recover dramatically following an epoch of sleep. This positive functional model, in which sleep would be shown to reverse a process that declines progressively in waking, has never been successfully applied to any functional question.

Even if one were successful in completely preventing sleep and effectively controlling the inadvertent side effects of deprivation, one would then have to move to a molecular or cellular neurobiological approach to understand the positive effects of such deprivation. Researchers have convincingly demonstrated that sleep loss can be fatal. Sleep-deprived rats fail to regulate their energy and literally consume themselves metabolically. Now the question is: How are such effects mediated? This example shows clearly that sleep deprivation per se is only an instrumental tool; it is not an analytic probe. It may help us to ask the right question, but it can never, by itself, give us the answers we seek.

From J. Allan Hobson, *The Dreaming Brain.* © 1988 by Basic Books, Inc.

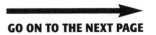

GO ON TO THE NEXT PAGE

37. The passage suggests that sleep researchers' inability to establish "convincing functional hypotheses" indicates that

    (A) the hypotheses of Freud and his predecessors must still be considered potentially valid.

    (B) the theory that the purpose of sleep is to allow the organism to rest must be eliminated.

    (C) researchers have experienced difficulty devising an appropriate experimental approach.

    (D) sleep may not have any particular function aside from rest.

38. Which of the following, if true, would most weaken the author's argument against the theory that the sole function of sleep is simply to provide passive rest?

    (A) Folk wisdom and science seldom agree in their explanations of natural phenomena.

    (B) Selective deprivation of sleep during each of its component phases has varying behavioral effects.

    (C) Some species of mammals spend over 50 percent of their awake time at rest.

    (D) Measures of attention and memory remain stable regardless of time spent in sleep.

39. On the basis of the author's comments in the second paragraph about our subjective experience of sleep, it is reasonable to conclude that the author believes that

    (A) subjective experience can stand alone as sufficient evidence to prove a theory about bodily functions correct.

    (B) dreaming subserves some sort of physiological restorative function.

    (C) a lack of scientific evidence for a theory does not automatically invalidate it.

    (D) subjective experience can always be relied upon as an accurate source of information.

40. Although no supporting evidence is provided, the author claims that

    (A) the function of sleep cannot be determined simply by observing the effects of sleep deprivation.

    (B) brain activity is at a low and monotonous level during sleep.

    (C) many organisms spend a good deal of their wake-state time at rest.

    (D) sleep deprivation can be fatal.

41. According to the passage, sleep deprivation is difficult to study for all of the following reasons EXCEPT:

    (A) Appropriate rooms for such study are unavailable.

    (B) It is difficult to keep subjects awake for long periods of time.

    (C) It is painful.

    (D) Subjects tend to doze off easily.

42. Suppose that a medical resident, who must stay awake during work shifts of 36 hours' duration, is given a simple memory test at the beginning and the end of one such shift. Her score is found to be significantly lower at the end of the shift. Which of the following responses is most consistent with the passage?

    (A) The experiment establishes that sleep deprivation affects memory function but doesn't provide information as to how this occurs on a molecular level.

    (B) The reason memory capacity decreased is that the resident was required to retain a lot of new information and wasn't able to review and reorganize it during sleep.

    (C) Because many factors could have affected the resident's memory capacity over the course of the shift, it cannot be concluded that the memory deficit was the result of sleep deprivation.

    (D) The resident's memory should have been tested during the work shift as well as before and after.

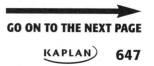

43. The author believes all of the following concerning the positive functional model EXCEPT:

    (A) Brain functioning would decrease in direct correlation to the number of hours a subject is awake.

    (B) Sleep reverses that which occurs to the brain during an active day.

    (C) It should be successfully applied to a functional question.

    (D) Recovery of behavioral capabilities would occur very slowly after a full night's sleep.

44. Which of the following would be the best example of the successful application of the author's "positive functional model" to a sleep-function question?

    (A) A subject's mood is evaluated before and after sleep deprivation and is found to have been improved by deprivation.

    (B) The overall level of brain electrical activity in a subject is measured over a 24-hour period and is found to oscillate regularly.

    (C) The concentration of a neurotransmitter in a subject's brain is found to decrease over the course of the day but is restored after sleep.

    (D) A subject's reading speed is tested after a night of sleep and is found to be nearly identical to the previous day's rate.

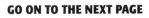

GO ON TO THE NEXT PAGE

Acute asthma attacks, which consist of shortness of breath, wheezing, and coughing, are known to be triggered by environmental allergens such as dust or pollen. Exposure of the asthma sufferer to these allergens precipitates an immune reaction, which rapidly leads to bronchospasm (contraction of the smooth muscle in the airways) and increased mucus secretion, with the result being the obstruction of airways. Treatment of acute attacks focuses on relaxing the constricted airway: patients are given beta-adrenergic agonists to inhale during an attack.

It was recently recognized, however, that asthma consists of more than just intermittent, acute attacks. The asthma patient's airways are in fact persistently inflamed, and this inflammation exacerbates the hyperresponsiveness of the airways to the allergens. Many chemical mediators found in the airways are believed to play a role in the process of inflammation. Research on some of them, particularly leukotrienes, has been carried out in the hope that new anti-inflammatory therapies for asthma patients could be developed.

Leukotrienes are synthesized by cells in the airways in response to an allergen. First, the enzyme 5-lipoxygenase acts upon arachidonic acid to generate leukotriene A4. The 5-lipoxygenase does not work alone; arachidonic acid must be bound to the membrane-bound protein 5-lipoxygenase-activating protein (FLAP) for 5-lipoxygenase to work. Then, leukotriene A4 may be converted to any of the sulfidopeptide leukotrienes (LTC4, LD4, LE4) or to leukotriene B4. Finally, the cell secretes the leukotrienes into the extracellular fluids, where they seem to have a number of effects that contribute to inflammation.

Inhibitors of both 5-lipoxygenase and of FLAP have been developed by pharmaceutical companies, and early clinical studies indicate that they do indeed mitigate the severity of the symptoms of asthma. The question of their safety remains, however, since the normal physiological role of leukotrienes is not known. It may be possible that using inhibitors of leukotriene synthesis to treat chronic asthma would have the undesirable side effect of knocking out an important physiological mechanism.

45. Based on the passage, what is the primary cause of asthma?
    (A) Airway obstruction
    (B) Airway constriction
    (C) Spirometry
    (D) Shortness of breath

46. Cells in the airways respond to allergens by
    (A) increasing the heart rate
    (B) deactivating 5-lipoxygenase.
    (C) secreting eosinophils.
    (D) producing leukotrienes.

47. Which is NOT a sulfidopeptide leukotriene?
    (A) LTB4
    (B) LTC4
    (C) LD4
    (D) LE4

48. 5-lipoxygenase inhibitors mitigate the severity of asthma symptoms because they
    (A) relax constricted smooth muscle.
    (B) inhibit the production of arachidonic acid.
    (C) inhibit the synthesis of leukotrienes.
    (D) prevent allergens from causing an immune reaction.

STOP

QUANTITATIVE ABILITY

Questions: 48
Time: 40 minutes

Directions: Choose the **best** answer to each of the following questions.

1. If $f(x) = x^5 + 2x^2 + \dfrac{3}{x}$, then $f(-1) =$

   (A) -11
   (B) -2
   (C) 2
   (D) 6

2. If $(0.06\%)x = \dfrac{\frac{3}{20}}{\frac{4}{5}}$, find x.

   (A) 312.5
   (B) 250.0
   (C) 187.5
   (D) 52.2

3. Frozen vegetables usually cost 19 cents a package. They are on sale at 6 packages for 90 cents. How much will you save if you buy 2 dozen packages at the sale price?

   (A) $2.25
   (B) $1.10
   (C) $1.00
   (D) $0.96

4. Last year, the ratio of juniors to seniors at a certain college was 8 to 7. If the number of juniors this year is 30% greater than last year and the number of seniors this year is 20% greater than last year, what is the ratio of juniors to seniors this year?

   (A) 26:21
   (B) 3:2
   (C) 12:7
   (D) 96:91

5. Find y if $\dfrac{4\frac{3}{4} \times 9 \times 3}{9\frac{1}{2}} = \dfrac{9}{y}$.

   (A) $\dfrac{1}{36}$
   (B) $\dfrac{2}{34}$
   (C) $\dfrac{11}{15}$
   (D) $\dfrac{2}{3}$

6. If the probability that it will rain sometime on Monday is $\dfrac{1}{3}$ and the independent probability that it will rain sometime on Tuesday is $\dfrac{1}{2}$, what is the probability that it will rain on both days?

   (A) $\dfrac{1}{6}$
   (B) $\dfrac{1}{5}$
   (C) $\dfrac{1}{3}$
   (D) $\dfrac{2}{5}$

7. $\dfrac{8}{5} \times 2\frac{1}{4} \times 1\frac{1}{6} =$

   (A) $\dfrac{43}{11}$
   (B) $\dfrac{21}{5}$
   (C) $\dfrac{61}{15}$
   (D) $\dfrac{17}{4}$

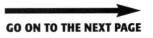

GO ON TO THE NEXT PAGE

8. Which of the following is equal to cos 59°?

    (A) sin 31°
    (B) cos 31°
    (C) sin 59°
    (D) $\cos\left(\frac{1}{59}\right)^{\circ}$

9. Using the definition of the definite integral as the area under the curve, compute $\int_{0}^{6} 2x - 2\,dx$.

    (A) 36
    (B) 18
    (C) −18
    (D) 24

10. If there are 12 women in a group of 18 adults, what fraction of the group is men?

    (A) $\frac{1}{6}$
    (B) $\frac{1}{4}$
    (C) $\frac{1}{3}$
    (D) $\frac{2}{3}$

11. Let $f(x)=x^{3}\,4\,x+2.$ If h is the inverse of f, then $h\theta(2)$ could be

    (A) $\frac{1}{26}.$
    (B) $\frac{1}{4}.$
    (C) $\frac{1}{2}.$
    (D) 2.

12. The integers c and d are positive, and the ratio of $6d$ to V is equal to the ratio of $3c$ to 4. Which of the following is equal to V?

    (A) $\frac{8d}{c}$
    (B) $\frac{8c}{d}$
    (C) $8cd$
    (D) 8

13.

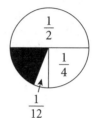

What part of the above circle is shaded?

    (A) $\frac{1}{12}$
    (B) $\frac{1}{6}$
    (C) $\frac{1}{4}$
    (D) $\frac{1}{3}$

14. Evaluate the expression $\frac{6 \times 10^{-4}}{30 \times 10^{5}}$.

    (A) 2×10^{-1}
    (B) 5×10^{-10}
    (C) 2×10^{-10}
    (D) 5×10^{-9}

15. If $\dfrac{x}{\frac{35}{7}-y} = \dfrac{1}{7x}$ and $x = 1$, what is the value of y?

    (A) $\frac{19}{17}$
    (B) −2
    (C) $-1\frac{6}{7}$
    (D) $-\frac{17}{14}$

16. A store sells one brand of candy for 3¢ and another for 4¢. How many combinations of these two brands can a boy buy with a quarter and receive no change?

    (A) 0
    (B) 1
    (C) 2
    (D) 3

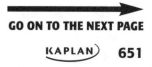

GO ON TO THE NEXT PAGE

17. There are 7 orange disks and 5 green disks in bag X, and there are 5 orange disks and 15 green disks in bag Y. If one disk is selected at random from each bag, what is the probability that both disks selected are green?

    (A) $\dfrac{5}{48}$

    (B) $\dfrac{7}{48}$

    (C) $\dfrac{5}{16}$

    (D) 0.046

18. If 2 cubic feet of liquid weigh 160 ounces, approximately how many ounces does a cubic inch of this liquid weigh?

    (A) 13.33
    (B) 1.11
    (C) 0.092
    (D) 0.046

19. Find $x - y$ if $\dfrac{x}{y} = \dfrac{1}{7}$ and $x + y = 1$.

    (A) 6

    (B) $-\dfrac{5}{7}$

    (C) $-\dfrac{3}{4}$

    (D) $-\dfrac{5}{6}$

20. Let $f(x) = x^3 - x + 2$. If h is the inverse of f, then $h'(2)$ could be

    (A) $\dfrac{1}{26}$.

    (B) $\dfrac{1}{4}$.

    (C) $\dfrac{1}{2}$.

    (D) 2.

    (E) 26.

21. What is the value of the expression $\dfrac{|6 - 12| - |-5 + 14|}{|-7 + 1|}$?

    (A) $-\dfrac{3}{2}$

    (B) $-\dfrac{1}{2}$

    (C) $-\dfrac{1}{3}$

    (C) $\dfrac{1}{2}$

22. Four letters mailed today each have a $\dfrac{2}{3}$ probability of arriving in two days or sooner. What is the probability that exactly two of the four letters will arrive in two days or sooner?

    (A) $\dfrac{4}{81}$

    (B) $\dfrac{16}{81}$

    (C) $\dfrac{6}{27}$

    (D) $\dfrac{8}{27}$

23. If $s''(t) = (t + 1)(t - 3)\sin^2 t$, then the function $s(t)$ has inflection point(s) at

    (A) $-1, 3$.
    (B) -1 only.
    (C) 3 only.
    (D) $n\pi$, where n is an integer.
    (E) $-1, 3$, and $n\pi$, where n is an integer.

24. Of the following pairs of numbers, which has a sum that is 5 less than its product?

    (A) $5 + \sqrt{7}, 5 - \sqrt{7}$
    (B) $4 - \sqrt{3}, 4 + \sqrt{3}$
    (C) $5, 0$
    (D) $6, 2$

GO ON TO THE NEXT PAGE

25. A marksman hits an average of 17 targets out of 20 for each of the first three rounds in a five-round shooting tournament. What must the marksman average for the last two rounds to bring his overall average up to 18?

    (A) 18
    (B) 18.5
    (C) 19
    (D) 19.5

26. In a barrel, there are 60 pints of a solution that is 20% alcohol. How many pints of pure alcohol must be added to produce a solution that is 40% alcohol?

    (A) 12 pints
    (B) 20 pints
    (C) 24 pints
    (D) 50 pints

27. The graph of the differentiable function $y = f(x)$ is shown below. Which of the following is true??

    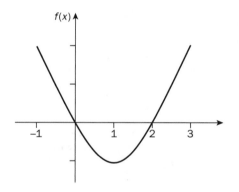

    (A) $f'(0) > f(0)$
    (B) $f'(1) < f(1)$
    (C) $f'(2) < f(2)$
    (D) $f'(1) = f(0)$
    (E) $f'(2) = f(2)$

28. If 42 rolls cost w dollars and 36 doughnuts cost x dollars, what is the cost, in dollars, of 17 rolls and 25 doughnuts?

    (A) $17\left(\dfrac{w}{42}\right) + 25\left(\dfrac{x}{36}\right)$

    (B) $17\left(\dfrac{w}{42}\right) + 25\left(\dfrac{36}{x}\right)$

    (C) $17(42)(w) + 25(36)(x)$

    (D) $42\left(\dfrac{w}{17}\right) + 36\left(\dfrac{x}{25}\right)$

29. Carmen is playing a game in which she draws marbles from a box. There are 50 marbles, numbered 01 to 50. Carmen draws one marble from the box and sets it aside, then draws another marble. If both marbles have the same units digit (such as 14 and 24), then Carmen wins. If the first marble she draws is numbered 25, what is the probability that Carmen will win on her next draw?

    (A) $\dfrac{1}{50}$

    (B) $\dfrac{1}{25}$

    (C) $\dfrac{2}{25}$

    (D) $\dfrac{4}{49}$

30. $\log_{10}(1{,}000) - \log_{10}(100) =$

    (A) 1
    (B) 10
    (C) 90
    (D) 900

31. The mass of the sun is approximately 1.99×10^{30} kg and the mass of the earth is approximately 5.98×10^{24} kg. Approximately how many times the mass of the earth is the mass of the sun?

    (A) 3.0×10^{-6}
    (B) 3.3×10^{5}
    (C) 3.0×10^{6}
    (D) 3.3×10^{6}

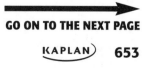

32. A six-sided die is thrown twice. What is the probability that both the sum and the product of the two numbers thrown will be even?

    (A) $\frac{1}{2}$

    (B) $\frac{4}{9}$

    (C) $\frac{1}{3}$

    (D) $\frac{1}{4}$

33. Evaluate $\int_{41}^{2}\left(3x^2\ 4\ 4x+2\right)dx$.

    (A) -2

    (B) 14

    (C) 9

    (D) 18

34. Which of the following includes all solutions to the equation $\sqrt{x^2-7}=7-x$?

    (A) 4

    (B) 7

    (C) 4, 6

    (D) $1+\sqrt{13}, 1-\sqrt{13}$

35. What is the value of x if $\sqrt{0.0036}=0.3+x$?

    (A) -0.24

    (B) -0.30

    (C) 0.06

    (D) $1+\sqrt{13}, 1-\sqrt{13}$

36. If $\frac{2}{5}$ of the animals in a pet store occupy 10 cages, how many animals are in the pet store? (Assume one animal per cage.)

    (A) 20

    (B) 25

    (C) 30

    (D) 40

37. What is the value of y if $\sqrt{\dfrac{3}{y}}-5=10$?

    (A) $\frac{1}{75}$

    (B) $\frac{1}{35}$

    (C) $\frac{1}{25}$

    (D) $\frac{1}{2}$

38. If two fair dice are tossed, what is the probability that the two numbers that turn up are consecutive integers?

    (A) 0.14

    (B) 0.17

    (C) 0.28

    (D) 0.33

39. Consider a continuous function f with the properties that f is concave up on the interval $[-1, 3]$ and concave down on the interval $[3, 5]$. Which of the following statements is TRUE?

    (A) $f''(2) > 0$ and $f''(4) < 0$.

    (B) $f''(2) < 0$ and $f''(4) > 0$.

    (C) $f''(3) > 0$ and $x = 3$ is a point of inflection of f.

    (D) Both (A) and (C) are true.

40. If 40 slices of pizza were divided among three people in the ratio of 1:4:5, how many slices were in the largest portion?

    (A) 4

    (B) 8

    (C) 16

    (D) 20

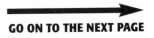

GO ON TO THE NEXT PAGE

41. If c is a positive integer, how many integers are greater than c and less than $2c$?

    (A) $\dfrac{c}{2}$

    (B) c

    (C) $c-1$

    (D) $c-2$

42. If x and y are positive and $10x + 6y = 7x + 8y$, which of the following is equal to $\dfrac{x}{y}$?

    (A) $\dfrac{2}{3}$

    (B) $\dfrac{3}{4}$

    (C) $\dfrac{6}{7}$

    (D) $\dfrac{7}{8}$

43. If $\dfrac{m}{2} = 15$, then $\dfrac{m}{3} =$

    (A) 5.

    (B) 10.

    (C) 15.

    (D) 30.

44. If $x^2 + 2x + 1 = 121$, then x could be equal to

    (A) 10.

    (B) 11.

    (C) 12.

    (D) 120.

45. If $2a - b = 1$ and $4a + b = 17$, then $a =$

    (A) $\dfrac{8}{3}$.

    (B) 3.

    (C) 6.

    (D) 8.

46. If $x < 0$ and $\dfrac{4}{x} < -2$, then x could equal

    (A) -4.

    (B) -3.

    (C) -2.

    (D) -1.

47. If r is positive, r is 30% of s, and s is 40% of t, what percent of t is r?

    (A) 1.2%

    (B) 2%

    (C) 5%

    (D) 12%

48. Suppose $f(x)$ is a differentiable function with $f(1) = 2$, $f(2) = -2$, $f'(2) = 5$, $f'(1) = 3$, and $f(5) = 1$. An equation of a line tangent to the graph of f is

    (A) $y - 3 = 2(x - 1)$.

    (B) $y - 2 = (x - 1)$.

    (C) $y - 3 = 5(x - 1)$.

    (D) $y - 2 = 3(x - 1)$.

STOP

WRITING

1 Topic
Time: 30 minutes

Discuss a solution to the problem of an increased high school dropout rate over the past five years.

---

*Please note: Due to the variable and subjective nature of the possible answers, an explanation is not available for this section of the exam.

STOP

CHAPTER FORTY-THREE

Final Exam Explanations

VERBAL ABILITY

Sentence Completion

1. **C** The context clue *but* after the comma indicates that a contrast is coming. At the beginning of the sentence, you're told that "many" think jazz improvisation first occurred in the 20th century. The second part of this sentence will no doubt dispute this belief.

   A good prediction is: "But it is believed that improvisation has its beginnings in the 17th and 18th centuries."

   Beginning with the choices for the second blank, (**A**) and (**C**) are the closest matches. (**A**) can be eliminated because the first word, *unlikely,* is the opposite of what you're looking for. (**C**) seems to fit both blanks well. Hold onto it and check the others. (**B**) is out because it is idiomatically incorrect to say that improvisation had its "past" in the 17th or 18th centuries. (**D**) doesn't work because the second word, *future,* is illogical. (**E**) also doesn't make sense because the second word, *unity,* is unsupported in the sentence.

2. **A** From key phrases in this sentence, you know that the whales are "peaceful," yet are "savagely hunted." From the tone, you can assume that the author disapproves of the situation. The blank, then, will be filled with something that suggests man's "superior need" is not a real one.

   A prediction for this sentence: "Whales are savagely hunted by man, who argues for superior need or believes he has superior need."

   Choice (**A**) looks good because *assumes* matches the tone and content of this sentence. Choice (**B**) does not work because nothing in the sentence tells you how long this has been going on. Choices (**C**) and (**E**) can be ruled out because they are not consistent with the author's tone. The author thinks it is bad that the whales are hunted. The author would not agree that man "retains" or "manifests" superior need. Both of these answers imply that man has a right to hunt the whales. Choice (D), "assimilates," is not logical in this context. What would the phrase "man assimilates superior need" mean?

3. C   The context clue *yet* between the clauses indicates that there will be a contrast in this sentence. You are told that his "unbridled curiosity" resulted in his exploration of every field, which is a positive thing. The contrast comes when, after the word *yet,* you find out something negative. He wanted to be acknowledged by a society that was "devout." The second blank, describing his stances, must be filled with a word that would not be acceptable to a devout society. Since *devout* means "devoted to religion," the word will have to mean "antireligious." For the first blank, any word that conveys the idea that he explored many different subjects would work.

You can make a pretty definite prediction for the second blank in this sentence, but the first blank could be filled with various words. A partial prediction is "yet his sacrilegious stances kept him at odds with a devout society."

Checking the second word, you are immediately drawn to (**C**) and (**D**), both of which have the meaning of "against accepted religious beliefs." Choice (**C**) looks good for both blanks because "every field of thought" conveys the idea of a wide array of subjects. Choice (**D**) doesn't work for the second blank because "field of hope" doesn't relate to the breadth of his explorations but more to expectations; besides, it's not really clear what the phrase "every field of hope" is meant to signify. Choice (**C**) seems correct, but review the others. There is no reason in (**A**) that his "interesting stances" would be objectionable to a devout society, and "field of science" is too limited. He may have explored much more than just science. In (**B**) and (**E**), *interest* and *study* work for the first blank, but *common* and *optimistic* don't make sense for the second. A devout society would not necessarily reject a common or optimistic stance.

4. D   The blank in this sentence needs a word that describes Harry's personality. He doesn't want a job that will be a "travail." Since travail means hard work, something that is extremely difficult, the missing word will reflect that disposition. Harry doesn't like to work hard.

A good prediction is: "Due to his laziness, Harry avoided jobs that might be a travail."

Choice (**D**), indolence, is perfect because it means "laziness," but look at the others to double-check this answer. Choices (**A**) and (**B**), impudence and insolence, are incorrect because they both describe someone who is disrespectful. Harry just doesn't like to work. Choice (**C**), eminence, means "high rank" or "high repute," neither of which works here. It doesn't make sense that Harry's eminence would make him want to avoid work. Choice (**E**), integrity, can be eliminated. It means honesty and has nothing to do with the desire or lack of desire to work.

5. B   The first blank in this sentence will describe Pacheco's "treatise." (A treatise is a detailed, formal writing.) Later in the sentence, you find out that this treatise contains information on iconography, technique, and contemporary painters. Already this sounds like a broad and significant treatise. This is confirmed after the second blank, when you're told that the treatise is "our most comprehensive information" on these subjects. The word in the first blank will definitely be a positive one.

You can't predict specific words, but you know you're looking for a positive word in the first blank and that the second has to describe how the information is used now.

Looking for a positive word in the first blank leads to (**B**), (**E**), and possibly (**C**). Choice (**C**) does not look very promising because *historical* is neither positive nor negative, and the second word, *lacks,* definitely rules this answer out. It's not logical that a treatise filled with so much information would now lack our most comprehensive information on these topics. Choice (**B**) looks good for both blanks. Even though *important* is a good selection for the first blank in (**E**), the second word, *excludes,* does not make sense. An important treatise, filled with so much information, would not exclude our most comprehensive information. *Choices* (**A**) and (**D**) can be eliminated—the first word in both is negative.

6. **A**   Two important context clues help in this sentence—the semicolon between the clauses and the word however. The semicolon indicates that the two clauses will contain similar thoughts; the second half of the sentence goes on to explain or elaborate upon the first. The word however indicates that even though the second clause will discuss the same topic as the first, something new or different has been brought in. In the first clause, you're told that not much is known about this writer. The second clause tells you that even though you don't know much about him, his writings are "eclectic," which indicates something about him. Since the word eclectic means "drawn from various sources," you can get a sense of what should go in the second blank. Some way or another, Theophilus was exposed to a lot of different information.

A prediction: "From his writings, we can presume him to be well traveled, well educated, or well versed."

Choice (**A**) looks like a good match right away, although (**D**) seems to work as well. Both words in (**A**) are logical and sound correct in the sentence. In (**D**), *expect* is fine for the first blank, but *exposed* doesn't work in the second. It is idiomatically incorrect to say that he was well exposed. Since we can eliminate (**D**), (**A**) looks like your answer. Choices (**B**), (**C**), and (**E**) can be rejected because the second word in each is not consistent with the meaning of *eclectic*. It is from his "eclectic writings" that you can make an assumption about him. So the second blank must be filled with a word that underscores the meaning of eclectic.

7. **D**   The first blank describes the aspect of life that was rewarded by "her systematic approach." From the key phrase, it is likely that this aspect will be found in her work life as opposed to her home life, but confirm that with the other information in the sentence. The word *but* after the comma is a context clue, indicating that there will be a contrast between the two clauses. So her approach is helpful in one aspect of her life but is detrimental in her personal life. The first blank will describe her life at work. The second blank will be filled with a word that describes her mind. You already know from the beginning of the sentence that she has a systematic approach to her research. The second missing word must be a descriptive word that is consistent with this systematic approach.

A prediction: "Her systematic approach was rewarded in her work life but was disastrous when her analytical mind examined every flaw in her friends and family."

Starting with the first blank, two choices fit perfectly, (**A**) and (**D**). Choice (**C**) might seem okay at first, but a public life does not necessarily mean "work." Since there are other selections that are more precise, you don't need one that is not a strong match. Choice (**A**) can be eliminated because the second word, *disorganized,* is contradictory to the sentence. Choice (**D**) is perfect for both blanks. (**B**) and (**E**) can be eliminated because the first word in each is the opposite of what you're looking for. The first blank describes her work life, not her private or family life.

8. **E**   The semicolon is a context clue that this is a sentence with continuity. The second half must agree with the first. If "personal correspondence" reflects the spirit of the age, then "Swift's epistles," or letters, must reflect the spirit of his. That is, whatever quality that is represented by the first blank must also agree with the quality represented in the second blank.

(**E**) works best: *vitriol* is abuse, so this would mirror his society's love of "elegant disparagement." Choice (**A**) can be eliminated because there is no link between profundity and ditties (songs). Choices (**B**), (**C**), and (**D**) can also be eliminated because the words in each are not necessarily linked.

9. C   The context clue *but* before the blank indicates that a contrast is coming. The spokesperson seems unsure of a victory but feels something about facing the alternative. After the comma, you get an idea of what that something is. Apparently, the spokesperson doesn't want to admit it, due to a superstition that just saying it would make it happen.

A good prediction is: "The spokesperson is afraid to face the alternative, as if admitting the possibility would make it happen."

Choice (**C**) is a perfect match. For (**A**) to work, the context clue before the blank would have to be *and*, indicating that the two things are closely linked. The spokesperson is unsure of the victory and unsure of facing the alternative. Even that doesn't make great sense, but *unsure of* will definitely not work with the contrast context clue *but* before the blank. Choice (**B**) is unacceptable, since *complacent* means unconcerned. Choices (**D**) and (**E**) are contradicted in the sentence. If the spokesperson is "uncertain" of the victory, he couldn't be certain of facing the future. And if the spokesperson is fearful of something, as we're told at the end of the sentence, then it's unlikely that he'd feel helped by it.

10. E   Taking a creative work like a play and moving it into another medium is an act of adaptation, so having seen adapted among the choices you might have been drawn right away to correct choice (**E**). And vehicle should not have been problematic for you—the sentence refers to vehicle not as a means of conveyance but as a means of display or expression. We can infer that *La Tosca* was Bernhardt's vehicle in the sense that it was created for her, to display her particular talents. (The purpose of any "star vehicle" is to showcase that star.)

It is incorrect to say that a play is written as a role (**A**)—written "to provide a role" would be more acceptable grammatically—and a work is not *reincarnated* from one medium into another, that verb being best reserved for the reembodiment or rebirth of living entities. The idea of *La Tosca*'s being a biography (**B**) for Bernhardt doesn't make sense (if the play were about her life, *biography of* would work), so this choice is out even though *changed* isn't bad in the second blank. A metaphor (**C**) is a poetic or figurative representation of something, and though we might call a play a metaphor for some event or idea, we would not be likely to do so for a human being; *edited* provides a further complication, in that the process of editing requires pruning and revision, whereas changing a play into a musical drama requires a great deal more firsthand creativity. And while M. Sardou might well have offered *La Tosca* as a present to Mme. Bernhardt (**D**), *fictionalized* won't do; a real-life event can be fictionalized—into a play or an opera—but that verb cannot apply to something that is already fiction.

11. E   If the requirement is that the verdict be a "definite determination," then a judge is pressured to consider a verdict to be definitely determined even when there is some room for doubt. (This analysis is supported by the author's use of the phrases *as if*, meaning something hypothetical, and *when in fact*, meaning that which is actually true.) Thus, if the evidence in a case is not conclusive (**E**), if there is room for doubt as to the guilt of the accused, a verdict based upon it probably will not be self-evident but will have to be treated as such by a judge (in the face of law and custom, that is).

Certainly if the evidence in a case is not persuasive (**A**), if the conclusion stemming from the evidence is debatable, it surely does suggest there's room for doubt. But pressure for a definite determination would hardly force a judge to view a verdict as negotiable, that is, open for debate among the interested parties and possibly subject to revision. On the contrary, the more negotiable the verdict, the less "definitely determined" it's likely to be. *Justified* (**B**) works well—the judge might have to consider this verdict warranted even if the evidence didn't support it—but *accessible* in none of its meanings (easily approached;

obtainable; open to influence) fits the context. Similarly the first words of (**C**) and (**D**), *unassailable* and *incontrovertible* respectively, give us what we need—a verdict that must be seen as a "definite determination"—but their respective second words shoot the choices down. Evidence that's not insubstantial is substantial, and there's no contradiction between an unassailable verdict and one based on substantial evidence. *Admissible* plays on your associations with real-life law, but the issue of whether or not something may properly be brought into evidence is far removed from the author's central point.

12. **A** The author mentioned in this sentence believes that businesspeople are models of some quality; "whatever qualities they may lack" implies that whatever bad points they possess, there's this one particular good thing about them. All of this should lead you to (**A**)—if an author's main characters are businesspeople, and if they're all paragons of ingenuity (meaning inventively talented), one could easily be led to the presumption that the author thinks all businesspeople are clever.

     Several of the wrong answers play off your possible biases about people in the business world, (**B**) being the most blatant in that regard. That choice is tempting only because an author's use of many greedy characters might suggest that that author thinks all businesspeople are covetous. But labeling businesspeople as greedy contradicts the sense of "whatever qualities they may lack"—as we noted, we need a positive quality. (Also, "paragons of greed" is awkward.) One who is morally upright or virtuous (**C**) would hardly be a paragon of deceit (lying, falseness). Characters possessing great ambition (**D**) wouldn't necessarily make one presume that the author believes all such people are successful, since ambition and success in a field don't always go hand in hand; and there's even less connection between characters who demonstrate great achievement (**E**) and a conclusion that, in the creator's opinion, all businesspeople are cautious.

13. **E** The first blank describes what type of budget the film had. The context clue *and* after the word *budget* tells you that the budget and the rate at which the film was edited are either both positive or both negative. Consequently, since the editing was done at a hectic pace, the budget must have been restricted in some way. The context clue *nonetheless* indicates contrast, suggesting that what you would expect after reading the first part of the sentence does not prove to be true. Instead of the negative reaction you would expect from the first part of the sentence, a positive word must describe the critics' responses. The critics must have liked the film even though the budget and editing were done under severe constraints.

     A good prediction for this is: "Filmed on a low budget and edited quickly, the film nonetheless was well received by the critics."

     Starting with the first blank because it is more precise, you are immediately drawn to (**A**) and (**E**). Although in (**A**) *low* works perfectly for the first blank, *disappointed* in the second blank is contrary to the sense of the sentence. Choice (**E**) looks good for both blanks. Choices (**B**) and (**D**) can be eliminated because the second word in each is negative. The second word in (**C**), *pleased*, looks good, but the first word doesn't make sense in describing the budget. How could a budget be "ludicrously uneven?"

14. **D** The "submissions" described must be manuscripts: apparently Ginnie is an author who believes she'll strike gold every time she sends in a story or play. The structural signal *and* suggests that her expectations are going to be taken a step further. Now her optimism will be vindicated (**D**) and she'll be published. That structural signal, by the way, is what keeps (**C**) from being correct: if the signal were *but,* then we'd need a contrast, and Ginnie's "dampened enthusiasm" would contrast strongly with her usual expectations of success. Since Ginnie

always figures that her stuff will be accepted, there's no reason for the sentence to point to her anticipation being piqued (**B**) on this particular occasion: her anticipation is always piqued (aroused, excited). Nothing in the sentence refers to or even hints at Ginnie's habit of speaking frankly, so it would be improper to conclude with a reference to her candor (**A**), dispelled or not. Similarly, Ginnie's perennial optimism about her chances at publication really has nothing to do with her awareness (**E**), but even if you justify it as a reference to "awareness of her chances to be published," a clouded awareness would suggest she's going to get shot down this time and would require a contrast signal like *but* rather than *and.*

15. **B**   No candidate would be pleased at an opponent's "solid support from the voting public," but any candidate would become mighty frustrated if such support continued despite overwhelming reasons why it should cease. In this instance, we can infer that the popular governor remains popular despite the fact that he either doesn't understand "significant issues" or has made foolish choices as to what the "significant issues" are. In line with that analysis, only (**B**) works: if the governor misapprehended, or misunderstood, the issues, how frustrating it would be to his opponent when the public seemed not to care.

You might have been tempted by (**C**) or (**D**), and both are wrong for pretty much the same reason—each is too neutral in tone. The other choices are a good deal worse. It's not clear how a candidate would exaggerate (**A**) significant issues, nor why public support would be expected to erode as result of such overstatement; and a candidate's acknowledgment (**E**) of the key issues—recognition of their existence, perhaps even of their significance—would probably have an effect opposite to the erosion of voter support.

16. **A**   We're told that the fundamental (blank) between cats and dogs is a myth, that the species actually coexist quite (blank). We need a contrast, and we find it in (**A**)—*antipathy* means aversion or dislike, and *amiably* means agreeably.

In (**B**), if the members of the species coexisted uneasily, their disharmony wouldn't be a myth. In (**C**), both *compatibility* and *together* imply that dogs and cats are good friends. In (**D**), it doesn't make sense to say that the relationship between dogs and cats is a myth. In (**E**), no one could claim that there's no difference between dogs and cats.

17. **E**   The clue is the signal *rather than*: we need a contrast between what the speaker intended and what he achieved. The word *monotonous* clues you into boredom, and *bore* in (**E**), followed by *convince,* makes the contrast we need. In (**A**), *enlighten* and *inform* are similar. *Interest* and *persuade,* (**B**), don't show contrast. In (**C**), *provoke* and *influence* don't express a contrast. *Allay* in (**D**) means to relieve, which is similar to *pacify,* which means to calm or to make peace. No contrast here, and again, it's (**E**) for this question.

18. **E**   The blank is part of a cause-and-effect structure as the key word *that* indicates. Because government restrictions are so (blank), businesses can operate with nearly complete impunity. There's an absence of restrictions, so we need a word that cancels out restrictions. Would a traditional restriction, (**A**), be canceled out? No. (**B**), *judicious,* means wise or having sound judgment, but a wise restriction would probably be effective. In (**C**), *ambiguous* means unclear, but though ambiguity might interfere with the effectiveness of restrictions, it doesn't cancel them out. Choice (**D**), *exacting,* means very strict, which is the opposite of what we want. Choice (**E**), *lax,* means loose, careless, or sloppy. This describes restrictions that aren't very strict, and it's correct for this question.

Analogies

19. B The bridge is: a CONDUCTOR oversees the performance of a COMPOSER's work. This fits well with choice (B): a DIRECTOR oversees the performance of a SCREENWRITER's work. (C) and (A) are both tempting but wrong once you look at them.

20. C To become FLUSTERed is to lose your COMPOSURE, just as to become CORRUPTed is to lose your INTEGRITY. (D), *eminence*, means "a state of superiority."

21. D A SWORD holder is called a SCABBARD. Likewise, a GUN holder is called a HOLSTER.

22. D If you can identify ASSENT in this question as a noun meaning "agreement," the bridge is simple: a NOD is an expression of ASSENT. Analogously, a SHRUG is indeed a sign of INDIFFERENCE. Notice the root **bene**, or "good," in (A), *beneficence*, which means "kindliness." (B), *capriciousness* means "Aunpredictability."A

23. D A PERSON is an individual member of a CROWD, just as a STAR is an individual member of a GALAXY.

24. D AMNESIA is loss of MEMORY, just as BLINDNESS is loss of VISION. (A), insight, and (B), *perception*, are synonyms, meaning "the capacity to discern the true nature of a situation."

25. D To WINCE is to flinch. If you feel PAIN, you WINCE. In a similar way, if you feel EMBARRASSMENT, you BLUSH.

26. C The bridge is: "something INFLAMMABLE is easily IGNITED." So, too, something FRAGILE is easily SHATTERED. This question is tricky only if you thought *inflammable* meant "not flammable." However, *inflammable* and *flammable* in fact mean exactly the same thing.

27. C GLASS breaks into SHARDS, just as WOOD breaks into SPLINTERS. None of the other choices is functionally similar to the stem pair.

28. A To DESICCATE is, by definition, to remove the MOISTURE from something. To DEBILITATE is to weaken, or to remove the STRENGTH from something. (B), *augur*, means "to predict the future." (C), *exonerate*, means "to clear of blame."

29. D An ANODYNE is something that brings RELIEF. Aspirin might be said to be an ANODYNE, because it relieves pain. In (D), a SOPORIFIC is something that brings SLEEP.

30. A DILUVIAL means "having to do with a FLOOD," just as CARDIAC means "having to do with the HEART." In (B), *biological* means "pertaining to life." Only in a loose sense would you call a heart biological.

31. B Here the relationship between the two words in the stem is one of degree: someone extremely ATTENTIVE is RAPT. None of the answer choices works except (B): someone extremely CRITICAL is DERISIVE.

32. **C** This question's filled with words from Greek mythology that have taken on more general meanings. In the stem, a sphinx is a mythical winged monster who kills passers-by that attempt and fail to answer her riddle. A sphinx can also be a mysterious person. So the bridge here is "a SPHINX acts in a way that PERPLEXES you." This fits best with (C), because a SIREN acts in a way that LURES you. In mythology, sirens are half-woman, half-animal creatures that lure mariners to their deaths with their seductive songs. The word has now come to mean a woman who sings sweetly or who is seductive.

33. **D** A PIG lives in a STY, just as a HORSE lives in a STABLE.

34. **D** BASEBALL is played on a DIAMOND; BASKETBALL is played on a COURT.

35. **A** A person who is SHACKLEd is a PRISONER, and a person who is CHARGEd, or accused, is a SUSPECT.

36. **B** An ATLAS is a book made up of MAPs; a COOKBOOK is a book made up of RECIPEs.

37. **B** HOWLing is a characteristic noise of WIND; RUMBLing is a characteristic noise of THUNDER.

38. **C** A BRIGAND is an individual member of a BAND; a PERFORMER is an individual member of a TROUPE.

39. **C** If you are PENNILESS, you lack MONEY; if you are CALLOUS, or insensitive, you lack COMPASSION. (B), *haughty*, means "arrogant."

40. **C** Something ASYMMETRICAL is not in BALANCE; something CHAOTIC is not in ORDER.

41. **D** Something NUPTIAL has to do with a WEDDING; something NATAL has to do with a BIRTH.

42. **A** Here's another question where you might look for answer choices that are functionally similar to the words in the stem pair. In the stem pair, to FILTER is to remove the IMPURITY from something. To filter water, for instance, means to remove dirt and sediment from it. Analogously, to EXPURGATE is to remove the OBSCENITY from something, usually from a piece of writing. (B) doesn't fit the bridge because to whitewash is to cover up. In (C), *perjury* is lying during testimony when you've sworn to tell the truth.

43. **B** Note that the two words in the stem pair are rough opposites. If you PARAPHRASE something, it, by definition, will not be VERBATIM, or word for word. Likewise, if you ESTIMATE something, then by definition, it will not be PRECISE.

44. **C** An OSTRICH is unable to FLY; an ELEPHANT is unable to JUMP.

45. **B** To HONE is an extreme form of to SHARPEN; to BURNISH something is an extreme form of to WIPE.

46. **B** HEPATITIS is an inflammation of the LIVER; ENCEPHALITIS is an inflammation of the BRAIN. Word roots can give you clues about the meaning of encephalitis: **en-** (inside), **cephal-** (head), **-itis** (inflammation).

47. **A** Something done in a MINIMALIST style could be described as SPARTAN; something done in a MANNERIST style could be described as OSTENTATIOUS.

48. **B** HIERATIC means relating to the priesthood and thus RELIGIOUS. DEMOTIC means relating to the populace and thus SECULAR.

BIOLOGY

1. **B** This question asks you to identify the aspect of cellular respiration that is correctly paired with its location in the cell. The Krebs cycle enzymes and intermediates are located in the mitochondrial matrix.

    (A) is incorrect because glycolysis occurs in the cytoplasm of the cell, not in the outer mitochondrial membrane. (C) is incorrect because coenzyme A formation occurs in the mitochondrial matrix, not across the inner mitochondrial membrane. (D) is also incorrect because ATP synthesis occurs across the inner mitochondrial membrane, not in the cytoplasm.

2. **A** (A) is true because the superior vena cava and inferior vena cava route deoxygenated blood from systemic circulation into the right atrium.

    Let's review the flow of blood through the heart. Deoxygenated blood from systemic circulation enters the right atrium via the superior and inferior vena cavae. From there, the blood is pumped to the right ventricle, which sends the blood through the pulmonary arteries to the lungs, where it is oxygenated. After the blood is oxygenated in the lungs, it returns to the left atrium via the pulmonary veins. From there, the now-oxygenated blood is pumped into the left ventricle, whose powerful muscle mass propels the blood through the aorta to the systemic circulation.

    Thus, (B) is incorrect because in adults, blood can only pass from atrium to ventricle; it cannot flow between the atria. In the fetus, however, blood can pass between the atria via the foramen ovale. (C) is also incorrect because the tricuspid valve lies between the right atrium and ventricle. The mitral, or bicuspid, valve is located between the left atrium and ventricle. Both of these valves function to prevent backflow of blood into the atria. (D) isn't the correct answer either; the pericardium is the tough connective tissue sac that surrounds the heart, not a network of blood vessels.

3. **B** According to the endosymbiotic hypothesis, chloroplasts may once have been free-living prokaryotic autotrophs that entered into and established symbiotic relationships with primitive eukaryotic host cells. An autotroph is an organism that has the ability to synthesize organic nutrients from an external energy source (sunlight or chemical energy) and simple inorganic material. In time, a symbiotic relationship developed between the two organisms: the host cell provided protection to the bacterium in exchange for the capacity to carry out photosynthesis. Eventually, they became completely dependent upon one another, and the symbionts (now known as chloroplasts) lost the ability to exist outside of their eukaryotic hosts.

    Choices (A), (C), and (D) are all incorrect because they are not in accordance with the endosymbiotic hypothesis.

4. **D** The genetic material of both prokaryotes and eukaryotes is DNA.

   Prokaryotes do not have membrane-bound organelles, so (A) is incorrect. Plasmids are found in prokaryotes only, so (B) is incorrect. Cell walls made of peptidoglycan are found in prokaryotes only, so (C) is incorrect.

5. **A** The kidney is the main organ involved in balancing the inorganic ion level in the body.

   (B) is incorrect because in the kidney, water is moved by the passive process of osmosis. Osmosis is the diffusion of water across a semipermeable membrane; the water molecules tend to move from a region of low-solute concentration to a region of high-solute concentration. (C) is incorrect because the descending loop of Henle is permeable to water, whereas the ascending loop is not. (D) is not the correct answer because glucose, amino acids, and vitamins are reabsorbed in the proximal, not distal, convoluted tubule.

6. **D** DNA replication is semiconservative, which means that with each replication, both daughter DNA molecules contain one old strand and one new strand. So after one molecule of DNA replicates, each daughter molecule would contain 50 percent of the original DNA (each daughter molecule contains an original strand). After a second replication, the original DNA would constitute 25 percent of the total DNA present in the daughter cells (2 of 8 total daughter strands are original DNA). After a third replication, the original DNA would constitute 12.5 percent of the total DNA present in the daughter cell (2 of 16 total daughter strands are original DNA).

7. **D** When you inhale, air enters your body through the external nares (nostrils) and then travels through the nasal cavity, where it is filtered by nasal hairs and mucous. Next the filtered, warmed air travels through the internal nares to the pharynx (throat) and then into the larynx, or voice box. After the larynx, the air travels through the trachea, or windpipe, until it flows into the right and left bronchi. The air then flows into the bronchioles and ultimately into the alveoli, where gas exchange occurs.

8. **C** Enzymes increase the rate of a spontaneous reaction by lowering the activation energy of that reaction.

   (A) is incorrect because enzymes are very selective; they may catalyze only one reaction or one specific class of closely related reactions. (B) is incorrect because reactions that are normally catalyzed by enzymes are able to proceed without enzymes but at a much slower rate. (D) is incorrect because enzymes decrease, not increase, the activation energy of a reaction.

9. **C** This question asks you to identify the statement that is part of the modern evolutionary theory—also called neo-Darwinism—that is a fusion of Darwin's original theory of evolution with modern genetic theory. Darwin's original theory states that the following factors contribute to evolutionary change: 1) Organisms produce more progeny than will survive to reproductive maturity; 2) Heritable chance variations exist between different individuals of a population. The variations that give an individual an advantage are called favorable variations; and 3) If an individual has inherited favorable variations, that individual will live longer and will produce more offspring than others; thus, favorable variations become more common from generation to generation—this theory is also known as natural selection. The modern evolutionary synthesis includes these three factors but also maintains that the source of hereditary variation lies in both mutation and genetic recombination. Some novel gene combinations increase chances of survival, whereas others do not. This leads to differential reproduction, in which individuals with favorable genetic combinations produce more offspring.

(C) is correct because it is part of the modern view of evolution. Individuals who have inherited some trait that allows them to be more successful with respect to the environment (favorable characteristic) are more likely to live longer and produce more offspring than others who have not inherited that trait. This is known as "survival of the fittest."

10. **C** A ribosome is composed of protein and RNA. The two ribosomal subunits are manufactured in the nucleolus, a region within the nucleus. The fact that ribosomes are partly composed of RNA could have clued you in to the correct answer.

Choices (A),(B), and (D) are all incorrect because they refer to organelles that are composed of phospholipid membranes and protein, so they are not manufactured in the nucleus. Rather, they are synthesized in regions of the cell—specifically the smooth endoplasmic reticulum and the ribosomes.

11. **A** Hydrostatic pressure is defined as the force per area that blood exerts on the walls of the blood vessels. A capillary has a higher hydrostatic pressure at the arteriole end and a lower hydrostatic pressure at the venule end. As blood flows from arterioles to capillaries, blood pressure gradually drops because of friction between the blood and the walls of the vessels and the increase in cross-sectional area provided by numerous capillary beds. Thus, (A) is correct, and (B) is wrong.

(C) is incorrect because the pumping force of the heart through the blood vessels creates hydrostatic pressure. (D) is incorrect because blood plasma in the capillaries has a higher osmotic pressure than the osmotic pressure in interstitial fluid. This is a result of the greater amount of dissolved solutes in the blood plasma of the capillaries.

12. **C** During glycolysis, two net molecules of ATP are produced by substrate-level phosphorylation, and two molecules of NAD^+ are reduced to form NADH.

(A) is incorrect because glycolysis is an anaerobic process. Thus, oxygen plays no part in glycolysis. (B) is incorrect because during glycolysis, glucose is partially oxidized, not reduced. (D) is also incorrect because two molecules of pyruvic acid are formed for each molecule of glucose that undergoes glycolysis.

13. **C** When the sperm and egg cell membranes fuse, an electrical response is initiated across the ovum cell membrane. A special membrane called the fertilization membrane forms around the zygote to protect it from the entrance of other sperm.

(A) is incorrect because the sex of an individual is determined at the moment of fertilization, not when the zygote has implanted in the uterus. (B) is incorrect because the sex of an individual is determined by the sperm, not the egg. The egg cell always donates an X chromosome to the offspring, whereas a sperm can donate either an X or a Y chromosome. (D) is incorrect because it states that once an egg is fertilized, the egg cell decreases its rate of oxygen consumption. In actuality, once an egg is fertilized, its rate of oxygen consumption and, subsequently, ATP production, is increased because of the extensive synthesis and division that it undergoes.

14. **D** This question asks you to identify which of the substances listed in the answer choices are not reabsorbed back into the body from the tubules of the nephron. Proteins are too large to filter through the glomerulus of the nephron, so they remain in the blood and never enter the tubules. Thus, the proteins can never be reabsorbed from the nephron tubules.

Choices (A), (B), and (C) all refer to substances that are reabsorbed from the tubules of the nephron and returned to the body. Water is reabsorbed from the proximal tubule, the descending limb of the loop of Henle, the distal tubule, and the collecting duct via osmosis. Glucose is reabsorbed from the proximal tubule by active transport. Amino acids are reabsorbed by active transport from the proximal tubule.

15. **B** Lambda phage has two methods of reproduction, the lytic cycle and the lysogenic cycle. In the lytic cycle, the phage attaches to a host bacterial cell and injects its DNA into the bacterium. The virus uses the nucleotides, enzymes, and ribosomes of the host bacterium to replicate and organizes the DNA and coat proteins into new phages. The host cell bursts, releasing the phages. In the lysogenic cycle, the phage attaches to a host bacterial cell and injects its DNA into the bacterium. The phage DNA is integrated into the genome of the bacterial host, and when the bacterium divides by binary fission, the viral DNA is passed on to daughter cells. (B) is correct since it correctly describes the events of the lysogenic cycle.

(A) is incorrect because it describes the lysogenic cycle, not the lytic cycle. (C) is incorrect because viral DNA is integrated into the host genome in the lysogenic cycle, not the lytic cycle. (D) is incorrect because it describes the lytic cycle, not the lysogenic cycle.

16. **B** Let's first define the alleles in this problem. Let T = tall height and t = short height. Next let's define B = brown eye color and b = blue eye color. The father is described as homozygous tall and homozygous blue-eyed, so we know his genotype is TTbb. The mother is described as heterozygous tall and heterozygous brown-eyed, so her genotype is TtBb. This question asks you to determine the probability that these parents could produce a tall child with blue eyes. Remember, the genes for height and eye color are unlinked. Now, the father can only contribute the T and b alleles, so all of his gametes will have both the T and b alleles. On the other hand, the mother can contribute either T or t and either B or b, so her gametes are the following, all in equal amounts: TB, tB, Tb, or tb. Thus, the possible genotypes of the offspring are: TTBb, TTbb, TtBb, Ttbb. Half the offspring are tall and brown-eyed, and the other half are tall and blue-eyed. Therefore, the probability of a tall child with blue eyes is 1/2 (one of two), or (B).

A shorter method involves calculating phenotype ratios for height and eye color separately and then combining them. The mating of TT × Tt produces 100 percent tall. The mating of Bb × Bb produces 1/2 blue and 1/2 brown. Multiplying 1 tall × 1/2 blue gives us 1/2 tall blue, or (B).

17. **D** The lymphatic system is a secondary circulatory system distinct from cardiovascular circulation. Its vessels transport excess interstitial fluid, called lymph, to the cardiovascular system, thereby keeping fluid levels in the body constant. Lymph capillaries are closed at one end and lead into other lymph vessels that have valves to prevent the backflow of lymph. These lymph vessels then converge in the region of the upper chest and neck where they return lymph to the circulatory system via the thoracic duct, which empties lymph into the jugular vein.

(A) is incorrect because the function of lymph veins is to carry lymph (clear fluid derived from blood plasma) from one lymph node to the next under low pressure. (B) is incorrect because there is no such thing as a lymph artery. (C) is incorrect because lymph nodes are structures along lymph vessels where lymph is filtered by phagocytic leukocytes.

18. **A** During the light reactions, water is broken down into hydrogen ions and oxygen gas molecules.

(B) is incorrect because the light reactions involve two major classes of pigments—

chlorophyll and carotenoids. Chlorophyll is the green pigment responsible for collecting photons. The carotenoids are yellow pigments that act as auxiliary photon collectors; they absorb photons and pass them on to chlorophyll. (C) is incorrect because the light reaction forms NADPH. (D) is incorrect because oxygen, not carbon dioxide, is released.

19. **A** During prophase I of meiosis, homologous chromosomes pair tightly with each other. At this stage, because each chromosome actually consists of two sister chromatids, each synaptic pair consists of four chromatids; therefore, each synaptic pair is called a tetrad. During metaphase I, the tetrads align at the equatorial plane of the dividing cell; during anaphase I, the homologous pairs separate and are pulled to opposite poles of the cell. Thus, (A) is correct because tetrads are present in the same nucleus during metaphase I.

    (B) is incorrect because there are no tetrads present in the same nucleus during interkinesis. Interkinesis is the rest period between meiosis I and meiosis II during which the chromosomes partially uncoil. Choices (C) and (D) are incorrect because there are no tetrads present in the same nucleus during any part of meiosis II. During prophase II, the centrioles migrate to opposite poles, and the spindle apparatus forms. During metaphase II, the chromosomes line up along the equatorial plane, and the centromeres divide, separating the chromosomes into pairs of sister chromatids.

20. **D** This question asks you to identify the enzyme that breaks down two-sugar (disaccharides) molecules into their component one-sugar (monosaccharides) molecules. Lactase hydrolyzes lactose, a disaccharide, into its components, glucose and galactose.

    (A) is incorrect because pancreatic amylase hydrolyzes starch, a polysaccharide, into maltose, a disaccharide. (B) is incorrect because carboxypeptidase hydrolyzes the terminal peptide bond at the carboxyl end of a protein. (C) is incorrect because maltose is a disaccharide composed of two glucose molecules. It is not an enzyme, so it does not have the ability to hydrolyze two-sugar molecules into their component one-sugar molecules.

21. **D** For each glucose molecule that undergoes glycolysis, two pyruvate molecules are produced. You can remember this because glucose is a six-carbon molecule and pyruvate is a three-carbon molecule.

    (A) is incorrect because the Krebs cycle must turn twice to oxidize completely each molecule of glucose that enters the glycolytic pathway. Each molecule of glucose that enters the glycolytic pathway produces two pyruvic acid molecules. In turn, those two pyruvate molecules are decarboxylized, and coenzyme A is added, forming two acetyl CoA molecules that enter the Krebs cycle separately. Thus, the Krebs cycle must turn twice to oxidize completely one molecule of glucose. (B) is incorrect because all specific reactions in the Krebs cycle are catalyzed by specific enzymes, not the same enzyme. Remember enzyme-substrate specificity here—enzymes catalyze only one reaction or a group of closely related reactions (the reactions of the Krebs cycle are not closely related). (C) is incorrect because one acetyl CoA molecule is produced per pyruvic acid molecule.

22. **C** Chitin is a component of the cell wall found in fungi, so chitin is an ideal target for a drug that is specific for fungal cells as opposed to prokaryotic cells. Both fungal cells and prokaryotic cells contain DNA and RNA, so a drug that targets either of these cellular components would be toxic to both fungal cells and prokaryotic cells. (A) and (B) are therefore incorrect. Peptidoglycan is a component of the cell walls of prokaryotes, so (D) is incorrect.

23. **C** Because purines only bond with pyrimidines in double-stranded DNA (and vice versa), the total amount of purines must always equal the total amount of pyrimidines.

(A) is incorrect because adenine and guanine are purines; thymine and cytosine are pyrimidines. An easy way to remember which nitrogenous bases are the pyrimidines is with the mnemonic CUT the PY: **C**ytosine, **U**racil, and **T**hymine are the **PY**rimidines. (B) is also incorrect because RNA is usually single stranded, not double stranded. (D) is incorrect because during complementary base-pairing, thymine always forms two hydrogen bonds with adenine, whereas guanine forms three hydrogen bonds with cytosine.

24. **D** The sarcomere, the unit of contraction in skeletal muscle, is composed of thick and thin filaments. The thick filaments are composed of myosin, and the thin filaments are composed of actin. The sarcomere is divided into different bands and zones, depending on the presence or absence of thick or thin filaments. The A band contains the entire length of the thick filaments and any thin filaments that overlap with the thick filaments. The I band is located between the A bands and is composed of thin filaments only. The H zone is located at the center of the A band and contains thick filaments only. The Z-lines define the boundaries of a single sarcomere and anchor the thin filaments.

If you examine the diagram, you will see that (A) represents the Z-line, (B) represents the I-band, and (C) represents the H-band. Thus, (D) is correct.

25. **B** The question stem asks you to identify the cross of ABO blood types that cannot produce type O offspring. The cross in (C), AB × O, cannot produce type O offspring. In humans, blood type is determined by three different alleles, I^A, I^B, and i. Individuals who are homozygous $I^A I^A$ and heterozygous $I^A i$ have blood type A, meaning that they have the A antigen present on the surface of their erythrocytes. Individuals who are homozygous $I^B I^B$ and heterozygous $I^B i$ have blood type B, meaning that they have the B antigen present on the surface of their erythrocytes. Individuals who are homozygous ii have blood type O or have no antigens on their erythrocytes. Finally, individuals who are heterozygous $I^A I^B$ have the blood type AB, which means that they possess both A and B antigens on their red blood cells. Therefore, you should construct a Punnett square for an AB × O mating. (If you don't know how to construct a Punnett Square, turn to Chapter 9.)

	i	i
I^A	$I^A i$	$I^A i$
I^B	$I^B i$	$I^B i$

The Punnett square reveals that half the offspring will have the $I^A i$ genotype, so phenotypically, they will have type A blood. The other half of the offspring will have the $I^B i$ genotype, so they will have type B blood. As you can see, this mating can't produce type O offspring.

(A) is incorrect because an A × O mating could produce an O offspring if the type A parent was heterozygous ($I^A i$). (C) is incorrect because an A × B mating could produce a type O offspring if the parents had the genotypes $I^A i$ and $I^B i$. (D) is incorrect because an A × A mating could produce a type O offspring if both parents had the heterozygous $I^A i$ genotype. If you are still confused by this, go back through the question, and draw out Punnett squares for each type of mating.

26. **B** Remember, sex-linked traits are located on the X chromosome; therefore, affected females always have two copies of a sex-linked trait—one per X chromosome—whereas affected males carry only one copy of the trait, located on their single X chromosome. Because red-green color blindness is a sex-linked recessive trait, let's define it as X^a and define the normal allele as X^A. The male parent in this problem is normal, which means that he carries the normal allele on his one X chromosome. Thus, his genotype is $X^A Y$. The female parent in this problem is a carrier, which means she is heterozygous for that trait, so her genotype is $X^A X^a$. So construct a Punnett square for this cross:

		female parent	
		X^A	X^a
male	X^A	$X^A X^A$	$X^A X^a$
parent	Y	$X^A Y$	$X^a Y$

The genotypes of the offspring are as follows: $X^A X^A$, $X^A X^a$, $X^A Y$, and $X^a Y$. So as you can see, half of the male offspring will possess the genotype $X^a Y$ and will therefore be red-green color-blind.

27. **A** Cholecystokinin (CCK), a hormone secreted by the duodenal mucosa, stimulates the release of bile from the gall bladder. (B) is incorrect because CCK does not stimulate the pancreas to secrete lactase. The hormone secretin is primarily involved in causing the pancreas to release enzymes such as pancreatic amylase, trypsin and chymotrypsin (both of which are secreted as the zymogens trypsinogen and chymotrypsinogen), carboxypeptidase, and lipase. Lactase is not a pancreatic enzyme. Lactase, the enzyme responsible for the breakdown of lactose into glucose and galactose, is secreted by the intestinal mucosa. (C) is incorrect because it is the hormone gastrin that stimulates the gastric glands to release gastric juices. (D) is incorrect because enzymes (proteases) such as pepsin, trypsin, and chymotrypsin hydrolyze peptide bonds and break down protein molecules into their constituent amino acids.

28. **B** Although you don't have to know the exact amount of ATP that each nutrient yields, you should know that fat yields the most energy per unit weight. Many molecules of acetyl CoA can be formed from each long fatty acid chain. As acetyl CoA subsequently enters the Krebs cycle and undergoes normal aerobic respiration, a large amount of energy can be obtained in the form of ATP.

(A) is incorrect because carbohydrates do not yield the most energy per unit weight. Polysaccharides are converted to monosaccharides, most of which can be converted to glucose or glycolytic intermediates. Then, the monosaccharides undergo normal aerobic respiration. (C) is incorrect because protein is the least efficient energy source per unit weight, and the body degrades protein only when not enough fat and carbohydrates are available. First, proteins are hydrolyzed into amino acids, which subsequently undergo transamination reactions to be converted to a usable form. During transamination, the amino acid loses its amino group, forming an alpha-keto acid. Then the alpha-keto acid is converted to acetyl CoA, pyruvate, or a Krebs cycle intermediate. (D) is incorrect because cellulose is a polysaccharide (a long chain of repeating glucose units), so its energy yield matches that of carbohydrates per unit weight.

29. **D** In this problem, a homozygous red flower was crossed with a homozygous white flower, and the resulting heterozygote was pink. In other words, a cross between contrasting homozygotes yielded progeny with an intermediate phenotype. Incomplete dominance is defined as a genetic effect in which the phenotype of a heterozygote is a reflection of both alleles at a particular locus. Thus, the cross in the question stem illustrates incomplete dominance, so (D) is correct.

   (A) is incorrect because Mendel's Law of Segregation is not being illustrated in the question stem. The Law of Segregation states that every diploid organism has two alleles for every trait and that during meiosis, these alleles segregate, forming gametes that carry only one allele for a given trait. (B) is incorrect because a testcross involves mating of an unknown individual with one who is recessive. The progeny are then examined, and the genotype of the unknown parent is determined. Finally, (C) is incorrect because the cross does not provide an example of nondisjunction. In nondisjunction, homologous chromosomes fail to separate during meiosis, so the resulting zygote will have either three copies of the affected chromosome or just one.

30. **B** Most of the ATP generated in cellular oxidation is produced by the electron transport system. If we recall that 36 molecules of ATP are produced per molecule of glucose, 32 out of the 36 molecules of ATP are produced by the electron transport system.

   (A) is incorrect because oxygen does participate in the electron transport system as the final electron acceptor. (C) is incorrect because the electrons carried by $FADH_2$ do not yield the same number of ATP molecules as do the electrons carried by NADH. Rather, each $FADH_2$ generates 2 ATP, and each NADH generates 3 ATP, except for the two NADH reduced during glycolysis, which generate only 2 ATP. (D) is incorrect because the enzymes of the electron transport system lie in the inner mitochondrial membrane.

31. **A** (A) is correct because it describes skeletal muscle accurately. Skeletal muscles contain many nuclei per fiber and striations, and they are the voluntary muscles that produce intentional physical movement.

   (B) is incorrect because it describes smooth muscle as having cross-striations when, in fact, smooth muscle does not have any striations. Cross-striations are alternating light and dark bands visible under the microscope because of the arrangement of thick and thin filaments in the sarcomere. Smooth muscle is the involuntary muscle found in the visceral systems. (C) is incorrect because it describes cardiac muscle as having many nuclei per fiber when, in fact, cardiac muscle has only one or two nuclei per fiber. Cardiac muscle is the muscle that forms the heart. (D) is incorrect because a correct answer choice can be determined.

32. **C** The three primary germ layers (ectoderm, endoderm, and mesoderm) are responsible for the differential development of the tissues, organs, and systems of the body at later stages of growth. The musculoskeletal system, circulatory system, excretory system, reproductive system, and the connective tissues, including blood, are all derived from the mesoderm. Thus, the heart arises from the mesoderm.

   (A) is incorrect because the intestinal mucosa arise from the endoderm. Endoderm derivatives comprise the lining of the digestive system and the associated glands and organs, including the pancreas and liver. The lungs are also derived from the endoderm, so (B) is incorrect as well. (D) is incorrect because the peripheral nerves arise from the ectoderm. The ectoderm gives rise to the epidermis and nervous system, including the sense organs.

33. **D** The lysosome is a membrane-bound organelle that stores hydrolytic enzymes. A cell may "commit suicide" by rupturing the lysosome membrane and releasing its hydrolytic enzymes, which will digest the cellular contents; this process is referred to as autolysis, and it is an important process during development.

    (A) is incorrect because the Golgi apparatus is an organelle that aids in the packaging and secretion of proteins and other molecules produced intracellularly. (B) is incorrect because the ribosome is the site of protein synthesis. (C) is incorrect because the mitochondrion is the site of aerobic respiration.

34. **B** A nuclear membrane is not found in prokaryotes, since prokaryotes have no nucleus and no membrane-bound organelles. (B) is the correct answer.

    Prokaryotes do have a cell membrane and a singular circular chromosome. Many prokaryotes have rigid cell walls. In contrast, eukaryotes have both a nucleus and membrane-bound organelles. Ribosomes and DNA are found in both prokaryotes and eukaryotes, so (A) and (D) are incorrect. (Note that prokaryotic ribosomes are smaller and simpler than eukaryotic ribosomes.) (C) is incorrect since a prokaryote might have a cell wall.

35. **C** Small, charged molecules, such as calcium ions, are usually able to cross plasma membranes through protein channels in the membrane. Thus, calcium ions require assistance when crossing the plasma membrane.

    As a result of its lipid bilayer structure, a plasma membrane is readily permeable to small nonpolar molecules, such as oxygen, and small polar molecules, such as water. Therefore, (A) and (B) are incorrect because oxygen and water do not require assistance when crossing the plasma membrane. Carbon dioxide is a small polar molecule, so it doesn't require assistance when crossing the cell membrane either. Thus, (D) is incorrect.

36. **A** A tRNA anticodon is a three nucleotide sequence that is complementary to the corresponding mRNA codon. Thus, if the tRNA anticodon for the amino acid valine is AAC, the mRNA codon for valine is UUG.

    The function of tRNA is to bring amino acids to the ribosomes in the correct sequence for polypeptide synthesis; thus, tRNA needs to "recognize" both the amino acid and the mRNA codon. The tRNA anticodon is precisely for this purpose—during translation, the anticodon hydrogen bonds to the mRNA codon.

37. **A** ADH (antidiuretic hormone, vasopressin) increases the permeability to water of the nephron's distal tubule and collecting duct, thereby promoting water reabsorption and increasing blood volume. ADH is secreted from the posterior pituitary in response to an increase in plasma osmolarity or a decrease in blood volume.

38. **C** The cerebellum is the region of the brain that is responsible for coordinating motor impulses.

    (A) is incorrect because the hypothalamus controls visceral functions such as hunger, thirst, sex drive, water balance, pain, blood pressure, and temperature regulation. Higher intellectual functioning is controlled by the cerebral cortex, so (D) is incorrect as well. (B) is incorrect because the medulla controls autonomic, homeostatic activities such as breathing, heart rate, and gastrointestinal activity.

39. C Erythrocytes (red blood cells) are formed in the bone marrow where they lose their nuclei, mitochondria, and membranous organelles.

Choices (A),(B), and (D) are all incorrect because they refer to cells that contain nuclei.

40. D Viruses can only express their genes and reproduce within a living cell, since they lack the structures necessary for independent activity.

(A) is incorrect because not all viruses carry DNA as their nucleic acid. Some viruses carry single-stranded and double-stranded RNA. Similarly, (B) is incorrect because not all viruses carry RNA as their nucleic acid. Some viruses carry single-stranded and double-stranded DNA. (C) is incorrect because viruses do not lack protein; the capsid that encloses the nucleic acid is composed of protein subunits.

41. A Recall that the ribosomes of prokaryotes differ from those of eukaryotes. (A) is the correct answer.

Lysosomes and endoplasmic reticula are only found in eukaryotes, so a drug that targets these cellular components would be toxic to eukaryotes, not prokaryotes. Eliminate (B) and (C). (D) is incorrect, since a drug that targeted amino acids would be toxic to both prokaryotes and eukaryotes.

42. A The first complete cleavage of the zygote occurs approximately 32 hours after fertilization. The second cleavage occurs after 60 hours, and the third cleavage after approximately 72 hours, at which point the eight-celled embryo reaches the uterus. As cell division continues, a solid ball of embryonic cells, known as the morula, is formed. Blastulation begins when the morula develops a fluid-filled cavity called the blastocoel, which by the fourth day becomes a hollow sphere of cells called the blastula. The blastula implants in the uterine wall five to eight days after fertilization. Once implanted, cell migrations transform the single-cell layer of the blastula into a three-layer structure called a gastrula. These three layers of cells are known as the primary germ layers, which are responsible for the differential development of the tissues, organs, and systems of the body at later stages of growth. By the end of gastrulation, regions of the germ layers begin to develop into a rudimentary nervous system: this process is known as neurulation. Thus, (A) clearly demonstrates the correct order of developmental events.

43. B In humans, most chemical digestion occurs in the duodenum (first section of the small intestine), where the secretions of the intestinal glands, pancreas, liver, and gall bladder mix together with the chyme (partially digested food).

(A) is incorrect because only about 2 percent of total digestion occurs in the mouth (carbohydrates are broken down by salivary amylase). (C) is incorrect because chemical digestion does not occur in the liver. The liver is responsible for the production of bile, the regulation of blood glucose levels, and the production of urea. (D) is incorrect because chemical digestion does not occur in the large intestine, either; the large intestine functions in the absorption of water and salts and in the storage of feces.

44. B Gas exchange between the lungs and the circulatory system occurs across the very thin walls of the alveoli.

(A) is incorrect because ventilation (breathing rate) is controlled by the medulla, not the cerebellum. (C) is incorrect because the rate of breathing is increased by sympathetic stimulation, not parasympathetic stimulation. Remember, the sympathetic nervous system is responsible for the "fight or flight" reaction that prepares the body for a stressful situation. Increasing the breathing rate prepares the body for a stressful situation by increasing available oxygen to the tissues. (D) is incorrect because contraction of the diaphragm *increases* the volume of the thoracic cavity. This increase reduces the intrapleural pressure, causing the lungs to expand and fill with air.

45. **B** Retroviruses contain reverse transcriptase, an enzyme that transcribes DNA from viral RNA.

    (A) is incorrect because reverse transcriptase does not transcribe DNA from RNA. (D) is incorrect because retroviruses are not capable of metabolism or reproduction outside of a host cell.

46. **C** Active transport is the use of energy (ATP) to move a substance across a membrane against a concentration gradient. The key to answering this question correctly is that the question stem mentions ATP—an instant signal for you to think of active transport.

    Choices (A), (B), and (D) all refer to transport processes that do not use energy. (A) is incorrect because simple diffusion is the passive movement of substances from a region of high concentration to a region of low concentration. (B) is incorrect because facilitated diffusion is the movement of a substance down the concentration gradient using a carrier molecule but not using ATP. (D) is incorrect because osmosis is the diffusion of water over a membrane from an area of greater water concentration (less solute) to a region of less water concentration (more solute).

47. **A** Because there are 4^3, or 64, different codons possible based on the triplet code, and since there are only 20 amino acids that need to be coded for, the triplet code contains "synonyms." Most amino acids have more than one codon specifying them, although each codon specifies only one amino acid. This property is referred to as the degeneracy or redundancy of the genetic code, so (A) is indeed correct.

48. **D** Of all the answer choices, the only one that does not deal with bacterial infection of other organisms' cells is choice (D). While the ability of bacterial cells to exchange genetic information through pili make help antibiotic resistance spread, all the other choices are more direct causes of increased virulence within a given organism. Look out for answer choices such as (D) that do not fit with the pattern given by all the other choices.

CHEMISTRY

1. **C** The acid dissociation constant, K_a, is really a type of equilibrium constant, and when a weak acid, HA, dissociates into H^+ ions and A^- ions, the K_a is equal to $[H^+][A^-]/[HA]$. Consequently, a strong acid will have a large K_a, and a weak acid will have a small K_a. The strength of an acid is usually expressed in terms of pK_a, rather than K_a, where $pK_a = -\log K_a$. Therefore, a strong acid will have a small pK_a, and a weak acid will have large pK_a. If the pK_a of the acid is equal to 7, the K_a will be equal to antilog -7, or 10^{-7}.

2. **B** Boiling occurs when the vapor pressure of a liquid is equal to the ambient (atmospheric) pressure. The vapor pressure is the pressure exerted by the gas phase molecules (the vapor) that exist in equilibrium with its liquid or solid phase.

3. C This potential gas law problem can be solved faster through reasoning. First, if the temperature is higher while the pressure and number of moles are the same, it follows that gas A must occupy a larger volume than does gas B, so (A) can be removed. Secondly, since 30°C is only slightly higher than 20°C when we convert to the (mandatory!) Kelvin scale by adding 273, it follows that the volume of gas A will be only slightly larger than that of gas B. (C) is thus the only sensible answer. The full calculation is as follows:

Rearranging the ideal gas law, we get $V_a = \dfrac{n_a R T_a}{P_a}$ and $V_b = \dfrac{n_b R T_b}{P_b}$. Therefore, the ratio of

$V_a{:}V_b$ is $\dfrac{V_a}{V_b} = \dfrac{n_a R T_a / P_a}{n_b R T_b / P_b}$. Because $n_a = n_b = 1$, R is a constant, and because $P_a = P_b = 1$ atm,

all these factors cancel, so $\dfrac{V_a}{V_b} = \dfrac{T_a}{T_b}$, or $V_a{:}V_b = T_a{:}T_b$. This is actually Charles's Law.

When we convert to the Kelvin scale, gas A is at $(30 + 273) = 303$ K, whereas gas B is at $(20 + 273) = 293$ K. Hence $V_a{:}V_b = 303{:}293$.

4. D We should be both wary of excessive time spent on calculations and on the lookout for logical shortcuts. As far as logic is concerned, note that we are asked about the ΔH when SO_2 is "burned." We are therefore talking about a combustion reaction, which is exothermic. The answer should thus be negative. Furthermore, since SO_2 and SO_3 will be one to one in terms of stoichiometry, the answer should be a simple combination of the two numbers given, either a sum or a difference; $3{,}600 + 1{,}300 = 4{,}900$ or $3{,}600 - 1{,}300 = 2{,}300$. More rigorously, note that the reaction in which sulfur burns to form the SO_2 is:

$$S(s) + O_2(g) \longrightarrow SO_2(g)$$

However, this is also the formation reaction of SO_2 since the reactants, sulfur and oxygen, are elements in their standard state. The enthalpy change of this reaction, $-1{,}300$ cal (negative because this heat is released), is therefore the heat or enthalpy of formation of SO_2 (i.e., $\Delta H_f(SO_2, g) = -1{,}300$ cal/mol). Similarly, when we burn sulfur to form SO_3, the reaction, $S(s) + \frac{3}{2}O_2(g) \longrightarrow SO_3(g)$, is also the formation reaction of SO_3, and so $\Delta H_f(SO_3, g) = -3{,}600$ cal. We are asked to determine the enthalpy change for the reaction:
$SO_2(g) + O_2(g) \longrightarrow SO_3(g)$.

From Hess's Law, we know that the enthalpy change of this reaction can be expressed as $\Delta H = \Delta H_f(SO_3, g) - \Delta H_f(SO_2, g) - \Delta H_f(O_2, g)$. The last term, the heat of formation of oxygen, is zero because it is an element in standard state. So $\Delta H = \Delta H_f(SO_3, g) - \Delta H_f(SO_2, g) = -3{,}600 - (-1{,}300) = -2{,}300$ cal.

5. A From the Aufbau principle, atomic number 16 corresponds to an electron configuration of $1s^2 2s^2 2p^6 3s^2 3p^4$. All the electrons up through the $3s$ subshell are paired, but the four electrons in the $3p$ subshell must occupy the three available orbitals in this subshell. Since no more than two electrons can occupy a single orbital, we have two electrons which must remain unpaired:

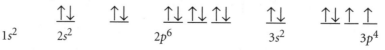

6. **C** A saturated hydrocarbon is one that contains only single bonds. If it is noncyclic, its formula will conform to that of alkanes: C_nH_{2n+2}. Only (C) satisfies this.

7. **B** The best way to solve this problem quickly is to apply the titration formula: $V_AN_A = V_BN_B$. We are given the volume of acid and the concentrations of both the acid and the base, but we must convert the given volume to milliliters and the concentrations from the given molarity (M) to the corresponding normality (N) before applying the formula. One liter is 1,000 mL. Acetic acid is monoprotic; thus its normality is the same as its molarity, and N_A equals 0.01 N. Calcium hydroxide provides two OH– groups per formula, so its normality will be twice its molarity; V_B thus equals 2(0.10), or 0.20 N. With these conversions complete, we can now rearrange the equation and solve for the volume of basic solution required:

$$V_B = V_AN_A/N_B = (1000 \text{ mL})(0.01 \text{ N})/(0.20 \text{ N}) = 50 \text{ mL}$$

8. **C** In one mole of NaOH, there is one mole of sodium, one mole of oxygen, and one mole of hydrogen. Because the molar masses of sodium, oxygen, and hydrogen are 23 g/mol, 16 g/mol, and 1 g/mol, respectively, there are 16 g of oxygen, 23 g of sodium, and 1 g of hydrogen in one mole of sodium hydroxide. Therefore, the percent composition by mass of oxygen in sodium hydroxide is equal to the mass of one mole of oxygen, 16 g, divided by the mass of one mole of sodium hydroxide (23+16+1) multiplied by 100. This is equal to $16/40 \times 100 = 40\%$.

9. **B** The molecular formula of a compound gives us the exact number and type of atoms in a molecule, whereas the empirical formula of a compound gives us the simplest integral ratio of atoms to each other but not necessarily the exact number that is present in a molecule. Only when the molecular formula of a compound equals the empirical formula does the empirical formula tell how many atoms are in the compound. In this case, the molecular formula is equal to $C_6H_{12}O_6$. The ratio of carbon to hydrogen to oxygen is 6:12:6. However, this is not the lowest ratio possible; if we divide by the common denominator 6, we get the simplest ratio of atoms to be 1 carbon to 2 hydrogens to 1 oxygen. Therefore, the empirical formula is CH_2O, and (B) is the correct response. (D) can be eliminated because this is the molecular formula of glucose, not the empirical formula, and (C) can be eliminated because this is not the simplest ratio of elements in glucose. (A) can be eliminated because we have established that there are 2 hydrogens to every 1 oxygen and 1 carbon.

10. **D** The –COOH group is the carboxylic acid group. The ether functionality is represented by the formula R–O–R', and in this case R is the ring and R' is the methyl (CH_3) group.

11. **B** When an acid reacts with a base, a salt and water are formed. In this case, the salt is sodium chloride, so the missing product, X, is water, and (B) is the correct response. This reaction is a neutralization reaction—the hydrogen ions from the acid combine with the hydroxide ions from the base; and the combination of hydrogen ions with hydroxide ions always results in the formation of water, so again (B) is the correct response.

12. **C** The heat capacity of water is the amount of energy needed to raise the temperature by 1°C and is equal to the specific heat capacity multiplied by the mass of water—4.184 J/g•°C multiplied by 100 g, or 418 J/°C. The starting temperature of water is equal to 5 °C, and the final temperature of water is equal to 75 °C. If 418 Joules of energy is needed to raise the

temperature of water by 1°C, then (75 – 5) × 418 Joules—approximately 28,000 Joules or 28 kJ—is needed to raise the temperature from 5°C to 75°C. The answer closest to this value is (C), the correct response.

13. A   Benzene was originally thought to be a cyclic, six-membered ring that contained an alternating system of double and single bonds. However, it was found that all the carbon-carbon bonds were of equal length. Hence, benzene is a cyclic, six-membered ring that has delocalized pi electron clouds above and below the ring (these delocalized pi electrons overlap to give benzene its unique chemistry). A system of delocalized pi electrons is identified by a circle within the six-membered ring; therefore, the most accepted structure of benzene is that shown in (A). (B) can be eliminated because each carbon exceeds its octet (remember, carbon can only form a maximum of four bonds), and (D) can be eliminated because this is the structure of cyclohexane, not benzene.

14. B   When studying gas behavior, scientist Robert Boyle noticed that when the temperature is held constant and the total pressure applied to a gas increases, the volume of the gas decreases. Conversely, if the temperature is held constant and the applied pressure decreases, the volume of the gas increases. Choices (A) and (D) can be eliminated because these laws state that at constant pressure, the volume of a gas is proportional to the temperature—that is, when a gas is heated, it expands, and when it is cooled, it contracts. Avogadro's law, choice (C), states that at constant temperature and pressure, the volume of a gas is directly proportional to the number of moles of gas.

15. C   When the volume of a gas decreases at constant temperature, the pressure increases. Because PV over nT is constant and the temperature and number of moles of gas are kept constant, we can derive the relationship, $P_1V_1 = P_2V_2$, where P_1 and V_1 are the original pressure and volume and P_2 and V_2 are the new pressure and volume. We need to find the new pressure of the gas, P_2, so rearranging the equation $P_1V_1 = P_2V_2$, we get: $P_2 = P_1V_1/V_2$. By substituting numbers into this equation, we get, $P_2 = (700 \times 500)/100$, or 3,500 mmHg (C).

16. D   The half-life of a radioactive isotope is defined as the time it takes for one half of the substance to decay. The general equation relating time elapsed to substance remaining is $A/A_o = (1/2)_n$, where A is the amount of substance present, A_o is the original amount, and n is the number of half-lives gone by. From this equation, one can predict the fraction of material remaining after any number of half-lives have passed. After one half-life, $A/A_o = (1/2)^1 = 1/2$; after two half-lives, $A/A_o = (1/2)^2 = 1/4$; etc. If the physicist begins with 320 grams of substance, he will have half as much, or 160 grams, left after one half-life has elapsed. The passing of another half-life will reduce the 160 grams to 80, and so on. Applying either the equation or some quantitative reasoning, it follows that if 320 grams becomes 20, or one-sixteenth of the original amount, then four half-lives have elapsed. Since we are told that 20 minutes actually passes, it follows that 20 minutes is four half-lives, or that one half-life is five minutes.

17. D   Substituted cycloalkanes are named as derivatives of their parent cycloalkane, which in this case is cyclohexane. Thus, choice A can be ruled out immediately. Then the substituents are listed in alphabetical order and the carbons are numbered so as to give the lowest sum of substituent numbers. This cyclohexane has an ethyl and two methyl substituents; it is therefore an ethyl dimethyl cyclohexane. All of the remaining answer choices recognize this; they only differ in the numbers assigned. To give the lowest sum of substituent numbers,

the two methyl substituents must be numbered 1 and 2, and the ethyl substituent must be numbered 4. The correct name for this compound is thus 4-ethyl-1, 2-dimethylcyclohexane.

18. **D**   Because chlorine has an atomic number of 17, it possesses 17 electrons in its neutral state. According to the Aufbau principle, electrons fill orbitals so that the atom is in its lowest energy configuration. Therefore, the order of filling is: $1s$, which can hold a maximum of two electrons; $2s$, which can hold a maximum of two electrons; $2p$, which can hold a maximum of six electrons; $3s$, which can hold a maximum of two electrons; and $3p$, which can hold a maximum of six electrons. Because chlorine possesses 17 electrons, the electron configuration is $1s^2 2s^2 2p^6 3s^2 3p^5$, and (D) is the correct response. (A) can be eliminated because this electron configuration contains 18 electrons and would, in fact, be the configuration of the Cl^- anion, not neutral chlorine. Choices (B) and (C) can be eliminated because these electron configurations disobey the Aufbau principle—the $4s$ orbital does not fill before the $3p$ orbital, and the $3p$ orbital does not fill before the $3s$ orbital.

19. **D**   To determine which compound has the lowest boiling point, we have to look at the intermolecular forces. When a liquid boils, the molecules become separated as they enter into the gas phase. Therefore, the stronger the intermolecular forces, the more difficult it is bring the liquid to boil; in other words, the stronger the intermolecular forces, the higher the boiling point. Ethane is a nonpolar hydrocarbon; therefore, the only type of intermolecular forces it can experience are dispersion forces. These forces are weak and short-lived and arise when the random fluctuations of electron density result in a temporary dipole moment and induce temporary dipole moments in other molecules. Ethanal is an aldehyde with formula CH_3CHO, a polar molecule: the oxygen in the carbonyl bond is electronegative, and there is a net dipole moment in the direction of the oxygen. Since part of the ethanal molecule is positively polarized and part of the molecule is negatively polarized, ethanal can undergo intermolecular dipole-dipole interactions. These interactions are stronger than dispersion forces; therefore, ethanal will have a higher boiling point than ethane. Ethanol, (C), contains a hydrogen attached to an electronegative atom. Therefore, ethanol can form hydrogen bonds to other ethanol molecules or to water. Hydrogen bonds are stronger than dispersion forces and dipole-dipole interactions, so ethanol will have a boiling point higher than either ethane or ethanal. Ethanoic acid, (A), has a carboxyl group; therefore, it can form dimers—two carboxylic acid molecules held together by two hydrogen bonds. Since ethanoic acid can form two hydrogen bonds per molecule and ethanol can form only one hydrogen bond per molecule, ethanoic acid will have a higher boiling point than ethanol. Therefore, the order of boiling points increase as follows: ethane < ethanal < ethanol < ethanoic acid.

20. **A**   This question about solubility and K_{sp} can be answered using the relationship $Ksp = x_2$, where x is the solubility of the salt in moles per liter, M. This expression is valid for any MX salt, including the silver iodide of this question. Because there is exactly one silver cation and one iodide anion per formula of salt, it follows that for each mole of AgI that dissolves, there will be one mole of $Ag+$ and one mole of $I-$ in solution or, in other words, $x = [Ag+] = [I-] = \sqrt{Ksp}$. Thus, we can solve for x from the expression for K_{sp} (i.e., $x = \sqrt{8.5 \times 10^{-17}} = \sqrt{85 \times 10^{-18}} \approx 9 \times 10^{-9}$).

21. **A**   In a many-electron atom, the energy of the orbitals within the principal quantum numbers is as follows: $2s < 2p$; $3s < 3p < 3d$; $4s < 4p < 4d < 4f$. From this ranking it is clear that the correct choice is (A).

22. **C**   While we might be tempted to apply the ideal gas law to this problem, this attempt would lead to frustration and wasted time. Simply put, if 3 moles (the stoichiometric quantities referred to) of gaseous reactants produce a pressure of 12 atm, it follows that 1 mole of gaseous product will produce 1/3 the pressure, or 4 atm, at the same temperature and in the same volume.

    As a semiquantitative approach, we could rearrange the ideal gas law, $PV = nRT$, into $P = n(RT/V)$ and, noting that R, T, and V are all constant, "delta" each side, then rearrange:

    $$\Delta P = \Delta n(RT/V) \implies \Delta P/\Delta n = \text{constant}$$

    From this semiquantitative rearrangement, we may be more easily able to see that if n triples, then P will triple and so on.

23. **A**   In this case, the pressure and temperature are held constant, and we are asked to find the change in volume as the reaction proceeds. Because complete reaction means that 3 moles becomes 1 mole, and since volume is proportional to the number of moles (Avogadro's Law), it follows that the volume will be one-third as large after the reaction as it was before the reaction. Thus, 30 liters becomes 10 liters.

24. **D**   The ionization energy of an atom is defined as the amount of energy required to remove an electron from a gaseous atom in its ground state. The first ionization energy is the energy required to remove an electron from a neutral gaseous atom, and it increases from left to right across a period and upwards in a group. When an electron is removed from a gaseous atom, the result is the formation of a positively charged ion, as shown in (A). The energy required to remove a second electron is called the second ionization energy, and this reaction is shown in (B). The reactions involving third and fourth ionization energies are shown in choices (C) and (D). Now, as each electron is removed from the atom or ion, the number of electrons remaining decreases; consequently, the effective nuclear charge—or the attraction of electrons towards the nucleus—increases. Therefore, with each ionization, it becomes increasingly difficult to remove electrons, and the highest ionization energy will be that required to remove an electron from a +3 ion (the fourth ionization energy) as shown in (D).

25. **A**   The simplest type of sugar is a monosaccharide—this contains one carbohydrate unit. Because the monomer shown contains two monosaccharide subunits, (B) can be eliminated. (C) may appear to be a viable answer since a disaccharide is a sugar consisting of two monosaccharide subunits; however, these subunits repeat 2,000 times (according to the subscript outside the brackets shown in the diagram so there are, in fact, 4,000 monosaccharide subunits in the molecule. Any carbohydrate that contains more than 10 monosaccharide subunits is called a polysaccharide. (D), oligosaccharide, is a carbohydrate that contains two 10 monosaccharide subunits.

26. **B**   Boron is a group IIIA element; therefore, its valence electron configuration is $2s^2 2p^1$. These electrons form covalent bonds with three fluorines—the result being the formation of three bonding electron pairs around the central boron. According to the VSEPR theory, pairs of electrons repel each other and arrange themselves in such a way as to achieve maximum separation. Since there are three bonding electron pairs in BF_3, the bond angle that results in maximum separation is 120°, and the geometry is trigonal planar. Therefore, (B) is the

correct response. Nitrogen and arsenic are Group VA elements; therefore, their valence electron configurations are $2s^22p^3$ and $4s^24p^3$, respectively. Since nitrogen and arsenic have five electrons in their valence shell, they will form three bonds to hydrogen (hence AsH_3 and NH_3 contain three bonding electron pairs) while a lone pair of electrons around the central atom remains. Again, based on the VSEPR theory, the geometry that would allow for maximum separation of three pairs of bonding electrons and one lone pair of electrons is trigonal pyramidal. Therefore, choices (A) and (D) can be eliminated. Finally, (C) can be eliminated because the central atom in $AlCl_4^-$ is surrounded by four pairs of bonding electrons, and the geometry that allows for maximum separation of four pairs of bonding electrons is tetrahedral.

27. **B** The carbon in CCl_4 is sp^3-hybridized; consequently, carbon has four sp^3 orbitals that can overlap to form four sigma bonds. Each carbon-chlorine sigma bond contains two electrons; therefore, CCl_4 contains four bonding pairs of electrons. The bond angle associated with an sp^3-hybridized central atom surrounded by four pairs of bonding electrons is 109.5°, and the resulting molecular geometry is tetrahedral. Therefore, (B) is the correct response. (C) can be eliminated because a bond angle of 120° is associated with an sp^2-hybridized central atom and three pairs of bonding electrons. (D) can be eliminated because a bond angle of 180° is associated with an sp-hybridized central atom and two pairs of bonding electrons. Finally, (A) can be eliminated because a bond angle of 90° is associated with inorganic compounds that have a square planar, octahedral, or trigonal bipyramidal geometry.

28. **B** Carbon occurs in nature in either of two forms, or allotropes: graphite and diamond. The two allotropes differ in how the carbon atoms are bonded to one another. In diamond, each carbon atom is sp^3 hybridized and thus forms four single bonds to adjacent carbon atoms; the tetrahedral arrangement of atoms in the crystal leads to one large three-dimensional lattice in which the strong, directional, and localized single bonds make diamond very hard as well as thermally and electrically insulating. A perfect diamond has an uninterrupted carbon crystal lattice, while flaws and impurities lead to the refractive planes and color found in most natural diamonds. In graphite, on the other hand, all the carbon atoms are sp^2 hybridized and are thus each bonded to three neighboring carbon atoms in a trigonal planar array composed of fused six-membered rings with alternating (conjugated) single and double bonds. The planar arrangement of the carbon atoms results in the formation of two-dimensional sheets; these sheets are stacked like a deck of cards and can slide over each other leading to the softness of graphite and its applicability as a lubricant. The conjugated nature of the π system gives graphite a high electrical conductivity, and these loosely held π electrons absorb light at all visible wavelengths, giving graphite its characteristic black color. Choices (C) and (D) are incorrect based on the facts above. (A) is wrong since naturally occurring carbon is mostly ^{12}C in both allotropes, with trace amounts of other isotopes present.

29. **C** The –CO–NH– linkages that arise between individual amino acids are known as amide linkages or, more specifically, peptide linkages. These linkages form when the carboxyl group (the *C*-terminal) of one amino acid reacts with the amino group (the *N*-terminal) of another, and when these peptide bonds link amino acids together, a polypeptide and, eventually, a protein can form. This linking together of amino acids through peptide bonds constitutes the primary structure, or sequence of amino acids, of a protein, so (C) is the correct response. (A) can be eliminated because dipole-dipole interactions occur between

polarized species, and this type of interaction contributes to the secondary structure and tertiary structure of a protein. (B) can be eliminated because hydrogen bonds are a specific type of dipole-dipole interaction that contributes to the secondary structure of a protein (it can assist in the formation of an α-helix or a β-pleated sheet) and the tertiary structure of a protein. (D) can be eliminated because dispersion forces occur between nonpolar molecules. These forces would occur between nonpolar groups on the interior of a protein that has been exposed to an aqueous environment and, therefore, would contribute to the tertiary structure.

30. A Phase diagrams show the conditions of temperature and pressure under which a substance exists as a solid, liquid, and gas. Region *a* corresponds to the solid phase, region *b* corresponds to the liquid phase, and region *c* corresponds to the vapor phase. The lines on the graph correspond to *phase boundaries,* in which the different phases coexist in equilibrium: the line between regions *a* and *b* corresponds to the solid-liquid equilibrium, the line between regions *b* and *c* corresponds to the liquid-vapor equilibrium, and the line between regions *a* and *c* corresponds to the solid-gas equilibrium. Point *d* is known as the triple point and represents the point where the solid, liquid, and vapor phases exist together at equilibrium.

31. B In a double-bonded carbon, *sp*2 hybridization occurs (i.e., one *s* orbital hybridizes with two *p* orbitals to form three *sp*2 hybrid orbitals). Therefore, the correct choice is B. Note that the *sp*2 orbitals take part in *s* bond formation, making choice (D) incorrect. The third *p* orbital of the carbon atom remains unhybridized and takes part in the formation of the *p* bond of the double bond.

32. D The first task in balancing an equation is to ensure that both sides contain equal numbers of atoms. Both sides do contain the same number of silvers (3), nitrogens (1), and oxygens (3), but they do not contain equal amounts of hydrogen (there are X hydrogens on the left-hand side and 4 hydrogens on the right-hand side). Therefore, to balance out the equation, X must be equal to four, and (D) is the correct response. By the way, you must make sure that the charges on both sides are equal. If X equals four, you can see that the charges on the left-hand side add up to +3 and the charges on the right-hand side also add up to +3, so again, (D) is the correct response.

33. D The carbon atom and the nitrogen atoms are connected by a triple bond in CN⁻.

$$:N \equiv C:^-$$

A triple-bonded atom is *sp* hybridized; one *s* orbital hybridizes with one *p* orbital to form two *sp* hybridized orbitals. The two remaining unhybridized *p* orbitals take part in the formation of two *p* bonds. The correct choice, therefore, is (D).

34. D The rate law for a reaction is experimentally determined, and the rate law tells us the order of a reaction (how the reaction rate is affected by varying concentrations of reactants). The overall order of a reaction is equal to the sum of the exponents to which the concentration of each reactant is raised. Since the concentration of A is raised to the power 1 and since the concentration of B is raised to the power 2, the overall order of the reaction is equal to 2 + 1, or 3—(D). (C) is the order of the reaction with respect to B only, and (B) is the order of the reaction with respect to A only. (A) can be eliminated because a zero-order reaction would not depend on the concentrations of A or B—the rate of the reaction would be equal to the rate constant, *k*.

35. B The reactant molecules (A and B) must have a minimum energy—called the activation energy—to collide and react. On a reaction profile, this activation energy is shown by the "hump." Catalysts work by lowering the activation energy; therefore, there is an increase in the number of reactant molecules that can "climb the energy hill" and react to form products. Consequently, catalysts increase the rate of a reaction. When a catalyst is added, the only feature of the profile that should change is the "hump"—it should be smaller. Therefore, (B) is the correct response. (A) can be eliminated since this reaction profile corresponds to the uncatalyzed reaction profile. Choices (C) and (D) can be eliminated because the energy of the products (C and D) should not change.

36. B A reducing agent is the species that gets oxidized in a REDOX reaction. Using the mnemonic OIL RIG, we remember that oxidation is loss of electrons and an increase in oxidation number. In (A), the chromomium goes from +6 in $Cr_2O_7^{2-}$ to +3 in $Cr(OH)_3$, so it is an oxidizing agent (it gets reduced). In (B), the chlorine goes from +1 in ClO^- to +5 in ClO^{3-}, so is a reducing agent (it gets oxidized). Choices (C) and (D) are products of the reaction, so cannot be the answer.

37. B Each molecular orbital, like an atomic orbital, can contain a maximum of two electrons with opposite spins.

38. B The pH and pOH of any aqueous solution must add up to 14, so if the pOH equals 4, the pH must equal 10. Now, the pH is equal to –log of the hydrogen ion concentration; therefore, the hydrogen ion concentration must be equal to the antilog of –10, or 10^{-10} M.

39. C The atomic weight of an element is calculated by multiplying the atomic mass of each isotope of that element by the relative abundance of that isotope. In this example, there are only two isotopes of boron, so the calculation setup goes: $(x)(10.013) + (1 - x)(11.0093) = 10.811$, where x = the relative abundance of $_{10}B$, and thus $1 - x$ = the relative abundance of $_{11}B$. Approximating the mass of the isotopes to be 10 and 11 respectively, the calculation gives:

$$10\,x + 11 - 11\,x \approx 10.811$$
$$-x \approx 10.811 - 11 \approx -0.2$$
$$x \approx 0.2 = 20\%$$

So a naturally occurring sample of boron would contain about 20 percent of the 10-amu isotope, with the rest (100 – 20 = 80%) being the 11-amu isotope.

40. A Let's call our acid HX, where X in this case is a halide ion. When the acid dissociates, it forms H^+ and X^-; therefore, a strong acid is characterized by the tendency to dissociate into hydrogen ions, whereas a weak acid remains undissociated. If the conjugate base is strong (i.e., it likes to donate electrons), HX will form readily (the acid will be weak), whereas if the conjugate base is weak (i.e., it does not like to donate electrons), the acid will readily dissociate. Base strength decreases down a group; therefore, F^- is the strongest conjugate base, and I^- is the weakest conjugate base. Since I^- is the weakest conjugate base, it will readily accept protons, and HI will dissociate into H^+ and I^-. Consequently, HI is the strongest acid, and (A) is the correct response.

41. A The rate law for any reaction, A + B $\longrightarrow$ C, is given by:

rate = $k[A]^x[B]^y$

where k is the rate constant at the temperature at which the reaction is carried out, [A] and

[B] are the concentrations of the two reactants, and x and y are the reaction orders with respect to A and B, respectively. This question asks us to find x from the experimental data provided. To simplify the tabulated rate data, we can rewrite the table as small whole-number multiples of the smallest entry in each column:

Trial	$[A]_o$	$[B]_o$	rate
1	1	1	1
2	1	2	4
3	2	4	16

Looking at lines 1 and 2, where the concentration of reactant A is held constant, we see that a doubling in the concentration of B results in a quadrupling of the rate; therefore, the reaction is second order with respect to B. We can now look at lines 2 and 3 (or 1 and 3) to determine the required reaction order. From line 2 to line 3, the concentration of B is doubled; the reaction rate should thus quadruple due to the influence of the concentration increase of second-order reactant B. We can divide out this quadrupling effect and create a hypothetical line 4:

line #	$[A]_o$	$[B]_o$	rate
1	1	1	1
2	1	2	4
3	2	4	16
4	2	2	4

From this revision of the experimental data, it can be seen (lines 2 and 4) that a doubling of [A] results in no change in the rate (i.e., $2^x = 1$). Therefore, the reaction is zero order with respect to A.

42. **B** This question is based on the same reaction and can be answered quickly based on the results outlined above. As determined in the explanation above, the reaction is zero order in A; as a result, changing the concentration of A will have no effect on the reaction rate. The original entry labeled as trial 1 has the same initial concentration of B, 3×10^{-3} M, as that offered in this question. The answer will thus be that the rate is the same as that in trial 1, or 2×10^{-3}.

43. **A** Each single bond has 1 σ bond, and each double bond has one σ and one π bond. In this question, there are five single bonds (5 σ bonds) and one double bond (one σ bond and one π bond), which gives a total of six σ bonds and one π bond. Thus, the correct choice is (A).

44. **A** This question deals with a colligative property, freezing-point depression in particular. Recall that the number, not the nature, of particles in solution affects the freezing-point depression. Since the freezing-point depression is equal to the freezing-point depression constant, K_f, multiplied by the molality of the solution, the solution that will possess the greatest freezing-point depression and, therefore, the lowest freezing point, will be the one with the highest molality. In (A), Na_3PO_4 dissociates into 3 Na^+ ions and a PO_4^{3-} ion; therefore, the effective molality is 0.4 m. In (B), H_2SO_4 dissociates (at most) into two H^+ ions and an SO_4^{2-} ion, so the maximum effective molality is 0.3 m. In (C), glucose does not

dissociate into ions, so the molality remains at 0.1 *m*, and in (D), NaCl dissociates into an Na$^+$ ion and a Cl$^-$ ion, so the effective molality is 0.2 *m*. Since sodium phosphate has the highest molality of particles in solution, this solution will have the greatest freezing-point depression.

45. **D** An amide is a carboxylic acid derivative, in which the –OH group of the carboxylic acid has been substituted by an –NR$_2$ group, where one or both of the R groups can be a hydrogen atom. In this case, the amide nitrogen is attached to three carbons, so this compound is an *N,N*-disubstituted amide, and (D) is the correct response. (A) can be eliminated because an aldehyde contains a terminal carbonyl group (CHO), not a carbonyl group and a nitrogen-containing group. (C) can be eliminated because an amine doesn't contain a carbonyl group. Amines fall into three classes: primary, where the nitrogen is attached to one carbon (RNH$_2$); secondary, where the nitrogen is attached to two carbons (RNHR'); and tertiary, where the nitrogen is attached to three carbons (RNR'R"). If an additional alkyl group or hydrogen atom is added to the nitrogen, a quaternary ammonium salt is formed (R$_4$N$^+$), where R is any alkyl group. Therefore, (B) can be eliminated.

46. **B** The carbons in ethyne, or acetylene, are *sp* hybridized: the carbon 2*s* orbital hybridizes with an empty 2*p* orbital to form two *sp* orbitals and two 2*p* orbitals. One of the *sp* orbitals from each carbon then overlaps to form a carbon-carbon sigma bond, while the second *sp* orbital of each carbon overlaps with a hydrogen 1*s* orbital, and two carbon-hydrogen sigma bonds are formed. Therefore, the ethyne molecule contains three sigma bonds, and (B) is the correct response. Let's confirm (B) as the correct answer by establishing the number of pi bonds in the molecule. Each carbon atom contains two unhybridized *p* orbitals. If two atoms lie adjacent to each other and they each possess a *p* orbital, these orbitals undergo sideways overlap to form a pi bond. Since each carbon contains two unhybridized *p* orbitals, two pi bonds form between the carbons; therefore, one sigma bond and two pi bonds form between the carbons, and a triple bond is formed.

47. **B** Beta-minus or β^- decay involves the breakdown of a neutron into a proton and an electron. Therefore, in β^- decay, the atomic number increases by 1, but the mass number remains the same while an electron is emitted. Positron or β^+ decay occurs when a proton decays into a neutron and a positively charged electron. In this case, the atomic number decreases—not increases—by 1. (D) is an example of positron decay, so it can be eliminated. (A) can be eliminated since this reaction is an example of gamma decay, the emission of high-energy gamma rays from a high-energy parent nucleus (hence there is no change in atomic number or mass number). Finally, (C) can be eliminated since this reaction is an example of alpha decay. In alpha decay, a helium nucleus is emitted, so the atomic number decreases by 2, and the mass number decreases by 4.

48. **B** The carbon-carbon bond in ethane is a single bond; the carbon-carbon bond in ethyne is a triple bond; the carbon-carbon bond in ethene is a double bond; the carbon-carbon bond in benzene is intermediate between a single and a double bond. Triple bonds are the strongest among the different kinds because they are of the highest bond order. By the same token, they are also the shortest because they hold the two carbons atoms together most tightly. Therefore, the carbon-carbon bond length in ethyne—an alkyne—will be the shortest. The carbon-carbon bond length decreases in the order: ethane > benzene > ethene > ethyne.

READING COMPREHENSION

Passage I (Questions 1–7)

1. **D** Paragraph 4 discusses that the maintenance of the respondents' smoking habits was most related to their proximal social environment. The passage says that a young woman's "closest female friends" most influence the duration of her smoking habit.

    Because (D) is correct, (A) is logically eliminated. Nowhere in the passage does it say, or infer, that a young woman's friends encourage heavy smoking; thus, (B) is eliminated. Paragraph 2 indicates that the initiation of smoking is most related to the influence of the respondents' mothers, not the woman's closest friends. Therefore, (C) is also incorrect.

2. **D** Information contained in the final sentences of the third and fourth paragraphs and the last two sentences of the fifth paragraph indicates male smoking behavior does not account for female smoking habits, (D). Choices (A) and (C) contradict this information. (B) is wrong because nowhere in the passage is there anything suggested about the effect of male smoking behavior on other males.

3. **D** If further study confirmed that mothers have influence over their daughters' early smoking careers, (A), this would strengthen Smith's argument. (B) would also tend to strengthen Smith's argument, as it coincides with Smith's conclusions that female friends affect maintenance while mothers affect the frequency of women's smoking.

4. **C** This passage is primarily concerned with describing the results of Smith's study, so it is a summary of recent research findings. (A) is wrong because no earlier hypothesis about female smoking behavior is ever mentioned in the passage, let alone "refuted." There is no indication anywhere in the passage that this study is either "popular" or "controversial," so choices (B) and (D) are wrong.

5. **D** The second sentence of the first paragraph indicates that in the early 1970s, the percentage of males smoking leveled off at 19 percent.

6. **B** Nicotine is discussed in the second sentence of the third paragraph, which indicates that nicotine does not become a factor in determining smoking behavior until after the initiation of smoking. The next sentence then tells us that the smoking of mothers is significantly associated with the initiation of smoking in daughters. In other words, nicotine has less effect than maternal influence on the initiation of smoking, (B). Choices (A) and (D) contradict information in the third paragraph. The first sentence of the third paragraph tells us that nicotine does have effects on smoking behavior, but these effects come later, after the initiation stage of smoking. Because the passage does not discuss the effect of nicotine on male smoking behavior, we have no basis for concluding that nicotine affects female smokers more than male smokers, (C).

7. **A** The fact that the author has chosen to write about a paradoxical situation—increased smoking among young women at a time when smoking has become less popular in the United States—does, itself, suggest that he is interested in Smith's study. (B) is wrong because the author unemotionally lays out Smith's data and conclusions. "Dismissive," (C), and "flippant," (D), are wrong because they imply that the author has a negative attitude toward Smith's conclusions or takes the subject very lightly.

Passage II (Questions 8–15)

8. **B**   When determining the main idea of a passage, identify the author's purpose for writing the passage. The first and second paragraphs introduce stress ulceration as a serious medical condition, especially in individuals who possess many of the risk factors. Therefore, (B) is correct. Choices (A) and (C) are true statements; however, they do not capture the main idea of the entire passage. These choices refer to specific details within the passage. (D) is too strong a statement. The passage never states that *all* patients in intensive care need ulcer prophylaxis.

9. **B**   In paragraph 3, the author states, "the most important nonpharmacologic method for the prevention of stress ulceration is to remove the patient from the stressful environment." None of the other choices offers a better treatment plan for ulceration. (A) is incorrect because an alkaline pH can lead to bacterial colonization, even pneumonia, in some individuals. (B) is incorrect; total inhibition of gastric acid secretion would not be the goal of antiulcer treatment. (D) is incorrect because it refers to a highly specific treatment; sulcrafate is administered to patients at risk for developing pneumonia.

10. **C**   The author refers to pneumonia as an example of a side effect of antiulcer therapy. (A) is too broad a statement. The passage does not imply that *all* patients in the intensive care setting need ulcer prophylaxis. (B) is incorrect; the author states that sulcrafate is less effective in treating ulcers than H2-antagonists. (D) is incorrect because paragraph 3 states that "the stressor cannot always be removed, making pharmacologic ulcer prophylaxis necessary."

11. **D**   Since the patient is at risk for pneumonia, the patient should be treated with a cytoprotective agent. (A) is incorrect because the patient is at risk for developing an ulcer and some form of prevention therapy should be instituted. The patient is at risk for pneumonia; therefore, the patient should not be treated with high doses of antacids, (B). (C) is incorrect because the passage focuses preventing ulcers, not treating ulcers after they have developed.

12. **A**   Paragraph 5 states that patients at risk for pneumonia should take cytoprotective agents over antacids or H2-blockers. (B) is incorrect because nowhere in the passage does the author say that *all* intensive care patients need prophylactic ulcer therapy. (C) is also too strong a statement. The author believes that the appropriateness of each prophylactic regimen needs to be assessed so that an optimal patient outcome can be achieved. (D) is beyond the scope of the passage. The author does not recommend one of these treatments over the other.

13. **D**   H2-antagonists do, in fact, potentiate bacterial colonization. If these bacteria are aspirated, pneumonia can develop, making (C) a true statement. H2-antagonists inhibit parietal cell activity, so (B) is a true statement. H2 antagonists are mentioned as a method for stress ulcer prophylaxis, so (A) is also a true statement.

14. **C**   The author would agree with (A) because the author does feel that antacids provide short-term relief, not long-term relief. The second sentence of paragraph 4 mentions that antacids need to be administered frequently, so the author would also agree with (B). Paragraph 4 implies that H2-antagonists would work well with antacids since they compensate for antacids' inability to prevent acid production, so (D) can be inferred from this statement.

15. C The author discusses many different options for the prevention of stress ulceration. Based on the information presented in the passage, the author considers stress ulceration as a preventable condition if the patient is treated properly, making (C) correct. In the second paragraph, the author states, "substantial ulceration can cause potentially life-threatening bleeds." Thus, the author considers ulceration to be fatal, eliminating (A). (B) is incorrect because there is no mention or inference that stress ulceration is a condition that needs further research. If ulceration can be life-threatening, then it is a serious condition, and (D) is incorrect.

Passage III (Questions 16–22)

16. C Pupillary dilation, hallucination, and convulsions all can occur after ingestion of high doses of atropine. In paragraph 2, pupillary dilation is described as an effect of atropine administration. Paragraph 1 describes that high doses cause both hallucinations and convulsions. Paragraph 3 states that products of the deadly nightshade inhibit lacrimation; therefore, lacrimation would not occur as a result of atropine overdose.

17. B If *Atropa Belladonna* causes pupillary dilation, the iris must decrease in size.

18. D Paragraph 2 discusses the etymology of *Atropa Belladonna. Bella* and *donna* both refer to the historical use of atropine as a beauty enhancer. (B) may be tempting because it is mentioned in the passage. *Atropos* is the Greek word from which *Atropa* is derived. Thus, *Atropa*, not *Atropos*, is the part of the botanical name that refers to the toxic nature of the plant.

19. D The first sentence of paragraph 3 states that atropine is an anticholinergic, thereby acting as an antagonist to the parasympathetic nervous system. The paragraph continues by explaining that anticholinergic medications prevent congestion due to their "drying effect." Constipation, urinary hesitancy, and dry eyes are all described as side effects of atropine. Thus, these symptoms do illustrate atropine's effect on the parasympathetic nervous system.

20. B If extracts of the deadly nightshade act as cardiostimulants *and* as antagonists to the parasympathetic nervous system, it follows that the parasympathetic nervous system normally causes the heart rate to decrease.

21. B If you have no knowledge of the various conditions listed in the answer choices, then you can identify the correct answer by process of elimination. Increased heart rate, dry mouth, and hallucinations are all mentioned in the passage as side effects of the extracts of the deadly nightshade. Therefore, these conditions would not be treated with its extract.

You could also arrive at the correct answer by noting that the extracts inhibit defecation and sometimes even cause constipation. Thus, this would be beneficial in treating diarrhea.

22. C There is no evidence in the passage that would lead the reader to believe that the author doubts the folklore stories of the belladonna plant. Thus, (A) is incorrect. (B) is wrong: the author repeatedly describes the potency of the plant's products. The author does not suggest using alternative medications in the passage. So (D) is also incorrect.

Throughout the passage, the author expands upon the importance of the plant's extracts in medicine but also describes the toxicity. Therefore, their author would definitely promote the use of belladonna products with caution.

Passage IV (Questions 23–29)

23. **D** The first sentence of paragraph 2 mentions that the method of treatment depends on many factors, not just the blood calcium level.

    A is stated in paragraph 1. (B) is evident after reading the passage. (C) is mentioned in paragraph 2.

24. **C** Paragraph 2 discusses that loop diuretics are usually effective in lowering calcium levels. Paragraph 2 also mentions that loop diuretics lower blood potassium levels, causing hypokalemia, in turn causing a rebound hypercalcemia. Thus, loop diuretics can decrease and increase blood calcium levels.

25. **D** Treatment should be based on blood levels *and* clinical presentation. (A) is incorrect because a blood calcium level that high indicates severe hypercalcemia and some form of treatment would definitely be administered. Choices (B) and (C) may be correct, but not enough information is given in the question stem to indicate which of these treatments would be used.

26. **C** If calcium levels decrease with the administration of EDTA and EDTA forms an EDTA/calcium complex, then the complex must be eliminated more frequently than free calcium.

    The passage does not indicate whether or not EDTA-bound calcium is toxic; therefore, choosing (A) is unfounded. (B) is incorrect because EDTA does have a toxic side effect profile, as indicated in the last sentence of the passage. (D) contradicts information in the passage.

27. **D** (D) is mentioned in the last sentence of paragraph 3. The passage mentions nothing of renal failure, making (A) and (B) beyond the scope of the passage. (C) is a nonsense statement.

28. **B** If asymptomatic individuals have a higher incidence of mortality than symptomatic patients, then asymptomatic individuals should be treated as, if not more, urgently than symptomatic patients. This would refute the statement in the question stem.

    Choices (C), and (D) have nothing to do with the question stem. Choice (A) would support the idea, not weaken it.

29. **D** The nature of hypercalcemia dictates that there is an increased calcium level in the blood. If calcitonin is supposed to lower blood calcium, it seems unable to do so in hypercalcemic patients. So (D) is correct because calcitonin cannot do its job and prohibit calcium release into the blood.

    (A) is not mentioned and, in fact, is contradicted in paragraph 4. It is mentioned that testicular cancer patients are treated with agents that lower blood calcium, not raise it. Thus, these patients have the opposite result of those who might have calcitonin suppressed.

    (C) is wrong because hypercalcemia is caused by cancer or hyperparathyroidism, both of which cause massive release of calcium into the blood. Calcitonin could still operate correctly and be overwhelmed by calcium release. In fact, this is exactly what happens.

Passage V (Questions 30-36)

30. **D** In paragraph 3, the author states that aloe vera gel stunts bacterial growth. (A) is true, as mentioned in paragraph 1. Choices (B) and (C) are also both true statements.

31. **D** Paragraph 3 states that aloe weakly stunts bacterial growth; therefore, it would not be useful in treating an infection. If you didn't know that bacteria cause infections, then you could arrive at the correct answer by process of elimination.

    (A) is supported by paragraph 4. (B) is supported throughout the passage. (C) is true because Native Americans use aloe to treat skin irritations just like modern non-Native practitioners.

32. **C** The last sentence of paragraph 2 recommends that aloe be used for skin conditions. (A) is a true statement, supported by the fact that aloe is used to treat sunburns and eczema, human ailments. Nothing in the passage indicates that the author would disagree with (B). (D) is supported by paragraph 2.

33. **D** Paragraph 4 indicates that aloe causes gastrointestinal problems; therefore, it would not be very effective in treating colonic irritation. Choices (A), (B), and (C) are all supported by paragraph 2.

34. **C** The beginning of paragraph 3 describes the prostaglandins' role in the inflammatory response. The bacteriocidal, bacteriostatic, and anesthetic properties of aloe are unrelated to prostaglandins. Thus, choices (A), (B), and (D) are incorrect.

35. **B** Today, lanolin is used as a buffer against the acidic properties of the aloe gel. Native Americans directly applied the aloe extract to their wounds; therefore, they would have felt the acidic effects of aloe's low pH.

    Paragraph 3 states that aloe only weakly stunts bacterial growth; thus, it would not instantly kill bacteria, (A), or stop bacterial growth, (D). Weak anesthetic properties would not cause total numbness; (C) is incorrect.

36. **C** The passage describes two uses of aloe, as a skin treatment and as a laxative. Because of its potency on the gastrointestinal system, it is not recommended as a laxative. The quotation in the question stem reinforces the fact that aloe is preferably used as a skin treatment.

    (A) is never mentioned in the passage. (B) contradicts the information in the question stem. (D) is beyond the scope of the passage.

Passage VI (Questions 37–44)

37. **C** The author says that the researchers' inability to establish functional hypotheses has been due to methodological problems, which we learn about in the last three paragraphs. Sleep-deprivation experiments are difficult to carry out and give only limited information, and the ideal alternative approach has not proved successful.

    The author never suggests that the failure to establish functional hypotheses has any implications regarding Freud's hypotheses (A) or the passive rest theory of sleep, whether it be for the theory (D) or against it (B).

38. D The author offers several reasons in the first four paragraphs that passive rest is probably not the sole function of sleep: 1) sleep is too complex and has different component phases, 2) you don't need sleep to rest, and 3) sleep is probably associated with the active processes of restoring efficiency to attention and memory and of reviewing acquired data.

The question is: Which one of the answer choices contradicts one or more of these reasons and thus weakens the author's argument? (A) doesn't. The fact that folk wisdom and science seldom agree (but do in supposing that the sole function of sleep is rest) has nothing to do with the author's argument. (B) and (C) are wrong because they both support the author's argument. If selective deprivation of REM sleep has a different effect from that of selective deprivation of non-REM sleep, then this implies the component phases have different functions—just what the author says. The author also says that some animals get plenty of rest when they're awake, implying that sleep must provide more than just rest; therefore, (C) strengthens the author's argument as well. (D) is the one that weakens the author's argument. If measures of attention and memory are stable regardless of sleep-time, then the author's idea that attention and memory is restored during sleep seems to be wrong. This strengthens the possibility that rest actually is the sole function of sleep.

39. C The author's point in the second paragraph is that our subjective experience of sleep as restful and restorative should "more powerfully motivate us to seek physiological or behavioral explanations" of this phenomenon, even though there is no physiological evidence. From this you can infer that the author thinks that a theory—in this case, that sleep is physiologically restorative—may be true even if there isn't any scientific evidence for it (C).

The author never says that subjective experience can prove a theory correct all by itself (A); he thinks that subjective experience should prompt scientists to move in a specific direction. Nor does the author link dreaming to physiological restoration (B) or state that subjective experience is always accurate (D).

40. C The best way to approach this question is to run through the choices quickly to see whether one of them jumps out as a claim the author makes but doesn't support with evidence. (A) is wrong because the author spends all of paragraphs 5 and 7 arguing that the sleep deprivation approach is flawed. (B) is labeled a "naive notion" by the author, so it's out as well. (C), on the other hand, is a statement made by the author at the end of the third paragraph for which he never gives any supporting evidence or statistics. As for (D), the author mentions the results of experiments with sleep-deprived rats to back up this statement.

41. A (A) is correct because it is never mentioned in the passage.

42. C This is essentially a sleep deprivation experiment in which the resident goes without sleep and then is tested for signs of a memory deficit. Remember what the author says in the fifth paragraph about such experiments: there is no way to know whether the memory deficit is the result of sleep deprivation or other factors, such as the things the subject did to keep herself awake.

(A) is tricky because the author does say that sleep deprivation doesn't provide information on a molecular level; however, the experiment does *not* establish that sleep deprivation affects memory function. (B) is wrong because the author never directly states that if you don't review and reorganize information during sleep, your memory will decrease. Finally, (D), testing the resident's memory during the work shift may have made it possible to get a better look at the resident's memory capacity over the course of the shift, but the author would still object by saying it's not clear that her memory is being affected only by sleep deprivation.

43. **D** (D) contradicts the author's statement that "behavioral capabilities … (would) recover dramatically following an epoch of sleep."

44. **C** Review the sixth paragraph to understand what a "positive functional model" is: a measure of brain function or behavioral capability or psychological process that could be tested around the clock and show deterioration as the subject stayed awake longer yet recover after sleep.

    (A) doesn't fit the model because the subject's mood doesn't show deterioration. (B) doesn't fit either, because it doesn't show the subject's brain electrical activity deteriorating prior to sleep and then recovering. (D) is incorrect for similar reasons: reading speed does not deteriorate or recover and is not tested around the clock. (C) is the best example of the successful application of the author's model, since the concentration of neurotransmitter decreases the longer the subject is awake but recovers after sleep (unfortunately, such a neurotransmitter has not been discovered).

Passage VII (Questions 45–48)

45. **B** Airway inflammation is the central cause of asthma (B). It is believed that when the airways become inflamed, they lead to obstruction (A) and shortness of breath (D). The last sentence of paragraph 1 claims that treatment focuses on "relaxing the constricted airway."

46. **D** The first sentence of paragraph 3 states that cells in the airways produce leukotrienes (D) in response to allergens.

47. **A** The sulfidopeptide leukotrienes are LTC4 (B), LD4 (C), and LE4 (D). LTB4 (A) is not a sulfidopeptide leukotriene.

48. **C** This question could appear to be a bit tricky. An immediate response would be to believe that inhibitors "prevent allergens from causing an immune reaction." Careful examination of paragraph 3 and the first sentence of paragraph 4 will lead us to the correct answer. 5-lipooxgenase inhibitors specifically work at the step before production of leukotrienes. However, we still need to be careful—paragraph 3 never states that the inhibitors block production of arachidonic acid (B). Therefore, choice (C) is correct. Choice (A) has nothing to do with the drug's mode of action.

QUANTITATIVE ABILITY

1. **D** We first rewrite f with negative exponents instead of denominators and use the power rule, the sum and difference rule, and the constant multiple rule to differentiate f:

$$f(x) = x^5 - 2x^2 + \frac{3}{x} = x^5 - 2x^2 + 3x^{-1}$$

$$f'(x) = 5x^4 - 2 \cdot 2x + 3 \cdot (-1)x^{-2} = 5x^4 - 4 - \frac{3}{x^2}$$

   We can now substitute $x = -1$ into $f'(x)$ to get $f'(-1) = 5(-1)^4 - 4(-1) - \frac{3}{(-1)^2} = 6$.

2. **A** To answer this question, you must simplify the fraction $\dfrac{\frac{3}{20}}{\frac{4}{5}}$. This can be re-expressed as $\dfrac{3}{20} \times \dfrac{5}{4}$. The 5's cancel out, and the product of the remaining fractions is $\dfrac{3}{16}$.

$$0.06\% \, x = \frac{3}{16}$$

$$\frac{6}{10,000} \, x = \frac{3}{16}$$

$$x = \frac{3}{16} \times \frac{10,000}{6} = \frac{1}{16} \times \frac{10,000}{2} = \frac{5,000}{16} = \frac{1,250}{4} = 312.5$$

3. **D** The first thing that you must do is find out how much each sale item costs ($\frac{90}{6} = 15$ cents). To find how much you save per package, subtract from the normal price (19 cents) the sale price (15 cents). The total savings is 4 cents per package: 4 cents times 24 packages = 96 cents.

4. **A** The question can be solved by picking an appropriate number for the number of juniors. Notice that the percents appearing in this question are 30% and 20%. The fractional equivalent of 30% is $\frac{3}{10}$, and the fractional equivalent of 20% is $\frac{1}{5}$. Since the number of juniors increased by 30%, which is $\frac{3}{10}$, we want the original number of juniors to be a multiple of the denominator 10 of $\frac{3}{10}$. Since the number of seniors increased by 20%, which is $\frac{1}{5}$, we want the original number of seniors to be a multiple of the denominator 5 of $\frac{1}{5}$. Since 10 is a multiple of 5, we can let both the number of juniors and the number of seniors be multiples of 10. Since the original ratio of juniors to seniors was 8 to 7, the original number of juniors must be a multiple of 8, the original number of seniors must be a multiple of 7, and, of course, the original ratio of juniors to seniors must be 8 to 7. Let's let the original number of juniors be 80. Then the original 8 to 7 ratio of juniors to seniors will require that the original number of seniors be 70. Notice that our selection for the original number of juniors, 80, and our selection for the original number of seniors, 70, are both multiples of 10.

The original number of juniors, 80, increased by 30%, or $\frac{3}{10}$, over last year, so the number of juniors this year is $80 + \frac{3}{10}(80) = 80 + 3(8) = 80 + 24 = 104$. The original number of seniors, 70, increased by 20%, or $\frac{1}{5}$, over last year, so the number of seniors this year is $70 + \frac{1}{5}(70) = 70 + 14 = 84$. So the ratio of the number juniors to the number seniors this year is 104 to 84, which can be reduced to 26 to 21 by dividing each member of the ratio 104 to 84 by 4. Choice (A), 26 to 21, is correct.

5. D The easiest way to approach this problem is to apply the rules of simplification and cross multiplication. First convert the mixed numbers to improper fractions $\left(4\frac{3}{4} = \frac{19}{4} \; ; 9\frac{1}{2} = \frac{19}{2}\right)$. Cross multiply the fractions: $\frac{19}{4} \times 9 \times 3 \times (y) = \frac{19}{2} \times 9$. The 9's cancel. So simplify by multiplying to get: $\frac{57}{4} y = \frac{19}{2}$. Solving for y gives you $y = \frac{38}{57}$ or $\frac{2}{3}$.

6. A The probability of independent events occurring is the product of the separate probabilities: $\frac{1}{3} \times \frac{1}{2} = \frac{1}{6}$.

7. B The way to approach this problem is to convert the mixed numbers to fractions $\left(\frac{8}{5} \times \frac{9}{4} \times \frac{7}{6}\right)$, then cancel where appropriate. The 4 and 8 can be canceled, yielding $\frac{2}{5} \times 9 \times \frac{7}{6}$. The 2 and 6 can be canceled, yielding $\frac{1}{5} \times 9 \times \frac{7}{3}$. Doing the same thing with the 9 and the 3 gives you $\frac{1}{5} \times 3 \times 7$. Multiplying what's left gives you $\frac{21}{5}$.

8. A Using a simple mnemonic and some common sense, this question can be answered quickly. Recalling the mnemonic SOH CAH TOA, $\sin \theta = \dfrac{\text{opposite}}{\text{hypotenuse}}$ and $\cos \theta = \dfrac{\text{adjacent}}{\text{hypotenuse}}$.

From this, it is easy to see that the functions sine and cosine are not inversely related. The true relationship is $\cos \theta = \sin (90 - \theta)$. Therefore the $\cos 59° = \sin 31°$.

If you were not sure of the relationship between the sine and cosine functions, you can still get this question correct by eliminating answer choices. Answer choices (B) and (D) can easily be eliminated—the only cosine function that can equal the cos 59° is the cos 59°. Answer choice (C) can also be eliminated—since the functions of sine and cosine are different, the cosine of an angle cannot equal the sine of the same angle.

9. D The definite integral is the area under the curve, where the area under the axis is negative. If we graph this function, we can see that there are two regions of area; a small triangle below the x-axis and a large triangle above the axis.

$$\int_0^6 2x - 2 \; dx$$

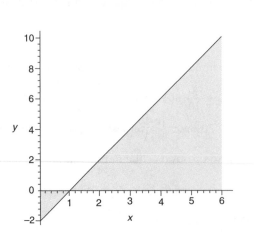

The area of the small triangle is $\frac{1}{2} \cdot 1 \cdot 2 = 1$. The area of the big triangle is $\frac{1}{2} \cdot 5 \cdot 10 = 25$.

We count the area of the small triangle as negative so $\int_0^6 2x - 2 \, dx =$

$-$ (area of the small triangle) + (area of the big triangle) $= 1 + 25 = 24$.

10. C The women comprise $\frac{12}{18}$ of the group; therefore, $\frac{6}{18}$, or $\frac{1}{3}$, of the group is comprised of men.

11. C If h is the inverse of $f(x) = x^3 - x + 2$, then, according to the formula for the derivative of an

inverse: $h'(2) = \dfrac{1}{f'(h(2))}$. To compute $h'(2)$, we must evaluate $f'(h(2))$, so we need find

$f'(x)$ and $h(2)$. The function $f(x) = x^3 - x + 2$ is a polynomial; we compute its derivative using

the power rule, the constant multiple rule, and the derivative of a constant: $f'(x) = 3x^2 - 1$.

Because h is the inverse of f, to find $h(2)$, we solve the equation
$2 = x^3 - x + 2 \Rightarrow x^3 - x = 0 \Rightarrow x(x+1)(x-1) = 0 \Rightarrow x = 0, -1, 1$.

Therefore, $h(2) = 0, -1$, or 1. We plug each of these options into the formula for $h'(2)$ above:

$h(2)$	0	−1	1
$f'(h(2))$	−1	2	2
$h'(2) = \dfrac{1}{f'(h(2))}$	−1	$\dfrac{1}{2}$	$\dfrac{1}{2}$

Because -1 is not one of the answer choices, the correct answer is $h'(2) = \dfrac{1}{2}$.

12. A Let's rewrite the ratios as fractions, write down an equation showing the equality of the two equal

ratios written as fractions, and then solve that equation for V. The ratio of $6d$ to V is the fraction

$\dfrac{6d}{V}$. The ratio of $3c$ to 4 is the fraction $\dfrac{3c}{4}$. The two fractions are equal, so $\dfrac{6d}{V} = \dfrac{3c}{4}$. Now solve this

equation for V.

$$\frac{6d}{V} = \frac{3c}{4}$$

Multiply both sides by $4V$: $\quad 4V\left(\dfrac{6d}{V}\right) = \left(\dfrac{3c}{4}\right)4V$

Simplify each side: $\quad 24d = 3cV$

Divide each side by $3c$: $\quad \dfrac{24d}{3c} = V$

Simplify the left side: $\quad \dfrac{8d}{c} = V$

So $V = \dfrac{8d}{c}$, and choice (A) is correct.

13. **B** The figure is a geometric representation of the algebraic equation:

$$\frac{1}{2} + \frac{1}{4} + \frac{1}{12} + x = 1$$

where x is the fraction of the circle that is shaded. Solving for its value, we get:

$$x = 1 - \frac{1}{2} - \frac{1}{4} - \frac{1}{12} = \frac{12}{12} - \frac{6}{12} - \frac{3}{12} - \frac{1}{12} = \frac{2}{12} = \frac{1}{6}.$$

14. **C** This is a simple arithmetic problem, as long as you remember the rules for handling exponents and scientific notation:

$$\frac{6 \times 10^{-4}}{30 \times 10^{5}} = \frac{6}{30} \times 10^{-9}$$

$$= \frac{1}{5} \times 10^{-9}$$

$$= 0.2 \times 10^{-9}$$

$$= 2 \times 10^{-10}$$

15. **B** This question looks a great deal tougher than it really is. First of all, substitute 1 for x. Further, the fraction $\frac{35}{7}$ can be simplified to 5. So we're left with $\frac{1}{(5-y)} = \frac{1}{7}$. These equal fractions have equal numerators, so the denominators must be equal. Then $5 - y = 7$, $-2 - y = 0$, and $y = -2$.

16. **C** For this question, start with the maximum number of 3¢ candies the boy can buy. Then subtract the total cost of these 3¢ candies, and see if the remaining change will divide by 4. If it does, then the purchase is exactly equal to $0.25. The boy can buy a maximum of eight 3¢ candies (with a penny left over) for a quarter. Remember, you want no remainder, so the combination of eight 3¢ and zero 4¢ candies does not work. Seven 3¢ candies cost $0.21 and leave a remainder of 4 cents, which will buy one 4¢ candy for exactly $0.25. That's one combination that works. If you try six 3¢ candies, you have 7 cents left, which doesn't divide evenly into 4. Five 3¢ candies leaves 10 cents remaining, which also has a remainder when divided by 4. Four 3¢ candies doesn't work, as it leaves 13 cents remaining. Three 3¢ candies leaves 16 cents remaining, which *does* divide by 4. The combination of three 3¢ candies and four 4¢ candies is the second combination to work. If you try the other possible combinations in the same way, you'll see that they don't work. Thus, there are 2 possible combinations.

17. **C** In bag X, there are 5 green disks among a total of $7 + 5 = 12$ disks. The probability of choosing a green disk from bag X is $\frac{5}{12}$. In bag Y, there are 15 green disks among a total of $15 + 5 = 20$ disks. The probability of choosing a green disk from bag Y is $\frac{15}{20}$, or $\frac{3}{4}$. Since the selections of the disks from the bags are independent, the probability that both disks selected are green is $\left(\frac{5}{12}\right)\left(\frac{3}{4}\right) = \frac{15}{48} = \frac{5}{16}$.

18. **D** If 2 cubic feet weigh 160 ounces, then 1 cubic foot weighs 80 ounces. Remember, we're asked for a cubic *inch*, but we're given cubic feet. To convert, remember that since 1 foot =

12 inches, 1 cubic foot = 1 foot^3 = (12 inches)^3 = (12 × 12 × 12) inches^3, or 1,728 cubic inches. So the weight per cubic inch is:

$$80 \frac{\text{ounces}}{\text{per cubic foot}} \times \frac{1 \text{ cubic foot}}{1,728 \text{ cubic inch}} = \frac{80}{1,728} \text{ ounce per cubic inch} \approx 0.046 \text{ ounce per cubic inch.}$$

If this math is too daunting, note that $\frac{80}{1,728}$ is a bit less than $\frac{80}{1,600}$, which is 0.05. The only answer choice even close to this is (D).

19. C This is a straightforward question involving two variables and two equations. Cross multiplying $\frac{x}{y} = \frac{1}{7}$ gives $y = 7x$. If you substitute $7x$ for y in the equation $x + y = 1$, you obtain $x + 7x = 1$, $8x = 1$, and $x = \frac{1}{8}$. Now you can find the value of y. $y = 7x = 7\left(\frac{1}{8}\right) = \frac{7}{8}$. The question stem asks for $(x - y)$, which is $\frac{1}{8} - \frac{7}{8}$ or $-\frac{6}{8}$. This is the same as $-\frac{3}{4}$.

20. C If h is the inverse of $f(x) = x^3 - x + 2$, then according to the formula for the derivative of an inverse:

$$h'(2) = \frac{1}{f'(h(2))}$$

To compute $h'(2)$, we must evaluate $f'(h(2))$, so we need find $f'(x)$ and $h(2)$.

The function $f(x) = x^3 - x + 2$ is a polynomial; we compute its derivative using the power rule, the constant multiple rule, and the derivative of a constant:

$$f'(x) = 3x^2 - 1$$

Since h is the inverse of f, to find $h(2)$, we solve the equation:

$$2 = x^3 - x + 2 \Rightarrow x^3 - x = 0 \Rightarrow (x + 1)(x - 1) = 0 \Rightarrow x = 0, -1, 1$$

Therefore, $h(2) = 0, -1$, or 1. We plug each of these options into the formula for $h'(2)$ above:

$h(2)$	0	−1	1
$f'(h(2))$	−1	2	2
$h'(2) = \dfrac{1}{f'(h(2))}$	-1	$\dfrac{1}{2}$	$\dfrac{1}{2}$

Since −1 is not one of the answer choices, the correct answer is $h'(2) = \frac{1}{2}$.

21. B The absolute value of a number is the number without its sign. Thus, $|3| = 3$, $|-7| = 7$, $|0| = 0$, and $|-134.5| = 134.5$. Zero is the only number with an absolute value of 0. The absolute value of any other number is positive. (The absolute value of a number can also be thought of as the distance of that number from 0 on the number line. Absolute values, like distances, are never negative.)

Now let's find the value of the expression.

$|6 - 12| = |-6| = 6$

$|-5 + 14| = |9| = 9$

$|-7 + 1| = |-6| = 6$

Then $\dfrac{|6 - 12| - |-5 + 14|}{|-7 + 1|} = \dfrac{6 - 9}{6} = \dfrac{-3}{6} = -\dfrac{1}{2}.$

22. **D** You can start by counting the number of ways this outcome can occur. There are $\dfrac{4!}{2!(4-2)!}$

$= \dfrac{4!}{2!2!} = \dfrac{(4)(3)(2)(1)}{(2)(1)(2)(1)} = \dfrac{12}{2} = 6$ ways that exactly two of four letters will arrive in two days

or sooner (the first and second letters, the first and third, the second and fourth, etc.).

The probability of a letter failing to arrive in two days or sooner is $1 - \dfrac{2}{3} = \dfrac{1}{3}$.

So the probability of the first two letters arriving in two days or sooner, and the other two arriving later than that is:

$$\dfrac{2}{3} \times \dfrac{2}{3} \times \dfrac{1}{3} \times \dfrac{1}{3} = \dfrac{4}{81}$$

The probability of any other pair of letters arriving in two days or sooner, and the other two arriving later than that is the same. The probability of any of those outcomes occurring is the sum of all of them. Since they are the same, the probability of exactly two arriving in two days or sooner is

$$\dfrac{4}{81} \times 6 = \dfrac{24}{81} = \dfrac{8}{27}.$$

23. **A** The only possible points where the second derivative could change sign are places where it equals zero. We solve the equation $s''(t) = (t + 1)(t - 3)\sin^2 t = 0$ to find $s'' = 0$ at $t = -1, 3,$ $n\pi$, an integer. Notice that since the factor $\sin^2 t$ in the equation of s'' appears to the second power, it is always positive (i.e. $\sin^2 t > 0$). Therefore, the sign of s'' does not depend on the sign of this factor, and the second derivative will not change sign at $n\pi$ (the roots of $\sin^2 t$); we only need to include $t = -1, 3$ in our sign analysis of the second derivative.

Interval	$t < -1$	$-1 < t < 3$	$t > 3$
Test Point	$t = -2$	$t = 0$	$t = 4$
Sign of s''	$s''(-2) = (-2 + 1)(-2 - 3)(+)$ $= (-)(+)(-) = (+)$ positive	$s''(0) = (0 + 1)(0 - 3)(+)$ $= (+)(+)(-) = (-)$ negative	$s''(4) = (4 + 1)(4 - 3)(+)$ $= (+)(+)(+) = (+)$ positive
Concavity	up	down	up

Since s'' changes sign at both $t = 3$ and $t = -1$, both of these points are inflection points. This can also be phrased in terms of concavity.

There is a point of inflection at $x = -1, 3$, since s'' changes concavity at both $t = 3$ and $t = -1$. Both of these points are inflection points.

24. **B** This question is simply a matter of solving a problem by process of elimination. You're trying to determine which two numbers have a sum (addition) 5 less than their product (multiplication). The simplest one to assess first is choice (C). The sum is $5 + 0 = 5$, and the product is $(5)(0) = 0$. This may appear correct, but remember the product must be 5 more than the sum, not the other way around. So choice (C) is incorrect. Choice (D) is also easy to eliminate—the sum is 8; the product is 12. Choice (A) is also incorrect; the sum (10) is not 5 less than the product: $(5 + \sqrt{7})(5 - \sqrt{7}) = 5^2 - (\sqrt{7})^2 = 25 - 7 = 18$. Finally, choice (B) must be correct (by process of elimination). Verifying this, you can see that the sum (8) is 5 less than the product $16 - 3 = 13$ using the same expansion as in choice (A). So choice (B) is correct.

25. **D** There are five rounds. To have an average of 18 per round, he must hit $18 \times 5 = 90$ targets. In three rounds, he hit a total of $17 \times 3 = 51$ targets; therefore, in the last two rounds, he must hit $90 - 51 = 39$ targets or an average of $\frac{39}{2} = 19.5$ targets per round.

26. **B** Twenty percent of the 60-pint solution is pure alcohol. So $20\% \times 60 = 0.2 \times 60 = 12$ pints of this original solution are alcohol. Let's try solving the question both algebraically and by backsolving. First let's set up the algebra. If we add x pints of pure alcohol, the total volume of the solution will be $(60 + x)$ pints. The amount of pure alcohol in the new solution will be $12 + x$ (the 12 pints in the original solution and the x pints of pure alcohol we've added). If the new solution is 40% alcohol, the following relationship must be satisfied:

$$0.4(\text{total volume}) = \text{volume of pure alcohol}$$
$$0.4(60 + x) = 12 + x$$

Solving for x, we get:

$$24 + 0.4x = 12 + x$$
$$0.6x = 12$$
$$x\frac{12}{0.6} = \frac{12 \times 10}{0.6 \times 10} = \frac{120}{6} = 20$$

With the backsolving approach, we try solving backwards until the ratio of alcohol pints to total pints equals 0.4, or the solution becomes 40% alcohol. Start with choice (C). If you add 24 pints of alcohol, you have a total of 84 pints, of which 36 are alcohol. $\frac{36}{84}$ is approximately 43%, which is too high. Choices (C) and (D), can be eliminated because these both will give concentrations higher than 40%. Choice (C) was slightly too high, so looking at choices (A) and (B), choice (B) is probably correct, since it's just a little smaller than (C). Adding 20 pints of alcohol will give 80 pints total and 32 pints of alcohol. $\frac{32}{80}$ is equal to 0.40 or 40%.

27. **D** (D) True: $f'(1) = 0$ and $f(0) = 0$
   (A) False: $f'(0) < 0$ and $f(0) = 0$
   (B) False: $f'(1) = 0$ and $f(1) < 0$
   (C) False: $f'(2) > 0$ and $f(2) = 0$
   (E) False: $f'(2) > 0$ and $f(2) = 0$

28. **A** Because 42 rolls cost w dollars, 1 roll costs $\frac{w}{42}$ dollars. So the cost of 17 rolls is $17\left(\frac{w}{42}\right)$ dollars. Because 36 doughnuts cost x dollars, 1 doughnut costs $\frac{x}{36}$ dollars. So the cost of 25 doughnuts is $25\left(\frac{x}{36}\right)$ dollars. Finally, the total cost of 17 rolls and 25 doughnuts, in dollars, is $17\left(\frac{w}{42}\right) + 25\left(\frac{x}{36}\right)$.

29. **D** Remember that the probability of something happening is the number of desired outcomes over the number of possible outcomes. Once Carmen has drawn a marble, there are 49 marbles left, so there are 49 possible outcomes. Now of those 49, how many are desired outcomes? Carmen must draw a marble with a 5 in the units digit. How many of the remaining marbles will have a 5 as the second digit? 05, 15, 35, 45. Remember that Carmen has already drawn the 25. So there are 4 desired outcomes. Therefore the probability that Carmen will win is 4/49. The answer is (D).

30. A Recall that the definition of log is such that if $\log_b x = y$, then $b^y = x$. In this case, you're dealing with powers of 10. $\log_{10} 10 = 1$, since $10^1 = 10$, and $\log_{10} 100 = 2$, since $10^2 = 100$, etc. Therefore, $\log_{10} 1{,}000 - \log_{10} 100 = 3 - 2 = 1$.

31. B To find what number multiplied by the mass of the earth equals the mass of the sun, divide the mass of the sun by the mass of the earth. So the number we're seeking is $\dfrac{1.99 \times 10^{30}}{5.98 \times 10^{24}}$. Next, let's simplify this, approximating where it is appropriate.

First, group the numbers 1.99 and 5.98 together and group the powers 10^{30} and 10^{24} together. Then $\dfrac{1.99 \times 10^{30}}{5.98 \times 10^{24}} = (\dfrac{1.99}{5.98}) \times (\dfrac{10^{30}}{10^{24}})$. Now 1.99 is approximately 2 and 5.98 is approximately 6. So $\dfrac{1.99}{5.98}$ is approximately $\dfrac{2}{6}$, which is $\dfrac{1}{3}$, and $\dfrac{1}{3}$ is approximately 0.33. To work with $\dfrac{10^{30}}{10^{24}}$, you need to know a law of exponents: whenever you divide powers with the same base, you subtract the exponents and keep the same base. Algebraically, $\dfrac{b^x}{b^y} = b^{x-y}$. So $\dfrac{10^{30}}{10^{24}} = 10^{30-24} = 10^6$. Now $\dfrac{1.99 \times 10^{30}}{5.98 \times 10^{24}}$ is approximately 0.33×10^6. None of the answer choices is 0.33×10^6. Let's rewrite 0.33×10^6. We have $0.33 \times 10^6 = (0.33 \times 10^1) \times \left(\dfrac{10^6}{10^1}\right) = 3.3 \times 10^{6-1} = 3.3 \times 10^5$.

32. D For both the sum and product of two numbers to be even, both numbers must be even. There is a 3 in 6 chance for an even number to occur on any die throw. The probability that each number is even is $\dfrac{3}{6} = \dfrac{1}{2}$. Because both dice must have an even number, you multiply the two probabilities: $\dfrac{1}{2} \times \dfrac{1}{2} = \dfrac{1}{4}$.

33. C You must evaluate the definite integral. If you differentiate instead of integrate and then plug in the limits of integration, you'll wind up with answer (D). Other mistakes, like not keeping track of your signs properly, will lead to other incorrect answers. Carefully taking the antiderivative of the integrand and then plugging in the limits of integration will yield the correct answer, (C).

34. A This question requires the use of the FOIL (First, Outer, Inner, Last) method of polynomial expansion. You need to solve for x. To remove the square root from the equation in the question stem, square both sides. This gives you $(x^2 - 7) = (7 - x)^2$. Use FOIL on the right-hand side to get $x^2 - 7 = 49 - 14x + x^2$. The x^2 terms cancel, and solving for x, we get $-14x = -56$, or $x = 4$.

35. A The positive square root of 0.0036 is 0.06, so the given equation becomes $0.06 = 0.3 + x$. Solving the equation gives you $x = -0.24$.

36. B If $\frac{2}{5}$ of the animals occupy 10 cages (at one cage per animal), then 10 animals are $\frac{2}{5}$ the total in the store. Dividing 10 by $\frac{2}{5}$, gives you the total number of animals. Therefore, $\frac{10}{\left(\frac{2}{5}\right)} = 10 \times \frac{5}{2} = \frac{50}{2} = 25$.

37. B Solve the equation $\sqrt{\frac{3}{y} - 5} = 10$ for y.

$$\sqrt{\frac{3}{y} - 5} = 10$$

Square both sides:
$$\left(\sqrt{\frac{3}{y} - 5}\right)^2 = 10^2$$

Simplify each side:
$$\frac{3}{y} - 5 = 100$$

Add 5 to both sides:
$$\frac{3}{y} = 105$$

Multiply both sides by y:
$$3 = 105y$$

Divide both sides by 105:
$$\frac{3}{105} = y$$

Divide the 3 and the 105 on the left side by 3:
$$\frac{1}{35} = y$$

Thus, $y = \frac{1}{35}$.

38. C The total number of possible outcomes is $6 \times 6 = 36$. Of those outcomes, the following are consecutive integers:

1 and 2

2 and 1

2 and 3

3 and 2

3 and 4

4 and 3

4 and 5

5 and 4

5 and 6

6 and 5

That's 10 favorable outcomes:

$$\text{probability} = \frac{\text{favorable outcomes}}{\text{total possible outcomes}}$$

$$= \frac{10}{36} = 0.28$$

39. A This question requires you to know that a positive second derivative on an interval corresponds to the function being concave up on that interval, while a negative second derivative on an interval corresponds to the function being concave down on that interval. With this knowledge, choice (B) must be eliminated. To finish answering the question, you still need to understand what is happening at the point $x = 3$. From the question, it is apparent that the concavity of the function changes at that point. You may remember that such a point is called a point of inflection. If you know that $f''(3) = 0$ is equivalent to the point $x = 3$ being a point of inflection for f, you can eliminate choices (C) and (D). If you don't know this, you may be tempted to choose (C) or (D). But if you can think of a function you know that has the properties described in the question, for example, $f(x) = -(x - 3)^3$, and if you check the second derivative at $x = 3$, you'll get 0. Thus by thinking of a simple example, you can eliminate (C) and (D) and be left with the correct answer (A) as the only remaining choice. Having in mind some examples of simple functions and expressions can be handy in eliminating incorrect answers.

40. D Because the ratio of the number of slices is $1:4:5$, we can let the numbers of slices be x, $4x$, and $5x$. Then, $x + 4x + 5x = 40$; $10x = 40$; and $x = \frac{40}{10} = 4$. The number of slices are $x = 4$, $4x = 16$, and $5x = 20$. The largest portion contained 20 slices of pizza.

41. C The simplest way to solve this problem is to pick a simple number and find the integers between integer c and 2 times integer c. Let $c = 6$; then $2c = 12$. Because the stem asks you for the number of integers greater than c and less than $2c$, you don't count 6 and 12. Therefore, you have 7, 8, 9, 10, and 11, or a total of 5 integers between the numbers. Now substitute 6 for c into each answer choice. Any answer choice that does not equal 5 when $c = 6$ may be eliminated.

42. A Solve the equation $10x + 6y = 7x + 8y$ for the value of $\frac{x}{y}$.

$$10x + 6y = 7x + 8y$$

Subtract $7x$ from both sides: $\quad 3x + 6y = 8y$

Subtract $6y$ from both sides: $\quad 3x = 2y$

Divide both sides by 3: $\quad x = \frac{2y}{3}$

Divide both sides by y: $\quad \frac{x}{y} = \frac{2}{3}$

43. B If $\frac{m}{2} = 15$, you can multiply both sides by 2 to get $m = 30$. Because $m = 30$, $\frac{m}{3} = \frac{30}{3} = 10$.

44. A If you recognize that $x^2 + 2x + 1 = (x + 1)^2$, rewrite the equation as $(x + 1)^2 = 121$. The two square roots of 121 are 11 and -11, so $x + 1 = \pm 11$, so x is equal to either $11 - 1$, or $-11 - 1$ (i.e., $x = 10$ or -12). Because 10 is one of the answer choices and -12 is not, the answer is choice (A).

45. B The easiest way to find a in this question is to add the equations together. $2a + 4a = 6a$, $-b + b = 0$, and $1 + 17 = 18$, so you're left with $6a = 18$. Dividing both sides by 6 gives you $a = 3$.

46. D Simply plug in the answer choices and see which one works. Start with choice (C) because $4 \div (-2) = -2$. Because the question stem asks you to find a value that's less than -2, you have to find a value that gives you a smaller value. Because x is negative, in $\frac{4}{x}$, a larger denominator, (a denominator with a smaller absolute value) gives you a smaller fraction, and the only choice greater than -2 is -1. $\frac{4}{-1} = -4$, which is less than -2. Choice (D) is correct. We could also solve the inequality by multiplying both sides of the inequality by x. However, because it is given that $x < 0$, we need to reverse the direction of the inequality when we do this. So $\frac{4}{x}(x) > -2x$, and $4 > -2x$. We then divide both sides of the inequality by -2, but once again we have to reverse the inequality: $-2 < x$. Hence, x is less than zero but greater than -2. Among the answer choices, only (D) fits.

47. D A good way to solve this question is by picking a number. In percent questions, it is often good to pick 100. That is the case here. The variable whose value we should let be 100 is t. So let $t = 100$. Since s is 40% of t and the fractional equivalent of 40% is $\frac{40}{100}$, s is $\frac{40}{100}$ of 100, which is 40. Since r is 30% of s and the fractional equivalent of 30% is $\frac{30}{100}$, which is $\frac{3}{10}$, r is $\frac{3}{10}$ of 40, which is $\frac{3}{10}(40) = 3(4) = 12$. So t is 100 and r is 12. The fraction that r is of t is $\frac{12}{100}$. Now $\frac{12}{100}$ is 12%, so r is 12% of t.

48. C The equation of the line tangent to the graph of $f(x)$ at the point $x = a$ is given by $y - f(a) = f'(a)(x - a)$.

We are given information about three values of x: $x = 1$, $x = 2$, and $x = 5$. It is difficult to try to retrofit the answer choices to the equation of a tangent line, so we use the given data to write the equations of tangent lines. To find the equation of a tangent line at a, we must know both the value of the *function* at a and the value of the *derivative* at a. This is clear if we organize the given information in a table:

a	$f(a)$	$f'(a)$	$y - f(a) = f'(a)(x - a)$ equation of the tangent line at $x=a$
1	2	3	$y - 2 = 3(x - 1)$
2	-2	5	$y + 2 = 5(x - 2)$
5	1	?	not enough information

Now we can easily match the information on the table with the answer choices. Only one of the answer choices matches the equation of a tangent line on the table—(D).

NOTES

NOTES

NOTES

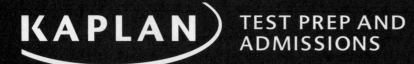

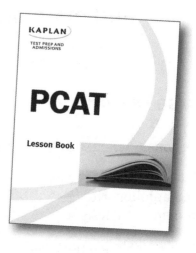